THE SUBTLE
ENERGY BODY

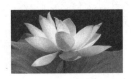

THE SUBTLE
ENERGY BODY
The Complete Guide

Maureen Lockhart, Ph.D.

Inner Traditions
Rochester, Vermont • Toronto, Canada

Inner Traditions
One Park Street
Rochester, Vermont 05767
www.InnerTraditions.com

Library of Congress Cataloging-in-Publication Data

Lockhart, Maureen.
  The subtle energy body : the complete guide / Maureen Lockhart.
      p. cm.
  Includes bibliographical references and index.
  ISBN 978-1-59477-339-6 (pbk.)
  1. Spirituality—Miscellanea. 2. Energy medicine. I. Title.
  BL624.L64 2010
  128'.6—dc22

                                                                2010032075

Printed and bound in the United States by P. A. Hutchison

10 9 8 7 6 5 4 3 2 1

Text design and layout by Priscilla Baker
This book was typeset in Garamond Premier Pro with Elegans Script and Agenda used as display typefaces

Color plates 4, 11, 32, 33, and 35 and images on pages 21, 29, 43 (right-hand image), 48 (left-hand image), 77, 90, 93, 94, 107, 127, 166, 171, 195, 200, 201, 202, 208, 209, 215, 243, 273, 274, 290, 307, and 333 copyright © by Eric Franklin

To send correspondence to the author of this book, mail a first-class letter to the author c/o Inner Traditions • Bear & Company, One Park Street, Rochester, VT 05767, and we will forward the communication.

Contents

PART TWO
Western Perspectives

Dedication

In memory of my late husband Peter Sandhu,
who would have been delighted to see this book
materialize out of my "mystical meanderings."

Acknowledgments

I am indebted to many people who, knowingly or unknowingly, have been involved in the production of this book. I would like to thank all students and clients, past and present, who have been my greatest teachers; my yoga tutor, Latvian poet Velta Snikere Wilson, for keeping the connection, and whose patience and forbearance through the trials and tribulations of exile have been an inspiration for over three decades; the many healers who shared their knowledge with me at just the right moments, including Dr. Ramakant Kenny, Dr. Vasant Lad, and Shrimati Shamala Chandran; the many friends who encouraged me to write a book that addresses their interests at an intelligent professional and academic level, for their patience in awaiting its arrival and their support through difficult times, among them Christine Meek, Carol Deans Shinwell, and Lady Ann Clyde; my spiritual brothers and sisters in the Yogic, Buddhist, and Tantric communities, particularly Dr. M. L. Gharote, Dharmacharyi Lokamitra, and my dear friend Swami Sivadhara Saraswati, with whom wide-ranging conversations and shared experiences, both spiritual and material, have been a "gift."

I would also like to thank my academic colleagues, especially Dr. James E. Robinson, who first gave me the opportunity to write about the Subtle Body and to teach it in a university master's degree program. A special thank you goes to Gyorgyi Byworth for bringing the resulting study module to the attention of Dr. Ervin Laszlo, whom I'd like to thank for enthusiastically recommending it to Inner Traditions Acquisitions Editor Jon Graham, and to Jon for his foresight in seeing its potential as a book; to my editor Laura Schlivek and the rest of the team at Inner Traditions for overseeing its "rebirth."

I would like to express my grateful thanks to Professor Olga Louchakova, Dr. Arielle Warner, David Osborn, and the other authors who generously permitted me to "borrow" from their books and articles; to Jon Moult for the picture of his yoga class; to Bob Clyatt for his kindness in permitting me to use the picture of his beautiful sculpture of Gandhi; and last, but certainly not least, to Eric Franklin for his huge contribution, hundreds of hours of dedicated work in producing the illustrations, the chapter "Science, Philosophy, and the Subtle Body," and his unflagging help and support throughout.

Preface

When I was six I had my first mystical experience. On my sixth birthday, my mother got me up at dawn to take a photograph in the garden. It was a typical summer morning in the highlands of Scotland, one of those days that starts with swirling grey mist and later gives way to balmy sunshine. As my mother was fiddling with the camera, which seemed to have jammed, I became aware of how patient and calm I felt. This was unlike me. I was a hyperactive child who did everything at high speed, so sitting still was usually torture for me. Then the mist began to clear, and suddenly from within the shrouds of grey, the Japanese cherry blossom tree in the center of the garden appeared like a vision out of a dream; I had an extraordinary sense of well-being, of connectedness, of being merged with the tree in its "beingness" and with the whole world that surrounded us.

I never forgot the feeling of that experience, although it only lasted minutes, perhaps even seconds. It became the archetypal sacred "place" to which I constantly returned whenever I needed peace, solace, guidance, or knowledge. In the spiritual life, however, I discovered that there are many ways of knowing.

The next significant experience came ten years later when I discovered yoga. When I was fourteen a TB patch had been found on one of my lungs, which explained the long and frequent bouts of bronchitis that had occurred throughout my childhood and had left me with breathing problems. I was still suffering from shortness of breath nearly two years later when I went to a badminton club with a friend and had to sit out some of the sets because I was so easily exhausted. At one point two women sat down next to me. The chairs were quite close together so I couldn't help hearing their conversation. They were talking about yoga, about which I had only the vaguest notion, but it seemed to have something to do with breathing. Just as they were going to join their friends in the next game, I found the courage to ask them if yoga could help me with my breathing problem. They said they were very sure that it could. However, as they were being called by their friends to start the next game, I didn't have time to ask how I could learn it.

Attempts to find a teacher or a class proved fruitless, so I searched the local library and, fortunately, found a do-it-yourself book written by Ernest Wood, also known by his Indian name, Shri Sattwikagraganya. Professor Wood was a Sanskrit scholar, a translator, and prolific author of works on yoga, with an interest in Buddhism and theosophy, who became the first "guru" of many an isolated yoga student like myself half a century ago. I say "fortunately" because he introduced me to the path of *rāja yoga,* which, as John Collins points out in his book on mysticism, is the path of the "spiritual warrior," requiring discipline and determination.[1] And discipline and determination were exactly what I required over the next year as I struggled with the roles of teacher and student. Still, thanks to Professor Wood's clear instructions, I succeeded in no small measure: when I went for my next x-ray, the patch on the lung had disappeared, and the breathing exercises I'd learned became an indispensable part of the "spiritual toolkit" that helped to keep me in reasonable health thereafter.

When I was twenty, I met my first husband at the newspaper where we both worked. Fortunately for me, he was a "spiritual warrior" with experience and knowledge of yoga, and much else, which exceeded my own.

Not only did he introduce me to meditation, but to many areas of spirituality, religion, philosophy, psychology, and, while he was writing his first novel, literature and creative writing. All of this not only opened a completely new world to me but stood me in good stead later when I worked in publishing as an editor, then eventually freelanced as a specialist in yoga, psychology, healing, and comparative religion for some of the leading London publishers at that time.

The other important skill I developed in this relationship came from the yoga and meditation that we practiced together daily, for most of the nine years we were together, whether we felt like it or not. If one of us was too tired, the other would cajole or persuade, and we would practice together even if it was late at night or early in the morning, or even if we were already late for work. When I went for an interview for a place in a yoga teacher training course, the tutor was so surprised that I had learned so much about yoga without having had a teacher or ever having been to a class that she was convinced that I had "remembered" from a past life. It was during this period, too, that I had other experiences, some through "grace," others through effort, and many a contemplative "knowing" that was mediated through dreams and meditative visions.

When I was twenty-one I had a serious accident. I fell down a whole flight of concrete steps and landed on my coccyx, fracturing seven spinal vertebrae and breaking my left arm on the way. As a result I was in pain most of the time, but the daily discipline of yoga and meditation helped me to survive, to work, to study, and eventually to teach. It was during this period that I met another important "guru," a very talented young chiropractor, who not only helped me back to health but also gave me many hours of his valuable time in discussing alternative medicine and lending me books to read. I was so enthused by his enthusiasm that I decided, after years of writing articles about healing and alternative medicine, that I should learn to do it myself. But after four years of studying and practicing different bodywork techniques I decided to take one tutor's advice and study homeopathy. She felt it would be far less demanding on me as I got older, when all the injuries I had suffered might reduce my stamina and make it difficult for me to work.

How farsighted that was. When I later went to India, met and married my second husband, and had to commute long distances from my rural mountain home to the intense heat and overcrowding of a major metropolis to work, I was so glad to be able to use my healing knowledge in difficult conditions in a way that didn't cost me valuable energy and end in "burnout."

At the age of twenty-four I had my first experience of kundalinī. In fact, my husband and I had the same experience at the same time. We were meditating late one night when, without warning, I felt a sudden rush, like a current of electricity, up my spine. I was "catapulted" into bright light, like clear moonlight. His experience was identical except that he seemed to be illuminated by sunlight. This was unnerving for both of us as there was little known about "spiritual emergence" in the West at that time. But, as always, when help was needed, it appeared. The next day we were still quite wobbly when we went to a friend's for dinner and were introduced to her spiritual guide, who had been a monk in Burma. We told him what had happened to us and he directed us through a simple Buddhist technique that we practiced for the next week until normality was restored and we lost the fear that it might happen again as traumatically.

There is a saying in Yoga that "when the pupil is ready, the teacher will appear," but not always in the form we expect. My next important "mystical" experience came in a dream some time during my early years in India. During a particularly bad bout of gastric illness, I had a dream that lasted three nights. On the first night, I was falling in space. It was dark, and I could see nothing and feel nothing other than the sensation of falling. On the second night, I was falling through space, then landed on the ground, but was still in blackness. On the third night, I was lying on the ground, aware that I'd just fallen through space but that I'd injured myself as I landed. As I lay there in the dream, wondering what to do, there appeared, softly at first, a bright, white light, illuminating my whole body. As I looked down at my body, I felt I was being lifted out of it so that I could see it from a few feet away. What struck me was that my body didn't appear to be made of bones and tissues, but seemed to consist of a finer, ethereal-like material with a network of fine vein-like channels. It had wheel-like areas of color up the center that, despite my rudimentary knowledge, I "knew" to be the chakras that I'd read about in yoga manuals.

Although I didn't at first know what to do with all this, I realized in a flash that I was supposed to manipulate these channels and centers somehow. Suddenly, I was back in my body looking down at the pattern of energy currents and I also "knew" that what I had to do was to breathe into them, drawing the breath upward and downward and opening any blocks that I encountered. I don't remember if I did this in a systematic way or even if I finished the dream, but the next day I got out of bed feeling extremely well and full of energy.

It was from this experience that I began to explore the subtle body, in meditation and out of it, through study and training, not only in Yoga with the great Hindu teachers like Sri Aurobindo and Swami Sivananda, who greatly influenced my early years "on the path," but by wandering down the byways of other traditions: Buddhist, Taoist, and Tibetan. I also learned other ways of understanding the energies and organs of the subtle body—the kośas, nadis, and chakras—through the techniques of pulse diagnosis, with Ayurvedic and Siddha medicine practitioners and my homeopathy "guru" Swami Narayani. But I had so many unanswered questions. What did it all mean? What do all these connections mean to us as human beings? What role does the subtle body play in our development as human beings, how does it affect our relations in and with the world? And why should one ancient culture appear to have developed such a system more than any other; or is it a universal phenomenon?

These questions plagued me for the next two decades, and what troubled me most was trying to understand the relationship between healing and spirituality and the attempt to integrate these two strands of my life. In India, where the main healing modality is the indigenous system of Ayurveda, nothing is "alternative." All branches of healing and spirituality are treated with equal respect. Through my training in homeopathy, naturopathy, and Yoga I was able to meet, learn from, and work with some of the most eminent and talented homeopaths and healers in the world. I also had complete freedom to develop a synthesis of the many skills I'd learned through working with people from all strata of society, from nomads to maharajahs, from nuns, priests, and Buddhist monks to professional men and women from many different communities, Indian and European.

It was only after I returned from India following the death of my husband that I had the opportunity to start the next phase of my search and to make some sense, in an objective way, of the many experiences that the spiritual life confers. Just as I was wondering what to do with the rest of my life, the strangest of teachers appeared. I was invited to join, as a lecturer, a university course exploring Eastern and Western perceptions of the body in all its facets, material and subtle. I welcomed the chance to delve into the academic treasure house of scholarly writings, and what I learned was fascinating: that the concept of the subtle body exists in virtually every culture in the world, that it has been written about from both secular and spiritual viewpoints, that it is beginning to be explored as a serious academic and scientific subject in the West, and that our own long tradition of esoteric and arcane spiritual teachings has much wisdom to offer us. Of greatest promise, perhaps, is the fact that researchers are beginning to realize that the subtle body's relationship to the human condition, not least as an indicator of health in its broadest sense, is of paramount importance to our well-being as we explore consciousness and, through "new frontier science," the connections between the human and cosmic energy fields.

What has emerged from this exploration is an important realization: that we *cannot* fully understand the subtle body from the "outside." Roger Walsh, psychiatrist and neuroscientist, who has spent a quarter of a century studying and practicing the world's great spiritual traditions, comments:

> Asian meditative and yogic states are now recognized as distinct states *sui generis* that may exhibit a variety of unique phenomenological, perceptual, electrophysical, and hormonal changes. Until recently, however . . . most researchers have had little direct experience of the states they investigate. Yet classical descriptions . . . and personal reports by Western trained researchers suggest that it may be difficult to comprehend fully without direct experience of them.[2]

And neuroscientist Richard J. Davidson also remarks:

> Some of these practices span thousands of years and [as Jacob Needleman and Professor Geoffrey

Samuel, too, have noted] some of mankind's best minds have also devoted themselves to their study. The meditative traditions almost invariably state that the intellectual understanding of the nature of the meditative process is dependent on an adequate base of personal experience. This seems to be borne out by [those] researchers who have themselves undertaken the practice and also in some cases by the quality of research . . . it is sometimes painfully apparent that researchers lack direct experience when statements are made and conclusions drawn that are markedly at variance with even a basic experiential understanding.[3]

A new paradigmatic approach has even appeared in areas that have traditionally demanded "hard" experimental data. It has been recognized, as John Collins reports in his study of mysticism, for instance, that while priority has been given by some researchers to experimentally generated data, there is available a "pool of valid data," including "much that orthodox psychology would reject without investigation," which constitutes a body of scientifically controlled introspective data. He points out that what we need now is an integration of the two approaches, hitherto regarded as contrary or opposite, so that we may explore all human possibilities.[4] This is a truly Yogic approach. As the Yoga historian Georg Feuerstein observes, both practice and study have always been integral aspects of Yoga, and the sage Patanjali listed both in his *Yoga Sūtras,* which detail his "ladder of being," the *aṣṭānga* or "eight limbs."[5]

In this book, I've tried to explore both the experience and the investigation of the *subtle energy body* in different cultures and from different perspectives, to enhance understanding of the whole phenomenon. I hope that you, the reader, will find inspiration in this book to help you to connect, or reconnect, with this great human enterprise. As it says in the philosophical poems of the sixth-century Tamil *Tirumantiram,* referring to the experience and the study of the esoteric bodies, although the soul may appear to be beyond our subtlest understanding and the path ahead shrouded in mist, "it is the beginning of limitless possibilities."[6]

Introduction

The idea that the human being is a complex—including a material body and a nonmaterial, or *subtle*, body—has persisted throughout the ages and is common to many cultures, though the term *subtle body* itself is of relatively recent origin. In many traditions, the entities considered to be parts of the subtle body constitute what we might today interpret as a map of levels of consciousness, or as a hierarchy of nonmaterial entities, each existing on its own plane of reality, while surrounding and enveloping the same visible and tangible physical form, the *gross body*. Schematic descriptions of the subtle body vary in the different traditions, but in most cases belong to a cosmology, a system of thought that attempts to discover the origin, purpose, and destiny of the whole universe, not merely of humankind within it.

An underlying tenet of all philosophical, religious, and mystical doctrines of the ancient world is that the subtle body is an energetic, psychospiritual entity of several layers or sheaths of increasing subtlety and metaphysical significance, through which the aspirant seeks knowledge of the self and the nature of God. The practices and disciplines that evolved to attain this goal form a coherent system of psychospiritual transformation, what religious studies professor David Gordon White calls a "mesocosm," a mediating structure, a bridge, between the human microcosm and the divine macrocosm.[1] In some traditions, that mediating structure was seen as including relationships between the human and the higher worlds through a hierarchy of demigods, angels, avatars, and discarnate teachers and guides who were believed to facilitate the mystical or altered states of consciousness experienced in meditation and prayer, and to lead the seeker to union with the source of all Being.

Author and homeopath David Tansley has written: "The ancient Egyptians, Chinese and Greeks, the Indians of North America, the Polynesian Kahunas, the Incas, the early Christians, the Vedic seers of India, and the medieval alchemists and mystics of Europe have all in one way or another seen man and the study of his anatomy, both physical and subtle, as a key to the nature of God and the universe."[2] Extant writings on the subtle body and its functions include the esoteric cosmologies of Gnosticism, Neo-Platonism, Kabbalah, and Sufism and, nearer our own era, of Rosicrucianism, Theosophy, Anthroposophy, and the "Fourth Way" philosophy of Gurdjieff and Ouspensky. Today, we have "New Age" philosophers who, from beginnings perhaps attributable to Helena Blavatsky, herself a founder of Theosophy in the later nineteenth century, include a new breed of holistic psychologist-philosophers such as Ken Wilber.

The teachings that have come to us from both Eastern and Western ancient sources are often expressed in a "secret" or "twilight" language, the meaning heavily veiled by visual or verbal symbolisms, or merely hinted at in ritual. This secretiveness arose from several synergetic motives. The message could be properly understood only by those whose insight was already sufficiently mature to perceive it for themselves when presented with it, while less mature people would, by misunderstanding, fail to benefit by it themselves and go on to purvey it to others in debased and therefore unhelpful forms. Further, it was felt that only those who had been initiated into a graduated series of practices and had proved themselves ethically as well as intellectually mature would use the knowledge wisely. Yet another reason for secrecy was that in some periods of history initiates were so grossly misunderstood, or even feared, that they were in serious danger of religious or political persecution.

1

Most of the writings on the subtle body include the teaching that the practitioner will escape the wheel of birth, death, and rebirth and avoid the misery of the human condition by climbing a threefold, fivefold, or sevenfold "ladder of being." The by-product of the attempt to become "perfected" (and so avoid the need to reincarnate) is enhancement of the quality of life and well-being even while living in the body. It is perhaps this aspect of immediate betterment that, in recent times, has attracted the greatest interest in these ancient practices. Today, the subtle body and its energy systems, the *chakras* (energy centers or vortices) and the *nadis* (energy currents or streams), are virtually household concepts in the West. This familiarity arose partly through the arrival of Yoga in Europe in the late nineteenth century and its ever-increasing popularity since that time, and partly through the revival of interest in the healing systems and esoteric philosophies that underpin the Holistic and New Age movements.

There is a long Western tradition of esoteric (inner) teachings and practices, the alchemical not least among them, having strong doctrinal parallels and many cultural contacts with the Eastern traditions, carried on in close secrecy by specialists, but the beginnings of a rapidly growing popular awareness of the subtle body in the West is seen in the work of C. G. Jung and Abraham Maslow. They, and more recently Ken Wilber, among others, adopt a transpersonal approach to psychology based on a hierarchy of "individuated" stages of growth that, while adapted to modern conditions and needs, shows marked similarity to the "ladder of being" through which the aspiring mystic, Western or Eastern, passes on the spiritual journey toward the Godhead.*

While the names of the scholars and translators—such as G. R. S. Mead, John Woodroffe (Arthur Avalon), W. Y. Evans-Wentz, and Mircea Eliade, without whose work the current revolution would not have occurred—are hardly known to the present generation of spiritual seekers, some Yoga students and teachers in the West are familiar with their translations of a few of the ancient texts that embody the early teachings: the Vedas, Upaniṣads, Tantras, and the *Yoga Sūtras* of Patanjali. However, a

great many are preoccupied only with the physical aspects of practice, the *āsanas* (postures), and remain completely ignorant of the foundations of the tradition to which they claim to belong. Worse, some healers claim to "balance" and "align" the chakras, the energy centers housed in the subtle body, despite having little or no experience of working on their own through disciplined and sustained practice of Yoga and meditation.

What was once secret knowledge, acquired by sincere practice under the guidance of wise teachers, has now been spread so widely by the huge proliferation of books, workshops, courses, and internet sites that the teachings are in danger of being no longer respected, recognized, or valued at true worth. However, the positive side of the present wide and free dissemination of knowledge is that it has opened up possibilities of engaging with the doctrines, practices, beliefs, or traditions that surround models of the subtle body. This offers everyone the opportunity to explore their spirituality and common spiritual heritage, whether or not as part of an organized religion, and to participate in a more open-minded, holistic approach to health and well-being.

This complete guide to the subtle energy body traces first Eastern then Western developments of paths to transformation in several traditions, ancient and modern. It draws together scientific and spiritual perspectives and discusses the potential that understanding of the subtle body offers for an integral model of healing. Readers should not be troubled to find themselves surrounded at times by what appear to be incompatible ideas, anomalies, and puzzles. In this regard it is important that the book be read as a whole; this will facilitate a general understanding that includes concepts already somewhat familiar from Western culture. When pondered alongside the Eastern concepts and descriptions they will reveal many mutually illuminating similarities. This process will enhance understanding of both the past and the future development of our quest as human beings to know ourselves (see plates 1 and 2). Stated far too briefly, the quest now is not to destroy humanity's past states of being but to embrace what we have been in the past, bringing those prior modes of consciousness into a new consciousness that integrates everything we are. The results of past analyses will become the recognized energies of a new mode of life in which everything is in place and everything functions as it should.

---

*In Genesis 28.10–19, for example, the Hebrew patriarch Jacob is granted a dream of a ladder from earth to heaven, with angels ascending and descending it, which causes Jacob to name the place where he experienced the dream Beth El, the House of God.

PART ONE
Eastern Perspectives

In this first part we shall explore some of the historical, philosophical, and practical aspects of the subtle body in Eastern traditions. We shall ask, and attempt to answer, some intriguing questions about the concept of the subtle body, such as the following:

What is the subtle body?

What are the earliest known textual references to the subtle body?

In which religio-spiritual traditions did the concept of a subtle body first appear and why?

What are the nature, purpose, and functions of the subtle body?

What cultural transformations have conceptions of the subtle body undergone and what have been the effects of these changes?

In the attempt to answer these questions we shall survey a range of ideas from the Eastern perspective, such as attitudes to the body and the concept of "embodiment," and attempt to see their essence by examining the "disembodied" and "embodied" practices found in different traditions. For example, we shall find "interiorized" correlates of exoteric (outer) rituals, a fact that alerts us to the need for empathy and contemplative insight if we are to grasp what the traditions have tried to say and to preserve for later generations.

Accordingly, we shall examine some key concepts relating to the subtle body, which include the following:

The relationship between body, mind, and spirit in ancient Indian, Tibetan, and Chinese thought

Ideas about visible and nonvisible aspects of Reality

The microcosm and the macrocosm

The "hidden," esoteric knowledge of various schools of thought

How the schema of the subtle body is integrated into the practices of some traditions such as Yoga, Tantra, and Qigong

The body itself as the locus of spiritual transformation

As we shall see, models of the subtle body vary in different traditions throughout the ancient East and Far East, but they share most of their major components and concepts. Nomenclatures and emphases vary, a fact that often obscures the underlying similarities of concept. Despite the variations in schematic representation, however, the different perceptions and understandings have a common *purpose*. A particular point to note is that many of the traditions share a belief in immortality and the continuity of the invisible, subtle part of the human being from life to life. Of course, much follows from all this.

A central realization was that the objective was the broadening, even the complete transcendence, of what we are as embodied beings living "down here." This should alert us to an important fact: the study of cultural symbols is not itself the attainment of the objects of the symbolism. To give a relevant example, to be dealt with in chapter 2, the complex process of conceptualization that saw parallels between trees and the human quest for self-transcendence, taken alone and as a cultural phenomenon, could provide lifetimes of fruitful study, but the grasping of *what it was in itself* that had been thus perceived and conserved in the tree symbolism is another matter altogether. A meditator might well arrive at that realization without the cultural study, which, though fascinating, could never by itself provide the enlightenment that the sages had experienced. The use of the tree symbolism enabled the sages to simultaneously hide what they had realized from those who could not benefit from their understanding and *reveal it* to those with eyes to see what the symbols meant.

Such symbolisms are analogous to a musical score, which is only an approximate map of a living reality, for the music is not the marks on paper, nor is it even the notes. No one prefers the printed score, let alone the mere verbal comment in the program notes, to *the living experience of hearing the music itself*. Spirituality is like this. As the subtle body seems to be a many-layered and largely *spiritual* entity, we should therefore recognize the need for empathetic discrimination between substance and mere symbol throughout our exploration.

ONE

The Spiritual Enterprise

The common theme of most of the major religions of the world is the striving for a lost unity. Religion always proceeds from an existential dichotomy between man and the world, between man and God or the gods. Man longs for unity, longs to overcome the dichotomy; wholeness rather than division seems to him necessary for living.

HANS JOACHIM SCHOEPS, *AN INTELLIGENT PERSON'S GUIDE TO THE RELIGIONS OF MANKIND*

The spiritual direction of the major religions of the East is toward the inward experience of enlightenment, and the process arises out of a desire to be united with the cosmos as an unrestricted spirit, free of the weariness of worldly life and its sufferings.

In his introduction to *Yoga: Immortality and Freedom,* Mircea Eliade states that, in Indian thought, the "normal" human condition is equivalent to bondage and the idea of the *jīvan-mukta,* the "liberated-while-living," expresses the nostalgia of the whole Indian soul.[1] In early Indian thought the means to immortality and freedom from *samsāra,* "the chain of rebirths," was believed to come through four main pathways: the understanding of reality, spirituality, integration, and liberation. Together, these pathways constitute the core of life in Indian society.

Foremost among the four paths is the quest for reality, states Troy Wilson Organ, professor of philosophy, in *The Hindu Quest for the Perfection of Man.* This is not an external reality that may be known discursively, but an inner reality to be known by direct insight. The attainment of *moksa* (liberation) is a creative achievement by which the finite self reaches an identity with the Supreme Reality through proper techniques. Hence moksa is the removal of confining perspectives that prevent the self from having an existential awareness of its true nature.[2] Further and most importantly, Organ observes that man seeks liberation in order to become what he is. The full realization of his nature is the goal of positive freedom. As he expresses it, moksa is the opportunity to become the "Perfected Man." A man does not become a superman, or an angel, or a god. He becomes himself.[3]

This enterprise has both clearly defined goals and methods to achieve them. The "proper techniques" referred to by Troy Wilson Organ are what the Yoga historian Georg Feuerstein calls "that enormous body of spiritual values, attitudes, precepts and techniques developed over five millennia, that may be regarded as the very foundation of the ancient Indian civilization."[4] *Yoga* is thus the generic name for the various Indian paths of self-transcendence, the methodical transmutation of consciousness to the point of liberation from the spell of the ego-personality. It is the psychospiritual technology that "yokes,"* harnessing attention, or consciousness, to

---

Yoga is etymologically derived from the verbal root *yuj,* meaning "to bind together" or "to yoke," and can have many connotations, including: "union," "endeavor," "occupation," "equipment," "trick," "magic," "aggregate," and "sum."

the point of reaching the ecstatic condition (*samādhi*) in which the mechanics of the mind are at least temporarily transcended. The word *yoga* also refers to the by-products of this process, such as "equanimity" (*samatva*), which literally means "sameness" or "evenness," "balance," and "harmony."[5]

The Six Systems of Traditional Indian Philosophy

The extensive field of traditional or orthodox Indian philosophical understanding is divided into six complementary *darśanas* or visions, which are linked in pairs:

- *Samkhya* (evolution from the dual principles of *puruṣa,* "spirit," and *prakṛti,* "nature") and *Yoga* (dynamics of the process of liberation)
- *Vaiseshika* (cosmology) and *Nyaya* (logic)
- *Mimamsa* (study of ritual action) and *Vedanta* (final truth or end, *anta,* of the Vedas)

The oral teachings of the lineage of profound ancient Yoga referred to as *rāja yoga* (royal path) were recorded and arranged by Patanjali (ca. 200 BCE) in the *Yoga Sūtras,* one hundred and eighty aphorisms that guide aspirants through physical, psychological, moral, behavioral, and spiritual practice to samādhi, transcendence. Rāja yoga is also known as *aṣṭāṅga yoga,* the "eight-limbed path" on the "ladder of being." The *Yoga Sūtras* reiterate the dualistic philosophy of Samkhya. Many later lineages or teachings (such as *agni yoga*) replace the philosophical dualism of the *Yoga Sūtras* with Tantric and nondual perspectives, while still using many of its practical teachings.

Like most philosophical and religious systems of the ancient world, Yoga has both exoteric (outer) and esoteric (inner) means of discovering the nature of the human spirit, soul, and body, and the nature of God. There are several Yogic paths through which the aspirant may experience self-realization or liberation. Many Westerners are at least superficially familiar with some of the major forms of Yoga, namely *rāja, hatha, karma, bhakti, jñāna, kriyā,* and *tantra,* the last often taken to include two further practices known as *laya*

and *kundalinī.* The yogas most widely practiced in the English speaking countries today are the classical system of Patanjali, which came into vogue in India in the sixteenth century CE, and hatha yoga, also a medieval development, which aims to strengthen the body for the rigors of the mystical experience (see plate 3). In addition, the unique modern approach of Sri Aurobindo's integral yoga, which favors an evolutionary synthesis, is gaining ground.

Transcendence as a process of emanation from the gross material body via invisible, hence "subtle," bodies is the central concept of many of these Yogic paths. The idea that the body itself is the means to transcendence of

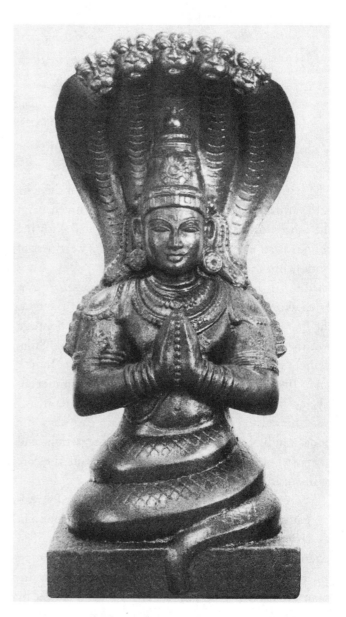

Fig. 1.1. Patanjali, author of the *Yoga Sūtras,* a prime classical Yoga text, lived ca. 200 BCE.

the body is perhaps best expressed by the Greek word εκ, meaning "out from." Thus we have the concept of the jīvan-mukta, the person who is liberated from the privations imposed by the gross material body, while still in that gross material body. The physical body (sthūla śarīra) is seen as the outer material form of a subtle body (sūkṣma śarīra), or of a series of such nonvisible bodies; it is through these interpenetrating forms that the aspirant becomes sensitive to the vital forces that connect the human soul (ātman) with the soul of the cosmos (Brahman). The subtle body is thus the arena of actions that, in the somewhat later and more Western Hermetic tradition,* are held to fulfill or demonstrate the formula "As above, so below."

In the Indic traditions the transformative methodology of the subtle body was not fully developed until the flowering of the esoteric tradition of Tantra,† about the middle of the millennium immediately before the Common Era, and it was the early Upaniṣads‡ (mystical spiritual treatises) that presented the earliest explicit model of five kośas (five "sheaths" or "layers of consciousness"), which surround the physical body. These are discussed in detail in chapter 3. However, Feuerstein points out that rudimentary descriptions of the subtle body had appeared as early as the *Atharva Veda,* in sections believed to have been composed between 3000 and 4000 BCE.[6]

The History of Consciousness

While all Yogic approaches aim at self-transcendence, it has always been recognized that some forms of Yoga are more suitable for particular temperaments than others, and at different stages of life. Furthermore, humanity as a whole has been involved in the spiritual enterprise. Consciousness itself has developed as human beings have evolved through different stages of awareness and

---

*The Hermetic tradition will be dealt with in part 2, beginning with chapter 10, and in greater detail in chapters 11 to 13.

†The word *tantra,* meaning "loom," is used to designate the ancient esoteric tradition as well as a sacred scripture of that tradition; Tantra gave rise to Tantrism, a many-branched religious and cultural movement that emerged in the early centuries CE and was at its height around 1000 CE.

‡The word *upaniṣad* literally means "sitting near," and is sometimes translated as "whispered."

cognition. While some believe that changes to our physical form may have come to an end, many hold that our subtle aspects will continue to evolve and expand.

The Swiss philosopher, linguist, poet, and mystic Jean Gebser (1905–1973) formulated a theory of consciousness in the story of the evolving soul. He recognizes five stages of development unfolded thus far in the ongoing history of human civilization after its emergence from what he calls the "Ever-Present Origin" or "Ground of Being." Gebser's stages of consciousness are also "cognitive styles."[7] Feuerstein claims that the progressing cognitive styles of this succession of civilizations have been the driving force behind the differing philosophies and practices of the Hindu, Jain, and Buddhist forms of Yoga.[8]

First is *archaic consciousness,** which is characterized by the state of deep sleep. According to Gebser's analysis, it is the cognitive basis out of which the urge to self-transcendence arose. It belongs historically to the age of *Australopithecus* and *Homo habilis* (3.9 to 2.9 million years ago). Out of this origin, the primal human being mutated from a state of "non-consciousness," of "spacelessness and timelessness," being part of the whole with a "full identity between inner and outer, expressive of the *microcosmic harmony.*"[9]

Next, *magical consciousness* arose, Gebser says, during the era of *Homo erectus,* over 1.5 million years ago. This consciousness structure is characterized by a sleep-like, semi-conscious state. Released from harmony, or identity, with the whole, human beings became "self-conscious" and able to "cope with the earth" through impulse and instinct. They distinguished the animal that threatened and gained power over it by drawing its picture. Here we see the appearance of "sympathetic magic" in "hunting magic." As part of the emerging ritual magic and ceremony, humans engaged in the "sacrifice of consciousness," which occurs in the state of trance and is a type of consciousness in which the person becomes so closely identified with someone or something that he or she becomes "spellbound," as in the ecstatic consciousness of the shaman immersed in the experience of the numinous.[10] Magical consciousness is the cognitive basis for intense inward concentration, and, in Yogic terms, those

---

*Archaic is from the Greek word *archē,* meaning "inception" or "origin."

Texts of the Vedic Revelation (*Śruti*)

The Four Vedas

The dates of composition of the four Vedas (collections of hymns), also known as the *Samhitās* (meaning "joined" or "collected"), range widely in estimates from approximately 3000 BCE to 1000 BCE. Originally transmitted orally, they were later recorded.

1. The *Ṛg Veda* (*Ṛg:* "praise" or "verse" and *veda:* "knowledge") consists of ten books of 1,028 hymns of 10,600 verses, essentially completed by about 1200 BCE although some were composed as late as the fourteenth century CE. They contain numerous passages of proto-Yogic ideas and practices derived from Indus-Saraswati rituals of sacrificial mysticism. To the authors of the verses, the poet-seers (*rishis*), they were not only prayers to petition the gods for health, prosperity, and cosmic harmony, but also a means of experiencing ecstatic self-transcendence through contemplation and inner recital of their symbolic and metaphorical expressions of the sacred.

2. The *Sāma Veda* (*sāma:* "contemplation" or "song" and *veda:* "knowledge") is next in liturgical importance to the *Ṛg Veda* and dates from around 1000 BCE. It is literally a "song book" of the hymns of the *Ṛg Veda* transposed and rearranged to suit the rituals sung by *udgātṛ* (singer) priests during the offering of the juice of the soma plant as a libation to various deities. These *mantras* (sacred sounds), which were said to have sprung from inner illumination, are still chanted by Hindus today.

3. The *Yajur Veda* (*yajur:* "sacrificial formula" and *veda:* "knowledge") is a compilation of 1,549 stanzas of the liturgical mantras of the *Ṛg Veda* for all sacrificial rites, not just the soma ritual, with commentaries in prose believed to date from 1400 to 1000 BCE. The use of mystical sounds later became a popular spiritual technique to attain salvation through the Yogic practice of concentration (*dhārana*) and the Tantric development of interiorized ritual.

4. The *Atharva Veda* (knowledge of the Atharvans) is a compilation of 760 hymns about 160 of which it has in common with the *Ṛg Veda*; other hymns are much older, collected by the fire priest and magician Atharvan and his followers. The first part of the six thousand verses consists mostly of spells and incantations for peace, protection, and healing, and is the first Indic text that deals with medicine. The second part is philosophical, speculating on the nature of the universe, anticipating the knowledge of the Upaniṣads. It not only contains hymns to Skambha ("support" or "First Principle") and on *prāna,* the "breath of life," but also cosmogonic hymns relating to the nectar of immortality and aspirations to transcendence within the body-mind of the seers. Many of the mystical passages are obscure, but there are also verses that refer to the chakras and nadis of the subtle body, giving clear indications of esoteric knowledge that preceded the development of Yoga.

Brāhmanas

The Brāhmanas are prose descriptions of ritual observances, explaining the Vedic hymns that are relevant to the practices of the brahmins, the priestly class of Hindu society.

Āranyakas (forest books)

In the Āranyakas the rituals were given symbolic meanings.

Upaniṣads

Upaniṣads are the esoteric, "secret" teachings that expound the metaphysics of nondualism (*Advaita Vedanta*), which is considered to be the last phase of the Vedic revelation. The oldest Upaniṣads were composed between 800 and 400 BCE, though some were composed as late as the fifteenth century CE.

practices that lead to loss of awareness of the physical body. The state is also sought in those schools of Tantra and Siddha (attainment) yoga that attempt to cultivate the magical or supernormal powers known as *siddhis*.

Gebser believes that this is the period when the soul came into being, "simultaneously with the sky," as Plato put it. The subtle body, therefore, began with the first acknowledgement of the cycles of time, of day, night, and seasons; it also heralded the "birth of imagination." The person was a unity yet able to recognize the world as a whole.[11] Out of this consciousness also arose alchemy with its law of correspondences. "Man replies to the forces streaming toward him with his own corresponding forces: he stands up to Nature. He tries to exorcise her, to guide her; he strives to be independent of her; then he begins to be conscious of his own *will*. . . . Witchcraft and sorcery, totem and taboo, are the natural means by which [magic man] seeks to free himself from the transcendent power of nature, by which his soul strives to materialize within him and to become increasingly conscious of itself."[12]

The third stage, *mythical consciousness,* arose during the Neanderthal era, 130,000 years ago, and during the Cro-Magnon era, 40,000 to 10,000 years ago. This consciousness structure is dream-like. It appeared before our consciousness of time *as such,* although humans previously had a time-sense closely attuned to natural cycles. We gradually became extricated from entanglement with nature through an increasing awareness of our individuation and an awareness of the external world, especially in the polarities and dualities of forms. Mythical consciousness is distinct from magical consciousness in that it bears the stamp of imagination rather than the stress of emotion. Feuerstein believes mythical consciousness to be a principal factor in the creation of the immense variety of sacred traditions, including Yoga.[13] Gebser describes it as a period in which "silent inward-directed contemplation . . . renders the soul visible so that it may be visualized, represented, heard, and made audible."[14]

Mythic consciousness is present in imagery and poetic expression and leads to an awareness of the psyche, the inner world. It is the cognitive basis of many forms of Yoga in which symbolism is the means toward transcendence, particularly traditional forms such as the classical and hatha yoga paths. Gebser terms it the "frequency" par excellence of the "Eastern Man"[15] and it

is exemplified in the Noble Eightfold Path of Gautama Buddha.

Fourth, *mental consciousness,* is what we in the modern West call "left-brain," rational, logical thinking. Gebser holds that this cognitive style, characterized by "wakefulness," has dominated European consciousness since the Renaissance, and has become a destructive force. However, it began as an emerging awareness of perspective, the visual, and of more "logical," self-examining and self-validating methods of thought. Feuerstein points out that at its best it produced the Patanjali *Yoga Sūtras* and other commentaries. He also notes that, while the intellectual process is often regarded as the enemy of spiritual progress, this limitation is not present in more integrative forms of Yoga in which the mechanisms of the mind are transcended by a process that combines them into an all-embracing awareness. This requires an understanding of the mind in both its lower processes (*manas*)* and its higher manifestations (*buddhi*)† and an acceptance of these as equally necessary parts of the intended Wholeness. This schema is similar to the idea introduced by Plato of body and spirit as "opposites," with the soul as mediator between them.[16]

Integral consciousness, Gebser believes, is what is emerging in our consciousness structure today. It represents an "intensification" of consciousness, that vital moment when thought turns toward itself. Integral consciousness is an awareness that we can change our way of being and thinking, and so help to bring balance to human civilization by integrating our inherent but disparate structures of consciousness. Many of the tools for this process, Feuerstein believes, are contained within the various paths of Yoga. Specifically, the philosophy of Sri Aurobindo, whom Gebser regarded as a "spiritual giant," is the most recognized path.[17] In his teachings, Sri Aurobindo spoke of "body consciousness" as part of the whole being, and of an "evolving soul." He postulated a central being, or "Psychic Being," as he called it, formed by a transcendent and eternal spirit, lying behind

Manas is the "lower mind." It is a "relay station" for the external sense organs and is itself one of the senses when operating as a faculty of *noninferential direct recognition,* as posited by Western philosophers such as Heidegger and, more specifically, Wittgenstein.
†*Buddhi* is the higher, intuitive mind, the faculty of wisdom, but the word is also used to denote "thought" or "cognition."

the veneer-like surface of consciousness. He believed that this Psychic Being can be contacted through spiritual discipline.[18] Much of his methodology was based on the awareness of planes of consciousness that emerged during the period of Tantrism.

Initially only one of these cognitive styles identified by Gebser was available to humanity; now, all are available, spontaneously, by choice, or after spiritual practice. Feuerstein believes that Gebser's "consciousness structures" represent an integral framework that can prevent a researcher from being caught within a single time, place, or mode of thinking or perceiving when studying a particular tradition. It makes it possible to simultaneously perceive, elicit, compare, and verify themes across the several modes of consciousness: archaic, magical, mythical, mental, and integral.[19]

Approaches to Liberation

Feuerstein distinguishes "verticalist, horizontalist, and integral approaches" to liberation, which he denotes by the Sanskrit terms *nivṛtti-marga* (the path of cessation),[20] *pravṛtti-marga* (the path of activity), and *pūrna-marga* (the path of wholeness), in each of which a different cognitive style dominates.[21]

The Path of Cessation

Nivṛtti-marga (the path of cessation) is essentially an ascetic approach followed by those who regard the body as an inconvenience, an obstacle to freedom. Feuerstein explains that philosophical verticalism views the body as a breeding ground for *karma** and an automatic hindrance to enlightenment. The common Sanskrit word for "body" is *deha,* which stems from the verbal root *dih* ("to smear" or "to be soiled"). It hints at the defiled nature of the body. Yet the same verbal root can also signify "to anoint," which gives the noun *deha* the far more laudatory meaning of "that which is anointed." The older Sanskrit word for "body" is *śarīra,* derived from the verbal root *śri* ("to rest upon" or "to support"), which has a more positive connotation: the body serves as the prop, or framework, by means of which the Self* can experience the world.

This notion led to the still more positive interpretation of the body as a temple of the Divine†—an idea intimated in the early Upaniṣads but not fully elaborated until the emergence of Tantra much later.[22]

However, the basic paradigm for the relationship between soul and body in Indian thought creates an enigma. On the one hand, the Vedantic perspective is that the phenomenon of embodiment is *dualistic.* The *Katha Upaniṣad,* described by Max Müller as "one of the most perfect specimens of the mystic philosophy and poetry of the ancient Hindus,"[24] states:

> [Like] light and shade [there are] two
>   [selves]:
> [One] here on earth imbibes the law (ṛta)
>   of his own deeds:
> [The other,] though hidden in the secret
>   places [of the heart],
> [Dwells] in the uttermost beyond.[25]
>   KATHA UPANIṢAD III.1

If the soul expresses itself through the body, this raises the question of whether the soul's true reality is impaired, reduced, restricted, or at the very least obscured by the body. Is the transcendental perspective of ātman as *pure consciousness* not similarly impaired, implying that the body must be seen as a prison and a tomb from which the soul longs to be released? The body therefore plays an ambiguous role. This ambiguity, as philosopher Debabrata Sinha points out, makes its appearance in the focus of reflection through the dialectical interplay of the mundane and extramundane consciousness, of the natural and the overnatural, of experience and transcendence. Paradoxically, it is that very ambiguity, that inexplicable dilemma, which helps us to attain an understanding of the total experience of the human condition.[26]

Recall, then, that the word *human* means "of the earth." So—in spite of the idea of the *wholeness* of human existence that is expressed in the *Katha Upaniṣad*—the

---

**Karma,* "action," is defined by Webster's English Dictionary as "the force generated by a person's actions, held in Hinduism and Buddhism to perpetuate transmigration and in its ethical consequences to determine his destiny in his next existence."

---

*In discussions of Hindu philosophy, Self (with a capital *S*) is used to indicate *ātman,* the transcendent, immortal Self, which is pure consciousness.

†The apostle Paul, in I Corinthians 6.19, expresses the related, if not identical, notion of the indwelling Holy Spirit, in arguing for cessation of immoral actions: "Your body . . . is the temple of the Holy Spirit."[23]

search for truth, which becomes the vehicle for liberation in Indian consciousness, seems to require separation from all that is human, from all that is of the earth. To "free oneself," according to Eliade, is equivalent to forcing another plane of existence, to appropriating another mode of being, thus *transcending* the human condition, "for India, not only is metaphysical knowledge translated into terms of *rupture* and *death* . . . it also necessarily implies a consequence of a mystical nature: *rebirth to a non-conditioned mode of being*."[27]

We should note here that while the "non-conditioned mode of being" to which Eliade refers seems to imply an inability to function in the mundane world, the study of mysticism and the transcendent state teaches us that the mystic process tends to be "enabling" rather than "disabling." In his study *Mysticism and New Paradigm Psychology,* for example, John E. Collins suggests that there are various stages in the transcendent process that eventually lead to an integrated understanding because "we are both mystical and scientific, introspective and empirical, spiritual and material."[28]

The following text indicates that while the Upaniṣadic conception of human existence is dualistic, *it is also holistic*:

> *Know this:*
> *The self is the owner of the chariot*
> *The chariot is the body*
> *Soul* (buddhi) *is the body's charioteer—*
> *Mind the reins [that curb it].*
> KATHA UPANIṢAD I.III 3–4[29]

This verse, Sinha believes, presents the entire psychophysical complex of the human reality, the microcosmic status of the body in the macrocosmic understanding of the universe at large. Coming directly to Advaita Vedanta,* he says that its recognition of the primacy of bodily reality is indicated in the very definition of *jīva* (individual soul) offered by Sankara: the word *jīva* indicates the conscious principle exercising supervision over the body and sustaining the vital airs. Sinha goes on to say that the body is not just a physical

lump, a mere complex of natural products, but rather the "matrix" of concrete human existence, and that this is borne out by the distinction between gross body (sthūla śarīra) and subtle body (sūkṣma śarīra). While the gross (visible) body is the locus of all experiences, the subtle (invisible) body is defined as the *means of* such experience.[30]

In Feuerstein's opinion, if the world is real the body must be real as well. If the world is in essence divine, so must be the body. If we must honor the world as a creation or an aspect of the Divine Power (*Sakti*) we must likewise honor the body. The body is a piece of the world and the world is a piece of the body. Or, rather, when we truly understand the body we discover that it is the world, which in essence is divine.[31]

The Path of Activity

Pravṛtti-marga (the path of activity) is, in Feuerstein's view of the three kinds of teachings, the "horizontalist" approach. He describes this approach as characterized by the typical extroverted lifestyle of the worldling (*samārin*) in which the experiences of the physical, material body of sensory gratification predominate.[32] Such a worldling is preoccupied with job, prospects, status, family, and belongings. However, there are a number of early Hindu texts that, if their teaching is assimilated, enable worldly minded people to live a better life in the pursuit of the first three goals of human existence, namely material welfare (*artha*), passionate self-expression (*kama*), and moral virtue or lawfulness (*dharma*). The best-known work on the last of these is the *Manava Dharma Sastra*, also known as the *Manu Smṛti*, consisting of 2,685 verses ascribed to Manu, the progenitor of the human race, who is believed to have divided the course of human life into four stages of twenty-one years within the full life-span of eighty-four years.

Pravṛtti means "action." Accordingly, karma yoga is the most suitable Yogic path for those of an active temperament and at this stage of development. The word *karma* is derived from the root *kri* ("to make" or "to do") and has many meanings. It can signify "action," "work," "product," "effect." Thus karma yoga is literally the "yoga of action." But here the term *karma* stands for a particular kind of action, denoting an inner attitude toward action in general. Such an attitude is itself seen as a form of action within the broad meaning of the word.

Advaita (nondual) is a subschool of Vedanta, the dominant school of Indian philosophy, the chief principles of which were consolidated by the monk-philosopher Adi Sankara (788–820 CE).

What this attitude consists of is spelled out in one of the essential philosophical texts of India, the Bhagavad Gītā, for example in the following verses:

> *"Just as the unwise act attached to action,*
>   *O Son of Bharata,**
> *the wise should act unattached, desiring*
>   *the world's welfare."*
>
> (3.25)

> *"Always performing all [allotted] actions*
>   *and taking refuge in Me,*
> *he attains through My grace the eternal,*
>   *immutable State."*
>
> (18.56)[33]

Feuerstein explains that the essence of karma yoga is being able to act in any given situation without being motivated by the ego; when the illusion of the ego as acting subject is transcended, then actions are recognized to occur spontaneously. Behind the action of the enlightened there is no author; or we could say that Nature itself is the author.[34] Here, Feuerstein highlights an important point that will be explored more fully in chapter 5, which is that through karma yoga, every action is turned into a sacrifice. This is true for those living the life of householders as well as those living an ascetic life. What is sacrificed is the self or ego (*ahamkāra*) that presumes itself to be the author of actions or inactions. When we act with this presumption, our actions or inactions have a "binding power"; they generate and accumulate karma from life to life. They reinforce the ego, thereby obstructing enlightenment.

Karma yoga goes even further, in a way that opposes the grain of human nature, by teaching that the quality of life on the earthly plane is controlled by the *intention behind the action* and therefore only *responsible* action can reverse the effects of existing karma. Mahatma Gandhi is perhaps India's best example of a karma yogi. Although he believed in the inevitability of karma, he also believed that human beings could change their destiny by responsible action through will.

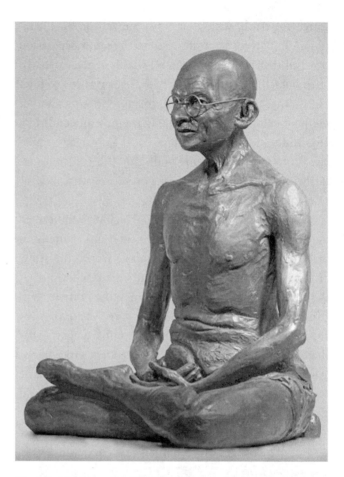

Fig. 1.2. Mahatma Gandhi seated in meditation in the lotus position. Although he was an advocate of nonviolent protest and lived an ascetic lifestyle, he is possibly India's best example of a karma yogi. (The figure is an original work by sculptor Bob Clyatt—bob@clyattsculpture.com. The photograph is reproduced here with the sculptor's kind permission.)

The Path of Wholeness

Feuerstein believes that pūrna-marga (the path of wholeness) is a synthesis of the highest cultural values of East and West; while technically it does not offer much that is new, its real significance lies in its overall holistic approach and its immense wealth of outstanding spiritual discoveries, which stand at the watershed of a new era of Yogic culture.[35]

The Central Goal

Many Upaniṣads assert that the most developed and wise are those who have no desires other than "the desire for the Self," which is a desire for under-

---

*Here Krishna, representing the Absolute, is speaking to Arjuna, whom he addresses as a son of *Bharata,* the Hindu name for India.

standing.[36] Chakravarthi Ram-Prasad, professor of comparative religion and philosophy, believes this is an important stage in the understanding of reality, because, as we saw earlier, the prevailing theme of Indian philosophy is that all life is suffering, and that realizing the Self (ātman) is essential in attaining the goal of mokṣa (freedom).[37]

But what exactly is ātman? And what is meant by "knowing the ātman"? In his article entitled "The Concept of the Spiritual in Indian Thought," P. T. Raju explains that the word ātman is related, perhaps, to the German word ātmen, "to breathe," and thus may be similar to "spirit" in its original connotation.[38] Perhaps it lost its first associations with wind and air in its later meanings. Both the *Taittirīya Upaniṣad* and the *Māndūkya Upaniṣad* offer helpful explanations of ātman. For example, in the *Taittirīya*, we read of five bodies and five ātmans, which together are interpreted as the five sheaths (kośas), as if the pure, original ātman were covered up with sheaths or enclosed within boxes. On the other hand, each ātman is thought of as a bird with wings, tail, and so on, because life is imagined to fly away from the body at death.

Paul Deussen (1845–1919), Orientalist and Sanskrit scholar, explains that the entire doctrine of the Upaniṣads is "the identity of the Brahman and the ātman, of God and the Soul" and he adds that "the original thinkers of the Upanishads, to their immortal honour . . . recognised our ātman, our inmost individual being, as the Brahman, the inmost being of universal nature and of all her phenomena."[39]

The kośas or sheaths arise from the ātman itself. Raju tells us that:

The *Taittirīya* says that ākāśa, space, or ether, is born out of ātman, air out of ākāśa, fire out of air, water out of fire, earth out of water, plants out of earth, food out of plants, semen out of food, and person (puruṣa) out of semen. Puruṣa here means the physical man. He is the essence of food. The physical body is not the ātman of anything else. Of this body, the vital principle (prāna) is the ātman: of the prāna, the mind (manas, not to be equated with the mind in Western philosophy and psychology) is the ātman; of the mind, intelligence (vijñāna, reason); of intelligence, bliss (ānanda); and of bliss, the pure ātman is not the body of anything else and the physical body produced by food is not the ātman of anything else.[40]

How did such an understanding of the kośas, the five sheaths, become the basis of the psychospiritual methodology required to attain liberation? We shall explore this further in chapter 3. How did human beings, separated from the source of being through ego-consciousness, discover how to become one with God? In chapter 2 we shall look at our place in the universe and our relationship with the God, the Great Being, with whom we attempt to become reunited through the great spiritual enterprise of transformation.

TWO

The Cosmic Person

The hidden dimension of macrocosmic existence, of the universe at large, has its precise parallel in the microcosm of the human body-mind. The "deep structures" of the body share in the "deep structures" of its larger environment. All esoteric traditions assume that there is a correspondence between inner and outer reality.

GEORG FEUERSTEIN, *THE YOGA TRADITION: ITS HISTORY, LITERATURE, PHILOSOPHY AND PRACTICE*

The human being is conceived in Indian thought as being the microcosm of all of creation, according to David Gordon White. Humans lie midway between the lower creatures, plants, and nonliving matter on the one hand, and the divine hierarchies and subtle beings on the other. But, more important than this, the human being has been seen, at least since the time of the Upaniṣads, as possessing an individual soul or spirit (ātman), which is a microcosm of the universal Brahman. Just as Brahman is seen as the hub of the cosmic round of creation, the axis of the universe, so ātman is seen as the center of the human body (see plate 4).[1]

In both Eastern and Western traditions introspection revealed distinct levels of being within the physical body's position in the world, and therefore, with or without the use of the term, these levels came to be thought of as the subtle body, existing at least approximately co-temporally and cospatially with the visible, gross body. "Correspondences" were conceived between the microcosm of the gross and subtle body system and the macrocosm within which it had its life, its movement, and its very being. In this chapter, we shall explore the microcosm and macrocosm in Eastern traditions, but show first that the two broad historical developments of

East and West share common ground and symbols, in particular the Tree of Life.

Symbolism and Knowledge

The great discovery of the Upaniṣads, Mircea Eliade tells us in his *Yoga: Immortality and Freedom,* was the identity between the ātman and the Brahman, the Upaniṣadic discovery that "immortality and absolute power became accessible to every being who made the effort to reach *gnosis* and thus acquire knowledge of every mystery, for the *Brahman* represented all that."[2] Among all of the nearly innumerable identifications and homologizations, Eliade says, "the *Brahman* was considered and expressly called the imperishable, the immutable, the foundation of all existence . . . the *skambha,* the cosmic pillar, the *axis mundi.*"[3]

Professor Eliade goes on to say that this primordial symbolic axis, always placed at the center of the world, is conceived of as supporting and connecting the three cosmic regions: heaven, earth, and underworld. However, it does not merely symbolize the manifestation of the cosmic as forms but also as that which contains them, as the *Atharva Veda* (X 8.2) says, "in the *skambha* is every-

14

thing that is possessed by spirit (*ātmānvat*), everything that breathes."[4]

The Being identified in the axis of the universe is found again, on another level, in the individual's spiritual center, in the ātman. "To know the *skambha* . . . is to possess the key to the cosmic mystery and to find the 'center of the world' in the inmost depths of one's being. Knowledge is a sacred force because it solves the enigma . . . of the Self."[5] The leitmotif of post-Vedic texts, says Eliade, is the claim that one becomes Brahman through knowledge of Being and by the acquisition of the highest of powers, *sacred* power.

Implicit to the Indian worldview, from the earliest traditions down to the present, there has been an understanding of reality as being ordered hierarchically, with correspondences existing between different or "parallel" hierarchical orderings. This is present in nearly every Indian realm of thought and practice, from the correspondences between the hierarchical social orders (*varnas*) and cosmic epochs (*yugas*) to those between the senses (*indriyas*) and the elements (*bhutas*). The same understanding is inherent in the concepts of the hierarchically ordered qualities (*gunas*), the aims of life (*puruṣarthus*), the stages of life (*asramas*), the arrangement of the concentric islands (*dvipas*) of the earthly disc around the central axis of Mount Meru, the vertical arrangement of heaven, midspace, earth, and the subterranean worlds, the planets, and so on, ad infinitum.

Such systems of hierarchies and correspondences exist in ritual practice as well as in conceptual systems. The *varna* system, for example, by which social relations and interactions are ordered in a ritual manner, has its origins in the sacrifice of the cosmic *puruṣa*, from which all creation emerged.* To this we might add the homologous vision of the parts of the body of a horse as the physical and divine universe in the royal

ritual of *aśvamedha* (horse sacrifice) described in the hymns of the *Ṛg Veda* (1.162–63), themselves known as aśvamedha. Another example is the naming of each of the bricks of the Vedic sacrificial altar (*vedi*) in which the five layers of bricks stand for the whole hierarchized universal order (see chapter 4).[6]

Essential to these corresponding systems of hierarchies, White believes, are the concepts of emanation or penetration (*vyāpana*),* and participation or absorption (*laya*).[7] In each hierarchical system, that which is superior penetrates (but cannot be penetrated by) and is capable of absorbing (but cannot be absorbed by) that which is inferior to it. Such hierarchical ordering is ultimately rooted in an understanding of cosmogony by which an original being or essence creates from itself, through emanation, something slightly different from itself, which is so by virtue of the fact that it is less essential and less original. Creation proceeds through a chain of emanations to the less and less essential, until all that has been created is located in the hierarchy.

While the writers of the classic Upaniṣads reacted to the earlier Vedic ritualism with metaphysics and contemplation, Eliade points out that the Yoga *ṛṣis* (sages) set out from "other premises," more technical, more mystical, believing that true knowledge of the cosmic mysteries could find expression in Yogic practice. They sought to identify the cosmos with their own body, by carrying to the extreme certain micro-macrocosmic homologies already attested in the *Ṛg Veda*: the cosmic winds "mastered" as breaths; the cosmic skambha (pillar) identified with the vertebral column; the "center of the world" found in a point (the "heart") or an axis (traversing the chakras) inside the body.[8]

Common to almost all religious thought was a belief that in some sense each person stood at the center of a world that extended upward into the beyond. At least the lower part of that upward extension was what we now call the subtle body, apparently nonmaterial, but perhaps not wholly consubstantial with the highest Being. Both mountains and trees were pressed into service as symbols for the concepts that arose. Mountains rose toward the heavens, trees had their roots in the earth, but grew up into the air. Of course, the adherents of the various beliefs acknowledged the inadequacy of

---

*In the Yoga and Samkhya traditions, *puruṣa* is the transcendental Self, spirit, or pure awareness (*cit*) as opposed to the finite personality (*jīva*). In the last (tenth) book of the *Ṛg Veda,* the "Hymn of the Cosmic Man" (verse 10.90) explains that the universe was created out of the parts of the body of a single cosmic man (puruṣa) when his body was offered at the primordial sacrifice. Out of this ritual came the four basic *varnas* (castes) of Hindu society: the Brahmins (priests) from his mouth, the Kshatriya (warrior princes) from his arms, the Vaishya (merchants) from his thighs, and the Shudras (artisans) from his feet.

---

*These concepts are also found in Neo-Platonism and many other philosophies.

the resulting symbols. The symbolic "Mount Meru" was one of these central axes of Being (see one of its representations in fig. 2.1 below).

It is essential to realize that Meru was not some impersonal entity but a vital force that became interchangeably identical with the Tree of Life and the Cosmic Lotus; it constituted the supreme organizing principle of Indian religious symbolism.[9]

Mount Meru became much more than a feature on the cosmographic map. A map is a misleading metaphor for a map is two-dimensional. Meru rose up in a third dimension; in doing so, it pierced the heavens; in piercing the heavens, it transcended time as well as space; in transcending time it became . . . a magical tool for the rupture of plane. This is evident in the many layers of symbolism that exchange Meru for the Cosmic Man, for the temple at the center of the universe, for the office of kingship, for the stupa, for the mandala, and for the internal ascent undertaken by the tantric mystic. Meru is not, we must recognise, a place, "out there," so to speak. It is "in here."[10]

To perceive this, we first need to survey and grasp the broad and many-leveled symbolism that took shape in the Eastern mind, while noting the wide geographical spread of similar ideas. Along with the concept of an axis-mountain around which visible and invisible heavens turned, tree symbolisms also arose (see plates 6 and 7). Once the (wooden) wheel had been invented, a tree was also seen as the axle around which the wheel turned (see plate 8). We still use the term *axletree*. Trees also showed a seasonal, cyclical, growth, loss, and regrowth of leaves, so multiplex symbolisms arose naturally in a prescientific and prototechnological world. The Tree of Life appears in Christian paintings, Indian carvings and architecture, and Islamic prayer rugs and marble screens.

In the Judeo-Christian traditions the Tree of Life (or Tree of the Lives) is mentioned in Genesis, the first book of the compilation known as the Bible, standing in the Garden of Eden together with the Tree of the Knowledge of Good and Evil, and it appears again in Revelation, also known as the Apocalypse, the last book of the Bible. The awakening of human consciousness provided metaphors that seemed to be handed down by

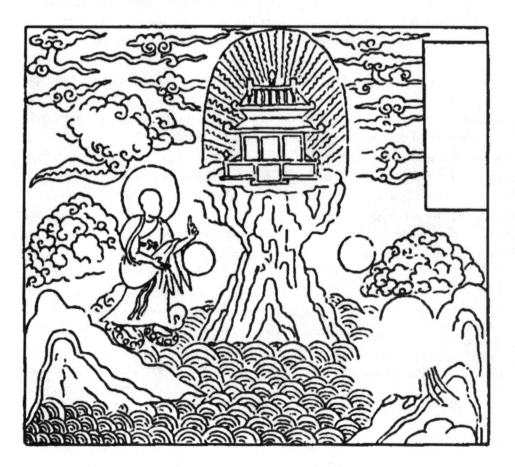

Fig. 2.1. Mount Meru, the world mountain, rises from the sea, surmounted by holy radiation, with sun and moon circling around it. The picture is from an ancient Buddhist cave sanctuary in Chinese Turkestan.

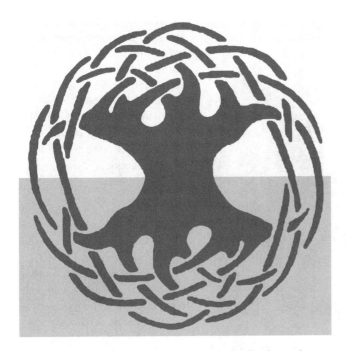

Fig. 2.2. This Celtic image of the Tree of Life elegantly suggests the wholeness and self-sustaining interconnectedness of the upper and lower worlds; in keeping with the Celtic character, it does not claim a place of importance for the human in either the terrestrial or the celestial world. Its form resembles that of a "strange loop," an enigmatic entity to be discussed in chapter 15.

God as our means of reunion with Him—perhaps the briefest possible description of what "religion" is. This concept is clearly relevant to any analysis of what our subtle body might be and what, above that subtle body, is to be distinguished as proper to the Great Being alone (see plate 5).

The question of where a line could be drawn between terrestrial being and heavenly Being puzzled many thinkers. Some thought there was no such distinction. Others thought it unbridgeable and absolute. In Genesis, we are told that the Elohim decided to expel Adam and Eve from the Garden of Eden once Adam had shown the hubris of eating of the Tree of the Knowledge of Good and Evil, thereby becoming "as one of us." He was expelled "lest he put forth his hand and eat of the Tree of the Lives and live for ever." Outside the Garden he (all humanity) would have "to till the ground from whence he was taken" until he returned to it in death, for "dust thou art, and unto dust thou shalt return." Many have felt there is sound reason to reject this materialistic, physicalistic view.

The Tree of Life, the Axis, Mount Meru, and the lingam are all names for a multifaceted and largely anthropomorphic entity at the center of the Vedic

Fig. 2.3. The Judaic Kabbalistic Tree of Life resembles the Hermetic schema and, even more closely, the Sufi, with humankind suspended between a material world, itself supported by God's presence, and the spiritual world. Humankind aspires toward Ein Sof, the unknowable Great Being, but not without God's gifts or assistance. The idea of the immortal soul was not part of early Hebrew belief, developing later, under foreign influences.

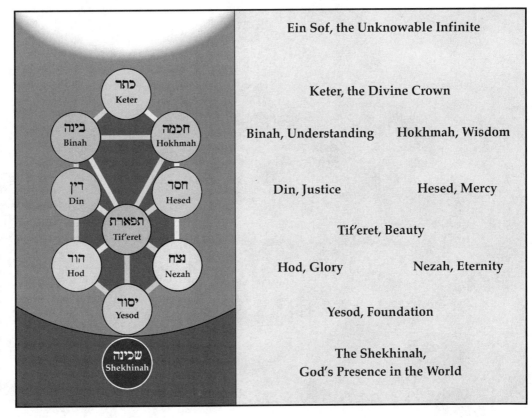

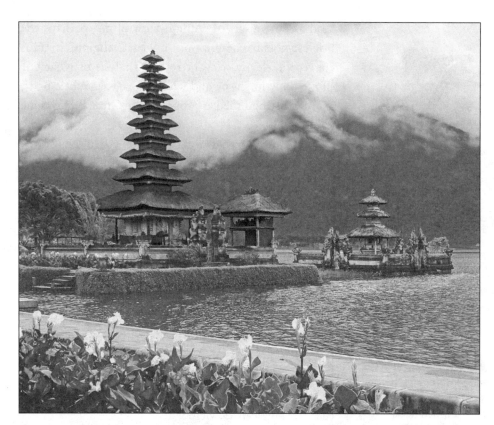

Fig. 2.4 (left). Hindu temple architecture often depicts Mt. Meru, the Tree of Life, the axis mundi, and the *lingam,* the male sexual organ, using similar forms. The fifteenth-century Hindu temple Tanah Lot (Land in the Sea) with its tiered *merus* is dedicated to the Balinese sea goddess, Dewi Laut.

Fig. 2.5 (below). The Muslim world developed from the same Abrahamic roots as the Judaic tradition, and the Tree of Life motif is found in Muslim prayer rugs of Turkey, Iran, and other countries. The fourteenth-century marble screen windows of the Sidi Sayyid Mosque in Ahmedabad, Gujarat, are probably the most exquisite examples of the Tree of Life motif in Indian art.

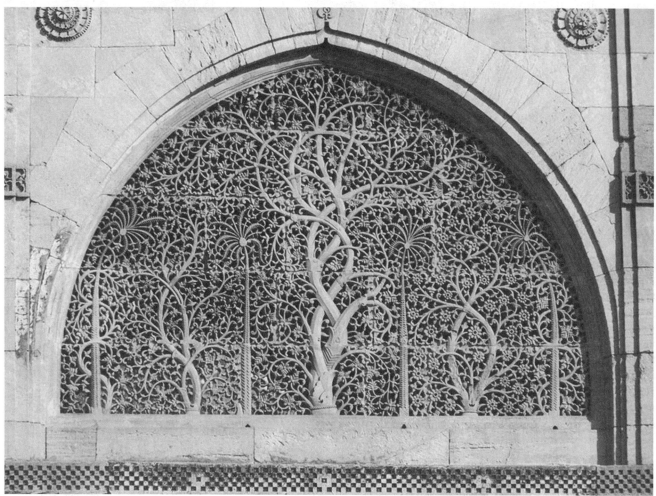

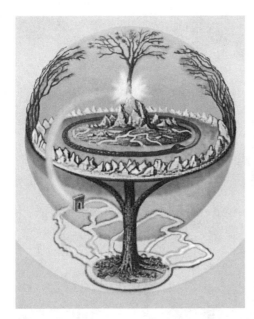

Fig. 2.6 (above). This picture shows Yggdrasil, the Norse Tree of Life. The god Odin is said to have found enlightenment not by meditating under a fig tree, like the Buddha, but by suspending himself in an ash tree, head downward, for nine days. The hanged man of the Tarot is an image of Odin and Yggdrasil. (Olufsen Bagge, 1847.)

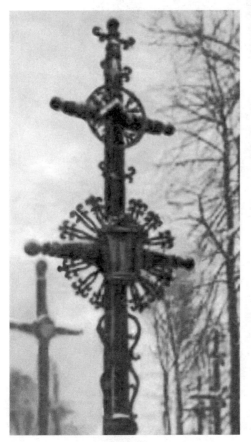

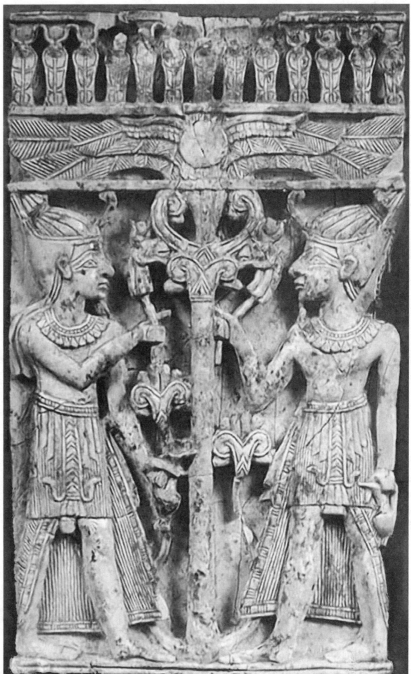

Fig. 2.7 (above). The feminine was included in the symbolism. This Egyptian sculpture is the Holy Sycamore of Hathor. The sycamore often grew, as if miraculously, by using invisible aquifers. After long periods of seeming to have died it produced figs even before the new leaves appeared. Humans naturally associated it with the cycle of life, death, and new life, and therefore with Hathor, goddess of the waxing and waning moon, which, after the cycle of day and night, was the most obvious periodicity in humankind's environment.

Fig. 2.8 (left). Yggdrasil is not the only manifestation of the Tree of Life in northern countries. This picture shows present-day Christianized versions of the Tree in Lithuania, and the ubiquitous "Christmas tree" is a relic, divested of most of its significance, of the same mythical imagination. The Druids also held certain trees to be sacred, as do today's Pagans.

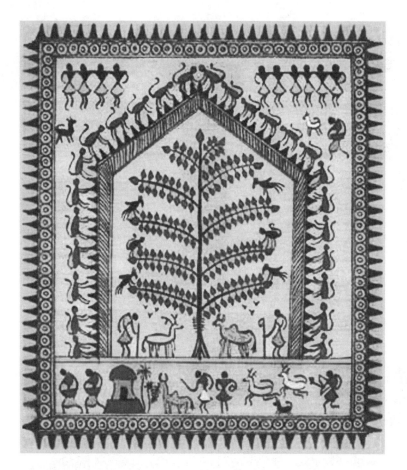

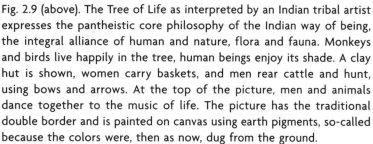

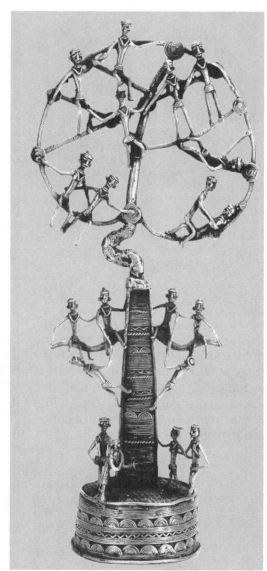

Fig. 2.9 (above). The Tree of Life as interpreted by an Indian tribal artist expresses the pantheistic core philosophy of the Indian way of being, the integral alliance of human and nature, flora and fauna. Monkeys and birds live happily in the tree, human beings enjoy its shade. A clay hut is shown, women carry baskets, and men rear cattle and hunt, using bows and arrows. At the top of the picture, men and animals dance together to the music of life. The picture has the traditional double border and is painted on canvas using earth pigments, so-called because the colors were, then as now, dug from the ground.

Fig. 2.10 (above right). This Tree of Life, in the form of a Dhokra art metal casting, was made recently by tribal craftsmen from Madhya Pradesh, North India, working in the traditional techniques, in this instance the "lost-wax" mold-making process.

Fig. 2.11 (right). The Tree of Life symbolism has an interesting variant. The *asvattha* tree is unusual in having aerial roots. In the Upaniṣadic era it seemed, at least partially, to be upside down, suggesting symbolically the two-way spiritual traffic of immanence and transcendence. Its roots are said to "rise on high" while its branches grow low, illustrating what was conceived to be a supreme principle, "As above, so below." This reminds us of the Kabbalistic Tree of Life, the Great Being reaching down to the mundane world, and so to us in our as-yet unenlightened state. With roots above and branches within our lowly reach, the asvattha seems to emanate from the world above, yet, for that very reason, all worlds also rest upon it.

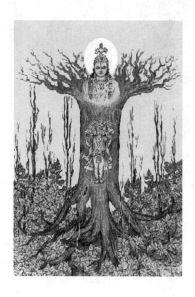

belief system, and they appear in many creation myths. The human being's awareness of itself as an identifiable, individual, indeed *nameable,* Being, distinguishable from all others and all-too-obviously finite, developed alongside consciousness of what the philosopher Martin Heidegger terms *der Umwelt,* roughly equivalent to "the environment" but probably best translated as "the world-about." In the outside world humans daily saw the heavens turn as if around an axis, and knew their place in the universe to be small. Unable to understand awesome experiences, their thought limited by their own nature to what we term anthropocentric thinking, humankind imagined gods, and thought them like themselves.

From the same anthropocentric awareness and myth-making came the correspondence in the Indian mind between internal experience and the grand conflation of notions that included the earth's axis, the columnar form of the life-initiating lingam, the growth heavenward of trees with their roots in the earth, and of ecstatic ascent in meditation from the microcosm of the body toward the macrocosm of the higher Self, and on, upward, to the gods. All Vedic spirituality expresses this multiplex axial alignment, and the Hermetic "As above, so below" was only one step in the future, to be conceived as soon as mental consciousness began to appear, augmenting, not supplanting, magical and mythical consciousness. It is not surprising that emotion-driven magical and mythical dreaming should produce such conflations, nor that religious longing directed toward the invisible but intuited "above" should be an integral part of the emotional whole, nor, again, that humans should invent deities in their own image and likeness to inhabit that "above." The imagined "axis" therefore combined, whether humans were fully aware of their synthesizing or not, sexual, anatomical, terrestrial, and transcendental components.

The naïveté of conflations of mountains, trees, the male (and female) organs, and the apparent rotation of the sky each day, on the one hand, with meditational awareness of pure being and of a Higher Being, on the other, gives no ground to reject the evidence from meditation or its many corroborations from medicine and science.

Meditation and other experiences seemed to reveal a multiplex of entities, approximately coextensive with

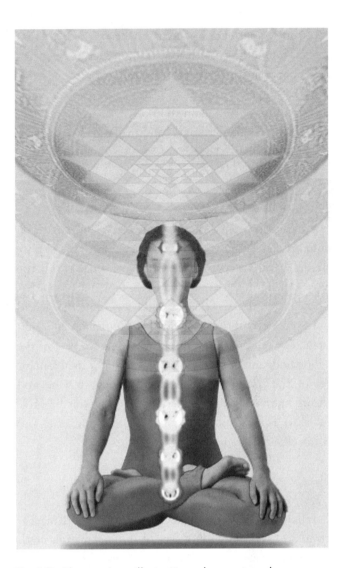

Fig. 2.12. The previous illustrations show external representations of the Tree of Life and related symbols. Here we try to illustrate the internal, meditative experiences that seemed to place the person at the center of an anthropomorphic universe. Yogic and Tantric mystics have recorded the rising of the kundalinī, describing it as a rush of energy up the spinal column, the vertical axis of the human being, and the same is experienced by adepts today.

the physical body, which we now call the subtle body. However, the seemingly higher meditative states also seemed to bridge a gap "upward, out beyond the body" into a "higher world" that could not be considered to be, or to be within, the body, except in the extreme anthropocentric view from the Hermetic tradition depicted in plate 5. A greater imaginative response to the experience would surely have "placed" this world of perception *no*where and *no*when, beyond the spatio-temporal experience of our human limitedness and therefore beyond the scope of our current language—hence the quotation marks around the word "placed," for nowhere and nowhen are better considered as a *state,* and *without* place or time.

But human beings have always made gods in their own image and, being limited in perception and imagination, many religious thinkers and meditators considered the Higher Being to be human, though writ large. Broadly, these were of the Advaitist persuasion, which presented a strongly monist view in some of its varieties. This was expressed by the claim *tat twam asi,* "thou art That."

Others saw that by no means could humans claim equality, let alone consubstantiality, with any Higher Being. While accepting the reality of what we in the West now term the subtle body, they took one or another of the huge variety of dualist views, regarding the "world out there beyond the bridge" as transhuman or suprahuman. They did not, however, deny that some part of the subtle body might survive death, and might then join, or rejoin, the Great Being. The range of views is wide, and shows myriad subtle distinctions, so it cannot be summarized. Each school of thought must be studied in and for itself, and its merits weighed.

The Primordial Substance

Parallels in language between microcosm and macrocosm are often found in a type of Indian creation myth in which the body of the Great Being, the "Cosmic Person," becomes the repository of the "original essence" that the "original being" creates.

The Three Humors (*Doṣas*) of Traditional Indian Medicine (*Ayurveda*)

In Ayurvedic philosophy the five elements are seen as interacting to form three dynamic forces or *doṣas* (that which changes):

- Vatam (wind)
- Pittam (bile)
- Kapham (phlegm)

These three governing principles are regarded as being responsible for health in the body when they are properly balanced, and for disease when they are out of balance.

In *Fluid Signs: Being a Person the Tamil Way,* a book that shows him to be a man of actual experience of the matters of which he writes, anthropologist E. Valentine Daniel tells us that the quest for the one undifferentiated, primordial substance of perfect equilibrium may be an extraordinary one, but the awareness of such a substance is neither extraordinary nor esoteric.[11] This is made clear by the following creation myth, told to him (and recorded in *Fluid Signs*) by an elderly villager in Tamil Nadu, South India, in the presence of a number of other villagers who threw in their own versions, corrections, and modifications as the narrative unfolded.

God (*Katavul*) was everything, the old villager said. In Him were the five elements of fire, water, earth, and ether (*akasam*), and wind. These five elements were uniformly spread throughout [the three humors] phlegm (*kapam*), bile (*pittam*), and wind (*vayū*). Let us say that they were in such a way that no one could tell the difference between them. Let us say they were nonexistent. Similarly, the three primordial qualities, or dispositions (*kunams*), or rajas, satvikam, and tamatam, neither existed nor did not exist. That is why we still call God Kunatitan [He who transcends all qualities]. Even the question as to their existence did not arise. Then something happened. The five elements started to move around as if they were not satisfied, as if they were disturbed. Now, as to who disturbed these elements or why they were disturbed, no one knows.[12]

Let us say that what disturbed the [elements] was their *talai eruttu* (codes for action, or, literally, "head writing").* When the elements started moving around, the humours started separating from one another and recombining in new proportions (*alavukal*). These new combinations resulted in the three kunams. Now the kunams and humours and elements all started to move hither and thither.

Head writing: Tamils believe that at the time of birth Katavul writes a script on every individual's head, and that the course each individual's life takes, to the very last detail, is determined by this script, known as *talai eruttu*. It is believed that even the particles that constituted the primordial being (Katavul) are subject to *talai eruttu*.

Then came the separation, as in an explosion, and all the jatis [types, castes, or categories of being] of the world, male jatis, female jatis, vegetable jatis, tree jatis, animal jatis, Vellala jatis, Para jatis, were formed, and they started meeting and mating and procreating. This is how the world came into being.[13]

At this point Daniel asked the old villager what happened to Katavul in the explosion. He replied that He is still there; not as before, but He is still there, more perfect than any of us. He has more equilibrium (*amai-tinilai*) than any of us. In Him the humors are more perfectly and uniformly (*camanilaiyaka*) distributed. That is why He does not fall ill, as we do. Our humors keep moving, running from here to there and there to here, all over our bodies, and into and out of our bodies.

But even in Him the elements, the humors, and the kunams move around, try as He might to keep them in equilibrium (*otamal atamal*). If he meditates for more than a certain number of years, the amount of satvikam begins to increase. So then Kamam [god of erotics; personification of desire] comes and disturbs him, and then he goes after Shakti* or the asuras.† This results in an increase in His rajasa kunam. When rajasa kunam increases beyond a certain limit, He must return to meditating. But most of the time He is involved in *lila* [sport or play]. All our ups and downs are due to His lilas. But that is the only way He can maintain a balance (*camanilai patuttalam*).[14]

This creation myth, in drawing on the worldview of the villager, reveals several cultural beliefs about the relationship between the "Cosmic Person" as macrocosm and the human as microcosm: all differentiated, manifest substantial forms evolved or devolved from a single, unmanifest, equilibrated substance, and the whole cosmos may be seen as a system capable of developing outward from or collapsing back into its essential cosmic original form. The "Tree of the Universe," the asvattha tree, is the perennial symbol of this cosmic hierarchy in which the five elements, the five gross senses, and the five subtle elements are seen as correspondences in mutual relationship:

With roots above and boughs beneath
This immortal fig tree [stands];
That is the Pure, that Brahman,
That the Immortal, so men say:
In it all the worlds are established;
Beyond it none can pass.
This in Truth is That.
K ATHA U PANIṢAD VI:1[15]

Daniel observes that what triggered the "first"* movement (action or *karmam*) of the generative process is an unknown, and therefore presumably an inner, property such as the codes of and for action that are "written" into all substances. This is like equating the "dissatisfaction" of the five elements that led to their movement with desire, which replicates the inception of other disequilibrated entities at a higher level of organization. In the West, the German philosopher Schopenhauer (1788–1860) and others have conceived something similar and called it "Will" and science would probably have to call it negative entropy. Different entities in the manifest world have different degrees of substantial equilibrium, Katavul's bodily substance being in a more equilibrated state than the bodily substance of human beings. As a result of disequilibration, humans and even gods must continue to strive to restore equilibrium to their bodily substance. This equilibrated state within the body is the key to health and well-being.[16]

The Mystical Body

Many practices that developed later in India with the aim of sanctifying or bringing equilibrium to the body, such as those of Tantra, are drawn from the cosmophysiology of the Vedas. Bodily organs and physiological functions were identified with cosmic regions, stars, planets, and gods.[17] Tantra, David Gordon White explains, is that Asian body of beliefs and practices that seeks to appropriate divine energy by ritual and channel that energy within the human microcosm, in creative and emancipatory ways, working from the principle that the universe we experience is nothing other than the concrete manifestation of the divine energy of the Godhead that creates and maintains that universe.[18]

---

*"Going after Shakti" means to indulge in sexual pleasure.
†"Going after the asuras [demons]" means to make war.

*Strictly speaking, as Hindu ontology is based on cyclical time, there is no absolute first event.

Eliade gives the example of a Javanese Tantric treatise that identifies each somatic element of the human body with a letter of the alphabet and a part of a *stūpaprāsād*, an architectonic monument within a shrine, usually in the shape of a dome or a pagoda, which, in turn, is assimilated to the Buddha and the cosmos. Several subtle bodies are here superimposed, explains Eliade: the sonorous body, the architectonic body, the cosmological body, and the mystico-physiological body (for the homology refers not to the organs of ordinary life, but to the chakras, the energy centers). This multilayered homologization must be "realized," "dilated," "cosmicised," transubstantiated.[19]

As Deussen,[20] Eliade,[21] White,[22] and others have pointed out, Tantric texts are often composed in a "hidden" or secret language. The enigmatic language designed to conceal the secrets of the universe from the uninitiated was an important part of the discipline for Tantric practitioners. It functioned to project the yogin into the "paradoxical situation" and the universe of convertible and integrable planes. In general, symbolism brings about a universal "porousness," opening beings and things to transobjective meanings. The disciple must constantly experience the mysterious process of homologization and convergence that is at the root of cosmic manifestation. As microcosm, he or she must become conscious of all the forces—now awakened within—which periodically create and absorb the universes.[23]

The practice of destroying and reinventing language, hiding profound meaning by substituting the profane for the sacred, is also found among the Tantric poets, and the Siddha poet-philosopher yogis of South India, whose alchemic system of medicine is expressed in a secret language of symbols and elaborately worked out ciphers.

Eliade states that ritual enigmas and riddles were in use from Vedic times and we can still find them in common usage today, for example, in Tamil proverbs.[24] Brenda Beck explains how it is usual to describe an inanimate object in human terms and human behavior in terms of the activities of the various body parts.[25] By this means, she points out, both common and abstract parallels are expressed, but in both cases the human body is the core descriptor on which the verbal codes rely and the yardstick by which other things are interpreted, measured, and understood. Beck gives an example from a much loved and revered fourth to fifth

century Tamil text, the *Tirukkural.* Two of the most famous *Tirukkural* passages describe life's tenuous relationship to the body:

> *The love of the soul for the body is like (the love of) a bird for its nest, which it flies away from and leaves empty.*
> (VERSE 338)

> *It seems as if the soul, which takes temporary shelter in a body, had not attained a home.*
> (VERSE 340)[26]

The *Tirukkural* states clearly that the body is merely a transitory physical repository for life's essence. This essence (*uyir*), often translated into English as "soul," leaves the body for an independent existence at death.

The Cosmic Winds

The methodology to maintain the equilibrated state came through the evolution of ideas about the breath, which, for early Indians, was the principal indicator of the presence of life; what humans breathed was seen as the motivating force of both the cosmos and of human existence within it. In the Samkhyan understanding of the unfoldment of the universe, *prāna* or the life force is the first evolute of prakṛti (nature); it is the power that exists in all matter at various levels.[27] The cosmic wind was humankind's vital breath (prāna), and therefore the principal observable manifestation and evidence of an immortal soul.

The association between human breath and atmospheric wind (*vāta, vāyu*) indicated in the famous "Puruṣa" hymn of the *Ṛg Veda* (10.90.13) is developed in the *Atharva Veda,* says Kenneth Zysk. He explains that wind is breath's principal link to the cosmos, for breath comes from wind and wind purifies breath. But the sun, the cosmic fire, is also seen as the source of breath because of its self-motivating and life-producing characteristics. Zysk goes on to say that the hymns of the *Atharva Veda* point to a fundamental connection

---

Tirukkural is an important work of Tamil literature written by the poet Thiruvalluvar in the form of *kural*, pithy couplets similar to *sūtras* (threads).

between life and the twofold breathing process of inhalation and exhalation, *prāna* and *apāna*. They are like two draft-oxen walking together, allies for maintaining a sound bodily condition and long life. He adds that, in his view, persistent meditation on the nature and function of breath eventually led to a bifurcation of opinions concerning bodily wind. While medicine concentrated on the physiology of bodily winds, Yoga focused on breath control.[28]

The old notion that prāna represented the atmospheric wind in humans and functioned as the animator and prolonger of all life was the starting point for the mystics' theory of respiration and the role wind played in the body. In their spiritual quest through meditation for the universal principle behind all existence, these ascetics realized that breath was the closest physical manifestation of the ultimate, unchanging, creative force in the human: the ātman, or soul, the embodiment of Brahman, or universal spirit. Prāna is the seat of Brahman and arises from the ātman.

It may be that some of the later systems adopted the "psychospiritual technology" first mentioned in the *Atharva Veda* in their attempt to balance the subtle and gross elements within the human body. This "psychospiritual technology" was based on the currents of the life force (*Atharva Veda* X 15.15.2–9) and the "eight wheels" of the deities (*Atharva Veda* X 10.2.31). In the next two chapters we shall explore the contention stated in the eleventh-century *Siddha-Siddhānta-Paddhati* ("tracks on the doctrines of the adepts," a text of 353 highly mystical verses ascribed to Gorakshanatha, the founder of kundalinī yoga, dealing with the esoteric nature of the inner bodies and the soul's union with Supreme Reality), that a yogin is someone who truly knows the psychospiritual centers (chakras) of the body, the five kinds of inner space, and so on.

THREE

The Ladder of Being

In certain religious traditions, models of the human body may transcend the visible order to postulate parallel "subtle" or "spiritual" bodies which function to mediate between the material and the transcendent realm. The concept of a "subtle body" provides an especially flexible and malleable field for mapping concepts of the human individual and relating these to wider metaphysical and ideological systems.

M. K. HERMANSEN, *SHAH WALI ALLAH'S THEORY*
OF THE SUBTLE SPIRITUAL CENTERS

The goal of self-transcendence requires "proper techniques," as Troy Wilson Organ calls them, for the methodical transmutation of ordinary consciousness in order to attain mokṣa, liberation. As we saw in chapter 1, liberation, in the Indian sense, means the unification of the individual soul (ātman) with the cosmic or universal soul (Brahman).[1] Some of the ancient scriptures recognize that there are stages on the path of self-transcendence. According to the *Yoga-Sāra-Samgraha,* sixteenth century CE, these stages are:

1. *ārukshu:* one who is desirous of spiritual life
2. *yunjāna:* one who is actually practicing
3. *yoga-arudha* or *yukta:* one who has ascended or yoked one
4. *sthita-prajñā:* one of steady wisdom[2]

What the yogin is actually practicing, that is, the techniques through which he or she becomes "one of steady wisdom," depends on the system of Yoga followed. The goal is to arrive at samādhi, the condition of ecstasy. Samādhi (literally "placing" or "putting together") is both the technique of unifying conscious-

ness and the resulting state of ecstatic union with the object of contemplation.[3] The impetus to connect with a greater reality, motivated by the desire to transcend the human condition, may be the same, but the paths are many. While each school has its own ideas as to how to arrive at this goal, they most frequently follow a graduated sequence of psychospiritual techniques, which the aspirant pursues at the pace most suitable for his or her own nature, well-being, and level of understanding.

According to Feuerstein Vedanta has greatly influenced the majority of Yoga schools. He states that Vedanta proper originated with the ancient Upaniṣads, which first taught the "inner ritual" of meditation upon, and absorption into, the unitary ground of all existence.[4] He notes that some schools deny that such a reunion is possible—because we are never separated from the Ground of Being—while others believe that it is more a kind of "remembering" or rediscovery of our eternal status as the ever-blissful transcendental Self. While the object of contemplation lies outside of or beyond the self in some traditions, it is found within the self in others. In the system of hatha yoga, for example, each journey takes the aspirant deeper into the body until, by what might seem a paradoxical process, the universe itself becomes a body for the liberated one. This will become clearer after the *kośas* have been discussed, below.

Some schools teach a dualist view based on the concept of gradual ascent from the material to the spiritual. The *yogin* or *yogini* (respectively, male or female practitioner of yoga) develops discernment (*viveka*) between the transcendental Self (ātman) and the non-Self (*anātman*) through withdrawal of attention, step-by-step, from the various objects of psychophysical existence in the phenomenal world until he or she becomes immersed in or identified with Brahman. This altered state of consciousness can be arrived at by two routes: the negative and the positive, encapsulated in the

Sanskrit phrases *neti, neti* (not this, not that) and *aham brahma asmi* ("I am Brahman," which is equivalent to "I am Siva"). Both can be seen, as complementary methods, in the *Nirvāna-Śatakam,* the didactic poem ascribed to Sankara, regarded as the greatest authority on nondualist Vedanta, which states:

> Om. *I am not reason, intuition*
> *(buddhi),*
> *egoity (ahamkāra), or memory. Neither*
> *am I*
> *hearing, tasting, smelling, or sight;*
> *neither*
> *ether nor earth; fire or air. I am Śiva*
> *in the form of Consciousness-Bliss. I am*
> *Śiva.*[5]

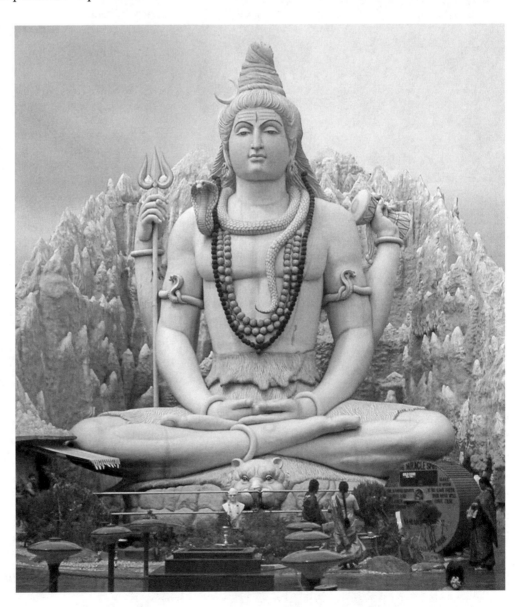

Fig. 3.1. Siva, usually identified as the Absolute principle, the Being-Consciousness of the universe, appears in many Tantras as the first teacher of esoteric knowledge. Among his many other names he is also called Sankara, the giver of joy or serenity. (Public statue at Bangalore, India.)

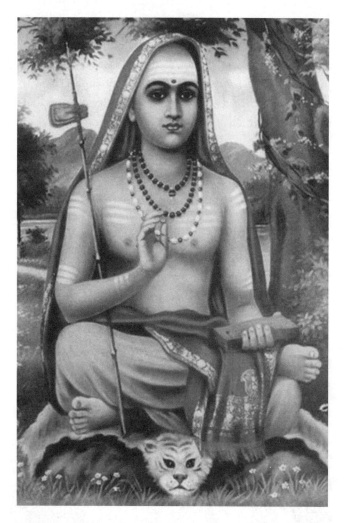

Fig. 3.2. Sankaracharya (*acharya* means "teacher"), also known as Adi Sankara (788–820 CE), was the first Indian philosopher to consolidate the doctrine of Advaita Vedanta (nondualism). The jīvan-muktas (liberated while living) were among the followers of Advaita, which, as an experiential philosophy, required the aspirant to practice throughout life even up to death. In Advaita there is no difference between the experiencer, the experienced (the world), and the universal Spirit (Brahman). (S. Vidyasankar.)

Various alternative routes to liberation developed through the centuries. The instructions were, in effect, initiations into spiritual realization given by enlightened teachers to their pupils, who were thereby rescued from the darkness of ignorance through knowledge. These instructions form the basis of many of the ancient scriptures from the Vedas to the Tantras, recorded over a period of some 5,000 years. Changes in the disciple's bodily, mental, and spiritual condition led to different conduct and behavior patterns depending on willingness and openness to change. Feuerstein describes the

process of change as a direct empowerment, in which the teacher effects in the disciple a change of consciousness, a metanoia or turnabout. By virtue of his or her advanced spiritual state, the body-mind of an adept teacher becomes a locus of concentrated psychospiritual energy, like a powerful radio beacon compared to the low-energy system of the ordinary body-mind. This is not a mere metaphor. Rather, it is an experiential fact recognized in many esoteric conditions.[6]

The Energy System

The conversion of a low-energy system to a high-energy system is accomplished through the energy system itself. This system is conceived as consisting of the kośas (sheaths), the chakras (energy centers or vortices), and the nadis (energy currents or streams). The model of the energy system that eventually evolved as a map of consciousness had its rudimentary beginnings in the Upaniṣads, which pose the question of why the Supreme Soul assumes a bodily form. "Whence does this *prāna* (the individual soul) originate, and how does it enter this body?"[7] Deussen points out that the answers to such questions given in the early texts seem unsatisfactory, but deeper insight is shown in the later texts, such as the *Maitrāyanīupaniṣad,* where the conclusion is drawn that the Self becomes twofold in order that it may "experience the illusion of a life in the world as well as eternal reality."[8]

It has been said that the entire creation is, in fact, manifested in our physical body and in the five layers of consciousness (kośas) that surround it. Though each tradition describes these layers differently, they are generally taken to be the emanations of consciousness ranging from the lowest, controlled by the crudest level of mind, to the highest: the Cosmic Mind or level of pure Spirit.

In its most basic form, states Buddhist writer Roar Bjonnes, mind exists on a cellular level, residing within the body as does oil in a seed. Mind is thus expressed as the most primitive cellular sensations and instincts. As it evolves to the human level, its capabilities radically expand through repeated experience. The human mind, as a culmination of this evolution, expresses itself through instincts, emotions, and rationality, and is thus capable of expressing everything from speech to logic, from creative imagery to spiritual bliss. The human mind, then, is a microcosmic potential or reflection of the Cosmic Mind, or the Mind of God.[9]

Tantra is the system that embodies the continuity of teaching on the energy system as a path to liberation. While the early Upaniṣads had already presented the concepts of the subtle currents of life energy (prāṇa or vāyu), the energy vortices (chakras), and the energy currents (nadis) some centuries before Tantra evolved as a great "spiritual synthesis," the *Atharva Veda* had, centuries even before that, mentioned the vital currents (15.15.2–9) and the chakras as the places where the deities reside (10.2.31).

Feuerstein points out that despite the similarities between the Vedic and the Tantric heritages, Tantra is a distinct tradition, meandering down India's history as a mighty companion to the Vedic stream of spirituality and culture. The interplay between the two traditions has been extremely complex and continues to this day. Despite the fact that some brahmins have branded Tantra as unorthodox, that is, as not affirming the truth of the Vedas, Feuerstein says that Tantra is a profoundly *Yogic* tradition.[10] Although the Tantras, the *sādhana-śāstras* (books of spiritual practice) of the Tantric tradition, were relative latecomers in the long history of Yoga, they represent a synthesis that embodies a spectrum of personal experimentation and experience. This spectrum embraces the archaic forms of ritual worship and meditation associated with the Vedic sacrificial cult (see chapter 5) and a hierarchy of male and female deities and ancestral spirits. It ranges through the intellectually and spiritually fertile period of India's great epic, the Mahābhārata, to the common era in which translations by Western scholars such as Sir John Woodroffe have revealed the inner world of Tantra to be a holistic approach. Tantra created a massive literature of its own in Sanskrit and vernacular languages, but apart from stray quotations and references in extant manuscripts most of it has been lost.

Although in many respects Tantra continued the Upaniṣadic metaphysics and language of nondualism, it often sought to express new meanings through them. In Tantra, for instance, One (*eka*) is not the life-negating singularity of some brahmanical teachers but the all-encompassing Whole (*pūrṇa*), which is present as the body, the mind, and the world, yet transcends all of these.* At its best, Tantra is integralism. This is hinted

*See chapter 15, where this schema is developed in detail and in the context of Western science.

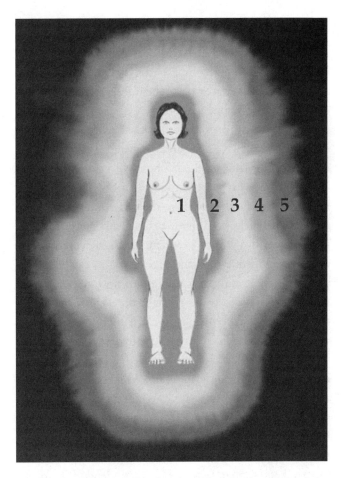

Fig. 3.3. The kośas are the sheaths or subtle coverings of the physical body, representing ascending planes of consciousness that have to be penetrated in meditation, as the meditator transcends the visible and invisible realms in order to realize the divine Self and the ultimate Reality.

at in the word *tantra* itself, which, among other things, means "continuum."

This continuum is what enlightened adepts realize as *nirvāna* (the "passing away" of desire and the extinction of the self in the Self) and what unenlightened worldlings experience as samsāra (the cycle of birth, death, and rebirth). These are not distinct, opposite realities, according to Feuerstein. They are absolutely the same essence. That essence is experienced as different by different people because of their differing karmic predispositions, which are like veils or mental filters obscuring the truth. To ordinary worldlings, the One remains utterly hidden. To spiritual seekers, it seems a distant goal, perhaps realizable after many lifetimes. To initiates, it is a reliable inner guide. To realized sages, it is the only One that exists, for they have *become* the Whole.[11]

The World of Inner Experience

As we have seen, and shall now see again, both Yoga and its interpretation are complex. Yoga includes not only a science of the body, a study of the mind and higher states of consciousness, and a philosophy of the structure and nature of the universe, but also the techniques to produce by experience a deep and meaningful realization of the wholeness thus implied. The way to this integration is a self-aware progress through the five "bodies," the kośas or sheaths that obscure the pure inner consciousness itself. The kośas provide a framework for coordinating the world of inner experiences, a structured space, or spaces, within which the yogi or yogini can meditate and so arrive at an understanding of how consciousness is organized. By focusing thought on each of the kośas, the meditator can influence the functioning of, and adapt his or her behavior to, each of these layers or levels so that energy increases and knowledge expands. This is, of course, a self-healing function. As a result, one is able to take control of personal growth and evolution.

But immediately a puzzling question arises. Our illustration (figure 3.3) shows an expansion, or ascent, from the physical body *outward and upward,* yet we have just spoken emphatically of *inner* experience. The problem is the universal one of how private inner experience is to be illustrated or verbally described. Is it not inherently and unavoidably incommunicable? If our illustration succeeds in making some kind of visual analogy with an upward and outward progress, it surely fails to illustrate the inward aspect of the experience. Indeed, one would think an inward "movement," as opposed to an outward one, utterly impossible to illustrate by any kind of diagram. Yet, strangely, if we explore this insoluble problem by such mental means as we have, it leads us to a far greater elucidation than we expect. Let us do this by placing a quotation from Swami Rama—philosopher, psychologist, former Shankaracharya (the highest spiritual post in India), and founder of the Himalayan International Institute of Yoga in Pennsylvania—in apparent opposition to our figure 3.3.

Consciousness is sometimes compared to a light, and the different bodies (the kośas) to lampshades that cover it, says Swami Rama. These shades surround the light, one inside the other, each of a different material. Each shade captures light to a certain degree and is illuminated by it. Each transforms the light and modifies

it according to the shade's own properties. The outer shades are the densest and let the least light through. If we remove each of them in turn, the light becomes brighter and brighter and is less obscured. Each is denser than the one just interior to it; in the terms of Yoga philosophy, each involves to a greater degree the principle of matter (prakṛti). The ancient philosophical writings often called these bodies "sheaths" because of the way they cover up and conceal the underlying consciousness (puruṣa).[12]

If we are not to misunderstand Swami Rama's description of a movement inward, rather than outward and upward, we have to realize first that all words such as *inner, higher,* or *more subtle* are spatial metaphors invented by our minds, which by nature think in spatial terms; these metaphors are applied to "worlds" in which our everyday sense of space, which is the basis of our language, cannot be relied upon. We humans invented the concept of the spiritual precisely because, as we became aware of it, it did not reveal itself as if it were a part of our everyday world, but as "something else." "Something else" needs, but lacks, a language of its own because spirituality is experienced as a world of its own, impossible to describe in the terminology of the ordinary world around us. All attempts to describe it and the approaches to it are unavoidably highly metaphorical, for either "the spiritual realm" is entirely without space and time or its space and time are not those of our everyday world, but something very different. There is, therefore, in addition to the difficulty of illustrating inner experience visually, the parallel risk of *verbal* confusion regarding the *metaphorical* "direction" of spiritual progress, whether "upward," "deeper," "inward," or "outward."

To make matters even more fraught, there is often a misleading conflation in our awareness of this progression with the more or less substantial, more or less subtle kośas themselves, the layers, or functions, of the physical body per se. Even though it leaves normal consciousness behind, the meditative journey always starts in normal consciousness, which includes consciousness of the physical or gross body. However, it is universally recognized, by Dvaitists (dualists) and Advaitists (nondualists) alike, that the spiritual "upward" journey does not reach its peak at the level of the "highest" kośa, but continues far beyond. To illustrate the verbal problem by just two serviceable phrases, we might ask whether the sitter, in meditation, "floats *upward* into a *spiritual realm*" or "enters more and more *deeply* into his or her *innermost space*"? The same meditative process is being described in each case. Either metaphor—for metaphors they are—will serve, but both will mislead unless we can imagine or, better, *recall* the experience *itself* that is being described but is in reality beyond the available words.

Even this does not exhaust the problems, for the Vedic Axis, as it rose "above" even the subtlest level that could rationally be considered still a part of the body, included *in one vertical, hierarchical system* both the sitter and the "higher" worlds revealed during meditation. The Vedas and, later, the Upaniṣads were therefore entirely the fruit of an introspective personal and private experience, the *telling* or *picturing* of which inevitably produced misleading impressions. As we shall see, one question that arose and caused a huge schism, which persists in a variety of forms even today, was that of where the sitter ends and a higher world begins. This is in effect what is in dispute when Advaitists claim that we can never lose touch with the Ground of Being while Dvaitists make the contrary claim that we are, as earth-dwellers, already estranged from that Great Being and need to seek reunion.

It is no wonder, then, that one person likens progress in meditation to a moving outward and upward from the body, and illustrates it in this way, as we have done in figure 3.3, while another sees it as entering more and more deeply into an "inner space," which, paradoxically, shows itself to be immensely larger than the body, as if it were a whole vast universe enclosing it. The words of a book such as this, and its illustrations, must, therefore, be taken as no more than guides to our own picturing of that which cannot be pictured. In understanding Swami Rama, quoted above, we should realize that in his conception it is the *innermost* being that is the *highest,* the brightest, the nearest to the light, but that it is obscured from normal human view, including even its own view, at least in the state of everyday awareness,* not only by the grossly physical body itself, but also by the other kośas. Naturally, meditators who hold an Advaitist conception are more likely to see the Highest as within themselves,

Dvaitists more likely to see the Great Being as separate, higher, to be reached only by a transcendence that carries the sitter up, out of the body, into a "sky-like" realm.

In the Tantric tradition, traversing the subtle dimensions of existence through the kośas is a practice that has its roots in the *Taittirīya Upaniṣad,* the third oldest Upaniṣad, written about 3,000 years ago. The *Taittirīya* teaches that there are degrees of bliss from simple pleasure to the ecstasy of union with the Absolute. This, too, is clearly compatible with the view that the kośas show a progression (whether seen as "inward" or as "upward") from the gross body toward more subtle "matter," and so constitute an approach to the experience of pure spirit—whatever that may prove to be—which only the experiencer of it will know.

Let us quote a passage from the *Taittirīya Upaniṣad* itself, which is not merely relevant to the present topic, but also to comments that we wish to make regarding the interpretation of such texts.

> He who knows Brahman, who is Truth, consciousness, and infinite joy, hidden in the inmost of our soul and in the highest heaven, enjoys all things he desires in communion with the all-knowing Brahman. From Ātman—Brahman—in the beginning came space. From space came air. From air, fire. From fire, water. From water came solid earth (*Taittirīya Upaniṣad* II.1).[13]

This text postulates a clear descent as the creation of the physical world "proceeded" from the "emptiness" of space (ākāśa) to the creation of substances that the protoscientific mind of the Upaniṣadic era saw as slightly more material at each downward step, until the solid earth, the "grossest" matter, was finally reached. Yet even for the writers themselves, this schema probably presented puzzling anomalies. Ice is just as solid as earth, but it should have been clear that it was, nonetheless, simply the element water, not the element earth, for it melted when the sun rose. Thus does modern science offer better explanations of the merely physical world than the fivefold system of "elements."

There is, of course, more to study in the passage quoted, but before continuing my general exposition I want to interpose a further quotation from Feuerstein that demonstrates the pitfalls of theoretical interpretation.

---

*Heidegger's philosophy, like science, is highly relevant, yet cannot be treated here without introducing a baffling complexity for the reader as yet unfamiliar with our subject. More will be said in chapter 15.

He states that, "In Tantra it is said that the five elements are created from the Cosmic Mind. This part of creation, which we may term 'the spectrum of cosmic-ness,' has yet to be clearly explained by modern cosmology or science. On the other hand, both the wisdom of Tantra and science agree that mind was created from matter. Tantra holds that because the entire mass of material structure has evolved out of the Cosmic Mind, the potentiality of mind will always remain latent in matter, and under the right conditions it will resurrect itself again."[14]

Analysis of this paragraph reveals a number of faults, from unjustified and conflicting claims to extreme vagueness. Feuerstein tells us:

1. The five elements were created from the Cosmic Mind.
2. This "spectrum of cosmicness" has not been explained by modern science.
3. Tantric wisdom and science agree that mind was created from matter.
4. Because matter evolved out of the Cosmic Mind, the potentiality of mind will always remain latent in matter, and under the right conditions will resurrect itself again.[15]

Read glibly, this might not alert one to any problems, but as soon as we begin to analyze the passage, asking what Feuerstein means, huge problems appear. His first claim risks serious contradiction with the third, though the third is ambiguous, not least because Feuerstein does not distinguish between Cosmic Mind and other mind or minds. However, since the human mind can be conceived either to be a part of the Cosmic Mind, which is the Advaitist view, in line with the tenet "Tat twam asi," or, at the terrestrial level, as a separate and distinct Being, which is approximately the Dvaitist view, it is important that some correction be made. However, Feuerstein himself gives us no resolution of the ambiguity and uncertainty his own words have introduced.

There are, in fact, three problems to clear up, and the key to them is to see that Feuerstein's statement that "Tantra and science agree that mind was created from matter" is incorrect. The conceptual change needed is large, but not difficult, and will be further illuminated in our chapter 15, "Science, Philosophy, and the Subtle Body," in which the harmony between dual-

isms and monisms will be shown. Shah Wali Allah, the eighteenth-century Islamic scholar and reformer, also harmonized monistic and dualistic views, as chapter 6 relates. Meanwhile, let us deal with the anomalies in the order in which they arise in Feuerstein's paragraph.

An Unjustifiable Demand upon Modern Science

Despite the comparability Feuerstein implies, without evidence of its validity, the hierarchy, or cascade, of created entities from "airiness" to "solidness" is *not* comparable with contemporary science of any complexion, for four of the five Upaniṣadic elements fall into just one class of entity within modern physics, namely that of matter. The normal *states of* matter under *terrestrial* conditions (please note our emphases) provide only three "levels," those of gas, liquid, and solid. These might be seen as analogous to air, water, and earth, but if any harmony were to be proved, five such terrestrial states of matter would be required so that fire and space could be included. Science cannot offer such a parallel. True, there are loose, almost "poetic," parallels, one being science's description of the "descent" through the era of radiation in the very early universe to the condensation of some of that energy into matter. Before the formation of the atoms that we terrestrial beings know, there was a plasma state that might be considered to parallel one of the more "airy" of the five stages required by the Upaniṣad, but since this plasma state is not natural on earth it is difficult to see how it could correspond to any terrestrial matter, let alone any layer of the body, no matter how subtle.

And, from that early moment in the universe's history onward, matter is *not* thought to have condensed into progressively grosser and grosser *kinds* of "stuff" (as the Upaniṣad states), but to have remained the same in essence, and (after supernova explosions had produced the heavier elements) in about a hundred different atomic arrangements, rather than the four material "elements" (plus space, ether, the void) postulated by the writers of the Upaniṣads.

Another parallel, again very loose, can possibly be seen between the Upaniṣadic schema and the fact, confirmed by Tonomura, of a field of potential underlying the visible physical world. This field, explained in chapter 15, could be the intuited space or ākāśa of the

Upaniṣadic schema. However, the two schemas still do not fit well, as we would then have space plus the other four elements grouped as one (matter), which gives only two downward steps, with nowhere to place the plasma state. Feuerstein cannot enlist today's science in a project of assimilation with Upaniṣadic science when the misfit is so obvious, nor in any venture that he cannot define with sufficient sharpness for our science to participate at all. The present-day successors of scientists such as Heisenberg, who struggled in the 1920s with the problem of defining sharply what was to be investigated regarding his famous uncertainty principle (see chapter 15) cannot be expected to show patience with the vague projects of scholars in other fields of study who are unused to such stringent requirements, nor to explain by their own metaphors an ancient scheme, even if it could be more sharply defined, which clearly does not fit.

No wonder, then, that Feuerstein complains that science has yet to explain what the writers of the Upaniṣads described, as though it were scientists' duty to do so. *Of course* today's science has not explained it, for science has, for the most part, no wish to explain it. It has neither wish nor duty to accommodate itself to, let alone confirm, any view more vague than its own. Rather, science has sought to create its own metaphors, as precise as possible, though equally anthropomorphic (as we shall show in chapter 15), but with *greater* explanatory power and corroboration from research, consistent with *its own* cosmology and the hundred or so denizens of the periodic table rather than with a naïve fivefold schema showing anomalies that could have been noticed even by the writers of the Upaniṣads.

Today's scientific hypotheses, their own limitations notwithstanding, have a far greater explanatory power for us than picturesque protoscientific writings, but this does not mean that important truth is not to be found in the Upaniṣads, or in Tantric Yoga. It is rather that the confirmations of the continuing validity of the Upaniṣadic insights from present-day and future science are probably not the confirmations Feuerstein demands.

Is Mind an Emergent Potential of Matter Itself, or an Independent Being?

Next, we have to question whether Feuerstein's third claim is correct, that "the wisdom of Tantra and science agree that mind was created from matter." Certainly, the

writer of the *Taittirīya Upaniṣad* thought otherwise, as a more careful examination of the text quoted a little earlier will show. For convenient reference, here it is again, with emphases added by means of italics:

> He who knows Brahman, who is Truth, *consciousness*, and infinite joy, *hidden in the inmost of our soul and in the highest heaven*, enjoys all things he desires in communion with the all-knowing Brahman. From Ātman—Brahman—in the beginning came space. From space came air. From air, fire. From fire, water. From water came solid earth.

Feuerstein claims that the Tantric belief is that the human being is made up of the five elements—ether, air, fire, water, and earth—but that the human is so constituted is precisely what the quotation from the *Taittirīya Upaniṣad* does *not* say. What it does say is that those five elements came *from the same essence as that from which the human essence also came,* for they both emanated from ātman-Brahman. *This* statement, the Upaniṣadic statement, not Feuerstein's, accords well (so far as it goes) with the Neo-Platonic views of many scientists of today, though it still fails to prove any parallel between the Upaniṣadic account of the descent from spirit into matter and modern physics.

The Upaniṣad itself claims that, *insofar as,* down here on earth, the human being develops through the five kośas, it lives within a *physical* system, which physical system did indeed emanate from the Great Being. However, the Upaniṣad says that the human essence *itself* is a *part of* that Great Being (this is the Advaitist view that we are never divorced from the Ground of Being); it is not only "hidden in the inmost of our soul" but is *also* (and apparently simultaneously) "in the highest heaven." The human *essence* is *not* said to be a part of the emanated world, for the source of the emanated, physical, world is said to be ātman-Brahman, while the innermost soul of the human being itself is stated to *be* Brahman *itself*: it is in *this* way that ātman *is* Brahman. This is a more direct link; indeed, it is an identity. Furthermore, it is a "spaceless" identity, not of this physical world at all, for it is *both* "hidden in the inmost of our soul *and* in the highest heaven." It is very important that the *duality* both of our Being and of our lines of dependence on the above, as Brahman *and* as physical bodies, be seen clearly. Duality then exists, of course, only at the level of terrestrial embodied life.

So Tantra cannot claim that mind was created from matter *in anything like the simplistic, emergent sense implied by Feuerstein.* To do so would be to deny a tenet that is fundamental for Vedic believers and others of both monist and dualist persuasions. The notion that matter creates mind implies a denial of "Tat twam asi." If it is asserted, there is nothing that scientists should be obliged to "explain," even if they feel that inclination, for everything in the world of our Being, including ourselves, is then merely physical, already largely explained by science, for science *is* precisely that which explains the *physical* (but nothing else). Here we almost think, as Feuerstein does, that science has not explained our Being, though not for the reason he states but for the opposite reason: that our Being, sharing the essence of Brahman, is *outside* physics. Far from having a duty to explain it, physics *cannot* explain it. An *extended* science may one day explain Tantra, but it surely has no concern to explain Feuerstein. That an expert such as Feuerstein seems to miscomprehend both the responsibilities of science and some points of Vedic teaching warns us to take extreme care to grasp with precision what both mystics and scientists are saying to us.

If a Truth and Its Domain Are Mutually Defining, Conflicting Truths Must Indicate Multiple Domains

One of the most resistant barriers to understanding is that—in their obsessive avoidance of the errors of Cartesian dualism—most of today's thinkers reject all dualisms without scrutiny, and therefore automatically miss a further important truth, that two distinct, even conflicting, descriptions of a single system may *both* be true, sometimes simultaneously, sometimes because each has a domain within the whole system in which it and it alone is applicable. There should be no intellectual difficulty in grasping this, or similar truths, especially as the current state of physics provides startlingly apposite examples.

Two major notions of today's science, field theory and quantum theory, scarcely impinge on one another, yet both provide accurate descriptions of observable realities, as we shall see in chapter 15. Field theory

recognizes that each unit of matter has an influence, known as "action at a distance," throughout the whole of space, while quantum theory acknowledges that all physical change occurs in discrete steps. They are compatible, but there is as yet no complete synthesis of these two parts of physical theory. The way reality can show itself as waves or as particles of "stuff" is another *real duality* with, again, no single theory to explain all the phenomena concerned. So if two descriptions, quantum and field, seem valid, which is true? Both are true, but both are partial; both are scientific experiences, but have not, as yet, been completely correlated by reason. Each is true in its own area of relevance, which depends on the aims of the experiment and on its sensing and measuring equipment. We can say no more here, but shall deal with such matters in greater detail in chapter 15.

If, as we believe, there is in the human constitution a duality having upper and lower domains, we would expect even stringently tested truths concerning those domains to differ, for if they did not differ, what evidence would we have of *two* domains? If an apparent truth survives scrutiny yet conflicts with another equally tested claim, the rational hypothesis is that there are indeed two domains, within each of which one and only one of the descriptions holds. Accordingly, if we fail to see anything but the domain of physical life we will reject a priori all evidence inconsistent with the hypothesis that only the physical exists. We will blind ourselves to the invisible, even when the evidence is staring us in the face. The difference between the "lived body," our own body, which we experience *as* our own, *as* we live in it, on the one hand, and the dead body, on the other, is a case in point, and highly relevant to our quest for the subtle body.

As we saw, Brahman is described in the *Taittirīya Upaniṣad* as being *hidden* "in the inmost of our soul" *and* as dwelling "in the highest heaven." Tat twam asi: you, living "down here," are That, the Great Above. The Great Above is invisible, but you, too, are invisible within your kośa-body. (This was Swami Rama's view, as we saw earlier.) A visible realm (the physical) and an invisible (the above) are, necessarily, two domains, at least when conceived or perceived on the basis of the physical body's sense of sight. One domain it sees, the other is invisible. Note, then, that what is being asserted in the Upaniṣad is not what Feuerstein claims, but the converse: at the level of our inmost being, our soul (which *must* be a domain of mind, not of gross body), we are of one nature with Brahman, not of one nature with the mere emanation that is the physical world of matter, which includes the gross body. So our mind was *not*, despite Feuerstein's assertion, created from matter. The Upaniṣad itself claims that mind exists independently of matter, being *a part of* the Being from which the whole physical world of matter is itself *only an emanation*. This, as we remarked earlier, is a strongly Advaitist view, in the sense that it denies any division between our Being and the Ground of all Being, Brahman.

However, the situation at the mundane, physical level is clearly quite different, for, according to the Upaniṣad, the world in which the human mind dwells is made up of the five elements (or the hundred atomic elements), which are not *essentially* Brahman but merely *emanations from* ātman-Brahman. We clearly have two domains, for what is true in the one domain is not true in the other. It follows that if the *very nature of* Brahman (i.e., not just an emanation from Brahman) is present in the invisible *inmost being* of the living human here on earth, then we humans are dual beings, for our gross bodies are parts of a world of mere emanation. This, by contrast, is a strongly Dvaitist view, similar to that advocated by Madhva.* Just as with field theory and quantum theory, might not *both* Dvaitist and Advaitist views be correct, but without conflict, *because each is true in, and only in, its own realm*? We are one with Brahman in the realm above, while our physical parts are parts of its mere emanation, the physical world around us "down here." Again, the evidence of the lived body and the no-longer-being-lived body stares us in the face.

This brings us to Feuerstein's final statement: "the potentiality of mind will always remain latent in matter, and under the right conditions it will resurrect itself again." While we know what Feuerstein means, he fails to say what he means, and his statement is misleading because it is so inaccurate, so vague; it is too unscientific to allow it to pass unchallenged (or, of course, to demand its corroboration by science). In the first place, the phrase "potentiality of mind" is hopelessly ambiguous, as a moment's consideration will show. Further, as we saw,

matter has, according to the Upaniṣad, *no* potential to give rise to mind, for *mind comes directly from Brahman*, not via the emanated physical world of matter. What Feuerstein should have said is that whenever matter is in a suitable state, as it is in the healthy body, mind can inhabit it. (This almost serves as a *definition* of bodily health, the state that allows a sound mind to inhabit it.)

Where, then, do we stand? The Vedic, Upaniṣadic, and Tantric view, *in broad outline,* is this: in the human body, the five elements are regulated and controlled by prāna (vital energy), which controls the vāyus (vital airs), interacting with the various organs and their processes: heart, lungs, excretion, circulation, and so on. The individual elements are also linked to the different psychospiritual vortexes, or subtle energy centers, the chakras, which are located along the spinal column and through which the psychospiritual kundalinī energy flows. Each of the first five chakras is conceived as controlling one of the elements. (See plate 9 where this is presented in a picturesque way.) Moreover, the chakras, which are associated with the glandular-endocrine system, which in turn is connected to the brain and thus to the mind, are chiefly governed by the five kośas or levels of consciousness.

In the Tantric laya yoga system, each of the five chakras from the base chakra, associated with earth, to the throat chakra, associated with space, is linked with one of the five elements and shows a simple correspondence with the function of the related part of the body. This "hypothesis" is not unscientific, being based on observation and reason, but is not well supported by today's analyses of phenomena. However, contemplation—which is not intended to make discoveries about the physical world but about the inner self—shows that the schema is serviceable in spiritual growth. This is sufficient validation, provided the two realms of thought are not conflated, and provided the result is not condemnation of the body on account of its "lower" functions. Wholeness accepts the necessity of bodily functions while we live "in the body."

The Kośas

The *Taittirīya Upaniṣad* presents a "world-affirming" philosophy: each level of self is described in a positive way, and Brahman is referred to emphatically as having the

---

*Sri Madhvacharya (1238–1317 CE) was the chief proponent of the Tattvavada (True Philosophy), or Dvaita (Dualistic) school of Hindu philosophy, and author of commentaries on the *Brahma Sūtras* and the Bhagavad Gītā.

nature of bliss (*ānanda*). However, the sages Guadapada and Sankara, the founders of the Advaitin spiritual tradition, promulgated the idea that all phenomenal existence is, if not literally illusory, then at least "false" (*mithya*) and ontologically inferior, and that only the Absolute is truly real. But that Absolute Reality (or Brahman) is totally devoid of qualities (*nirguna*).[16] As a result, Advaita Vedanta retained the *Taittirīya Upaniṣad*'s terminology, but overemphasized the accepted fact that the five "sheaths" or kośas veiled the light of the true Self (the ātman). The concepts underlying the world-accepting Upaniṣadic view were thus surreptitiously displaced.

The Three *Gunas*

Indic culture recognizes three major principles, or qualities, of energy:

- *Sattva:* pure lucidity
- *Rajas:* dynamism
- *Tamas:* inertia

In their adjectival forms (sattvic, rajasic, tamasic) these terms are widely used in Indian thought to describe states of being.

In the Vedantic version of how the individual mind (ātman) resides within the Great Mind (Brahman) the five sheaths are, in effect, the steps by which the yogin develops understanding and transcends the body, a process that might be illustrated by the emergence of a shoot from a seed. The sheaths are thus penetrated by progressively more powerful subtle energy, beginning with everyday gross physical energy and intensifying as meditation advances through etheric energy to mental, to intuitive, and finally to causal energy, which is seen as the level of steady wisdom already mentioned at the beginning of this chapter and elsewhere. These energies are correlated also with the five levels of expanding consciousness that result from the process:

1. The *anna-maya-kośa* (the body of food) is the physical body composed of the material elements, earth, water, fire, air, and space, through which we navigate in the material world. *Anna*

means "food," or "manifest matter"; *maya* means "full of."

2. The *prāna-maya-kośa* (the body of energy), composed of the life force, is the energy field that links body and mind and sustains all the physical functions. It is also associated with the emotions.

3. The *mano-maya-kośa* (the body of thought) processes sensory input. Also known as the "desire body," the lower manas or mind is driven by two of the three gunas (qualities) of energy, *tamas* (inertia) and *rajas* (dynamism); it alternates between doubt and volition, and between external consciousness and the inner world of imagination.

4. The *vijñāna-maya-kośa* (the body of intelligence) is a higher form of cognition and understanding that includes intuition, and discerns what is real from what is unreal. Controlled by the quality of *sattva* (pure being or lucidity), this layer of consciousness brings stillness, certainty, and faith.

5. The *ānanda-maya-kośa* (the body of bliss), through which we partake of the Absolute, is equated with the transcendental Self. The attainment of consciousness of the ānanda-maya-kośa removes the final "veil" that obscures Ultimate Reality from us.

Yogic Management of the Kośas

According to Yoga, the kośas are the five dimensions of existence into which all the other experiences fall, whether physical or emotional, whether in the realm of energy or that of mind. In order to deal with all the kośas, Yoga has developed different techniques. These techniques, says Swami Niranjanananda Saraswati of the Sivananda school, help us to experience the kośas as five layers of consciousness and to know the depth of the human mind.[17]

To experience optimum health in the different energies and functions of the physical body (anna-maya-kośa), Yoga teaches that we should practice āsanas (postures), *prānāyāma* (breath control), and the *ṣatkarmas* (six cleansing actions), which can help to purify and detoxify the body. To deal with prāna-maya-kośa, Yoga teaches the techniques of *prānāvidyā* (knowledge of prāna), *cakradhāranā* (concentration on the chakras), *kriyā* (dynamism, action, or ritual), and kundalinī (supreme power in the human body), which help to channel the flow of energy throughout the system, to stimulate and awaken the prāna.

To manage the activities and balance the agitations of mano-maya-kośa (body of thought), Yoga advocates the practice of *pratyāhāra* (sense withdrawal), *dhāranā* (concentration), and meditations on *mantras* (sacred sounds), *yantras* (geometrical figures), and *mandalas* (pictographs). To experience the power and force of vijñāna-maya-kośa, Yoga suggests the practices of *dhyāna* (meditation), laya yoga* (yoga of dissolution), and *nāda yoga* (yoga of subtle inner sound). To experience the state of ānanda-maya-kośa, it is necessary to attain the experience of samādhi, to awaken kundalinī. It is around these concepts that the entire system of Yoga evolved to manage the full range of human experience and existence.

Disconnecting from the Outer and Inner Mind

Swami Niranjanananda says that there comes a time when we need to dissociate our mind, attention, and awareness from the things that continually bombard us. Most of us are tamasic and rajasic by nature; we have not yet experienced the sattvic state. Sattva is not simple living or simple thinking, which are mainly outward and behavioral; it is the inner *direct awareness* of the true nature of the Self. Only a distorted and diminished self is seen and experienced when the whole life is lived under the influence of rajas and tamas alone. Only samādhi, only the awakening of kundalinī, only the understanding of absolute human potential, is the state of sattva.[18]

Swami Niranjanananda explains that, in order to come to the sattvic state, there has to be some form of disconnection, a dissociation from the world in which we live. When we go to sleep at night we disconnect from the outer world and connect with the inner mind. However, that is not enough. To experience the pure mind there also has to be a disconnection from the inner mind, which here simply represents an activity that we are not conscious of at present. If we try to "connect with our mind," we can become aware of our thoughts and emotions, the different qualities that manifest within the mind. If we go deeper,

*In his *Tantra: The Path of Ecstasy* (p. 179) Feuerstein defines *laya* as the "reabsorption of the elements into the pretemporal and prespatial ground of nature."

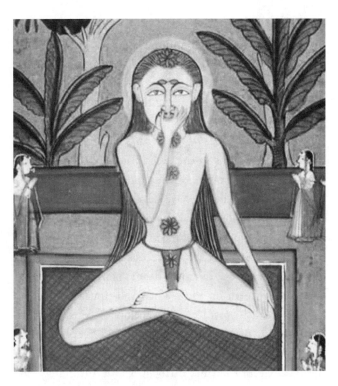

Fig. 3.4. Alternate nostril breathing (*prānāyāma*) is practiced to remove energetic blockages and restore balance in the subtle body channels. Rajasthan, 1858. (British Library.)

we may also become aware of deeper-seated *samskāras* (impressions) and karmas (actions) and identify them with our inner mind. But, as Swami Niranjanananda clarifies, what we are looking at is only the gross inner mind, "which functions in the third dimension, which is subject to the laws of time and space, which creates its own identity by looking at different forms, ideas, and names. These are the areas of the inner mind on which our mind projects itself."[19] He continues:

> Yoga says that there is another mind, the *pure* mind. This pure mind is experienced with the attainment of the *ānanda-maya* state, through *samādhi* and the awakening of *kundalinī*. *Samādhi* and *kundalinī* represent a state of being in which normal life events do not alter or affect our behavior, emotions or thoughts, and yet there is harmony in everything that we do. There is no effect from *tamas* and *rajas,* but only the experience of *sattva*. This is the proper aim of human life.[20]

Niranjananda concludes that the process is very simple, provided we do not deviate from it: "One has to move from the gross to the transcendental, from the impure, distorted, colored impressions to the experience of continuity of consciousness. . . . In *pratyāhāra* we observe the various experiences of the mind; and this is the first step in understanding the pure mind."[21]

Other Descriptions of the Kośas

There are variations in the descriptions of the five kośas or states of consciousness in different Indian religions. The Jains, for instance, have developed their own ideas of subtle physiology. Like the proponents of Samkhya, the Jains believe in the plurality of ultimate or spiritual entities, the *ātmans*. They are essentially infinite and pure consciousness, but they deem themselves confined to a certain form or body. Their self-limitation, which is regarded as a form of contraction of consciousness, results from the impact of karma (the effects of unenlightened actions responsible for rebirth); only through the reduction of karmic influences and, ultimately, the total obliteration of karma, can the jīva's consciousness be purified and transformed into the limitless transcendental consciousness.[22] The Jaina doctrine of the five bodies consists of:

1. *Audarika-śarīra* (the physical human body)
2. *Vaikriya-śarīra* (the transformation body), the size of which can be increased at will
3. *Āhāraka-śarīra* (the procurement body), which can be projected anywhere
4. *Taijasa-śarīra* (the indestructible body), which survives death and provides energy for the first three
5. *Karmana-śarīra* (the instrumental body), the innermost receptacle of karma.

The mystical treatise on the inner bodies, *Siddha-Siddhānta-Paddhati,* refers to six bodies. While these variations illustrate the metaphysical diversity of Tantra, we have to understand that, in Wilber's view, for instance, these energies are not the same as consciousness: consciousness cannot be reduced to these energies, nor can these energies be reduced to consciousness. Rather, these levels of energy accompany and support their correlative levels of consciousness (so that gross energy is the support of gross consciousness, subtle energy is the support of subtle consciousness, causal energy is the support of causal consciousness, and so on). In *Meditation: Classic and Contemporary Perspectives,* Roger Walsh, professor of psychiatry, philosophy, and anthropology, states: "*Every* level of both consciousness and energy higher than the lowest level (or 'matter') was completely *trans-material* (metaphysical, supernatural). These energies were said to form concentric spheres of increasing expanse, but they are themselves, in every essential way, *non-gross-material* (or ontologically pre-existing and separable from matter)."[23]

The philosopher, poet, and linguist P. R. Sarkar (Sri Sri Anandamurti), considered among the foremost twentieth-century teachers of Tantra and Yoga, suggests that there are seven levels of the body-mind-spirit complex:

1. *Anna-maya-kośa* (the physical body) is composed of the five fundamental factors or elements and controlled by the crudest layer of mind, the *kāma-maya-kośa*.
2. *Kāma-maya-kośa* (the desire body) is also known as conscious or crude mind. It has three functions: sensing stimuli from the external world through the sense organs of the body, having desires on the basis of those stimuli, and acting to materialize those desires by using the motor organs. This layer of the mind controls the motor organs and the instincts; it activates the body to satisfy the basic instincts of hunger, sleep, sex, and fear.
3. *Mano-maya-kośa* (the mental body) is also referred to as the subconscious mind. This state of mind controls the conscious mind. It has four functions: memory, rationality, experience of pleasure and pain based on reactions from past deeds, and dreaming.
4. *Atimanasa-kośa* (the supramental body) or subtle mind, is the layer of direct knowing, creative insight, and extrasensory perception. Although most people spend the majority of their lives in the kāma-maya- and mano-maya-kośas, sometimes this layer is accessed through deep contemplation, artistic inspiration, or intellectual discovery. In this layer a deep yearning for, and sometimes an experience of, Spirit is felt.
5. *Vijñāna-maya-kośa* (the higher mind) is also

called the "special knowledge" kośa. In this level of mind one is able to pierce through the veil of the gross, objective reality and get a glimpse of the world as it really is, simply Spirit. Many divine attributes are expressed through this state of mind: mercy, gentleness, serenity, nonattachment, steadiness, success, cheerfulness, spiritual bliss, humility, magnanimity, and more. This kośa has two main functions: discrimination (viveka) and nonattachment. True discrimination means to be able to discern between relative and absolute truth. True nonattachment does not mean to escape the world but rather to embrace it as Spirit, to see that all is divine.

6. *Hirana-maya-kośa* (the golden body) is the subtle causal mind. Here the feeling of "I" is only latent, only a thin veil separates the spiritual practitioner from the soul; the person has approached the dawn of true awakening in the all-pervading state of cosmic consciousness.

7. *Ātman,* being beyond mind, is the soul, the cosmic consciousness, the highest state of God-consciousness.[24]

I believe it may be useful here to state that we have covered, very briefly, systems of analysis of our being that differ, in some cases, only in their verbal descriptions, while in other cases the posited realities themselves differ.

The Three Bodies

The five sheaths or *kośas* grouped as three bodies or *śarīras*:

Body	Sheaths
Gross body (*sthūla śarīra*)	*anna-maya-kośa*
Subtle body (*sūkṣma śarīra*)	*prāna-maya-kośa*
	mano-maya-kośa
	vijñāna-maya-kośa
Causal body (*kārana śarīra*)	*ānanda-maya-kośa* (or "bliss body")

The Transpersonal Gateway

In the classical model of the five sheaths, they are grouped under three headings, as gross body (sthūla śarīra), subtle body (sūkṣma śarīra), and causal body (*kārana śarīra*). While the gross body is made up of gross matter (anna-maya-kośa), the subtle body is constituted of passions, desires, emotions, feelings, and thoughts. The bliss sheath is the causal body, consisting of *vāsanās* (latent impressions and energies) alone. The subtle body (sūkṣma śarīra)—composed of the prāna-maya-kośa, mano-maya-kośa, and vijñāna-maya-kośa—is also the realm where the chakras function. However, when the aspirant has been practicing sufficiently to have become "one of steady wisdom," it is believed that the formations of the subtle body change, and that the changes take place through the ānanda-maya-kośa (literally, "bliss sheath" or "bliss body").

When the hidden material in your causal body expresses itself as feelings and thoughts, it takes the form of your subtle body. The same material works out as perceptions and actions in the gross body. Let the causal body be instilled with the suggestion of health, the subtle body will entertain thoughts of health, and the gross body is bound to be healthy. Let the causal body be saturated with the suggestion of godhead, the subtle body will revel in the thought of godhead, the person is bound to be godly. You are the architect of your own personality inasmuch as it is your own causal body that is responsible for your behavior, movements, and environments. The substratum of your causal, subtle, and gross bodies is your real Self.[25]

The ānanda-maya-kośa, it will be noted, is the *highest* of the kośas in the five-tiered schema, and a person living at its level is only a single step from life without the body. Thus, the ānanda-maya-kośa is not a sheath in the same sense as the four other kośas, for it veils nothing, there being no embodied state above it. It is the soul itself, a body of light, also called the *karmāśaya,* or holder of karmas of this and all past lives. The ānanda-maya-kośa is that which evolves through all incarnations and beyond, until the soul is ultimately fulfilled by merging with the Primal Soul, *Parameśvara.* Then ānanda-maya-kośa becomes *Śiva-maya-kośa,* the body of God, Śiva. The lowest three kośas, the anna-, prāna-, and mano-maya-kośas, which animate all the activities of the sthūla śarīra (gross body), disintegrate at death, while the ānanda-maya-kośa persists.

Accordingly, the ānanda-maya-kośa was considered independent from the other four bodies, its ability to link to them in manifest existence notwithstanding. The ānanda-maya-kośa is independent of the patternings and distortions of the ego and the individual will. Rather, being the innermost sheath, it is the transpersonal gate, available here and now, to the causal level of consciousness that contains the causal body.

This, then, is the classical model of the kośas and the stages of consciousness associated with them. However, for the *spiritual adept* who, through Yoga and spiritual practices, has transmuted and purified his body, energy system, mind, emotions, will, and intellect, another model, having a downward extension, is applicable. Let us be clear as to the difference. The adept has, necessarily, already entered the high ānanda-maya-kośa state, but what is additional to that state as described in the classical model is the *downward* influence, while the "person of steady wisdom" is alive in the body, which operates *upon the body itself, upon its mind, its thoughts, its emotions, its will, its actions,* and which is exerted by the ānanda-maya-kośa state that now rules the person's whole being from its preeminent position as fully realized, indwelling soul.

A Note Concerning the Use of the Term *Bliss*

The term *bliss* is used to describe two distinct experiences occurring at two levels of mind, which are acknowledged by modern research to be divided into brain rhythms and the nature of consciousness. These are the so-called theta-wave and delta-wave states.

As noted above, the body of bliss, the ānanda-maya-kośa, consists of vāsanās (impressions) alone. When you are in deep, dreamless sleep, you are in the bliss sheath (the theta-wave state). When you cross the bliss sheath and move to other sheaths you experience the dream state (alpha) and waking state (mainly beta) of consciousness. Vāsanās are unmanifest in deep sleep, but

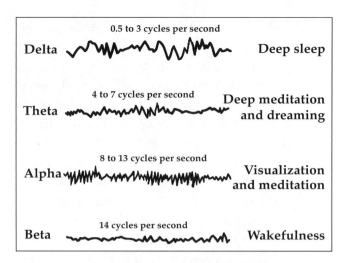

Fig. 3.5. Information on altered states of consciousness has been obtained by measuring the brainwaves of yogis on electroencephalographs. Brainwave activity has four wave patterns, designated alpha, beta, theta, and delta.

Alpha waves have a frequency of 8 to 13 cycles per second. They are associated with relaxed, detached awareness, visualization, daydreaming, and a receptive mind. They can also be seen as a bridge from the subconscious to the conscious mind.

Beta waves are produced at frequencies from 14 to 26 cycles per second. They produce the normal waking state of the brain, associated with logical thinking, concrete problem-solving, and active external attention.

Theta waves are those with a rate of 4 to 7 cycles per second and are related to awareness of the subconscious, dreaming sleep, creative inspiration, peak experiences, and deep meditation. It is from here that many of the spiritual "ah-ha" experiences occur.

Delta waves have frequencies from 0.5 to 3 cycles per second and are primarily associated with deep sleep. They can also be thought of as a kind of "radar" of empathic, intuitive, unconscious waves.

manifest in the form of thought in the dream state and in actions in the waking state. Consequently you experience mental agitations, great or small, as long as you remain in the dream and waking states. When, however, you enter the state of deep sleep, all your mental agitations cease and you experience undisturbed peace and bliss. Hence it is that this sheath is called the bliss sheath. But the bliss experienced in deep sleep is relative. It is not to be confused with the absolute bliss of Self-realization (*turīya*).[26]

FOUR

The Organs of the Soul

While Western science is still struggling to find explanations for such phenomena as acupuncture meridians, kuṇḍalinī awakenings, and Kirlian photography, yogins continue to explore and enjoy the pyrotechnics of the subtle body, as they have done for hundreds of generations.

GEORG FEUERSTEIN, *THE YOGA TRADITION*

Knowledge about the organs that the soul requires in order to exist in the world has been preserved and shared through the *śāstras,* which have been described as "the storehouse of Indian occultism."[1] The term *śāstra* (some Western authors give the word as *shastra,* others as *Śāstra*) means, approximately, "learned text," and is used by the Tantric schools as the generic title for their canon of written teachings. The śāstras contain both spiritual teachings on liberation and practices based on the teachings, which themselves arose out of mystical insights into the subtle dimensions of being, those multiple layers of reality, invisible to ordinary awareness, that exist between the material and spiritual realms.

As we have seen, those layers include the sūkṣma śarīra, the subtle body, described by Deussen as the "companion of the soul in its wanderings,"[2] as well as the sthūla śarīra, the gross body, which is sustained by prāna, meaning "wind" or "breath." However, there are said to be five "winds" or "breaths." Here we must therefore explain that the word *prāna* is used in two senses that overlap and can therefore be easily confused. It is used to name the whole group of five "winds" or "breaths," and it is also used specifically to denote *a particular one of* those five winds or breaths. During embodied life all five prānas penetrate the body and sustain its functions.

Hence the usage below, where the word *prāna* denotes only one of the breaths, because the other four are specifically named and their functions identified.

Deussen points out that, "According to Sankara, the *prāna* causes inspiration, the *apāna* expiration . . . the *vyāna* sustains life when the breath is arrested. The *samāna* is concerned with digestion. The *udāna* effects the departure of the soul from the body at death."[3] These five bioenergetic functions, the "bodily winds," are explained differently in different texts but there is unanimity about the prāna and the apāna whose incessant activity is believed to create mental restlessness and which, therefore, become the principal means of calming the mind through prānāyāma (breath control). Breath, the prāna and the apāna, is also the means of rousing the primordial energy or current, the kundalinī śakti, which ascends through the chakras (psychospiritual centers), speeding up the vibration of the physical body and transmuting it into the "divine body" (*divya-deha*).

The notion of respiration and bodily winds in the exegetical Samhitās, the Brāhmanas, and the philosophical and mystical Upaniṣads indicates a continuation of the conceptions advanced in the earlier Veda, but also demonstrates a further elaboration of breath in ritual and ascetic contexts. The internalization of ritual through

41

controlled breathing leading to meditation and ecstasy became the means through which ascetics believed they would attain longevity and immortality during embodied life. In his article "The Science of Respiration and the Doctrine of Bodily Winds in Ancient India," Zysk tells us that there can be little doubt that the ascetics of the Upaniṣadic age, through their long meditations on breath and its importance to the life process of a human being, conceived of a wind physiology codified according to the five fundamental bodily winds.[4] He refers specifically to the *Maitrī Upaniṣad* where prāṇāyāma, breath control, is referred to as one of the six, later to become eight, limbs of Yoga.

> By arresting both breath and mind through controlled respiration, the objects of the senses are restrained and a continued voidness of conception ensues, leading ultimately to the fourth superconscious condition (*turya, turīya*) in which one's soul (*ātman*) is free to dwell with the universal spirit (*Brahman*). . . . The texts on Yoga speak of numerous vessels which convey all the bodily winds: fourteen of them are most important, and three of these, *idā, piṅgalā* and *suṣumnā,* generally associated with the major vessels of the spine, convey *prāṇa.*[5]

The Wheels of Life

The structures of the subtle anatomy cannot be found, as Feuerstein points out, by dissecting the physical body, in spite of attempts by some writers to draw direct parallels between the subtle body and the organs and endocrine glands of the physical body. These structures are found only by entering a meditative state and experiencing the energy field from within.[6] To clairvoyant vision, the subtle body appears as a radiant, shimmering energy field that is in constant internal motion and is crisscrossed by luminous filaments, or tendrils (nadis). Feuerstein notes that the most stable structures of the subtle body are the chakras, because of their circular form and whirling motion and because of the way in which the prāṇa currents terminate at or issue from them.[7]

The chakras may be regarded as idealized versions of the actual anatomy and physiology of the subtle body, which are used as guides for visualization and contem-

plation. The yogin uses them purely as objects of focused contemplation to help him gain entry and insight into the particular states of being that are governed by the five kośas.

Textual Sources for the Chakras

The concept of the chakras has today entered public consciousness worldwide, and is widely viewed as an ancient and immutable element of the Indian worldview, says Dominik Wujastyk, writing about medicine in premodern India.[8] This view needs to be qualified in two directions. First, the idea of the chakras is a relatively recent development in Indian Tantric thought. It is datable only to the tenth century CE, making its appearance in texts such as the *Kubjikāmatatantra* and the *Maliniviyayottaratantra.*[9] Secondly, the chakras make no appearance whatsoever in Ayurveda. Notwithstanding the contemporary growth of various forms of massage and therapy focused on the chakras, there is no such theme in the classical Sanskrit literature on medicine. The chakras are an idea specific to Tantra and Yoga, and it is not until relatively recent times that this idea has been synthesized with medical thought and practice.[10] As we shall see, however, in the next two chapters, there are related ideas in Chinese Taoist practices that may have arisen in connection with similar spiritual goals.

According to David Gordon White, the earliest Hindu source of the chakras is most probably the *Bhāgavata-purāṇa,** in which six sites in the subtle anatomy are listed:

Mūrdha: the cranium
Bhruvorantara: the place between the eyebrows
Svatālumūla: root of the palate
Uras: breast
Hṛt: heart
Nābhi: the navel[11]

We show the list inverted so that the chakras appear in the correct positions relative to the physical body.

**Bhāgavata-purāṇa,* also known as *Śrīmad Bhāgavatam,* or simply *Bhāgavatam,* is one of the *Purāṇas,* a part of the literature of Hinduism. Its primary focus is the process of bhakti yoga (loving devotion to the Supreme Lord) in which Vishnu or Krishna is understood as the Supreme all-embracing God of all gods (Bhagavan).

The earliest Hindu source of the term *chakra* is the *Kaulajñāna-nirṇaya,* the most outstanding of the translated texts of Kaula, one of the oldest branches of Tantrism, attributed to Matsyendra Natha. However, the earliest text that documents the seven chakras is the eleventh-century *Kubjikamātatantra.* This text lists the centers known to later Yoga traditions, which are now widely regarded as the "standard" seven main chakras. Again, we have arranged the list in the proper order:

> *Sahasrāra:* the crown
> *Ājñā:* the brow
> *Viṣuddhi:* the throat
> *Anāhata:* the heart
> *Manipūra:* the navel
> *Swādhiṣthāna:* the genital region
> *Mūlādhāra:* the anal region

Among the earliest translations of Tantric texts that introduced Tantra to the Western world are the works of the British Orientalist Sir John Woodroffe (1865–1936), also known by his nom-de-plume, Arthur Avalon. John Woodroffe, son of the Advocate-General of Bengal, became Chief Justice of the Calcutta High Court in 1915. While serving on the bench he studied Sanskrit and Hindu philosophy. He was especially interested in the Tantric system and translated some twenty original Sanskrit texts. The first of these, the *Mahānirvāna Tantra,* published in 1913, was followed by *Shakti and Shākta* and *The Serpent Power* in 1918. The latter is still considered the most authoritative work on the *Ṣaṭ-Cakra Nirūpaṇa,* the *Description of and Investigation into the Six Bodily Centers,* believed to have been composed in 1576 and passed down through ten generations of a family of Tantric teachers.

Although Woodroffe describes the six centers discussed in this particular Tantric text, Feuerstein points out that, "many Tantric teachers speak of seven principal psychoenergetic centres . . . some schools list five, and others name nine, ten, eleven, or very many more."[12] Gavin Flood mentions that the *Kaulajñāna-nirṇaya* lists eight chakras and indicates that meditation and worship (*dhyanapuja*) of each in turn bestows different magical powers.[13] In his definitive work on *Layayoga,* Shyam Sunder Goswami describes thirteen chakras and refers to each one as a "power system," each with its individual concentration of energy and its specific life force activities.[14]

Feuerstein reminds us that the fact that different authorities have mentioned diverse numbers of chakras need not be taken as a sign of disagreement between them. The chakra models are just that: models of reality that are designed to assist Tantric practitioners in their inward odyssey from the many to the One.[15]

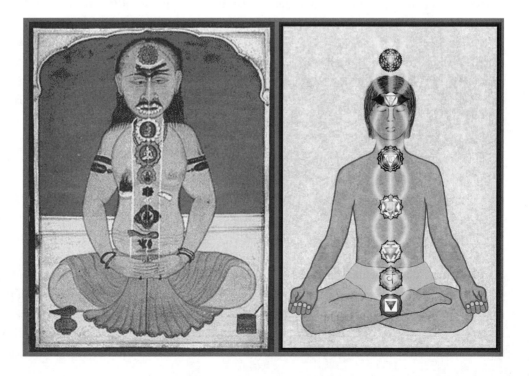

Fig. 4.1. The Tantric yogi (left), in this Rajasthani painting, ca. eighteenth century, shows the seven chakras that form the standard model of reality for meditation practice today (right).

The Seven Psychoenergetic Centers

Fundamentally, the seven chakras ("wheels" or "vortices") symbolize the relationship between the material world, the energy system, the mind, and the higher consciousness. At the outer circumference of a wheel there is more space, more material, more diversity, more movement. If you focus on the rim of the wheel, it flies by in a blur, like the variegated world of material phenomena. Moving inward, the spokes of the wheel converge, and the dizzying movement slows. At the center of each chakra is the center of consciousness, puruṣa, or Self.[16] Though it has many parts, it is all one wheel. Note how this description implies the concept of the Being-in-the-world as a wholeness that contains in itself both human (subject) and world (object) without any line of distinction between them, a dipole, not a duality.

Traditional representations of the chakra system depict them as distributed along the axis of the spine. Each is associated with an element, and has its own color and its own number of petals, each with its Sanskrit letter, its deities, and its mantras (see plate 10). The symbolism of each chakra represents a number of complex and intricate *experiences* that cannot be expressed in words or pictures. Only those who have the experiences know what the symbolism conveys.

Through meditation on each of the centers, aspects of life are brought to consciousness, enabling us to reflect on the outer and inner events that constitute the circumstances of our life. Swami Rama points out that, "like the wheel of fortune, they have a great deal to do with the shape and outcome of one's experience on its various levels. The spinning focus of energy and imagery experienced at each of these points reflects very concisely one's basic nature and contains the seeds of the fortune that awaits him."[17]

The energies focused at these centers are associated with the interaction of physiological, emotional, mental, and spiritual functioning. The intuitions and understandings of literature, of art, of mythology, of religious symbolism, physics, and metaphysics all come together at a central focus in the chakras. All understanding is distilled here. This is what is meant by saying that the microcosm reflects the macrocosm. Swami Rama says that "by immersing oneself in this inner experience, an understanding of the coordination between the various aspects of oneself and the universe begins to grow."[18] The

whole becomes whole*some*. The world and each person in it, no longer divided asunder, become whole, healthy.

Most Tantric authorities would agree with Feuerstein that in the ordinary person the chakras are functioning at a minimal level, leading them to be compared to drooping, closed lotus flowers. From a Yogic point of view, they can be said barely to exist. Through inner work, however, they automatically become more active, opening like lotuses in full bloom and extending upward toward the light (which is really omnipresent). Moreover, the chakras are not harmonized or mutually attuned with each other until, in the course of spiritual practice, they become so by a gradual progression; this state coincides with the balanced functioning of the body-mind.[19]

The Serpent Power

Two Sanskrit works on laya yoga, translated by Sir John Woodroffe and published under the title of *The Serpent Power*, deal with kundalinī, the microcosmic manifestation of the primordial energy, or Shakti. They present the process by which the primordial energy is polarized into potential energy and dynamic energy. Through regulation of the flow of prāna, that energy is withdrawn from the left and right nadis and forced into the central pathway, the suṣumnā (see plate 11). The dormant *kundalinī-śakti* is thus awakened, piercing the six chakras as it shoots up to the crown center, where, as Feuerstein puts it, "the blissful meltdown between Śakti and Śiva occurs."[20]

Although the network of energy currents or "filaments," the nadi system, is traditionally believed to be composed of 72,000 nadis, about fourteen of which are considered major, the three most important are the idā and pingalā, which spiral around the central channel, the suṣumnā, through which the energy travels upward, awakening the spiritual aspirant to a higher level of consciousness and ensuring self-control and harmony at all levels of human evolution and development. As Feuerstein points out, however, Western students of Yoga find it difficult to relate to the traditional model of the kundalinī process.[21]

Researchers have sought explanations for the phenomenon of the kundalinī process, but with uncertain results. A consequence of this is a plethora of vague and often misleading writing on related topics, sometimes hiding a large and increasing body of valid scientific research. Bill Schul Ph.D., researcher in mind expansion, creativity, and nonordinary states of awareness, for example, says the human can be viewed as a quadripolar magnet, and that all the laws of electricity and magnetism are at work in the human system.[22] He says that a potential difference between two poles always gives rise to a flow between them. Viewed in electrical terms, he continues, the potential difference is a *voltage* and the amount of flow between the poles can be considered as *current*. Whenever there is a flow of current, there is a magnetic field surrounding and at right angles to it. In a person, he says, the voltage and current between the polarity of root and crown produces a magnetic current, which is oftentimes referred to as the aura.

We acknowledge that this is vaguely correct, but it is misleading. Although he implies that these facts are unique to *Homo sapiens,* most of his statements apply to every animal and plant and inanimate object in the physical world. He therefore tells us nothing about human beings, let alone their spiritual experiences. The information is inaccurate, dealing with substantive ideas at a merely terminological level while purporting to make statements descriptive of deep nature. This is an example of the "bewitchment by language" of which Wittgenstein warns the unwary language-user, including writers and their readers.

To give an example, the "flow" (of electrons) referred to by Schul is not to be "considered as" current; it *is* the current, the flow of electrons under pressure from photons (which are the quanta of energy). In an alternative description, the current is electrons flowing because they are propelled by the electromotive force (EMF). This force or energy is not so much "a voltage," as Schul colloquially puts it, as it is a pressure (that causes movement), which is *measured in* volts; the volt is merely the standard unit of measurement for electrical pressure, or energy, as distinguished from current, which is in reality a numerical count of the number of electrons flowing in the circuit. One electron might move at great speed, or a large number of electrons, propelled by the same total energy, will move more slowly. The energy *per electron* relates in inverse proportion to the number of electrons and the speed at which they move.

Further, as it stands, Schul's statement that humans "work" using electromagnetic forces is a mere truism since it applies to everything in the physical world. The electromagnetic force is the *only* force other than gravity that is important in medium-scale physical phenomena such as ourselves, elephants, bacteria, and grains of sand, stones, and mountains. This force operates in both "living" *and* "nonliving" matter (if that distinction is valid at all within the physical world). Physicists such as Herbert Dingle, whom we shall quote in chapter 15, would point out that the laws of motion apply throughout the physical world, yet do not apply in anything like the same way to the living systems in it, so one must view with caution statements, purportedly based on "science" or the "laws of physics," including the laws of electromagnetism referred to by Schul, which do not provide a complete description of the phenomena of life, or even give information unique to them. One of Dingle's points, and one of ours, would be that while it may be possible to view a human as a quadripolar magnet, as Schul claims, this is an inaccurate and misleading picture because it is grossly incomplete. One would hardly expect all quadripolar magnets to experience kundalinī, an experience had by a few whole, living, human Beings, and usually when meditating. A Being is much more than a magnet. Of course, Schul is not deeply wrong, but what he tells us is misleadingly incomplete and, unsurprisingly, since it applies even to stones, also very far from a description even of kundalinī in itself. As an experienced meditator laconically remarked to me, many years ago in India, kundalinī is "only orgasm," and Freud would have added the adjective "sublimated." Others would hasten to affirm that the state of sexual abstinence is essential to spiritual growth, encouraging the occurrence of kundalinī, and yet others would emphatically deny this, perhaps most vehemently the Tantrics themselves. Clearly, an electromagnetic description of kundalinī, should it be possible at all, would be of little use since *all* our bodily states and processes are *electromagnetic* states and processes, and we are certainly not in a state of perpetual orgasm.

What we need to learn here is that description has many levels, no single one of them being complete, and that our goal is a way of looking out upon the world-about that comprehends all perspectives and all levels into one global grasp of reality so all-encompassing as to be *beyond* perspective, that is, in Gebser's terminology, *aperspectival* (which we will discuss further in chapter 15). For now, it is important to note that ill-understood

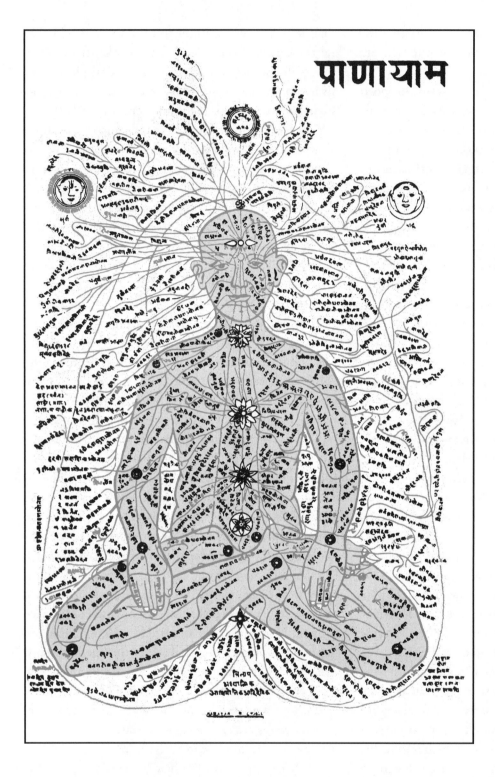

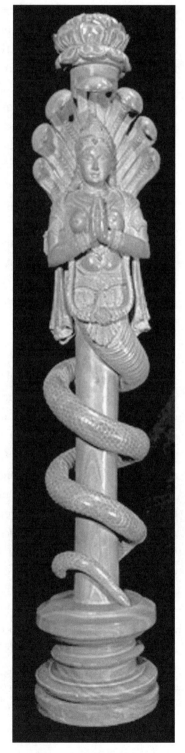

Fig. 4.2. The nadi system is the network of energy currents through which the life force circulates throughout the subtle body. (Tenth-century diagram.)

Fig. 4.3 (right). The Kundalinī Nagini goddess shown here symbolizes the hidden divinity within the subtle body, which is awakened as the rising kundalinī links human and divine consciousness. Although samādhi, immersion in universal consciousness (Siva), is said to bring effulgence or ecstasy, if the practitioner is not well grounded in yoga practice it can create a "spiritual emergency," physical and mental effects that are painful, debilitating, and disturbing, which may need specialist psychotherapeutic treatment. If "forcing" or "hurrying" of the practice is avoided, kundalinī will unfold safely, in its own time. Marble, South India, Shilpi Tradition. (Photograph © Chris Tompkins, Yoga Sculptures of India.)

science, as presented by many writers, does nothing but cloud understanding of ourselves, while well-understood science assists us in diagnosing our own Being.

In the actual experience of kundalinī the moment Feuerstein describes as "blissful meltdown" may be experienced differently by individual practitioners. Perhaps the most widely publicized kundalinī awakening was that of Gopi Krishna (1903–1984), whose graphic autobiographical accounts of kundalinī have become classic works on spiritual transformation. In his book, *Kundalini: Path to Higher Consciousness,* he describes his first experience in 1937 as a dramatic, unexpected, and uncontrolled burst of energy, culminating in his departure from the physical body, "entirely enveloped in a halo of light."[23]

The attempt to attain union with Brahman through the awakening of kundalinī is not always ecstatic, as the nature of the experience depends on the preparation and the perception of the meditator. The descriptions we have espoused in the past determine the understandings we bring to new experiences, and the interpretations we make of them. Gopi Krishna's experience exemplifies this, for, as he famously tells us in his book, kundalinī can be painful, producing debilitating effects over a long period of time if the aspirant is not properly grounded in Yoga practice.[24]

Sir John Woodroffe writes about a friend of his who unwittingly aroused kundalinī, but, not being a yogi, he says, "could not bring her down again." He had a fascinating experience in which he saw the idā and pingalā and the "central fire with a trembling aura of rosy light, and blue or azure light, and a white fire which rose up into the brain and flamed out in a winged radiance on either side of the head, fire . . . flashing from center to center with such rapidity that he could see little of the vision." Woodroffe reports that his friend was frightened by the rocking motion as the power seemed like something that could really consume him, but, most disappointingly, in his agitation his friend forgot to fix his mind on the Supreme, and so "missed a divine adventure."[25]

The Relationship between the Kośas, Chakras, and Nadis

As we saw earlier, the experience of the kośas that is gained in meditation helps us to know the depth of the human mind. Swami Niranjanananda introduces us to the relationship between the kośas (sheaths) and chakras

(wheels or vortices of energy) and explains how they interact as energy and consciousness.[26] The first dimension, he says, is the material body, the anna-maya-kośa (the body of food). Although, scientifically, we look at the physical body as a collection of systems controlling the bodily functions, Yoga teaches that these functions are nothing but manifestations of interaction between energy and consciousness. When we experience the inner bodies, energy and consciousness manifest in subtler form. Anna-maya-kośa is a mode of being in which we experience matter as a combination of energy and consciousness.

The prāna-maya-kośa (the body of energy), the next layer of experience, is movement of the pranic force directing our physical and mental activities. This movement flows through the nadis, which are conductors of energy controlled by the six chakras. All six chakras are dealt with when we are trying to manage prāna-maya-kośa. The mūlādhāra chakra controls the elimination of accumulated toxins from the body and mind. (Note in passing how this corresponds with the Freudian notion of anality.) In the physical process, what we eat is eventually excreted, but we derive nourishment and energy from it as it passes through the body. There is believed to be a parallel process of elimination of waste from the mind. However, Swamiji admits that we do not understand this process. He says that we tend to accumulate experiences in the form of what in Yoga are known as the five *kleśas* (disturbances), whether ignorance to begin with or fear of death to end with. We do not eliminate these disturbances from the mind, but retain them in the form of experiences or memory. Human consciousness revolves around those memories and experiences because of another factor, the ego. This is also reminiscent of Freudian and other Western psychologies.

The Five Kleśas

The five mental patterns or defects that cause all the miseries and afflictions in life are:

Avidyā (Ignorance)

Asmitā (Ego)

Rāga (Attachment)

Dveṣa (Aversion)

Abhiniveśa (Clinging to Life)

Swamiji goes on to say that we have to learn how to eliminate things from the mind and retain tranquillity and calmness. To help in the understanding of inner release, we have to work with swādhiṣṭhāna chakra, which represents the inner mind, the unconscious, the storehouse of experiences and memories in the form of samskāras or impressions. Samskāras can be eliminated or transformed when we learn how to work with our prāna-maya-kośa at the level of swādhiṣṭhāna chakra.

Dynamism of mind and aggression in our personality, whether physical, mental, or emotional, are controlled by the manipūra chakra. When we work with this chakra we transform the energies that are manifesting there, eventually experiencing the sattvic state of being. Anāhata chakra controls the manifestation and projection of feelings and emotions. It deals with the qualities of attraction and repulsion in our nature.

Viṣuddha chakra, behind the throat, is a center through which we learn how to interact in the world efficiently, effectively, and creatively. When we work with viṣuddha chakra we change our outlook, our vision of life, enhancing creativity, positivity, and optimism, along with improving communication.

The sixth chakra is ājñā, the doorway between the manifest energy and consciousness on the lower side and the unmanifest transcendental energy and consciousness on the higher. This chakra allows us to move from the manifest "dimension" to the unmanifest aspects of our personality.

Mano-maya-kośa, the dimension of mental awareness, is composed of two qualities, manas and buddhi. While manas is the rational, linear, sequential, thoughtful mind, buddhi is the quality of discrimination that comes after knowledge, after the removal of ignorance. The practices of pratyāhāra aim to realize, and to discover the nature of, our mano-maya-kośa. Harmony of mano-maya-kośa is attained by also balancing prāna-maya-kośa. We cannot say that mano-maya is different

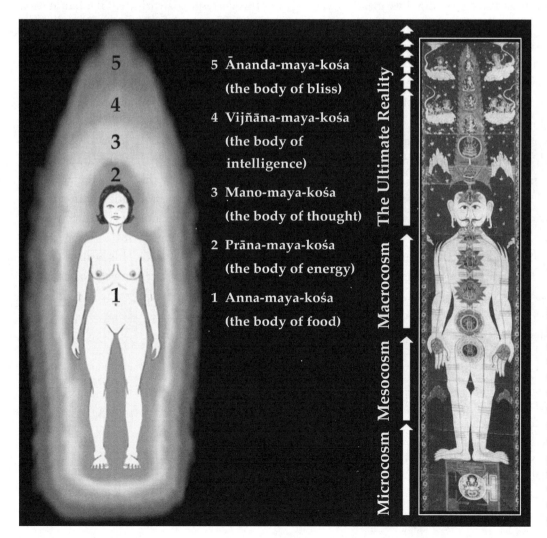

5 Ānanda-maya-kośa
   (the body of bliss)

4 Vijñāna-maya-kośa
   (the body of intelligence)

3 Mano-maya-kośa
   (the body of thought)

2 Prāna-maya-kośa
   (the body of energy)

1 Anna-maya-kośa
   (the body of food)

Microcosm Mesocosm Macrocosm The Ultimate Reality

Fig. 4.4. This composite picture shows the psychospiritual "map" of the "organs" needed by the soul for its ascent toward the Godhead, the five kośas, sheaths or subtle "bodies," that surround the physical form, and the chakras through which the energies of the subtle bodies are transformed.

from prāna-maya, or that prāna-maya is different from anna-maya; they are experiences and conditions of life that cannot be separated from each other. However, for our understanding and to define the sequence of our practice, yogis have defined the functions of anna-maya-, prāna-maya-, and mano-maya-kośa separately.

The name *vijñāna-maya-kośa* derives from *jñāna,* meaning "wisdom," or "knowledge," the prefix *vi* being a confirmation of the intensity of knowledge that is derived not only from experiences and memories gained in this lifetime but also in past lives. There is a storehouse of knowledge in every one of us, but we are not educated to experience that inner wisdom. Vijñāna-maya-kośa has the aspects of *citta* (consciousness) and *ahamkāra* associated with it. Citta means the ability to know, to become the observer of what is actually happening, to be able to live a reality rather than speculating or fantasizing about it. Ahamkāra is the ego aspect, in the real, not the gross, sense: knowledge of "I," becoming aware of the identity of the self. This understanding comes when we work with vijñāna-maya-kośa.

According to Swami Niranjanananda, "Once we have worked with and understood the identity of 'I,' the identity of the self which is manifest in the world in the third dimension and which experiences the pleasures and comforts, pains and sufferings of life, we move into the experience of *ānanda-maya-kośa,* the dimension of bliss, happiness, wholeness, contentment."[27]

FIVE

The Yoga of the Subtle Body

The lotus of spiritual enlightenment grows out of the mud of everyday life . . . a prettified and unrealistic picture of a religious tradition is of little use to anyone.

GEOFFREY SAMUEL, *THE ORIGINS OF YOGA AND TANTRA*

Although the common belief in Indian traditions is that the presence of ātman is in all life, and that all beings are subject to saṃsāra, the transmigratory process from life to life, human beings have a special and perhaps exclusive "soteriological qualification for liberative knowledge," as Gregory P. Fields puts it in his *Religious Therapeutics*.[1] The spiritual enterprise is uniquely human and the ability to experience and experiment within the interior of the body-mind, the very territory from which the aspirant desires to be liberated, represents an extraordinary feat in human development. An interesting point that Fields highlights is that human intelligence differs from that of animals in one particular respect: consciousness of the future. Our salvation lies in our ability to understand that certain ritual actions can define the limits of our potential unless we cultivate other paths to transcendence through self-development.

We have seen that different "maps" or models emerged in the pursuit of mokṣa (freedom); each attempted to encapsulate the process of union between ātman and Brahman. Here it is relevant for us to take a brief look at the tools or methods that evolved into the "yoga of the subtle body," into what Professor Samuel refers to in *The Origins of Yoga and Tantra* as the "disciplined and systematic techniques for the training and control of the human body-mind complex, which are also understood as techniques for the reshaping of

human consciousness toward some kind of higher goal."[2]

As some modern researchers observe, Indian societies have been particularly rich in these "technologies of the self," which have evolved over centuries through changing social, political, and religious conditions. Professor Samuel notes that there has been a historical development from simple to more complex approaches. These range from archaic forms of ritual worship and sacrificial cults to the "striking innovation" of the interiorized practices of the subtle body and its further development of the visualization of deities. The liberating insight, he observes, is not a logical proposition, but something akin to a patterning or attunement of the body-mind system as a whole to the wider universe of which it forms an indissoluble part.[3]

Yoga and meditation practices from a variety of traditions, some of which we are familiar with in the West today, constitute a synthesis of experience and experimentation evolved over centuries. These became the coherent mappings of highly disciplined skills of self-observation which, philosopher Jacob Needleman observed, may require longer training than any other skill we know. When we think about it, transforming the physical material body into a divya-deha, a "divine body," a *non*physical body, is no mean feat. Although we know that belief in the existence of a nonmaterial subtle body is an ancient one, we must wonder how the ancients learned that particular practices would give particular results and assure a transformation. We know that certain practices evolved from empirical evidence, tried and tested methods handed down orally from guru to disciple from one generation to the next. We also know that the first generation of gurus in some traditions attributed their knowledge to "divine inspiration," directly revealed by Brahman, by Siva, or by some other deity, but what is intriguing is how the ancient yogis were able to develop these techniques in such a way as to succeed in attaining the state of higher or "cosmic" consciousness required to "cross the abyss" between the human being in the world and the Great Being.

What were the physiological and psychological processes that took place that enabled aspirants to use the concept of the subtle body as both a goal and a path, a map and a vehicle in which to travel? It is only in recent years that researchers in the West have become interested in the phenomenology of the psychophysical practices they employed. What we have learned so far is that they relied on particular *types* of inner experiences and an embodied cognitive structure through which the yogi could learn about, make sense of, and repeat patterns that related to her experiences. She needed to be able to connect through her bodily experience, senses, and awareness to a multidimensional reality shaped by certain cultural, linguistic, and religious ideas that had been passed to her through the lineage of a particular tradition. Still she had to make her own journey, just as any practitioner has to do today, regardless of which tradition or "path" he or she may be following, or how wise the teacher.

It is believed that there was no unanimity as to which practices constituted Yoga until the development of Patanjali's eightfold path, about the second century BCE. Still there existed what John Brockington, professor of Sanskrit at Edinburgh University, calls "widely diffused" spiritual methodologies that are clearly indebted to Yoga.[4] It is worth stating here, however, as David Gordon White explains, that there is little in the *Yoga Sūtras* about yoga practice, in the sense of techniques involving fixed postures and breath control.[5] He also notes that there are no references to the subtle body, the nadis (energy channels), or chakras (energy centers). Nor are there any such references in the *Yoga-Bhāsya*, the fifth-century commentary on the *Yoga Sūtras* by Vyasa, author of the *Mahābhārata*. Some of the "widely diffused" practices that evolved into the "yoga of the subtle body" belong to the earlier period of the Vedic sacrificial tradition, which went through a process of "interiorization."

Interior Sacrifice

As Professor Yael Bentor explains, Hindu fire rituals already included not only external rituals in which libations were poured into a fire (see plate 12), but also internalized forms of these rituals.[6] What Bentor means by interiorization is a mental performance of the ritual, where the fire may be replaced with one of the continuing processes of life such as breathing or eating. He explains that in the Upaniṣads one of the most widespread forms of interiorization of the Vedic sacrifice considers life itself—together with the physiological functions that maintain it—as an unceasing sacrifice.

Professor Bentor goes on to say that the continuous employment of internalized fire rituals in India and Tibet appears to be part of a general process of interiorization that took place in both Hinduism and Buddhism, especially in their systems of Yoga and Tantra. The transformative power of the fire is especially significant in Tantric ritual, where the attainment of an inner transformation is the prime objective. The origins of such interiorization may be found, in the classical Vedic world, among the traveling brahmins who temporarily found themselves far from their sacred fires. The brahmins transformed the sacred fire into their breath, and when sacred fire was needed their breath would be used to sacralize any fire used for the ritual. The belief that some real effect is here described is supported by the fact that fire-eating, along with fire-walking, is practiced without suffering or harm by some groups to the present day.

The Brāhmana texts expanded the idea of the traveling brahmin, teaching that the *agnihotra* (fire ritual) is, in fact, breathing or life. It was believed that as long as one breathes, the agnihotra is being performed. According to the *Baudhaya Śrauta Sūtra* (29.5), a brahmin who is physically unable to perform the external agnihotra, after transferring the fire into himself, consumes the two agnihotra oblations himself, with the usual ritual. Such methods of expiation, of only incidental importance to the classical Vedic ritual, became central in Upaniṣadic thought, where they were interpreted as a continuous and uninterrupted inner agnihotra in accordance with the theories then current, which emphasized internal processes. Other brahmanical texts explicitly identify the sacred fires of the *śrauta* rituals with the three, or five, breaths. Such an interiorization of fire is related also to the notion of *tapas,* "inner heat," which, like breath, means life. The interiorization of fire serves to conserve inner heat, the life force. The conception of the body as a source of sacrifice through which suffering could be overcome is an important component of all Indic thinking concerning longevity, immortality, and health.

In presenting their new practices in terms of the Vedic sacrifice, the members of the renunciation movements characterized the ritualists of the earlier classical Vedic tradition by the word *devayajin,* "sacrificer[s] to the gods," while calling their own practitioners *ātmayajin,* "sacrificer[s] to one's self." Later Hindu schools developed the inner fire ritual still further, calling their own practices "inner sacrifice," while occasionally condemning the outwardly performed rituals outright, as in this example from the *Linga Purāṇa:*

> The aspirant who seeks salvation shall perform the nonviolent sacrifice. One shall meditate on the fire stationed in the heart and perform the sacrifice Dhyanayajna (meditation). After realising Śiva stationed in the body of all living beings, lord of the universe, he shall devoutly perform the sacrifice by Pranayama perpetually. He who performs the external Homa becomes a frog in the rock.[7]*

In the later Tibetan Buddhist practices, the entire ritual became an entirely interiorized process of contemplation, in which the worshipper follows in *imagination* the entire ritual procedure from the evocation of the deity to the final leave-taking. A Tantric at the highest stage of spiritual development depended almost

entirely on this mental *puja* (worship).[8]* Since it no longer required an "outer journey," the Vedic origin was gradually forgotten and the inner ritual came to be attributed to the Buddha. The significance of fire, Bentor explains, becomes the very embodiment of transformation because it contains a rich symbolism.[9] Both Buddhist and non-Buddhist schools of Yoga and Tantra have usefully drawn from its dualist manifestations of both localized internal heat and universal power, as an intimate personal experience that lives in the heart in the warmth of love, or even hidden in the body in dark recesses of hate and vengeance. In short, the fire rituals became a principle of universal explanation of the capacity to bring about the transformation from ignorance into enlightening wisdom "by consuming duality."

Reunifying Body and Mind

All these concepts—of breathing (prāna) as an interiorized fire ritual, of inner heat (tapas), and of controlling the breath (prānāyāma)—were combined in the yoga of the subtle body, which, Bentor notes, especially emphasizes inner experiences of nonduality as the basis for liberation. It is precisely because the human body is such an important *source* of suffering, according to general Buddhist theories, that it serves in the Tantra as both an instrument and a location for *overcoming* suffering.

Classical Yoga appears to be dualistic in nature in that it sees body and self as distinct,† and therefore teaches that only through independence from physicality can the spirit be free to attain transcendence.[10] It would be reasonable to ask, therefore, how the body could be the locus for liberation, and what practices could bring this about, especially since, as mentioned earlier, classical

---

*To be a frog trapped in a rock would indeed be a solemn fate, though there are anecdotes that some frogs have survived it, leaping free when a fortunate hammer blow clove their prison in two. So far as we are aware, no frog so released ever stayed to tell how it had come to be in the rock, nor how it had stayed alive.

*It is worth noting the strong parallel between Hindu interiorization and the rise of Christianity, which repudiated the Mosaic sacrifices, not by interiorizing them but by claiming that, after the crucifixion, they had become unnecessary, out of date. According to the Platonically minded Apostle Paul, the sacrifice of Christ fulfilled both prophecy and the Mosaic Law, and abolished the need for ritual, whether exterior or interior. There was to be, instead, a simple memorial meal each sabbath. However, Paul stressed the importance of a deep change of heart as much as, if not more than, his Judaic rivals in the Church. In some cases such change would go further than the interiorizations of the yogis.
†This view has, however, been opposed by Yoga scholars such as Ian Whicher.

Yoga had no concept of the subtle body. Such anomalies are common amid the huge range of beliefs and practices evinced by Yoga's long history.

Benjamin Richard Smith notes, in his paper on aṣṭāṅga yoga, "Adjusting the Quotidian," that there appear to be strong connections between Yoga's emphasis on the embodied self as inexorably tied to other aspects of personhood in patterns of thought and action, and the emotions and deeper structures of the self.[11] The process of revelation and transformation of the self centers on the way in which the body is encountered during the challenges of the Yogic practice of body postures (āsanas). He says that these moments of challenge almost always involve a confrontation, not only between the self and the limits of its own physical embodiment, but also with its emotional and mental reactions to such moments. Then the lack of awareness of embodiment, which philosopher Drew Leder calls "the body's usual absence from our consciousness," is replaced by an overwhelming experience of our physical embodiment.[12]

In āsana practice, the body confronts the self with a lack of cooperation that threatens the state of calm, controlled breathing and concentration that practitioners endeavor to maintain while simultaneously striving to achieve a controlled performance of each āsana. Over time, practitioners develop a greater facility to maintain their breathing and remain aware of and focused on the body. It is during the moments where concentrated awareness is brought to āsana practice that calm and equanimity are maintained and the patterns of the embodied self become visible.

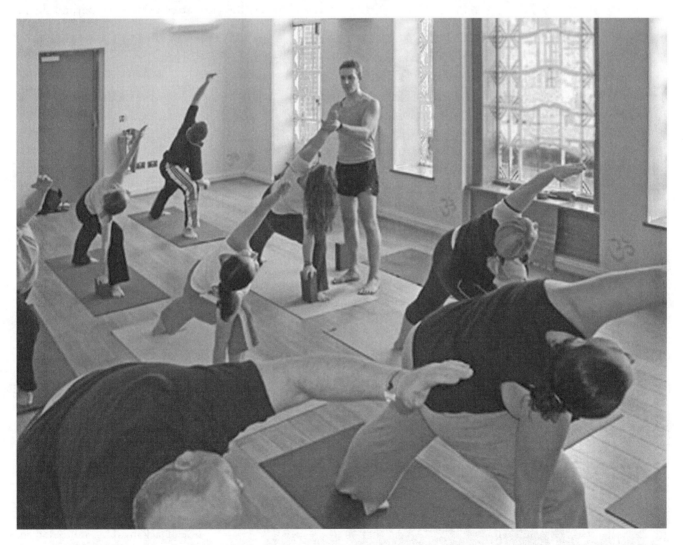

Fig. 5.1. Western yoga classes are more often perceived and experienced as a means to physical fitness than for spiritual development, but the practice of postures and breath control can, over time, increase awareness of the subtle aspects of the embodied state. (Courtesy of Jon Moult, jonlol@studio360.plus.com.)

Patanjali's Eight-Limbed (Aṣṭānga) Yoga

Classical Yoga is made up of eight interconnected limbs, which can also be viewed as eight rungs of a ladder.

1. *Yama:* restraints
2. *Niyama:* observances
3. *Āsana:* postures
4. *Prānāyāma:* breath control
5. *Pratyāhāra:* sense withdrawal
6. *Dhāranā:* concentration
7. *Dhyāna:* meditation
8. *Samādhi:* ecstatic union

Psychologist James Morley points to the habit of separating the "outer" body, which is in contact with the external world, from the "inner" body inside ourselves, which leads to feelings of alienation.[13] Prānāyāma, or breath control, integral to the practice of Yoga, prevails against this alienation: it is the concrete experience of the body as a relation between inside and outside. To breathe is to rhythmically pull external air into ourselves and release something of ourselves outward. It is in these moments of "inhabited, psychical space" that the "witness consciousness" emerges, and merges with what is observed, and that the practitioner becomes a totality.[14]

The spiritual as well as the physical aspect of yoga practice is much emphasized by practitioners. It seems likely that practitioners' experience of spirit is closely related to the bringing of awareness to the natural physical limits, and then attempting to go beyond them.

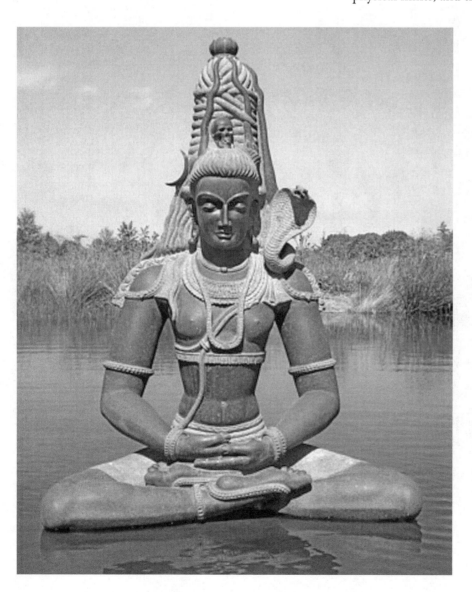

Fig. 5.2. Siva, Lord of Yogis, meditating in *padmāsana* (lotus pose). Yoga has been associated with divinity and spirituality since its first appearance in the *Ŗg Veda* ca. 1200 BCE. Black marble, South Indian. (Photograph © Victor Langheld, Spiritual Sculpture Park, Co. Wicklow, Ireland.)

Fig. 5.3. Siva in *ekapada urdhvāsana,* one of eighty-four āsanas (postures). Postures bring mind and body together through physical and mental control, and prepare the body for long periods of sitting in meditation by stretching, relaxing, and strengthening the muscles and tissues. (Photograph © Chris Tompkins, Yoga Sculptures of India.)

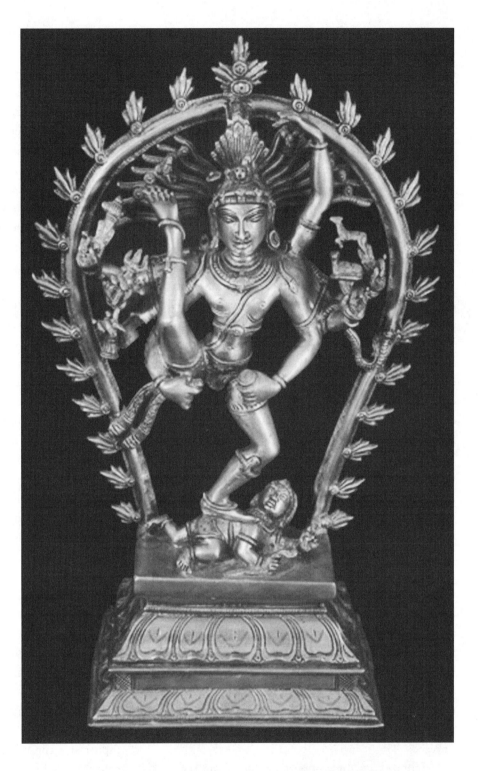

As author and former writer-in-residence at Madras University Inez Baranay, Ph.D., notes, difficult though the idea of the spiritual may be, it is hard to find another word to identify these moments of sublime immersion in practice that come when a person gains a sense of her own (potential) ultimate control and awareness of what the body is doing and what that is doing to her.[15]

As we see, the "basically flawed" state of human embodiment is understood differently in classical Yoga on the one hand and Tantric practice on the other. Tantrics would describe the sublime state as entering the ānanda-maya-kośa (the body of bliss), the ecstatic state that signifies union. Nevertheless, working from the body as the ground from which the deeper aspects of Yoga—including prānāyāma and the meditative practices detailed in the last four limbs of Patanjali's schema—are conducted, we see that the practices have the potential to reunify body and mind. Understood as one aspect of a wider Hindu religio-philosophical tradition, Yoga can be seen as a system of practices designed to compensate for the natural irregularities of the body-mind through the application of physical and mental control. Although a person may practice Yogic control and achieve a high degree of harmony, he or she is, nonetheless, not completely healthy until he or she has achieved Self-realization.[16]

The Phenomenology of Practice

We know from modern studies on meditation that certain methods of breathing have prompted thoughts about the relationship between the self and the cosmos. We can see from the following descriptions, for example, how the subtle experiences that arise out of continuous breathing would have given birth to particular ideas. For example, slow, controlled inhalation and exhalation can engender a state of "connectedness" by bringing calmness and a feeling of well-being. One meditator describes her experience as the "opening" and the "contracting" of the body. She notices how these two phases of the breath make her feel different at the beginning and end of practice. When her body feels open, she feels able to trust; when she feels worried and tense, her body contracts.

Gradually, as practice continues, there is a change in the body boundaries. The body seems to expand both vertically and horizontally. Inhalation, the ascending breath, opens the body boundaries toward the universe, toward the outer world, while exhalation, the descending breath, opens awareness to a deeper level of somatic connection.[17] Bringing the attention softly to the ascending and descending breath, some meditators have observed, maintains feelings of a higher "vibration" and of lightness. Some report feelings of being "merged" with the universe.

Here we have some important clues about how techniques that bring about strong subjective experiences in practitioners radically alter their perceptions of themselves, of others, and of the world around them. Morley gives a good account of the way the mechanism of proprioception makes this possible.[18] He says that proprioception, the stimulus related to the movement of the body, is an inverted, even an introverted, perception, the perception of the deep tissues of the body, of enclosed or encircled corporeal space. When we fall ill or experience extraordinary body sensations, perception becomes directed to the source of discomfort. Ill health makes us acutely aware of our potential for perceptual inversion: perception directed inward to the hollow of the body, rather than outward to the world. Unfortunately, in the case of illness, this is such an unpleasant experience that we tend to "depersonalize" our bodies, to distance ourselves or defend ourselves from the trauma of pain.

The Yogic practice of prāṇāyāma, on the contrary, gives us proprioception outside the context of illness. Through the practice of āsana together with prāṇāyāma, we develop an inverted sense of our muscles, tendons, heart valves, and lung cavities. We become aware of the opening and closing of these corporeal zones as we are of the movement of our external visible limbs. We experience the expansion of the chest in inhalation, the quickened tempo of the heart, and the blood's flow through the arteries. We incorporate the autonomic nervous system into the realm of the voluntary. We note how the lungs change tide between breaths and the movement of interior contraction as expiration moves outward only to pause between breaths before beginning the cycle again. In the context of āsana-prāṇāyāma, Morley observes, we focus on the rhythms of breathing; we take up what is involuntary and appropriate it into what Edmund Husserl, founder of phenomenology, would call "the sphere of ownness."

Looking at these sensory events in terms of the *subtle body* model, the levels or layers involved in this process are: the prāna-maya-kośa (the body of energy), composed of the life force, the template of and interface with the physical body (anna-maya-kośa), where sensation is perceived and which relates to the individual's emotional state; the mano-maya-kośa (the body of thought), which contains the thinking patterns, and processes sensory input; and the vijñāna-maya-kośa (the body of intelligence), a higher form of cognition and understanding capable of discerning what is real and what is unreal.

Yoshiko Matsuda, student of phenomenology observes in her doctoral thesis that in the Eastern traditions, knowledge is thought to be obtained only through the passage of personal cultivation, which involves bodily discipline, whereas Western traditions treat imagination as a mental capacity that produces and reproduces things that no longer exist or do not yet exist.[19] Imagination plays the role of the mediator between sensations (which the mind receives as something fragmentary and disappearing) on the one hand, and its capacity to reason on the other. In other words, the imagination bridges the inner and outer worlds, which are separated.

Besides the slow, rhythmic breathing practiced in Yoga there are several other gateways that open the body to the process of alteration of its boundaries. They can include the release, within a movement or exercise, of a tight muscle or a change of posture, or the freeing of a repressed emotion such as anger or fear, as we saw in āsana practice, or it can happen through certain kinds of therapy. For example, Matsuda describes an experience of sensing a different locus as the place where she "existed" after treatment by a Chinese doctor. She relates that when she stood up after treatment she felt as though she was looking at the doctor from an unusual perspective, as if she had suddenly became a foot taller. She also noticed that it was as if there were a large circular field on her shoulders, whose diameter was twice as large as her head. She wondered if this is what the ancient spiritual teachings meant when they spoke of higher consciousness, as if the sensations were first felt bodily, and then later interpreted as symbolic.[20]

This is a shrewd observation. It may explain how ideas about the siddhis ("powers" or "accomplishments") arose. They were first experienced bodily, then developed into symbols: recognizable patterns that could be used to recapture the original experiences by evoking changes in consciousness and awareness of inner sensations. These changes were mistakenly interpreted by those who had not experienced them as "magical powers," out of which evolved the stories and legends about the siddhas, the "accomplished ones," who had discovered these "secret" transformation techniques.

Metaphorical Projections and Image Schemata

The effective components of the stimuli that comprise meditation have been identified as quite sophisticated states of altered consciousness by some researchers in recent years. This has led them to a greater interest in the experience of such existential phenomena, which can only be understood by "doing yoga," rather than

through academic debate.[21] The alteration of consciousness has been observed to employ two particular modalities: *metaphorical projections* and *image schemata*. As we shall see, both are employed in the techniques practiced in the yoga of the subtle body.

Metaphor is a type of embodied imaginative structure, a mode of understanding by which we can have coherent, ordered experiences. In the cosmos of Yoga and Tantra, much of which, professor of religion G. A. Hayes believes, involves the imaginative structuring of experience, we can see, for example, how one domain of experience can accommodate to a domain of a different kind, creating a "mapping" of that region or locus through particular uses of language.[22]

Image schemata, Mark L. Johnson, professor of liberal arts and sciences, explains, are recurring, dynamic patterns of perceptual interactions and motor programs that give meaning and structure to our experiences, and are particularly useful in relation to our ideas of embodiment. One of the most common of these schemata is our relative valuation of the "up-down" experience, that is, verticality and direction. "Up" is more or better and "down" is less or worse. We saw an example of this in the experience of the meditator who described her body as "opening" and "contracting" in relation to her ascending and descending breath. The polarity of "inside" and "outside," Sunder Sarukkai, professor of Indian philosophy and science, believes, is a consequence of a duality found in many philosophical traditions.[23] To get beyond the concepts of transcendence and immanence we have to reflect on and understand the space where phenomenology and Yoga meet, and find other ways of using language to describe these phenomena.

In the context of Yoga and Tantra metaphorical projection has specific and significant implications. Firstly, both these systems have an entire inner world, a mystical model of reality derived from esoteric and, by implication, "secret" teachings, in which there is a subtle world system, a microcosm of complex meanings having special relevance for the understanding of the subtle body. Although it is difficult to understand how the material body of flesh and blood could be transformed into a divine (subtle) body, one possibility could arise from metaphorical projection upon our standard notions of direction and spatial relation (up, down, within, outside, and so forth). In such a method the physical body undergoes a transformation into the subtle body by being regarded as *both* "within" and "above" the body of flesh, thus able to become the divine body (divya-deha), despite having been born within the physical body.

The quality of the image schemata projected upon the physical body is also of importance in this process. In some traditions, the union between ātman and Brahman, or between the devotee and Buddha, comes through the help of deities or avatars, gods and goddesses with particular, desirable qualities that the devotee aspires to and that can help him or her become a perfected being. In the Tibetan Tantric traditions, such as Mahamudra and Dzogchen, a carefully detailed picture of the deity is built up bit by bit through consistent practice until the meditator can see the whole image at once (see plate 13). This practice serves to enhance awareness and improve memory so that the goal can be kept in sharp focus and the deity therefore can be experienced as *real*. Some practices have complex imagery, which the practitioner has to work up to gradually through a series of preparatory exercises that purify the "lower" chakras and attune the mind to the higher vibrations of the more subtle levels where the deities are believed to reside. In the Tantric and laya yoga traditions, we saw that the chakras each have their own deities presiding over them. Their individual mantras and letters of the alphabet are displayed on the petals of the lotus images representing the chakras, and the meditator progresses through months or years of daily contemplation of each in turn. (See chapter 4).

The culmination of this "inward odyssey" toward the deity comes when the divine presence is acutely felt and the meditator is able to "place" the deity anywhere in the body. The next step for the meditator is to be able to "become" the *devi* (goddess) or *deva* (god). The experience then becomes progressively transformed as these solid, seemingly real images are transmuted back into their universal abstract principles (see plate 14). For example, in the Dzogchen practice entitled "The Person of the Highest Mental Capacity," Padmasambhāva, the eighth-century teacher who brought Vajrayana (Buddhist Tantra) to Tibet, tells the practitioner that wisdom is to visualize the self as the deity in space, as visible while devoid of self-nature. Thus, he instructs, it is indivisible space and wisdom. The meditator is then guided through a series of steps until she can visualize herself as the deity, the body aspect visible yet devoid of

self-nature and therefore beyond age and decline. The speech aspect is perceived as unceasing and thus the essence (bijā) mantra is beyond cessation. The mind aspect transcends birth and death and is thus the continuity of dharmata.[24]

In the last step of the practice Padmasambhāva emphasizes that not being apart from the deity during the four aspects of daily activities—walking, moving about, lying down, or sitting—is the path of the person of the highest mental capacity. This achievement is considered extremely difficult, and is the domain of someone who possesses the residual karma of former training.[25] Drawing on his experience of Dzogchen, the scholar and teacher of Tibetan Buddhism Reginald Ray concurs, acknowledging the difficulty of this practice.[26] He finds that the experience of enlightenment is fundamentally and originally present in the body but, from the Tibetan point of view, he says, our experience of the body is a conceptualized interpretation rather than direct experience of embodiment, especially in relation to the chakras. Once you let go of your conceptual ideas of the body you discover that chakras comprise an ever-changing energetic body.

The Tantric tradition, Ray explains, is about working with the inseparability of form and emptiness, which is the open domain of your awareness. In the course of the path you discover deeper and deeper levels of your own nonexistence; inseparable from that in the experience of meditation is the welling up of energy. Working with physical embodiment, and the self and other, is transmuted through the "outer practice" which, Ray believes, can take ten or even twenty years. Then practicing visualization of Buddhas, and of the world as an expression of them, can lead to an understanding of form and emptiness represented in the most subtle energies of your being.

These practices are gateways to domains of energies represented by the chakras, which are uncovered in meditation, where you meet them more directly. The more profound the emptiness the more powerful the energy that arises. That energy has nothing to do with ego, Ray says, and is like being in a fire, for it "burns you up," taking you in the direction of greater presence. In his experience, life becomes more difficult because you are more open to its actual nature and to a realization of how astoundingly beautiful or horrific it is. At the same time you become more helpful and stronger because you are not trying to create a "secure nest." There comes a sense of the living out of the Buddha-nature rather than of some ego point of view.

An interesting theory of metaphorical projections and image schemata is put forward by Dr. Vasant Rele, physician and Vedic scholar.[27] His claim is that the Hindu scriptures are books of biology and the visual images of deities are imaginative ways of understanding the different centers of activity in the human brain and spinal cord. Rele points to the fact that in the pre-Upaniṣadic age, two great anatomists, Yajnavalkya and Aitareya, wrote their works in symbolical and allegorical language. He also refers to the great physician Sushruta, whose *Samhita* states that all gods mentioned in the Vedas have a permanent existence in the body. Here it is possible to see hints of an understanding or explanation grounded in sympathy and correspondence, as are many of the hypotheses of protoscience. Though sympathy and correspondence are much used in magic, they should not be set aside as fanciful simply on that account, as all understandings of reality are necessarily grounded in our way of being. Our power of imagination is limited by what we are as beings. This being so, it is unsurprising that there are also strong similarities between Dr. Rele's ideas and Western notions such as "psycho-neuro parallelism," which, briefly, sees a kind of duality-in-unity within our being in which our psychic, nonmaterial life is paralleled, instant by instant, by the physical, material processes taking place in the brain itself. The worldwide occurrence of such similarities between explanations from very different cultures should dissuade us from too readily dismissing either kind of explanation. All human explanation being in some sense "human-shaped," the ideas may have a greater "reality" than the skeptical Western mind would wish to concede.

At the root of Dr. Rele's schema is the parallel between the creation myth of the *Hiranyagharbha,* the cosmic egg that gives birth to the world, and the science of embryology, which deals with the origin, manner of growth, and eventual birth of an entirely new being. He reflects on the possibility that the ancient Indians were skillful physicians and had made considerable advances in biology, physiology, and anatomy, but kept this knowledge secret because of religious and caste taboos surrounding the handling of dead bodies. He gives as an example the parallels between metaphorical descriptions of the parts of the brain and their physiological functions.

He believes that the sacrifice of the horse (an ancient Vedic fire ritual to preserve the rule of kings), which is reprised in the opening mystical passage of the *Bṛhadāraṇyaka Upaniṣad,* is the sacrifice of "the horse-shaped mid-brain where all the important centers of sense in the form of the gods of the mid-heaven are located."[28] He reminds us that even in modern anatomy, this horse-shaped area is called the hippocampus (sea-horse) gyrus.* Rele states that the stimulation of the vital centers in the midbrain and medulla oblongata excites the "dawn of life" and causes the fetus to live.

We are advised to sacrifice our independence of action at the altar of Prajāpati, a supreme Vedic creator-god later identified with Śiva and the lords of time, fire, and the sun, in order to gain a higher conscious control over it. Such sacrifices, Rele tells us, are for regulating and modifying the working of this bodily universe so as to realize the powers of the higher god who is concerned with the creation of the cosmos. When this creative energy is excited in the body, he says, the individual establishes his connection with the cosmic energy outside and tries to gain his liberty by becoming one with it. The longed-for union between ātman and Brahman is then manifested in the microcosmic world of the human being. We notice throughout this understanding one of the myriad manifestations of the Vedic Axis.

Looking at a neurophysiological model of the effects of Yogic breathing techniques, Richard M. Brown, Associate Clinical Professor at Columbia University, found that some practices affected the hippocampus, which is associated with attention and orientation. The experimenters noted that two types of Yogic breathing techniques produced gamma rhythms, after the appearance of delta and theta rhythms, which are necessary in sensory integration and higher cognitive function.[29] Curiously, one of these was *bhastrika,* "the bellows," which has an excitatory effect during the practice but is

---

*We should note, however, that he is not referring to the hippocampus as we often do, describing it as horse*shoe*-shaped, rather than *horse*-shaped, but to the vertical section through the mid-brain, the shape of which, he says, does indeed resemble a horse's head.

followed by emotional calming with mental activation and alertness. So perhaps there are more layers of metaphorical parallelism yet to be discovered in the yoga of the subtle body.

Hayes believes that metaphors provide vital and dynamic ways of dealing with the abstract and sacred that are fundamental to the religious imagination.[30] Rituals and *sādhana* (practices) become enactments of symbolic and metaphorical structures that enable transformation from the material to the spiritual state. As an example, he reminds us that lotuses are not just static floral symbols. They float on fluids, draw fluids up by their roots, send scents out into the air, attract bees for pollination. They have both vertical dimensions, facing "up" to heaven and having roots going "down" to the mud, and horizontal dimensions, with rows of colored petals around a center. Only by taking all these images as metaphors and exploring their subtle, deeper meanings for our minds, and by sensing, and making sense of, the worlds outside and within the body, can transformation of both be realized and liberation so be attained.

SIX

The Subtle Body in Sufi Cosmology

Mysticism makes its appearance, as an inward dimension, in every religion, and any attempt to separate the mystical element from the religion which is its outward support is an arbitrary act of violence which cannot but be fatal to the mysticism, or spiritual path, concerned . . . nothing has suffered more from this vain procedure in recent times than Sūfism . . . one might as well try to purvey human life without a human body! To be sure, the body (though made in the image of God) is corruptible and mortal, while life is invisible and immortal. Nevertheless . . . it is only in the body that life finds its support and expression. So it is in the case of mysticism or spirituality; this is the inward or supra-formal dimension, of which the respective religion is the outward or formal expression.

DR. WILLIAM STODDART, *SUFISM: THE MYSTICAL DOCTRINES AND METHODS OF ISLAM*

In the section of his book *Sufism: The Mystical Doctrines and Methods of Islam* on the relationship between "exoterism" (the outward religion) and "esoterism" (the inward mystical path), Dr. Stoddart points out that "the Arabic word *ṣūfī,* like the word *yogi,* does not refer only to one who has attained the goal but is also often applied by extension to initiates who are still merely travelling towards it."[1] Tantra, with roots in the much older Vedic tradition, is nonetheless regarded as esoteric and therefore "non-Vedic" by orthodox Hindus. In the same way, despite its deep roots in Muslim culture, and despite being understood by scholars and Sufis themselves to be the inner, mystical, or psychospiritual dimension of Islam, Sufism or *tasawwuf* (in Arabic) is generally con-sidered by Muslims and non-Muslims to lie outside the sphere of Islam.[2]

The writings of Shaikh Ahmad Ahsai'i (1753–1826), founder of a nineteenth-century Shi'ite school, are described by historian Juan R. I. Cole of the University of Michigan as "one of the last great flower-ings of Muslim theosophy before the impact of modern European thought in the nineteenth century."[3] His fol-lowing rose to a quarter of the Shi'ites of Iran by the time of his death. His cosmology describes four levels of embodiment and four manifest worlds of existence. Corbin attributes to him the introduction of "creative imagination," for despite the Islamic tradition's discom-fort with myth, he painted colorful word-pictures as aids

61

to spiritual practice, which captured the imagination of adherents as far away as India.[4] His "spiritual enterprise" bears some resemblance to Sufism insofar as he seeks knowledge of the divine (*'irfan*) and accepts a view of the cosmos as made up of hierarchies running from the material to the intellectual, the latter coming closer to God. The believer's purpose is to move away from gross matter and animal instincts toward divine qualities and insights by means of spiritual and meditative exercises, dreams, and trance-states. The metaphor of the wayfarer traversing this metaphysical lattice is common to Shaikh Ahmad and the Sufis. Yet at several key junctures, al-Ahsai'i profoundly challenges the Sufism of the orders, especially in regard to social structure and conceptions of authority.

Nevertheless, Seyyed Hossein Nasr, one of the foremost scholars of Islam as a whole, in his article *The Interior Life in Islam,* contends that Sufism is simply the name for the inner or esoteric dimension of Islam. He states that the function of religion is to bestow order upon human life and to establish an outward harmony as the basis for an inward return to our Origin. This universal function is especially true of Islam "which is at once a Divine injunction to establish order in human society and within the human soul and at the same time to make possible the interior life, to prepare the soul to return unto its Lord and enter the Paradise which is none other than the Divine Beatitude. God is at once the First (*al-awwal*) and the Last (*al-akhir*), the Outward (*al-zahir*) and the Inward (*al-batin*). . . . By function of His outwardness He creates a world of separation and otherness and through His inwardness He brings men back to their Origin."[5]

Yet today there is evidence in many places in the world that the "outer form" has superceded the "inner form." For instance, Julia Day Howell, speaking of the Islamic revival experienced in Indonesia since the 1970s, points out that forms of religious practice and political activity that are concerned with what in the Sufi tradition is called the "outer" (*lahir*) expression of Islam include support for religious law and obligatory outer rituals.[6] As evidence of the Indonesian Islamic revival, several factors are commonly mentioned, including the growing numbers of mosques and prayer houses, the integration of daily prayers into the workplace, and increasing politicization in universities and financial

institutions. And yet, Howell states, there is a failure to call attention to the increasing popularity of Islam's "inner" (*batin*) spiritual expressions of the "Ṣūfī side," which, she believes, are as vital to the Sufi tradition as "scriptural piety." She contends that Sufi devotionalism is alive and well in country and city, among both old and young of an educated elite. It is regarded as a source of inspiration for contemporary religious practice and a component, if little noted, of both the "neo-modernist" and the traditionalist forms now enjoying prominence.[7]

"Sūfīsm is a spiritual phenomenon of tremendous importance," states the Islamic scholar Henry Corbin.[8] Essentially, he explains, it is the realization of the Prophet's spiritual message, the attempt to live the modalities of this message in a personal way through the interiorization of the content of the Qur'ānic revelation. What this means is that the *mi'rāj* or "ecstatic assumption," during which the Prophet was initiated into the divine secrets, is the prototype of the experience that each Sufi attempts to recapture for himself. The importance of Sufism, Corbin believes, is that it is "an entire metaphysical system that represents an irremissible testimony on the part of spiritual Islam against any tendency to reduce Islam to a legalistic and literalist religion."[9]

In an article on *Individualism and the Spiritual Path,* historian Juan Cole states that *mysticism* is a notoriously difficult word to define. Most often mysticism is discussed as a spiritual current differentiated from other sorts of religiosity, the high ritualism of the church and the egalitarian enthusiasm of the sect. In Islam, he says, mysticism has, of course, been taken to be synonymous with Sufism.[10] He refers to de Certeau's definition in his book *The Mystic Fable,* which suggests that we speak of the "procedures" of mysticism, which he considered "remarkably homologous with those of modern psychoanalysis." Among the procedures de Certeau sets out are "supposing that the body, far from being ruled by discourse, is itself a symbolic language and that it is the body that is responsible for a truth (of which it is unaware)."[11] In Corbin's words, the Sufi operates in a world "where the spiritual takes body and the body becomes spiritual."[12]

The core of Sufi thought is based on three concepts: a lower self called the *nafs* (corresponding to the Western concept of the ego), a faculty of spiritual intuition called the *qalb* (spiritual heart), and the *rūh* (spirit or soul).

In the human being they interact in various ways, producing the spiritual types of the tyrant (dominated by the ego, the nafs), the person of faith and moderation (dominated by the spiritual heart, the qalb), and the person lost in love for God (dominated by the spirit, the rūh). At death, the rūh is separated from the physical form and continues into the next life. The rūh can be made stronger by various spiritual practices in order to travel the path (*tarīqa*, "spiritual way") to God. These Sufi usages are said to be derived from the Qur'ān rather than from Indic sources, but the parallels are nonetheless notable.

The Sufi Orders

Undoubtedly influenced by its exposure to a variety of cultures throughout its long history, Sufism holds many features in common with other traditions. For example, at the structural level there are parallels between the orders of Sufism and the monastic and other orders of the Roman Catholic Church, particularly in that the various orders lay greater stress upon one discipline or another according to the personal experience and persuasion of the founder. This is a parallel development, not due to any relation of historical precedence or direct influence. The similarity with Hindu traditions, on the other hand, is one of direct causal influence, which has affected both fundamental doctrinal belief and, even more deeply, practice.

Sufism acquired a metaphysical philosophy through Arabic culture, and evolved its literature through Persian culture, but it learned the crucial techniques of contemplation and meditation from India (see plate 15). A prominent feature in common with India is that the spiritual master (*shaikh*) is the center of the organization. Followers gather around him or her and receive initiation through a lineage of masters descended, in the case of Sufis, from the Prophet and, in the Indian tradition, from the deity. In both systems, particular teachers have formed schools or orders that constitute the "branches" of the family "tree." They "in-form" or mold the aspirant on his or her path (*tarīqa*) to God. These orders have promoted particular practices and beliefs, and prohibited others, wherever they have settled throughout the world.

Four main Sufi orders came into being during the twelfth and thirteenth centuries and continue today. Having taken their names from their illustrious founders, they are the Qādirī, the Suhrawardī, the Shādhilī, and the Maulawī (Mevlevi in Turkish). The last of these is, perhaps, the best known in the West on account of its most characteristic feature, the whirling dance performed by the *fuqarā*, as the members of the order refer to themselves. *Fuqarā* is the plural of *faqīr*, meaning "poor in spirit," a phrase that naturally reminds Westerners of the Sermon on the Mount, and is also parallel to the statements of Indian ascetics. The Maulawī were founded by Jalal ad-Din Rumi (1207–1273), widely considered the greatest mystical poet of Islam, who was given the title Maulānā (our Lord) by his disciples. In addition, there are the Chishti (see plate 16), originating in India in the twelfth century, the Naqshbandī, and the Darqāwī, the last being a subgroup of the Shādhilī, founded in Morocco. The Sufi orders, Stoddart points out, should, despite their recognizable and distinguishable characters, not be regarded as "sects." He says "all the Ṣūfī orders are expressions of Islamic spirituality, and are only differentiated in that each one is 'perfumed' by the *baraka* ('blessing') of the founder and employs the spiritual methods taught by that particular master."[13]

In order to embark on the path to salvation the Sufi aspirant has to be a member of a religion that teaches that path and, on certain conditions, "guarantees" it. The form such a "guarantee" takes varies according to the spiritual destination in view. Religion and religious practice ordinarily embody the doctrine that salvation (however it is conceived) can only be attained after the death of the "gross" body. The spiritual or mystical path, on the other hand, is based on the belief, held with a conviction appropriate to certainty of knowledge, that the goal of salvation through self-realization is attainable within this, our embodied, life. The Sufi methods of achieving self-realization form different paths (*turug*) to *haqīqa*, the inward, divine reality, who is God himself.[14] Here there are parallels with both the Indic doctrine of the jivan-mukta and the teaching of Yahshua (Jesus) that certain believers have, already in this life, "passed from death into life" and so "do not come into judgment."[15]

The author and ethnomusicologist Habib Hassan Touma explains that in some Sufi orders initiation may take the form of rituals or ceremonies, involving recitation, singing, dance, drama, and meditation, which may induce ecstasy and trance. This illustrates the centrality for Sufis, just as for Buddhists, tantrics, yogis—indeed all mystics—of conscious states other than the everyday "mind."[16] The sharing of the concept of a center within our Being across traditions points, of course, to the relevance of the varied beliefs to the search for a subtle body, and for knowledge of what it is.

Dhikr Practice

The central spiritual practice, so important as to constitute a method, is *dhikr* (invocation), which begins to operate only when the Sufi has already achieved a symbolic understanding of the Five Pillars of Islam—faith (*īmān*); prayer (*ṣalāt*); fasting (*ṣawm*); religious tax

(*zakat*), which also includes almsgiving; and pilgrimage (*hajj*)—and has then learned to practice them in an inward manner. What this means, Professor Seyyd Hossein Nasr explains, is that the canonical prayers do not merely possess an interior dimension but also serve as the basis for other forms of prayer, which become ever more inward as the practitioner travels the spiritual path that leads finally to the "prayer of the heart." This is the invocation (dhikr), in which the invoker, the invocation, and the invoked unite into a single essence, and through which the person returns to the Center, the Origin, which is pure Inwardness.[17]

The invocatory prayer varies from one ṭarīqa to another, but always expresses the same three essential thoughts, each of which is recited one hundred times morning and evening. These three thoughts are: the believer first asks the forgiveness of God for his own

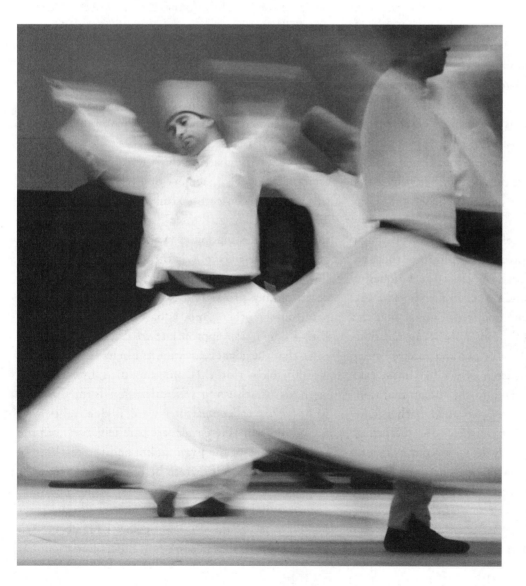

Fig. 6.1. The Mevlevi, "whirling dervishes," are the best-known of the Sufi orders, founded in Konya (present-day Turkey) by the followers of Rumi, the thirteenth-century Persian poet, jurist, and theologian. The *sema* (whirling) is a form of *dhikr* (remembrance of God), and represents "turning toward the Truth" on the mystical journey from which the *semazens* (whirlers) return "perfected," having transcended the ego and reached a greater maturity, ready to love and serve the whole of creation.

frailties, then asks God to bless the Prophet and give him peace, and finally attests the divine unity. Dr. Stoddart explains that the first formula symbolically represents the Sufi movement from outward to inward; from existence to Being; from human to the Divine.

The second concerns the Sufi's participation in the Muhammadan Norm, which is permeated and sustained by the divine blessing (ṣalāt) and peace (salām). It is a symbolic reintegration of the "fragment" (man) into the Totality (Muhammad), Muhammad being the personification of the whole creation, which some Sufis refer to as "Universal Man." Interestingly—and here we see parallels with the concept of the subtle body in the Indian traditions—"ṣalāt is performed not only by ordinary men, but also by prophets and even angels, and leads them into *invisible channels* [my emphasis] along which flow the blessings (ṣalāt) and the peace (salām) of God."[18]

The third formula (often expressed in the words "there is no reality other than the Reality") represents the extinction of everything that is not God. Here, Stoddart points out, are the three stages known to Christian mysticism, purification, perfection, union, and the three universal aspects of all spirituality, humility, charity, truth.[19]

The dhikr, as the tripartite invocation is known, is the most important spiritual practice of the Sufi. The meaning includes the notions of "remembrance" and "mention." Like all traditional metaphysics, says Stoddart, the dhikr teaches that human beings are trapped in manifestation, which is doomed to impermanence; it inevitably entails separation and consequently also suffering and death. The dhikr "reminds" the seeker that the Divine Name of Allah *is* liberation or, as Stoddart says, it directly "vehicles the Principle."[20] This means that the Divine Name of Allah invokes in the seeker the state of preparation to receive the holy power that will liberate the individual from the confines of the body. When the believer unites with it in fervent invocation, he frees himself inwardly from manifestation and its concomitant suffering. Through perseverance, this liberation becomes effective, and the grace of God is realized. Until liberation is achieved, overly fervent practice of the dhikr can present a mortal danger, hence the prohibition to practice it persistently unless initiated and under the guidance of a shaikh. However, all believers are permitted to practice dhikr from time to time, for short periods only.[21]

Parts of the Human Being in Sufism

Of particular interest to us in our quest for the subtle body is the Sufi belief that the wholeness of the human being contains distinguishable parts, which, of course, Sufism has named. Here, as so often in cross-cultural studies, especially those involving metaphysical concepts, we must negotiate problems of terminology. Even when translation has been done with care, accurate understanding is still not easily achieved by means of language. Nonetheless, we shall attempt to set out the Sufi understanding.

As we have seen, Sufism distinguishes a lower self called the nafs (ego), a faculty of spiritual intuition called the qalb (spiritual heart), and the rūh, a concept similar to the Western concept of the "immortal soul." The rūh never dies, but merely leaves the physical body behind at the event we call dying. Distinguishable from the rūh is the *nasma,* which is the subtle body, or one of the subtle bodies, in particular the entity known in many cultures as the "astral body." The nasma, like the rūh, is believed to survive the death of the physical body, though not necessarily permanently. Still, the nasma should not be confused with the rūh, which is considered to be eternal and to transcend not only the nasma but also all physical form. From a Western perspective, the rūh might be conceived as nonphysical, extraphysical, or supraphysical, while the nasma stands, in some sense, between the physical world and the beyond. It is not possible to speak meaningfully of the size, the place, or the date of a rūh, for it is dimensionless, as if it is both a point and of infinite extent, and also timeless, because it is "present at all times," eternal. The apparent irrationalities of such statements lie not in the concepts, which, with a modicum of word-free contemplation, become intelligible, comprehensible, and imaginable, but in the limitations of language.

Other terms are used to denote other "entities" in the Sufi schema. *Maqaam** is a person's level of spiritual development, the result thus far of her efforts to transform or, indeed, to transcend her selfhood (rather than to attempt to "improve" an inferior and inadequate

---

*Some authorities transliterate this word into English as *maqam.*

"thing"). Like other spiritual paths, the Sufi path invites a person to repudiate and surrender what, for millennia in the East and more recently in the West, has been characterized as the willful and assertive social or ego self, and, on thrusting it aside, to find the way toward the eventual achievement of the higher and infrangible true self. It is as if the true self is hidden behind a screen and denied development until the artificial, fragile, pride-protective ego is removed. As a person becomes aware of the true self and begins to live in it, he or she senses its nature as *security-of-Being-within-the-Ultimate-Being.* Words, of course, fail to express this adequately.

In Sufism a *haal* is a state of consciousness, the result, in a general sense, of spiritual practice. It is considered that, normally, particular states of consciousness will arise concurrently with each maqaam, that is, with each stage of growth along the rising spiritual path. The haal are thus the outward, sensible, states of consciousness that flow from the corresponding maqaam, which is achieved inwardly. A haal is regarded as a "gift," not a spiritual stature in itself, but its visible flowering in blessed experience, the experience of being conscious in an indubitably more joyful and peaceful way. Maqaam and haal go hand in hand. (We repeat that the limitations of language defeat the attempt to describe what can only be known truly in experience.)

Fundamentally, Sufism is not only intuitive knowledge but the wisdom of both inner and outer life. Like Indian yogis, Sufis, too, are advised to find a teacher and go through a long training to develop certain abilities or "spiritual technologies" that enable each aspirant to "become himself," to know his "true being." Many Sufi texts refer to stages or stations along the path to perfection, which measure the aspirant's achievements in inner transformation. They are achieved by *fanā,* "annihilation," similar to the Buddhist nirvāna.

Sufism asserts that there are seven planes of consciousness, known as *manzils,* along the path to God. The manzils are not in themselves the stages in the spiritual growth of the individual but rather the universal planes of consciousness relating to each of those stages. Each individual attains these stages one by one, arriving on each plane or manzil as his or her own personal growth proceeds, until *walāya,* "sainthood," is fully attained.

The number seven occurs frequently, as all who study these matters have noted, and questions arise from this, such as whether it is possible to discover meaningful mappings between the seven planes of consciousness and the seven main chakras in the body. To research such relationships in detail would be beyond the scope of this general survey.

The Perfect Man

One particularly interesting parallel between Sufism and Hinduism is Ibn al-'Arabi's concept of the "Perfect Man," *insān-i kāmil,* an idea that points to the final destination of the spiritual search. One of the great Islamic masters of gnosis, Ibn al-'Arabi, lived at the end of the twelfth and the beginning of the thirteenth century in Andalusia. He declared "I practice the religion of Love; whatsoever directions its caravans advance, the religion of Love shall be my religion and my faith." Islamic scholar Frithjof Schuon explains that what al-'Arabi means by this is a "truth that is lived" and that "spirit and love are here synonymous."[22]

In the Sufi tradition, the Perfect Man is the prototype of the self. This is not, of course, a prototype in the sense of an experimental version that needs to be improved, true though that undoubtedly is of all humans, but entirely the converse, a heavenly exemplar. This easily resolved linguistic ambiguity is not the only verbal problem, for nafs, meaning "the self," also means "soul," "psyche," "spirit," "mind," "life," and "person." It primarily refers to the animating principle of the body, the intermediary between the bodily constitution and the "spirit," here (used evidently in a different sense of the word) meaning the immortal aspect that can be perfected through the ascending stages of the spiritual life.[23] The concept of the Perfect Man is similar to that of the jīvan-mukta, the "liberated-while-living," whom we first met in chapter 1. However, as we are reminded by R. J. W. Austin, Arab scholar and translator, while a universalist approach can be extremely useful in illuminating fundamental principles and universal concepts such as the jīvan-mukta, there are always exoteric differences of perspective between the traditions that require careful evaluation if understanding of those fundamentals is to be enhanced by mutual influence rather than obscured.[24] The evident, but unexplained, difference between two usages of the word "spirit," just noted, provide a case in point.

Professor Masataka Takeshita at the University of Tokyo has identified three elements involved with the idea of the Perfect Man: man as divine image; as microcosm-macrocosm; and as "sanctity" (*walāya*). Unusually, since recent studies have devoted relatively little attention to the background of Ibn al-'Arabi's ideas, Takeshita has attempted to show their precedents in Islamic thought, noting that al-'Arabi employs more than forty other technical terms to refer to or describe the Perfect Man from various points of view.[25] In fact, the whole of the *Futūhāt al-makkiyya,* Ibn al-'Arabi's enormous magnum opus, revolves around this one concept. Al-'Arabi's mystical and philosophical ideas reshaped much of Sufi thought and, to a large extent, has shaped the language, if not always the content, of Sufi discussions since his time.[26] We add the thought that any such proliferation of language-based material for discussion, while unavoidable and necessary for the increase of understanding, should never be allowed to cloud conceptions of the entities themselves and so make itself the matter in hand. Philosophy is in constant danger of this decline from insightful contemplation of essence into argument about verbal description.

William Chittick, a professor of comparative studies and one of the world's leading translators and interpreters of Islamic mystical poetry, is clearly fully aware of this and other aspects of a complex of problems, and mentions them in the preface to his book *The Heart of Islamic Philosophy.*[27] Chittick explains that the concept of the Perfect Man is the ontological prototype of both the person and the universe—an idea similar to the Hindu concept of the person as ātman, the semi-divine, the microcosm within the macrocosm of Brahman.[28] In Sufism, the Perfect Man is regarded as God's first creation, the primordial and original theophany (*tajallī*), the first point in the descending arc of the manifestation of existence, which reaches its lowest point in the material world (*qaws-i nuzūlī*), the world of sensory perception (*ālam al-hiss, dlam al-shahādah*). At this point, the journey of the Perfect Man toward realization, his return to the Creator, begins as he infinitesimally turns Godward at "the bottom of the circle," on an ascending arc (*qaws-i ṣu'ūdī*).

The Eight Principles

There is another interesting parallel between the eight principles for practice in Sufism and the yama and niyama of classical Yoga. Yama includes restraints such as nonviolence, nonstealing, and truthfulness, and niyama includes observances such as cleanliness, self-study, and concentration on the Divine. In Sufism personal and social conduct is guided by the following eight precepts:

> Awareness in breathing (*hūsh dar dam*)
> Watching one's steps (*nazar bar qadam*)
> Journeying within (*safar dar waṭan*)
> Solitude within human society (*khalwat dar anuman*)
> Recollection (*yād kard*)
> Restraining one's thoughts (*bāz gard*)
> Watching one's thoughts (*nigāh dāsht*)
> Concentration on the Divine (*yād dāsht*)

These principles can be viewed in the context of the "spiritual technologies" that facilitate spiritual growth, the *kalimāt-i qudsīya* (sacred words), which came to characterize the Naqshbandiya, one of the dervish schools that rose in Central Asia and greatly influenced the development of the Indian and Turkish empires.* Central to the practices of the Naqshbandi is the belief that novice dervishes should join the order that is most suited to their inner nature, and should remain with their teacher until he has, through "special exercises," developed them as far as they can go. Different lists are given by different teachers of the qualities that the aspirant is expected to develop. As described above, progress is measured by reference to "stations," the maqaams, the aspirant's own efforts being rewarded, as each state is reached, with the associated haal or gift of God.

---

*The Naqshbandiya school, named after Khaja Bahaudin Naqshband (died ca. 1389), was regarded as one of the earliest "chains of admission," or Sufi lineages. After his death his followers were known as the "Designers," or "Masters of the Design." Only the Naqshbandi shaikhs have the authority to initiate disciples into any order of dervishes.[29]

The Subtle Centers in Sufi Tradition

The term *laṭīfa* (plural *laṭā'if*) arises from the Arabic adjective *laṭīf*, which means "tender," "subtle," "sensitive." The word was used to denote a *nonmaterial* part of a person's wholeness, which was believed to lie dormant until awakened by spiritual experience. Such experience can be deepened by practice, by spiritual exercises, by meditation. There is some uncertainty as to whether the use of the word *laṭīfa* in connection with the concept of a subtle body (*jism laṭīf*), is Qur'ānic in origin since it does not appear until the third century of the Islamic era. Over time, the concept was refined, but also became more complex, its main usage being in descriptions of psychospiritual progress, culminating in the annihilation of the self and its assimilation into the Divine Essence.

Having absorbed theoretical perspectives from other cultures, in particular the Indic traditions, Sufism elaborated certain spiritual doctrines and contributed to their scholarship. One of the most important areas of Sufi intellectual endeavor is the doctrine of the *Laṭā'if-e-Sitta,* the six subtle centers or "centers of subtle cognitions." Spiritual awakening is considered to take place by a sequential progress of "openings," or "awakenings" from the first, the lowest center, to the sixth, the highest. This scale provides an approximate parallel to the Indic notion of six main chakras within the body (the seventh being above the head), though the conceived locations of the centers within the Sufi body differ somewhat from those of the chakras.

Like the Indian chakras, the Sufi subtle centers or laṭā'if are thought of as faculties to be purified sequentially in order to bring the seeker's spiritual journey to completion. The picture held of these centers varies from order to order, but in each case each spiritual center is associated with a particular color and area of the physical body, and with a particular prophet. To activate the subtle centers, an aspirant is advised to take the help of a meditation teacher who has reached a certain kind of "completion," so becoming the "Perfect Man." The association of each center with a particular prophet is likely to have arisen from the natural tendency for a teacher to emphasize the aspect of humanness that has most impressed itself upon his or her awareness, as a result of his or her own imbalances of nature. We might coin the aphorism that humanity's thinking is always human-shaped, and always distorted by its own humanity.

While some of the laṭā'if have names or locations corresponding to body parts, they are not to be understood as identical with the organs. This is confirmed by many writers, such as Warren Fusfeld, for example, who points out: "Thus the distinction is clearly to be made between the physical flesh of the heart and the *laṭīfa* which is named 'Heart' (*qalb*). Rather, the *laṭā'if* are taken to be local manifestations of identically named parts of a higher realm of the cosmological structure which is above the realm of created things."[30] This expresses the universal belief in the Hermetic principle, "As above, so below," which first showed itself in the Vedas many centuries before either Sufism or Islam appeared.

The six centers or faculties—*Nafs* (the lower soul), *Qalb* (the heart), *Rūh* (the spirit), *Sirr* (the mystery or secret), *Khafi* (the arcane), and *Akhfa* (the super-arcane)—and the purificatory activities applied to them, might be said to "contain" the fundamental orthodox Sufi philosophy. The purification of the elementary

The Six Subtle Centers of Sufism

Name	Translation	Location	Color
1. Laṭīfa-e-Nafsi	Lower Soul	Slightly below the navel	Yellow
2. Laṭīfa-e-Qalbi	Heart	Left side of the chest	Red
3. Laṭīfa-e-Rūhi	Spirit	Center of the chest	Green
4. Laṭīfa-e-Sirri	Mystery or Secret	Right side of the chest	White
5. Laṭīfa-e-Khafi	Latent Subtlety	Between the eyebrows	Blue
6. Laṭīfa-e-Akhfa	Obscure Subtlety	Above the head	Violet

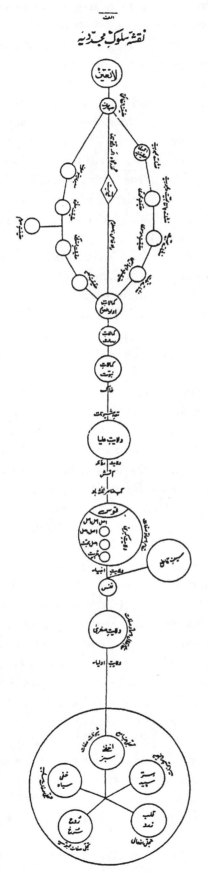

Fig. 6.2. Shah Wali Allah of Delhi, the eighteenth-century mystic and theologian, devoted an entire book to the concept of a subtle body with its spiritual centers, as well as referring to them in some of his other works. His map of the spiritual path (shown here schematically, with English annotations) includes the subtle centers, the laṭā'if, and was based on an original system attributed to the Mujaddidiyya branch of the Naqshbandi Sufis. The system was expanded and developed over time to include the nonmaterial component of the person that can be "awakened" through spiritual practices. The map of the laṭā'if, effectively of the psychological and spiritual journey of the aspirant toward fanā (annihilation in the divine essence), became increasingly refined and complex. Wali Allah's schema attempts to integrate two poles of Sufi thought: the Path of Prophetic Inheritance and the Path of Saintship, which, he believed, were alternative ways, suited to different personal character types, to produce "The Inspired Person." (You will notice that Wali Allah's particular color attributions for the spiritual centers do vary from the associated colors listed in the box on the facing page, which come from another branch of the tradition.) (Adapted from charts in Muhammad Dhauqi, *Sirr-i Dilbaran* [Lahore, 1974] and Aḥmad Sirhindī, *Maktubat-i-Imam Rabbani* [Lahore, 1964].)

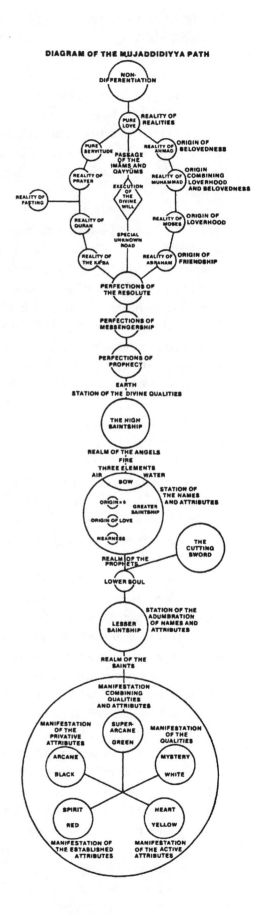

DIAGRAM OF THE MUJADDIDIYYA PATH

passionate nature (*tazkiya-i-nafs*) is followed by the cleansing of the spiritual heart so that it may acquire a mirror-like purity of reflection (*tazkiya-i-qalb*) and become the receptacle of God's love (*ishq*) and illumination of the spirit (*tajalli-i-rūh*). This process is facilitated and intensified by the emptying of egoic drives (*taqliyya-i-sirr*) and the remembrance of God's attributes (*dhikr*). The journey is completed by purification of the last two faculties, *khafi* and *akhfa*, the "deepest," most "arcane" of the centers.

The First Subtle Center: Laṭīfa-e-Nafsi

The *Laṭīfa-e-Nafsi* is located slightly below the navel and is associated with the color yellow. The word *nafs*, usually translated as "self" or "psyche," is etymologically derived from the word for "breath." In Genesis (2.7) God breathes into Adam's nostrils the breath of life; the word used in relation to this is *nephesh*, clearly cognate with the Arabic *nafs*. It is a child's breathing that first assures the mother that her baby has been live-born and has leaped its first great hurdle into embodied life, and it is the absence of breath that first signifies to the outside observer that death has occurred. Accordingly—and in common with virtually all universal concepts where the act of breathing is associated with life, such as *ātman* in Hinduism, *pneuma* in Greek, *spiritus* in Latin—nafs is usually identified with the basic visible process of physical breathing, and accordingly seen as the energizing, life-giving principle.

However, as mentioned earlier, Sufis of different schools show greater or lesser allegiance to the Qur'ān. Those whose doctrine is firmly, or solely, grounded in it believe that in addition to the physiological process of breathing per se, the nafs is also the whole of the "lower," egotistical and passionate human nature, which, along with *tab* (literally, "physical nature"), comprises the vegetative and animal aspects of human life. Some Sufis use the term with even wider reference, encompassing the whole range of psychological processes, that is, all mental, emotional, and volitional life. Synonyms for *nafs* then include even "devil," "passion," "greed," "avarice," and "ego-centeredness." In this we can see the imposition of moral teaching by powerful teachers, but these are of little concern to us, for our search is for what we are as living human beings rather than for how we ought to behave. It is, nonetheless, the central aim of the Sufi

path to transform nafs by the process of tazkiya-i-nafs (purgation of the soul), from its state of ego-centeredness through various psychospiritual stages to the purity of submission to the will of God.

The majority of the Sufi orders have adopted the schema mentioned earlier of seven maqaams (permanent stages) on the voyage toward spiritual transformation. The journey begins with *nafs-e-ammara* (the "self-accusing soul") and ends in *nafs-e-mutmainna* (the "satisfied soul"), although the final stage for some is described as *nafs-i-safiya wa kamila* (the "soul restful and perfected in God's presence").

The Second Subtle Center: Laṭīfa-e-Qalbi

The *Laṭīfa-e-Qalbi* is the second subtle center, situated in the left side of the chest and associated with the color red. The word *qalb* means "spiritual heart," a similar concept to the Tantric *hṛtpādma* (see plate 17). The function of this center is to remove everything that obscures *ishq*, God's divine love. Some Sufis also experience this center as the seat of beatific vision. Together, the nafs and the qalb form the *rūh-e-haivani*, the "animal soul." The nafs and the qalb are believed to engage in "spiritual battle" with each other, the higher part of nafs, the *'aql* (intellect or "rational soul") contending against the rūh. Here, as often before, we find the variety and flexibility of verbal usage a source of uncertainty, and, again, the individual's own discernment, if grounded in sufficient introspective experience, will surely be the best guide for appreciation of both subtle anatomy and personal growth.

Corbin explains that in Ibn al-'Arabi's teachings, the heart (qalb) is the organ that produces true knowledge, comprehensive intuition, disclosure, unveiling, or gnosis (*marifa*) of God and the divine mysteries, in short everything connoted by the term *esoteric science* (*'ilm al-Bāṭin*).[31] He observes that while love also is seen by Sufis as related to the qalb, it is the rūh, or spirit, that is usually regarded as the specific center of love. But what is being referred to here is "subtle [*sic*] physiology" elaborated "on the basis of ascetic, ecstatic, and contemplative *experience* [my emphasis] and expressing itself in symbolic language,"[32] for, we would add, it can express itself in no other way.

Clearly, while both al-'Arabi and Corbin see some kind of parallel between the physical and the "inner nonphysical," that parallel is difficult to map, and even more so to convey, not least on account of a conflation of emotional and cognitive experiences conceived as occurring at two existential levels, those of physiology and spirituality. The experiences themselves seem to inhabit a four-part complex (two types of experience at two levels of being). The "parallels" between physical and nonphysical are also felt, for if this were not so, the notion that they are "parallels" could not occur. Putting it the other way around, we would not find any parallel, but only a melee of sensations, if there were not something running alongside something else, drawing attention to the mapping of the one onto the other.

However, the attempt to communicate the intuited parallels between qalb and rūh is bound to face defeat, no matter what the language, for an organ that pumps blood is not obviously an organ that either "produces knowledge" or "feels love." The very phrase "produces knowledge" is not to be taken literally, physically, biologically, yet what is being referred to is certainly a felt experience: when realizations of a "spiritual" kind come, they are sensed in the qalb, in the left side of the chest, and perhaps, whatever their content, feel akin to the feeling of love. If this is not what al-'Arabi means, we have to wonder to what he was referring.

Perhaps because we cannot be sure we know his meaning, we assume the reality of the very phenomenon we want to show: that all spiritualities reflect the structure of the human being in its interconnected wholeness and at its various levels. However, this may indeed be the case for all humans, for Sufis just as for agnostic Westerners, for shamans just as for rationalist skeptics. We are what we are. The matter is one for simple *recognition that it is so,* not for independent or objective proof. To be independent of the feeling person is to lack all possibility of proving anything regarding her feelings; by the very nature of the inward experience, the only objective view of it is the subjective view, which only the experiencer has. All the experiencer can offer is testimony, words of description, and all we who hear her can offer is belief in her testimony, for the only proof of experience is the experience itself. However, we are not in fact arguing in a circle, impossible though it is to prove that claim. That there is such a thing as spiritual awareness, patently not "normally physical" or "normally physiological," is all too evident to a person who has it.

Its reality is confirmed when another to whom she wants to communicate shows by his incomprehension that he does not. The one party has the proof, for she experiences it, the other denies it is possible, because he cannot experience it. The claim of each is true, but only for the claimant herself or himself.

But we must make one further claim: it is *experience* that, were it possible, we should wish to prove, not *verbal descriptions of experiences.* No one can "prove" a verbal description of the personal experience of another, for a verbal description is totally unamenable to proof. Any bridge of words, on reaching midstream, leaves the reader or hearer struggling amid a raging torrent of mystifying, bewildering meaninglessness, unless he recognizes *for himself* what is being said, as if he is *building his own bridge out from his side toward the speaker.* This, too, it will be noticed, is itself an ostensive confirmation of its own truth. My account of my experience is meaningless, and will seem untrue to the hearer, unless the hearer has the same experience or something similar, enabling him to recognize that my reality is like his own. While some people do not see the need for the hearer to recognize the reality beyond the words, thinking the words themselves the reality, this is a mistake, and a serious one. The words are not enough, and it is this that other *experiencers* recognize, meeting one another safe above the troubled waters of *inexperience.*

No wonder, then, that al-'Arabi and all Sufis, like others of experience, fall back, because they must, upon the physical world for a means, however poor, of describing spiritual experience to others. No wonder that the parallels are recognized by those who share the experiences, for this is the universal experience of our physical-spiritual duality, within a certain range of personal variation, which is made the more treacherous to bridge by the semantic difficulties. Even when we share the same experience we may build our descriptive bridges using different words and phrases. Mircea Eliade has observed that "this does not mean that such experiences were not *real;* they were perfectly real, but not in the sense in which a physical phenomenon is real."[33]

In Sufism the heart is one of the centers of mystic physiology and al-'Arabi states that its importance lies in the fact that "the gnostic's heart is the 'eye,' the organ by which God knows himself . . . the power of the heart is a secret force or energy (*quwwat khafīya*), which perceives divine realities."[34] This is reminiscent of the Apostle Paul's words in I Corinthians 2.14, that "Spiritual things are spiritually discerned." No doubt al-'Arabi felt that his readers needed this information, as do all who seek to comment upon any of the world's spiritualities, for the very nature of what is being discussed is personal inner experience, making the attempt to convey something of its essence to others problematic. It might seem surprising, yet should not be so, that Einstein claimed his theoretical understandings of our physical world did not come in the form of words, but rather as pictures in his imagination. In our attempt to grasp the essence of all the subtle centers we should do as he did.

Corbin tells us that in the theosophy of Ibn al-'Arabi the qalb has, in practice, two aspects: the phenomena that today are the concern of parapsychology, such as telepathy, visions, and synchronicity; and the mystic perception of *dhawq* ("intimate taste" or "touch"), an epiphany of the heart, which is also an aspect of the gnostic's creativity through active imagination. The first is fulfilled through *intentions* and the second through *concentration,* which makes it possible to perceive the true knowledge of things, to know the Divine Being through intuitive vision. In this state of concentration, the Sufi "becomes" the Perfect Man as the microcosm of God.[35]

The Three Bodies or Souls Formed by the Six Subtle Centers

Body	English Name	Formed by the Subtle Centers
Rūh-e-haivani	Animal Soul	Nafs and Qalb
Rūh-e-insāni	Human Soul	Sirr and Rūh
Rooh-e-azam	Great Soul	Akhfa and Khafa

The Third Subtle Center: Laṭīfa-e-Rūhi

The third subtle center is the rūh, which is located in the center of the chest, and its color is green. Activation of this center results in knowledge of *alam-e-aaraf* (afterlife). The rūh, or spirit, is considered the second contender in the battle for human life. Some Sufis believe that it is "coeternal" with God; others consider it a created entity. For the Sufis who show gnostic lean-

ings (such as the Bektashi and the Mevlevi), the rūh is a "soul-spark," the immortal entity and transegoic *true self,* similar to the Christian concepts of *synteresis* or *Imago Dei* and akin to kabbalistic notions of the Divine within the body. It is also compared with the Vedantic jīva, the Tibetan Buddhist *shes-pa* (principle of consciousness), and the Taoist *shen* (spirit), but more orthodox Sufis regard it as a dormant spiritual faculty that needs to be worked upon by constant vigil and prayer in order to achieve the tajliyya-i-rūh, the "illumination of the spirit." Many believe that this spiritual center does not emerge or differentiate itself until it has been purified by strict religious observances in order to achieve illumination; until then it is to be regarded as similar to the nafs, nothing more than a "blind" life force.

The Fourth Subtle Center: Laṭīfa-e-Sirri

The *sirr* (secret) is the first of the "concealed" or "arcane" subtle centers. It is located at the right side of the chest and is associated with the color white. According to Dr. Alan Godlas, it is believed to "record the orders of Allah for the individual"[36] in a similar way as the original record in the preserved scriptures, which is known as the *loh-e-mahfooz.* Activation of the sirr results in knowledge of the *aalam-e-misal* (allegorical realm). The emptying of the sirr is known as taqliyya-i-sirr and requires a focusing upon God's names and attributes in perpetual remembrance or dhikr, through which the aspirant diverts his or her attention from the mundane aspects of human life and focuses on the spiritual realm. "Emptying" thus signifies the negation and obliteration of ego-centered human propensities, believed necessary for spiritual growth. Sirr and rūh together form *rūh-e-insāni,* the "human soul" or *ayan.*

Knowledge of this fourth center is believed to allow the aspirant to witness the record and plan of all that exists, written on the loh-e-mahfooz. However, that record can hardly be verbal, for all such descriptions are entirely divorced from the realities they attempt to describe; they are dependent upon the unreliable mappings and usages of a consensus as to their meanings, which may change. Such descriptions, being of the nature of the physical world, are utterly inadequate to their task. The very concept of a universal record is itself an instance of something entirely conceivable as a spiritual "thing," yet impossible, if its reality were as defined in verbal logic; this demonstrates yet again the utter inadequacy of words. Such a definition or description would be a lower-world symbol for an upper-world reality of timeless ever-presence. Of course, this leaves intact that ever-present eternal IS, which we, in our limitedness, name and refer to *as if* it were a *verbal* record. God is above words, but words are all humankind has when faced with the task of communicating the transcendent. We add, of course, that even via verbal statements truth is to be found, by the process of re-imaginative recognition described earlier. A part of the truth of the sirr is revealed in the biblical approval of those whose high principles are "written on the fleshy tablets of their hearts" (Proverbs 3.3 and 7.3., II Corinthians 3.3).

The Fifth Subtle Center: Laṭīfa-e-Khafi

The term *khafi* means "latent subtlety," "the mysterious," "the arcane." The Laṭīfa-e-Khafi is described as located between the eyebrows and is associated with the color blue. It is said to contain the *kitab-e-marqoom,* "the written book." The forehead is often seen as the seat of intellect, and it was on the forehead that Jewish clerics wore the phylactery, containing copies of short quotations from the writings of Moses. As the khafi is symbolized as a kind of book, it gives rise to a question regarding the distinction between it and the sirr, which is written upon the heart. The sirr is personal to the believer, his or her uniquely personal "karmic script" or "life script," a personal guide to what is required of that individual during life, while the khafi is a statement of universal truth. As might be expected, it is sited higher within the body just as, on account of its universality, it is nearer to God. However, we face here another possibility of confusion, for in Indic myth the karmic script or life script is called "head writing" or *talai eruttu,* concerning which we quoted E. Valentine Daniel in chapter 2.

The Sixth Subtle Center: Laṭīfa-e-Akhfa

Akhfa means the "obscure subtlety," the "most arcane," the "deeply mysterious." This center is located, like the Tantric seventh chakra, above the head, and is associated with the color violet. It is described as the *nuqta-e-wahida* (point of unity) in every human where the *tajalliat* (beatific visions) of *Allāh* are directly revealed. It is said to contain hidden knowledge of the universe. By meditating on and becoming one with this center,

the aspirant enters the system of the universe and attains knowledge of the universal laws of heaven and earth.

Akhfa and khafa form *rooh-e-azam,* the "great soul," which is also called *sabita,* which is described as a bright ring of light in which all the information pertaining to the invisible and visible cosmos is inscribed. The attributes of God that have become parts of the mechanism of the universe are collectively known as the *ilm-e-wajib* (incumbent knowledge); when they have been conferred on the aspirant through affinity and correlation they are styled *ilm-e-qalum,* the "knowledge of the pen." Again, the human scribes who first attempted to describe and define the centers naturally turned to their own experience and their own craft to provide a workable symbolism.

Correlations

The Sufi schema seems to combine Taoist and Hindu—more specifically, *qigong* (energy cultivation) and Tantric—understandings. The Taoist conception holds that there are three main "zones" within the body, which will be described in chapter 8. It is interesting that there are schools of Sufi thought that teach a doctrine of three bodily centers rather than seven. The similarity to the Taoist qigong schema invites speculation that proves fruitful, for the nafs (lower soul), the qalb (heart), and the rūh (spirit) of Sufism correlate precisely in both physiological location and spiritual character with the three zones of qigong, while the remaining three of the six Sufi centers that are placed within the body are the *hidden* or arcane laṭā'if, a designation that strongly suggests their correlation with the body is less obvious or even nonexistent. It is easy to imagine the generation of such schemata in meditation, when the sitter is still somewhat aware of the body, yet increasingly aware of spiritual imagery and experience arising and making, or not making, connections with the residuum of body consciousness still present. It is also easy to imagine how, according to personal nature and religious schooling, one teacher might conceive and teach a three-center scheme while another, perhaps more "spiritually aware," might come to "see" more centers, some of them entirely nonphysical. Note in passing the somewhat dualistic, or even multiplistic, tendency of many such conceptions.

Allowing ourselves the necessary flexibility of verbal

usage for our esoteric purpose, perhaps we might say of all such systems—Yoga, Tantra, Sufi, Taoist, and others—that they are the human spirit's self-commentary upon its Being-in-the-body, the world-about having been purposefully excluded from consciousness. The inner reality, freed of the outwardly directed consciousness that obscures the inward view, is then able to rise and show itself in consciousness. No wonder the schemata arrived at, despite the cultural differences, all seem bipartite, containing both a mapping onto the body and a world of consciousness that no longer relates to the body. This strongly suggests the validity of a description of our Being as partially bound to the body, but partially independent of it. Enquiry into the nature of these dependent and independent components is surely the central quest of this book, for it seems one and the same as the search for a subtle body. Perhaps, too, we might expect such an entity to show "layers" of increasing detachment from the body, of increasing "subtlety," that quality defined, if crudely and negatively, as "nonphysicality." This reminds us immediately of the layered kośas described in chapter 3. We offer this understanding tentatively at this point, for there is much to survey and describe before we attempt to draw conclusions.

The similarities between the teachings of the different traditions point, of course, to universal invariances inherent in human nature, and therefore to recurring thoughts about ourselves. The differences, on the other hand, point to the psychological, rather than physiological or anatomical, character of the whole system of understanding. The mapping onto the body is partly (though not wholly) schematic and conceptual rather than empirically observable; it is also ultimately personal and in any event very inexact. Naturally, the imposition of such conceptual mappings onto the already diverse existing languages, Sanskrit, Greek, Hebrew, Arabic, and the resulting scholastic nuances of verbal usage has produced a body of descriptions so complex and ambiguous that grasping the essence of any version is a reimaginative act. It requires an act of living re-cognition of what is being described by finding it within our own experience rather than the quasi-architectural erection of a dry intellectual edifice of verbal understanding within the mind (or within the scroll or codex on the shelf).

We thus need to wryly note that the greatest problem of Western philosophy, its disastrous tendency to fall into verbal analysis, is not uniquely its problem. War has always raged between Law and Spirit, and between Law and Grace. It is not just fundamentalist warring over ideologies—whose spiritual origins are betrayed as soon as they are made a cause for war—that should cease. The verbal warring also needs to come to an end, for it also far too easily hides the insights that alone are worthy of being sought out. Our search is for the subtle levels of what we are, not for descriptions, and we must each find the essential insights for ourselves.

SEVEN

The Bodies of Buddha

The coconut is the symbol of the body, since the coconut, like the body, has five sheaths. In the very centre of the coconut, ghee is poured . . . as an essence it corresponds to man's own essence, his jīvātmā, which flows freely from the paramātmā ("the universal soul," the Lord Ayyappan) only when the other body sheaths are torn asunder or broken, as in the case of the coconut which must be broken for the ghee to flow on, over, and with the deity.

E. VALENTINE DANIEL, *FLUID SIGNS*

As we saw in examining the Indian traditions, the goal of the many paths of Yoga is to attain mokṣa (freedom) from worldly existence and the chain of rebirths. We also saw that the subtle body with its five kośas (sheaths), seven chakras, and nadi system of energy streams or currents is the means of attaining the goal of freedom through the ascension of the subtle levels of existence, transforming consciousness by ritual, meditation, and other spiritual practices. However, in most Indian schools of thought, attention is focused on "other-world" concerns, whereas in the Chinese traditions, culture and spirituality are centered on this world. We can nevertheless find some common ideas, for example in the search for immortality and attunement with the cosmos. But while the Hindu seeks nothing less than *liberation,* the Taoist requires *rejuvenation;* while the former seeks release *from* the world, the latter attempts to function more effectively *in* the world. Between these two approaches lies the "Middle Way" of Buddhism, the path of "non-extremism," and within its later development we find Vajrayana, the Tantric "third vehicle" of Buddhism that attempts to integrate the threads of spirit and matter into a seamless whole.

In his book *Eastern Philosophy,* Chakravarthi Ram-Prasad states that there is no history of mutual discourse and debate between India and China.[1] The only truly pan-Asian tradition is the Buddhist religion, but its philosophy does not quite make that transition. Buddhist philosophy emerges in the specific context of the existing intellectual and social culture of the priestly brahmin class that we now see as the source of mainstream Hinduism. Some Buddhist schools are closer to Hindu schools on a variety of issues than to others of their own religion. The preoccupations of Indian Buddhism survived the spread to Tibet around the fifth century CE, but a change did occur: the Tibetans have seldom been interested in engaging with Hindu philosophies, as there are no Hindus in Tibet. Instead, the different Tibetan schools compete to interpret the same Buddhist materials. The Buddhism that spread to China initially carried native Indian theories and techniques, but soon the basic positions of the transplanted Buddhist schools were re-expressed in Chinese terms, doubtless expanding the Chinese philosophical vocabulary but nonetheless speaking to concerns that make sense only within China.

75

Although we cannot find exact parallels between the Indian and Chinese concepts of the subtle body because of different cultural attitudes and orientations, there are some points of comparison. Each tradition, Hindu, Buddhist, and Taoist, has a concept of the "mystical body" and uses mystical physiology in its own way. They each point to microcosmic relations and to certain truths about human nature as well as to a transformation of the body into a divine form, facilitated by a hypothetical "map" of the psychospiritual structures within the person that reaches beyond the ordinary level of awareness. All three traditions emphasize the necessity of experimentation and experience in realizing their goals, as well as an understanding of fundamental doctrines.

The Goal of Buddhism

The three major forms of Buddhism are three branches from the original trunk of Indian Buddhism. The first phase of Buddhism—known as the Hinayana (small vehicle) phase—developed in India over a period of roughly 1,500 years, from the time of the *parinirvāna,* the death of Buddha, to the beginning of the Christian era. Buddhist doctrine in this period was stated predominantly in ethical and psychological terms.

In the second phase, Chinese Buddhism produced a variant known as Mahayana (great vehicle) Buddhism. Mahayana is the more devotional and metaphysical expression of the Buddha's teachings and is based on the Chinese *Tripitaka,* the "three treasures," a compilation of all the Indian and the Chinese Buddhist scriptures available at the time.

The third phase, Tibetan Buddhism, about 500 CE to about 1000 CE, attempted the synthesis of Hinayana and Mahayana. The Hinayana ideal is the *arahant* who, according to the Mahayana, sought enlightenment only for himself, while Mahayana stresses the role of the *bodhisattva** (enlightened being) who, serving others, not himself, embodies the altruistic and compassionate aspects of Buddhahood.

---

*In Mahayana Buddhism the term *bodhisattva,* "enlightened being," refers to the spiritual aspirant who has committed himself or herself to the liberation of all beings.

The Three Schools of Buddhism

Name	Meaning	Country	Dates
Hinayana	Small vehicle	India	1500 BCE to CE
Mahayana	Great vehicle	China	200 BCE to 500 CE
Vajrayana	Adamantine vehicle	Tibet	500 CE to 1000 CE

Vajrayana, the third Buddhist school, known as the "adamantine" vehicle, is a Tantric form of Buddhism, which evolved out of Mahayana. The *vajra* is a small scepter-like ritual object that may symbolically represent "method" and is employed with a bell, which stands for "wisdom." These are abstracted symbols, almost metaphors for metaphors, for the vajra is also the male organ, and the bell the female, jointly symbolic of life itself or of a "life force."*

Vajrayana provides an esoteric, accelerated path to enlightenment, which does not claim to make other practices invalid but regards them as foundations for the attainment of enlightenment within one lifetime, a parallel concept to that of the jīvan-mukta of Hinduism. The earliest Vajrayana texts appeared around the fourth century CE. The main center for development of Vajrayana was Nalanda University in Northern India but it is believed that the university followed rather than led the Tantric movement that reached its height in the eleventh century CE.

Numerous schools and subschools of Buddhism have developed as it has spread across the world, par-

---

*The same bipolar symbol is found in the West, as the Wiccan "athame" and "grail." There are tantric forms of most religions, though not all use that adjective. While some use metaphoric ritual, others use the sexual act itself as ritual. These are the forms of religion that do not despise the body or condemn sexuality as sin. Indeed, they use life-affirming sexual symbols more or less knowingly and openly, and declare that an unshrinking embrace of sexuality is essential to human wholeness. These religions, neither puritanical nor prudish, nor unspiritually animal, but holding a balance between these extremes, are particularly pertinent to the theme of the body and important to the present movement toward holism and integral psychology.

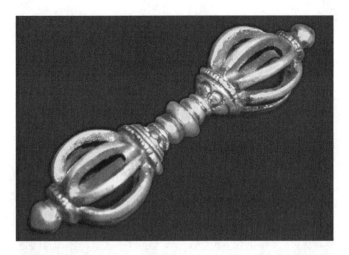

Fig. 7.1. The *vajra*, meaning both "thunderbolt" (irresistible force) and "diamond" (which can cut but cannot be cut) is an important symbol in Buddhism, Jainism, and Hinduism. Once used as a weapon, it is now purely ceremonial. Usually held by Tibetan lamas during religious ceremonies and in Tantric rituals, it represents firmness of spirit and spiritual power but has other symbolic meanings. In meditation on the vajra object, which has two spheres joined in the center like the two hemispheres of the brain, the meditator focuses on bringing the spheres together, joining two truths, the "absolute" and the "relative." This is said to result in a thunderbolt, a "bolt" at the center of the brain, which brings direct experience and a sudden awakening to Madhyamika, the "Middle Way."

ticularly in the East: Southeast Asian Buddhism spread into Sri Lanka, Burma, Thailand, Cambodia, and Laos; Chinese Buddhism into Japan, Korea, and Vietnam; Tibetan Buddhism into Mongolia, Bhutan, and Sikkim. This being so, Sangharakshita, founder of the Western Buddhist Order, advises, one should not mistake the part for the whole nor be content to understand a merely regional version of Buddhism, for it underwent continual transformation and development as it adapted its fundamental doctrines to the different needs of the peoples in the midst of which it found itself. In view of this, Sangharakshita says:

> One should approach the whole Buddhist tradition—whole in time and whole in space— and try to include, comprehend and fathom the essence of it all . . . we have to approach it as a means to psychological and spiritual wholeness, as a way to Enlightenment, as the instrument of the Higher Evolution.[2]

The goal of Buddhism, despite variations in doctrines and tradition, is always to know the inner experience of enlightenment for oneself, and Buddha's teachings are intended to shed light on the spiritual life. Buddhism abounds with universal symbols that are reminiscent of the Indian tradition and that have similar significance: the ladder between earth and heaven, the cosmic tree, and the image of a central point, the *bindu,* which represents a metaphysical, or transcendental "centrality," the "ground of being."

Meditation on the Four Phases of Buddha's Life

The influence of Tantra on Buddhist symbolism can be seen in allegorical tales of the Buddha's life relating to the subtle body and the inner processes of transformation. In Buddhism, contemplating and understanding the archetypal and symbolic content of the four phases of the Buddha's life, with its legendary and mythical elements, is one of the many paths to realization. Sangharakshita ventures to suggest that these four episodes of Buddha's life represent four archetypes of the unconscious that have to be integrated before liberation can be attained.

For example, in the last of the four episodes from Buddha's life we learn that in his seventh week of sitting beneath the bodhi tree there was a great storm. Out of the shadows appeared Mucalinda, the Serpent King, who "wrapped his coils around the Buddha and stood with his hood over his head like an umbrella." Sangharakshita explains that the symbolism pertains to the kundalinī experience, for in Indian mythology—Hindu, Buddhist, and Jain—the *nagas* (serpents) represent the forces in the depths of the unconscious in their most positive and beneficent aspect.

> The rain, we saw, falls at the end of the seventh week, and Mucalinda wraps his coils seven times round the seated figure of the Buddha. This repetition of the figure seven is no coincidence. Mucalinda also stands for what the Tantras call the *Chandali,* the Fiery Power (for which the Hindu word is the etymologically similar *kundalini*), and represents all the powerful psychic energies surging up inside a person, especially at the time of meditation, through the median

nerve. The seven coils, or the winding seven times round the Buddha, represent the seven psychic centers* through which the kundalinī passes. In the story, Mucalinda then assumes the form of a beautiful sixteen-year-old youth who represents the new personality born as a result of the upward progression of the kundalinī, the perfect submission of all the powers of the unconscious to the Enlightened Mind.[3]

Tri-Káya Buddha

As we can see, the Buddha himself is both the model for and the means of transcendence. The symbolic representations of his life and teachings embody different aspects of the *one* enlightenment experience, that is, different aspects of Buddhahood. The state that Buddhists aspire to through all spiritual practices is "unconditioned consciousness."

The spiritual process in Mahayana Buddhism is described as a combination of self-effort and graceful intervention. The agents of grace invoked in meditation and prayer are the great beings, the *mahā-sattva,* who embody the transcendental reality beyond space and time. For the Mahayana followers the human Buddha was a temporary projection of the Absolute. The true Buddha is the transcendental Reality itself, which is beyond space and time. This important notion is epitomized in the Mahayana doctrine of the triple body (*tri-kāya*) of the Buddha.[4]

The three "vestures" or bodies of Buddha are described as: the *dharma-kāya* (body of the law), the absolute or transcendental dimension of existence; the *sambhoga-kāya* (body of enjoyment), the psychic or inner dimension composed of numerous transcendental buddhas; and the *nirmāna-kāya* (body of creation), the flesh-and-blood bodies of the buddhas in human form, of which there have been many. A Buddha is considered to have such purity and "magnetic" power that he is able to manifest simultaneously in three worlds: in this world as a master of the wisdom; on his own plane as a bodhisattva; and as a *dhyāni buddha* (meditation

Buddha) on a yet higher plane. Yet the three are but one, even if the work he does seems to be the work of three separate existences.[5]

The cultivation of the dharma-body Buddha leads to a state of supranormality through "the three everyday actions [of body, language and mind] and are, in their origin, the three mysteries."[6] Yuasa explains that if one forms the *mudrās* (sacred gestures) with the hands, recites mantras with the mouth, and places the mind into a samādhi

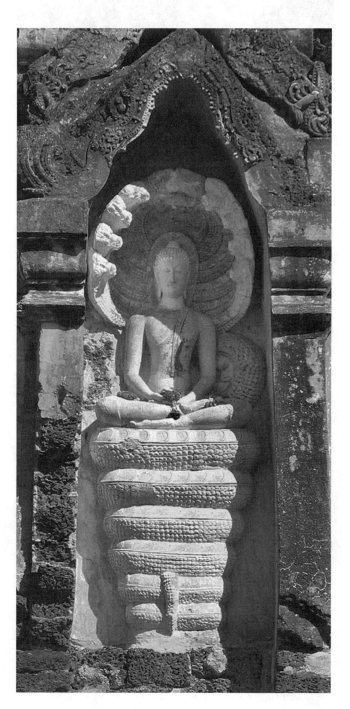

Fig. 7.2. Buddha sheltered by Mucalinda

---

*Traditionally, Buddhism is not concerned with the stimulation of the lower centers but only with the three highest, through which, in the course of meditation and other spiritual practices, the forces of the four lower centers are sublimated and transformed.

state, the three functions of body, mind, and intention reach a state commensurate with the Buddha's. "The grace of the three mysteries indicates cultivation's disclosure of the place hidden beneath the everyday world . . . originating in the metaphysical dimension."[7]

The visualization of the body of the Buddha is central to many Buddhist meditation practices. The ideal of Buddhahood is the attainment of *bodhi,* which can be translated as "knowledge," "understanding," or "awakening." Bodhi, that which makes the Buddha a Buddha, is a state of clear insight into the whole of nature, the universe in all its levels and the transitoriness of life. Bodhi is also a state of absolute freedom— from negative emotions, from the wheel of life and death—and is described by Sangharakshita as a state of uninterrupted creativity, especially spiritual creativity, and spontaneity. Having explained what he calls the cognitional and volitional aspects of bodhi he goes on to describe the emotional aspects: "*Bodhi* is also a state of positive emotion, or perhaps we should say of *spiritual* emotion. . . . Subjectively it consists in a state or experience of supreme Joy, Bliss, Ecstasy. Objectively, in manifestation, it is a state of unbounded Love and Compassion for all living beings."[8] Here we have a core element of Buddhist practice: the altruistic intention to become enlightened, to become a bodhisattva for the welfare of other beings.

The Five Dhyāni Buddhas

Symbolically, the three bodies became the basis for further development in both the Mahayana and the Vajrayana traditions. The image of the ideal Buddha, the archetypal Buddha of Truth, Infinite Light, and Eternal Life, acquired two more bodies, those of Love and Wisdom, as a result of developments in the Vajrayana, or Tantra.

The five dhyāni buddhas, or great buddhas of wisdom, are a central feature of Tibetan Buddhist belief and art. They are often found in Tibetan mandalas and *thangkas* (see plate 18).* Each buddha is believed to be capable of overcoming a particular evil with a particular good, and each has a complete system of iconographic symbolism. Each is associated with a direction, a color, a mudra, a mantra, a symbol, an element, a sense, and specific qualities.

---

*A thangka is a tapestry or wall hanging.

The Tantric Contribution

There is some argument among Buddhist scholars about the nature of the Tantric contribution. Some believe that Tantrism is a result of degeneration from high Buddhist practices of morality, compassion, and philosophical insight. They base this view on the "murky and macabre appearance" of early Tantric texts and sexual imagery. "We need to admit from the start," says Tantric Buddhist scholar Jeffrey Hopkins, "that the very vocabulary of some Tantric literature understandably creates the impression that the high moral and social ideals of Great Vehicle [Mahayana] Buddhism have been discarded for base pleasure-seeking."[9] But he goes on to explain in his article on *Tantric Buddhism* that:

> Both *sutra* and *tantra* rely on the same bases for practice and the distinction between the two vehicles occurs in the fact that there is [in Tantric Buddhism, which developed from Mahayana Buddhism] meditation on one's own body as similar in aspect to a Buddha's Form Body whereas in the sutra Great Vehicle [which, as its name attests, is a Mahayana text] there is no such meditation. In other words, in the Tantric systems, in order to become a Buddha more quickly, one meditates on oneself as similar in aspect to a Buddha in terms of both body and mind.[10]

Hopkins then points out that "deity yoga," the very heart and core of Tantrism, is a technique for enhancing the practice of compassion and wisdom. In this context, therefore, Tantrism seems not in the least a deviation from the high orientation of the sutra Great Vehicle. "Although the term *karunā* [literally meaning 'stopping bliss' and therefore implying that the torment of others interferes with one's own happiness] is sometimes used in Highest Yoga Tantra, [where it] additionally refers to orgasmic bliss without emission, [this fact] does not exclude its other meaning as the wish that all beings be free from suffering."[11]

Sexual frustration is indeed a "torment," but the question is why these two aims should ever be thought mutually exclusive. Perhaps it was thought impossible for an "impolite" matter to coexist with one of high unselfish moral tone. The condemnation of Tantra's use of the human body as a ladder for self-realization seems to be

THE FIVE DHYĀNI BUDDHAS

Dhyāni Buddha	Name	Direction	Color	Mudra	Vija (Syllable)	Symbol	Embodiment	Type of Wisdom	Cosmic element (skandha)	Earthly element	Sense
Vairocana	Supreme and Eternal Buddha; The Radiant One	Center	White	Dharmachakra (wheel-turning)	Om	Wheel	Sovereignty	Integration of the wisdom of all the Buddhas	Rupa (form)	Ether (space)	Sight
Akshobhya	Immovable or Unshakable Buddha	East	Blue	Bhumisparsa (witness)	Hum	Thunderbolt	Steadfastness	Mirror-like	Vijñāna (consciousness)	Water	Hearing
Ratnasambhava	Source of Precious Things or Jewel-Born One	South	Yellow	Varada (charity)	Trah	Jewel (ratna) or three jewels (triratna)	Compassion	Wisdom of equality	Vendana (sensation)	Earth	Smell
Amitabha	Buddha of Infinite Light	West	Red	Dhyana (chin mudra)	Hrih	Lotus	Light	Discriminating	Sanjñā (name or perception)	Fire	Taste
Amogasiddha	Almighty Conquerer or Lord of Karma	North	Green	Abhaya (fearlessness)	Ah	Double thunderbolt	Dauntlessness	All-accomplishing	Samskara (volition)	Air	Touch

based largely on the puritanical views of the Victorian colonial period. Yet many contemporary scholars held the Tantric works in great esteem, not least Woodroffe himself (see chapter 3). David Snellgrove, translator of the *Hevajra Tantra,* believed that while, in his view, defects were apparent in some of the texts, still more obvious and undeniable was the blossoming of human genius that they nourished. Scholars, saints, and artists of first rank appear throughout the succeeding centuries, and their works bear testimony to them to this day.[12]

Perhaps wisdom counsels that we take note of the Biblical saying "By their fruits ye shall know them." If the fruits are good can the tree be bad? Yahshua, claimed by the majority in the West during the very period in question, the nineteenth century, to be its spiritual leader, did not think so. If great saints, artists, and scholars flourished in the Tantric tradition, might not that tradition be more wholesome than the prejudices of its detractors? It is a cliché among artists that all art is erotic, and it is certain that at least one of the motivating energies of artistic creation is sublimated sexual energy, that out of which kundalinī itself also arises.

Those who seek the wholeness of the integral body and integral psychology have more to say, and to say strongly. Attitudes to other cultures are always colored by our own cultural predispositions, indeed prejudices, based on value judgments that are, on proper reflection, seen to be suspect. What could be more right than acceptance of our *entire* nature, as animals, but as animals capable of enlightenment and spiritual aspiration? We shall not find wholeness otherwise.

Tripitikamala, an Indian commentator on Tantra, believed that more evolved meditators did not need to use sexual union as a means to enlightenment. He felt that an "imaginary" consort was more appropriate in the higher stages and that physical enactment was only necessary for those attempting to conquer desire. This "sublimation," as Freudian terminology would describe it, is, of course, also an instance of interiorization, described in chapter 5. He is, however, reported to have believed that an actual consort is needed in the meditation practice of "emptiness," so that a practitioner could overcome the false sense that sex is "separate from" the scope of "emptiness."[13] This seems to show genuine recognition of a wholeness of some kind to be attained through Tantric meditation. However, Hopkins points out that there is no evidence that Tripitikamala was cognizant of the levels of consciousness manifested in orgasmic bliss and thus did not even conceive of utilizing them on the path.[14]

Such differing scholastic views do not detract, however, from the fact that Tantra, particularly Tibetan Tantra (Vajrayana), offered additional techniques to practitioners to enhance their capability to distinguish lower states from the higher, more subtle states of consciousness through focus on kundalinī, chakras, and nadis, the psychospiritual organs of the enlightenment experience. Without method, the means of progress on the spiritual path can be, literally, "painfully" slow and the desire to be of effective service to others therefore difficult to realize.

Deity Yoga

Hopkins calls "deity yoga," the fundamental practice of Tantra, "the very heart and core of Tantrism."[15] He describes a *deity* as a supramundane being who himself or herself is a manifestation of compassion and wisdom. In deity yoga, "one joins one's own body, speech, mind, and activities with the exalted body . . . manifesting on the path a similitude of the final effect."[16] Feuerstein believes that the Tantric worldview affirms the existence of deities, long-lived higher beings on subtle planes, who are endowed with extraordinary powers.[17] Tantric practitioners seek help from these deities (*yidam*) through invocation, ritual, meditative visualization, repetition of mantras, and the use of mandalas (see plates 19 and 20), which the Dalai Lama describes as "the celestial mansion, the pure residence of the deity."[18]*

Deity yoga is performed using the same ritual structure found in all Tantric traditions:

1. *Snana* (purificatory ablutions)
2. *Dehasuddhi* (purification of the elements within the body)

---

*A mandala is, literally, a "circle," a sacred area in which rituals are performed, or an "encircled" area of the body such as an element or chakra. The basic concept, prominent in the mind of earlier humanity on account of the wondrous discovery of the wheel, is found in early religions everywhere. It persists in a multitude of present-day concepts of "sacred space," such as Liverpool Roman Catholic cathedral with its emphasis on the circular form. Mandala has further conceptual links with such entities as the finite but unbounded universe.

3. *Nyasa* (divinisation of the body by imposing mantras upon it)
4. *Antara* (internal worship of the deity through visualization)
5. *Bahya* (external worship of the deity through offerings)

Feuerstein points out that these gods and goddesses are not yet fully mature spiritual beings. Powerful, but not yet liberated, they are equated with a particular energetic presence that helps practitioners accomplish the goal of transformation, blocking or dispelling negative forces and helping them to help others with their material or spiritual problems. "The masculine and feminine deities worshipped in the [Tantric] rituals are personifications of specific intelligent energies present in the subtle dimension."[20]

In his book *The Tantric Body,* Gavin Flood states that the purification of the body through dissolving its constituent elements into their cause seems to be a characteristically Tantric practice. Through symbolically destroying the physical or gross body, he explains, the adept can create a pure, divinized body (divya-deha) with which to offer worship to the deities of his system. He does this first only in imagination and second in the physical world for, as in all Tantric systems, only a god can worship a god. The textual representation of the *bhūtaśuddhi* is set within a sequence in which the physical or elemental body (*bhautika-śarīra*) is purified and the soul ascends from the heart through the body, and analogously through the cosmos, to the Lord Narayana* located at the crown of the head.[21]

In the Tantric tradition, the boundaries between energetic forces and symbolisms are often blurred and are simply regarded as different aspects of the one Reality. We see, for example, that the chakras, the energy centers of the subtle body, are each presided over by a deity and that Enlightenment is brought about by the union of the Goddess power, the Sakti, with the masculine universal force, represented by Siva, through the suṣumnā nadi, the "most gracious current," which is the royal road to freedom. The deities themselves can embody a symbolism within symbolism. For example, there are sixteen goddesses representing the sixteen phases of the moon

---

*Narayana, "that from which this whole cosmos has sprung."[22]

which, in itself, is associated with immortality and the path of cessation, the nivṛtti-marga, the Yogic process of reversal, introspection, and recovery of our true nature.[23]

When Tantric practitioners invoke a particular deity through visualization, mantra, or prayer, they are, says Feuerstein, mentally bridging the gulf between the personal and the impersonal, the concrete and the abstract. They are cognizant of "the singular Being looming large behind or shining through a specific deity" and it is the "radiant omnipresence of Being that imbues a deity with sacredness and special significance."[24] Despite understanding that the Godhead is beyond descriptive labels and categories, Tantric practitioners may draw on the mythology associated with Siva while being intellectually convinced of the featureless singularity of ultimate Reality.

Meditations from the Heart

The Tibetan metaphysical enlightenment path of Vajrayana has its roots in Indian Tantra, positing a similar subtle body of vayus or prānas (winds), chakras, and nadis, yet it retains the earlier model of just four chakras: navel, heart, throat, and head. Indian Tantra meditation begins at mūlādhāra, the base chakra, and moves upward. Tibetan Tantra starts at the head, considered the site of the lowest level of consciousness, and moves downward to the heart, considered the highest, and has no concern with centers placed lower in the body than the heart.

The heart center, the anāhata chakra, has particular significance in Tantra. The centers relating to lower bodily functions, mūlādhāra, manipūra, and swādhiṣṭhāna, which govern the processes of elimination, procreation, and digestion, can cause physical and emotional problems unless the heart center is awakened. The higher centers, too, can cause problems such as mental imbalance, psychic hypersensitivity, extreme susceptibility to mystical states (as opposed to the state of enlightenment), and hallucination or delusion, if not tempered by the heart qualities of kindness, compassion, empathy, and tranquillity.

Many teachers, says Feuerstein, prefer to work from the heart center, striving to live from this internal vantage point, with great passion but without attachment.

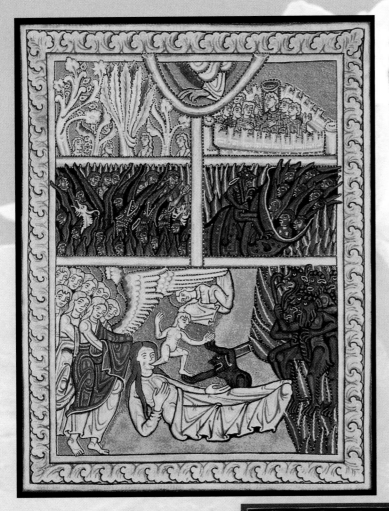

Plate 1. "Exit of the Soul from the Tabernacle of the Body" from a copy of Hildegard of Bingen's *Liber Scivias*, c. 1151, the first of three works relating her twenty-six religious visions, in which man is spiritually transformed. (St. Hildegard's Abbey, Eibingen. Photograph by Erich Lessing/Art Resource, New York.)

Plate 2. The *mandala* is an ancient device in many cultures, a sacred iconic space of esoteric, "hidden," knowledge of the self and the outer world, offering "spiritual tools" to transcend both. Its squares, circles, and triangles represent planes of consciousness experienced in meditation. Traditional Hindu, Buddhist, and Tibetan mandalas also contain images of deities who the aspirant seeks to "become," or from whom protection or healing are sought. Some mandalas preserve the lineage of teachers, lamas, buddhas, or bodhisattvas of long oral traditions. Mandalas exist in many forms, from Native American, Hindu, and Tibetan sand paintings to formal gardens and Gothic rose windows of European cathedrals. Jung saw mandalas as universal archetypes of wholeness and used them to interpret his patients' dreams and help them back to psychic stability.

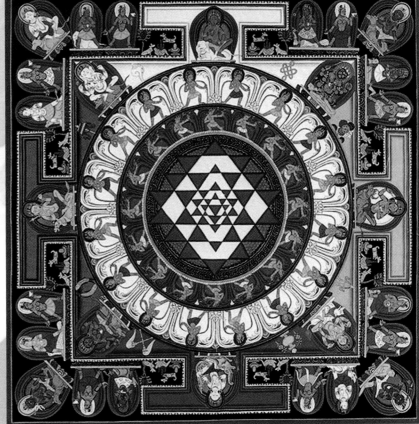

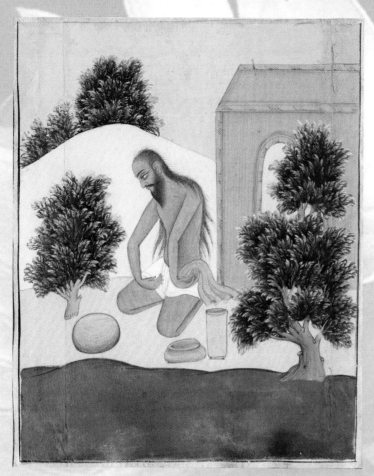

Plate 3. One of the miniatures of Yogic postures in the *Bahr al-Hayat* (The Ocean of Life), ca. 1718 CE. This text was copied from an earlier Arabic translation, ca. 1563 CE of an extremely popular Indian text originally known as the *Pool of Nectar,* which was widely circulated throughout the Islamic world. It is now in the Rare Book Collection of the Wilson Library at the University of North Carolina.

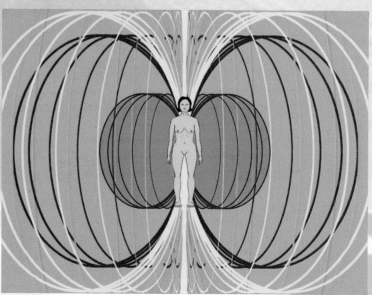

Plate 4. The human microcosm and greater macrocosm envisioned as fields of subtle energy.

Plate 5. The Hermetic view places man at the center of the microcosm, itself in the center of the macrocosm, while God is perceived as beyond even the macrocosm, just as Ein Sof is imagined above and beyond the Kabbalistic Tree of Life. (From a thirteenth-century copy of Hildegard's *Liber Divinorum Operum.* The Yorck Project, Berlin.)

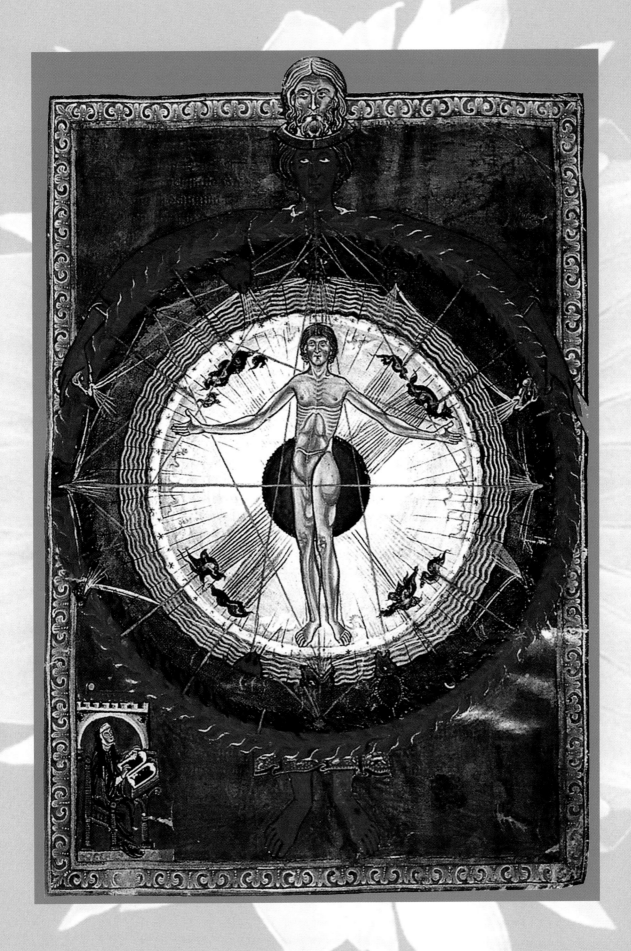

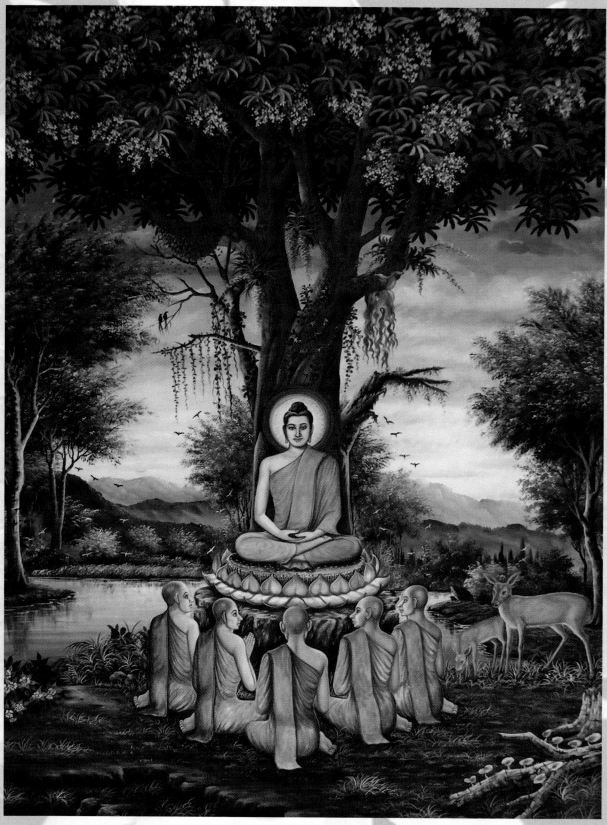

Plate 6. Gautama Buddha, under the bodhi tree, finds enlightenment, the final stage of spiritual development during embodied life. His attainment is shown by his halo of light, probably representing the physical phenomenon of the aura, visible to some, and now recordable by photography.

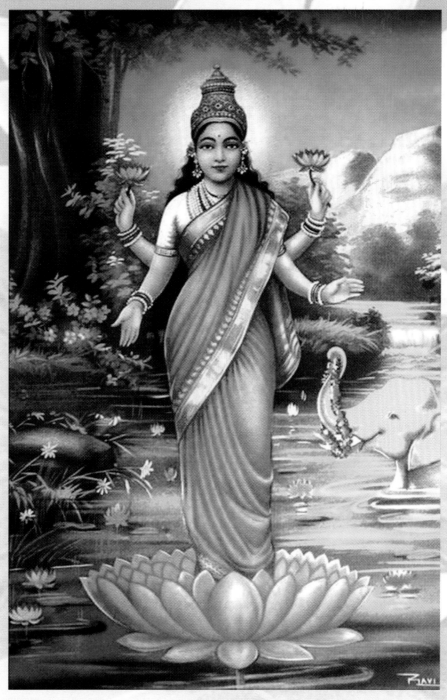

Plate 7. Lakshmi, Hindu goddess of wealth, love, and beauty, is also the Supreme Goddess, Mother Earth, and Sakti, the feminine aspect of Vishnu's divine power. In the creation myth "The Churning of the Milky Ocean at the Dawn of Time" (see plate 8), the *asuras* (demons), on the left shore, and the *devas* (deities), on the right, set up the axis mundi and with it churn the Milky Way to make the divine elixir of immortality. Lakshmi and other gifts to humankind emerge like butter from the ocean of churned milk. Accordingly, she is also known as the daughter of the sea, cognate with the Greek goddess Aphrodite, the Roman Venus, the Chinese Quan Yin, and the Buddhist Tara, the last the goddess of sea crossings as well as the Buddha's own consort. Lakshmi is always associated with the lotus, representing purity, spiritual perfection, and authority. She is the "lotus dweller," the "one whose face is as beautiful as a lotus," the "one who holds a lotus," the "one wearing a garland of lotuses." The lotus is also the *yoni*, the female sexual organ, complement of the lingam, which is symbolic of both the axis mundi, initiating life as it churns the milk sea of the yoni, and of the Tree of Life standing amid the lotus-filled Garden of Eden. (Raja Ravi Varma.)

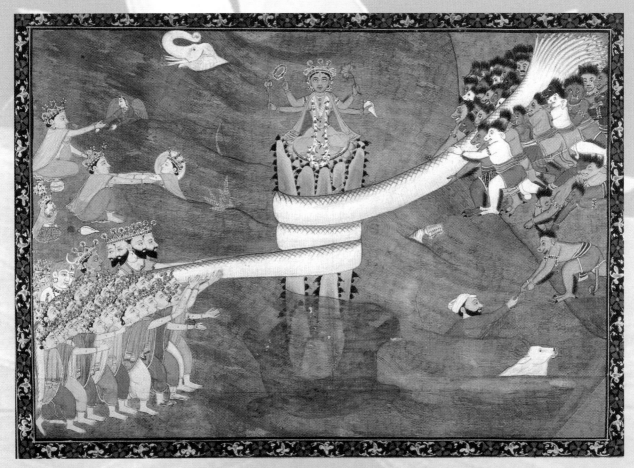

Plate 8. The myth of the setting up of the axis mundi, told in the Vedic classic "The Churning of the Milky Ocean at the Dawn of Time," is depicted here. In the naïveté of a still-limited consciousness humans imagined gods (seen on the left shore) and demons (seen on the right), all resembling themselves, cooperating to place and turn the axis, though the gods later cheated the demons of their share of the good results. Naive though the myth is, humankind's sense of the passage of time, psychological time, of the natural "time-liness" of our own consciousness, did in fact begin when we first dreamed and reflected upon what we had come to see as "our*selves*," *Beings-within-the-world-about*, as Heidegger put it, in and yet distinguishable from the world around us. Humans also observed physical time, most clearly in the daily journey of the sun and the monthly waxing and waning of the moon. The conflation of these two "times" bedeviled science until Einstein, and in the minds of most of us they are still not distinguished, though without detriment to everyday life. (Nineteenth-century painting. The Art Archive/Victoria and Albert Museum London/Eileen Tweedy.)

Plate 9. The yogi as microcosm embodies the elements of earth, water, fire, air, and ▶ space. Contemplation of the elements, the principles of the material world, is a method through which a yogi can find the doorway to understanding how the One can become many. In order to be liberated, the yogi must find the way back from the many to the One, the singular ultimate Reality. (Illustration © Pieter Weltevrede, www.sanatansociety.com, and printed by permission of the artist.)

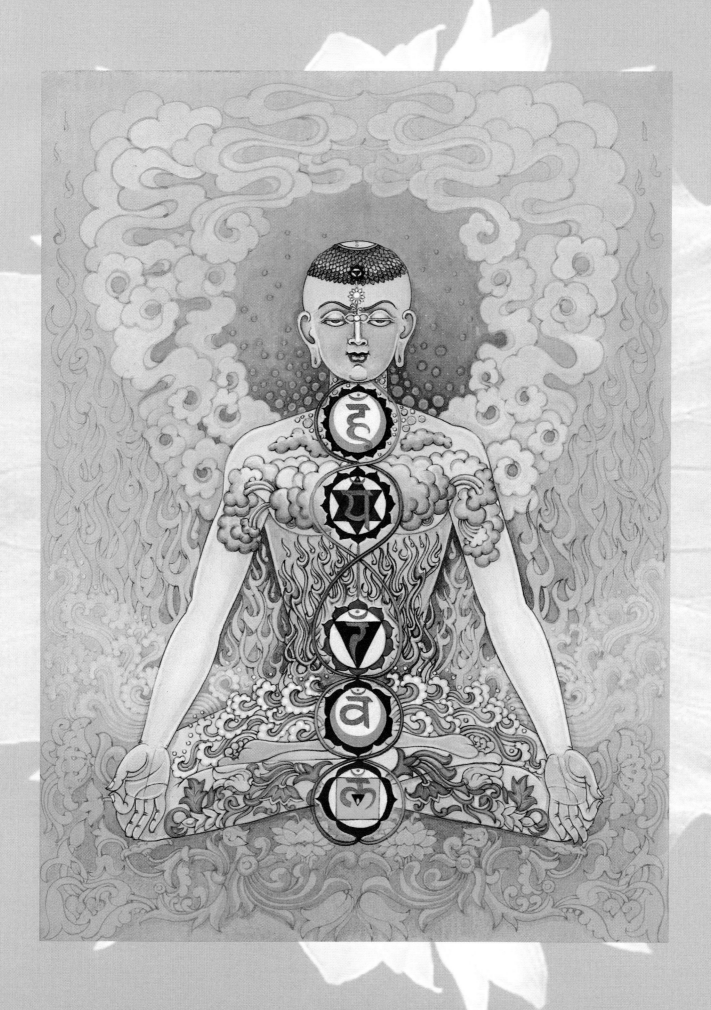

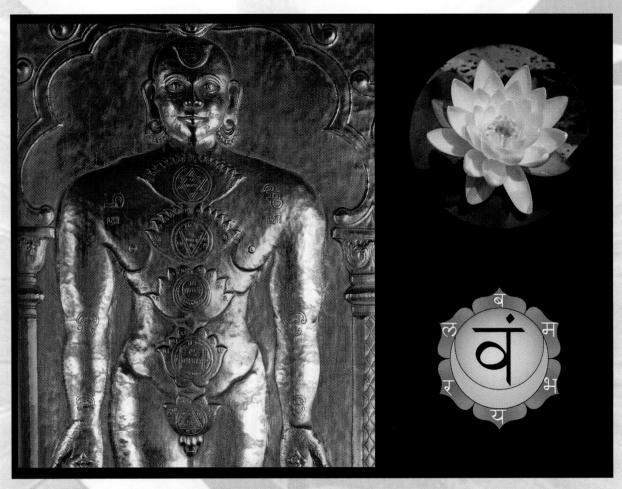

Plate 10. The notion of the golden body, immortal while in the physical world, is universal, found even in the Platonically influenced writing of the apostle Paul. We illustrate just one of the chakras, the basic structures of the subtle body. Each chakra is represented by a lotus (*padma*) with the sign of its specific seed sound, its *bīja mantra*, at its center. Each lotus has a specific number of petals, each of which is inscribed with a Sanskrit letter associated with the residing deity. The lotus is the symbol of spiritual unfoldment; through inner work each chakra is said to open like a lotus flower coming to full bloom. This statue is south Indian, ca. eighteenth century, cast in copper with gold wash.

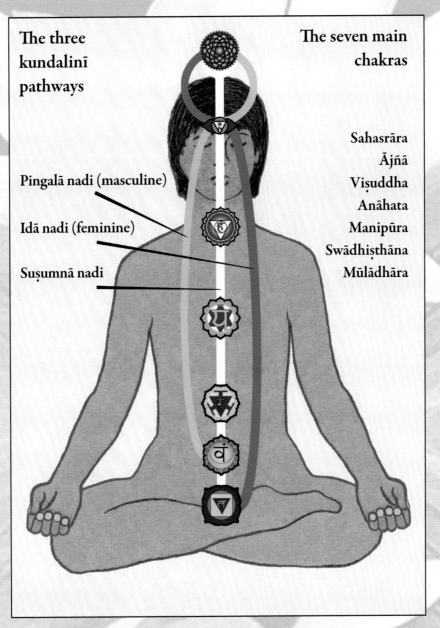

The three kundalinī pathways

The seven main chakras

Pingalā nadi (masculine)

Idā nadi (feminine)

Suṣumnā nadi

Sahasrāra
Ājñā
Viṣuddha
Anāhata
Manipūra
Swādhiṣthāna
Mūlādhāra

Plate 11. In this schematic attempt to show the kundalinī process the polarized masculine and feminine energies enter the pingalā and idā channels at the mūlādhāra and flow upward through the suṣumnā, to unite at the sahasrāra and merge with the Absolute, symbolically the peak of Mount Meru, in the center of the spinal column. Tantric practitioners aim at reuniting these two energies to bring about the enlightened state of ānanda (bliss).

Perceptions of the kundalinī process vary widely as do the number and placement of chakras. Here, for instance, the crossing over of the idā and pingalā energy currents at each chakra is not shown, since this illustration seems to represent a later stage of the kundalinī process when the cooling channel associated with the moon (and thought to be placed in the stomach) consumes the nectar of immortality (amṛta) oozing from the microcosmic moon stationed in the head. The yogi must gain control over the ambrosial fluid and distribute it over the entire body to bring vigor, health, and longevity.

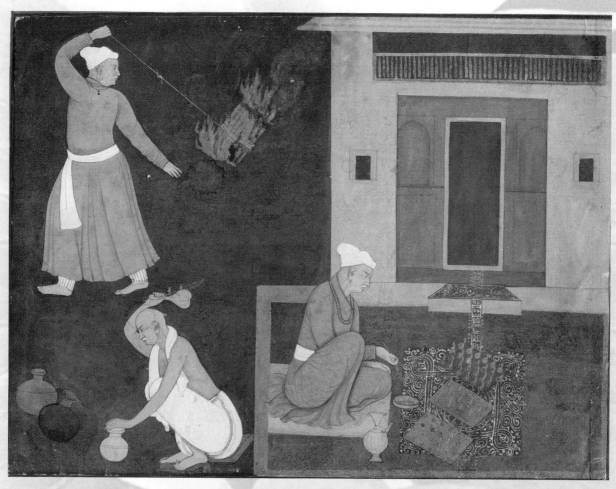

Plate 12. *Agnihotra* or *homa,* the purifying fire ritual shown in this painting—attributed to Nainsukh ca. 1735 CE—is one of the five duties of the Indian householder. Fire rituals are intended as an oblation or personal sacrifice, to honor the deities, to celebrate special occasions, and to unite family and community in a common bond. (Photograph © 2010 Museum of Fine Arts, Boston.)

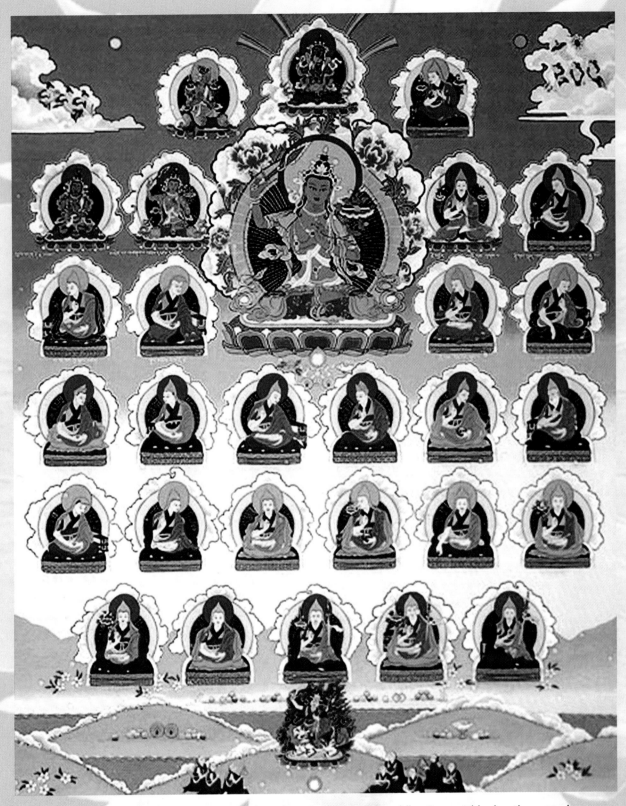

Plate 13. Dzogchen teachings are attributed to the Primordial Buddha, Samantabhadra, the central figure in this Tibetan thangka, and have been transmitted in an unbroken lineage from master to disciple to the present day.

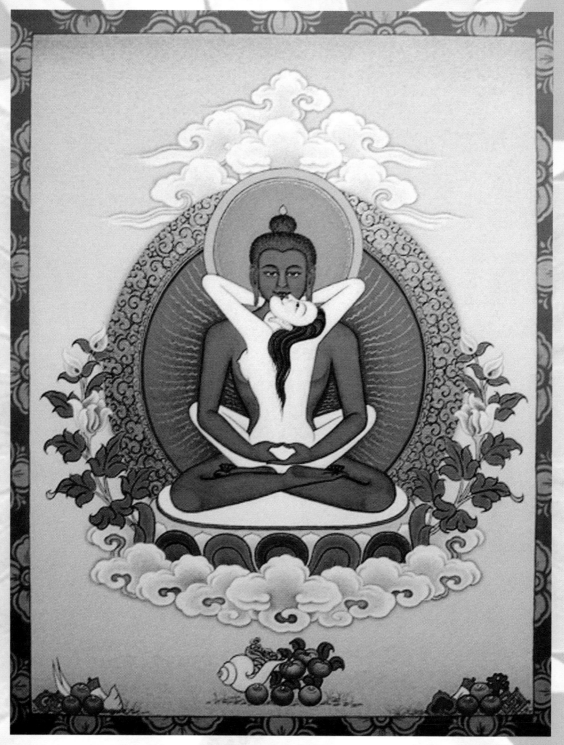

Plate 14. Intense concentration on the deity during normal activities is an advanced practice in Dzogchen, personified here by Samantabhadra with dakini (goddess). *Termas* (esoteric teachings known as "treasures") were hidden by Samantabhadra and his principal disciple in scriptures, images, and ritual articles, to be revealed at an appropriate time for the future benefit of Dzogchen practitioners.

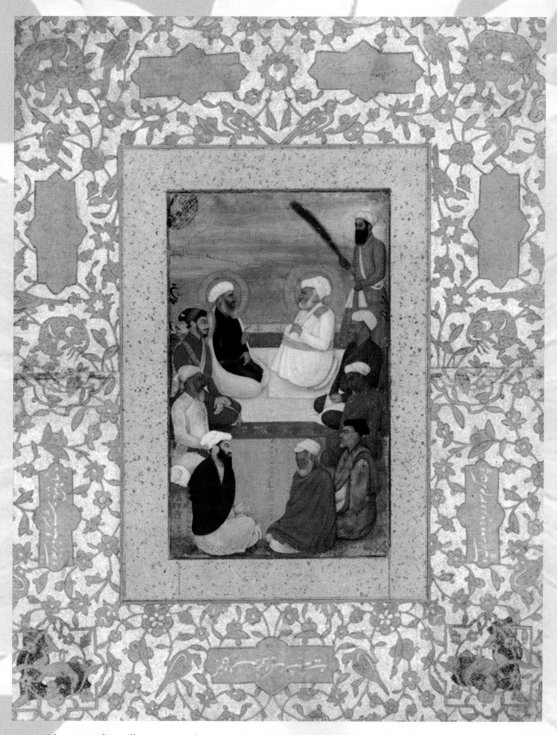

Plate 15. This silk painting depicts a meeting between Islamic and Hindu mystics who had a great influence on Muhammed Dara Shikoh, eldest son of the Mughal Emperor, Shah Jahan, who built the Taj Mahal. In his book *Majma al-Bahrain* (The Commingling of the Two Oceans), Dara argues that Islam and Vedanta are essentially the same under different names, a fundamental quest for unity with God.

Plate 16. In this painting the most famous Persian saint of the Chishti order, Hazrat Khwaja Moinuddin Chishti, is visited by Akbar the Great, who was emperor of India for almost half a century, from 1556 to 1605. Akbar initiated debates on matters of belief between Muslims, Hindus, Sikhs, Jains, and the Christian Jesuits. Moinuddin Chishti himself had traveled widely with his teacher throughout Asia and—after a dream that he had the Prophet's blessing to do so—he settled in Ajmer, North India, where he attracted a substantial following and established his order. His faith in *Wadat al-wujud* (unity of being) inspired him to promote emotional integration and guide those he lived among to spiritual transformation.

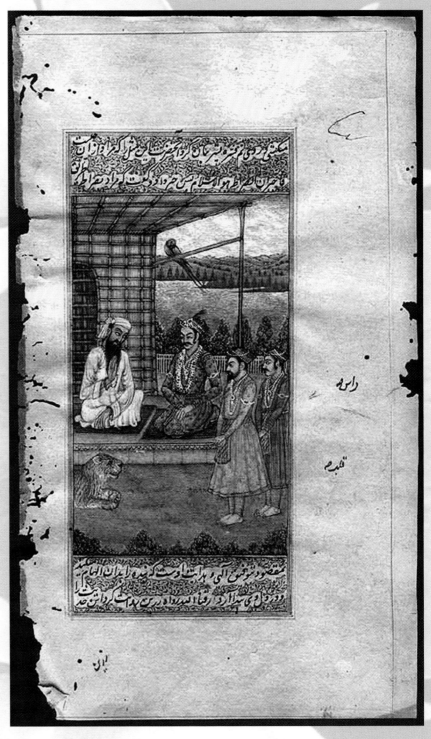

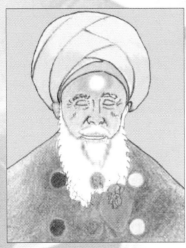

Plate 17. A Sufi meditating on the qalb, the "spiritual heart."

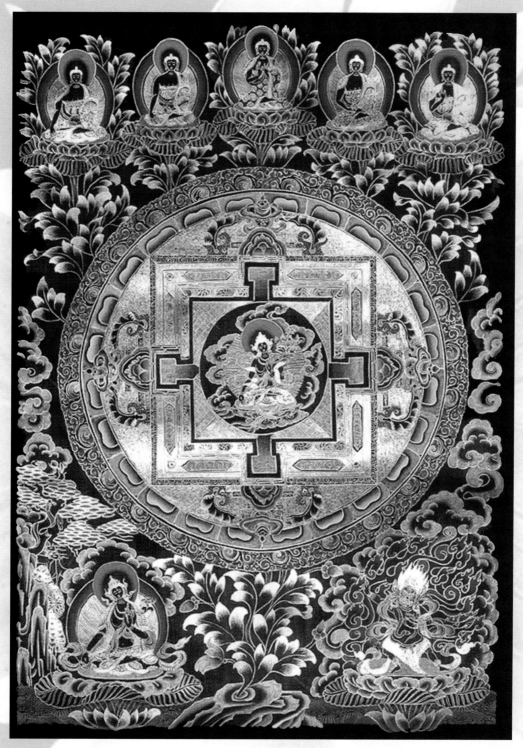

Plate 18. The Goddess Tara with five dhyāni buddhas. The black background indicates that the thangka painting is highly mystical and esoteric. Tara, from the root *tar,* to "traverse" or "cross over," serves as a bridge to carry devotees to immortality. Of her twenty-one emanations, two are particularly popular. As White Tara, representing purity and radiance, she is known as the "Mother of all Buddhas" and embodies compassion and the undifferentiated truth of dharma. As Green Tara she represents power, nature, and healing. The elements (details) of her bodily forms are important in Tantric practice as reminders that the body is the vehicle by which enlightenment is attained in the here and now. Different visualizations create a bond between practitioner and deity and, when the practitioner becomes the deity, are believed to lead the practitioner to the ecstatic experience of enlightenment.

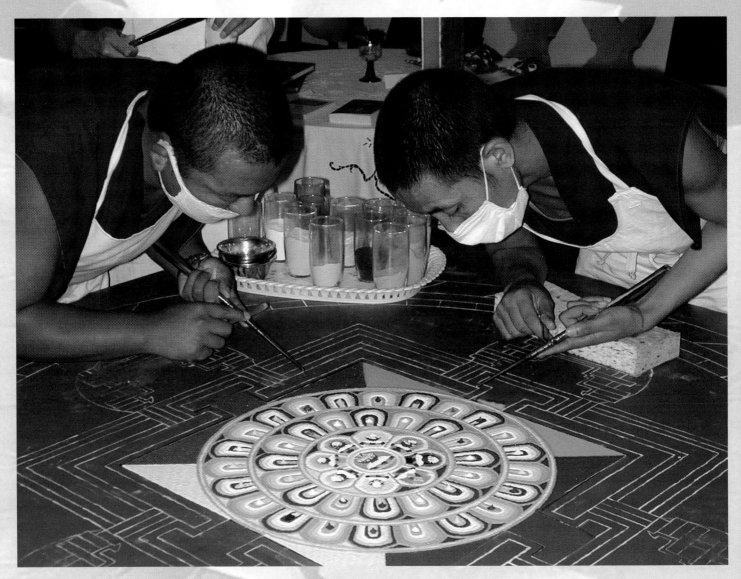

Plate 19. A group of Tibetan monks demonstrate mandala painting.

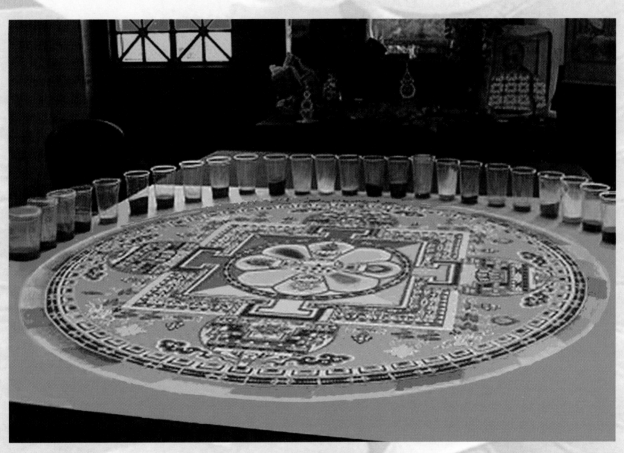

Plate 20. This figure depicts a *kalachakra* (wheel of time) sand mandala. Sand painting is a Tibetan Buddhist tradition in which a mandala is constructed using colored sand. When the mandala has been completed and its accompanying ceremonies and viewing are over, it is ritually destroyed to symbolize the Buddhist belief in the transient nature of life. Within its complex structure the kalachakra mandala contains 722 deities, which are removed in a specified order before the sand is collected in a jar and placed in the sea or a river to be returned to nature.[19] (See notes for chapter 7.)

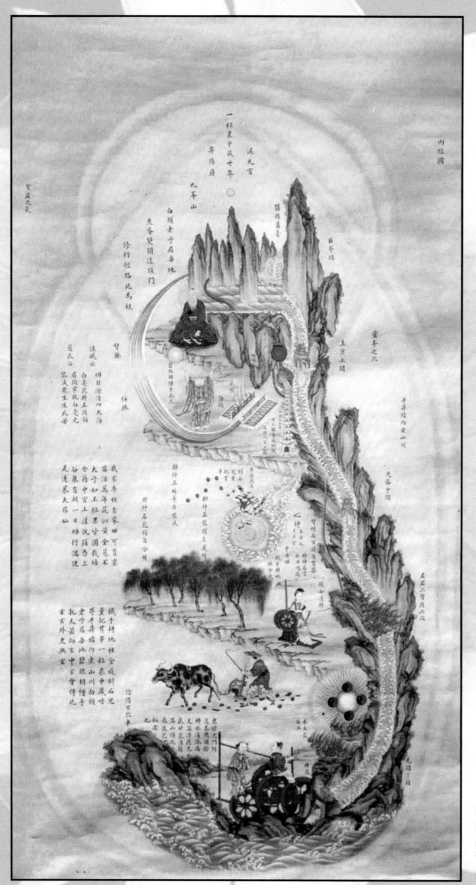

Plate 21. The Taoist inner landscape follows the shape of the spine, the "locus of each man's vital spirit."

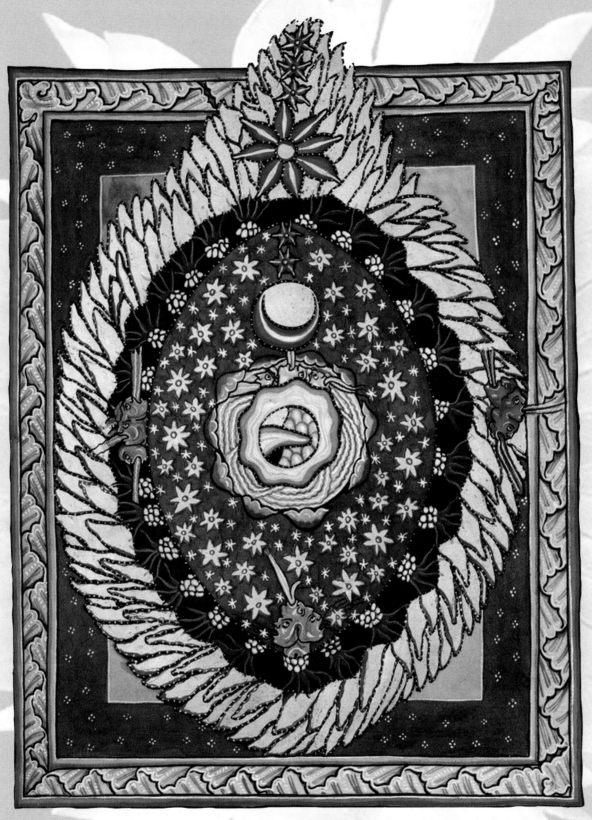

Plate 22. Models of the medieval world postulated correspondences between the human body and the cosmos. In the third of Hildegard of Bingen's visions she saw the universe as a layered structure symbolizing the mysteries of incarnation and the stages of human history. (*Liber Scivias,* ca. 1150. The Yorck Project, Berlin.)

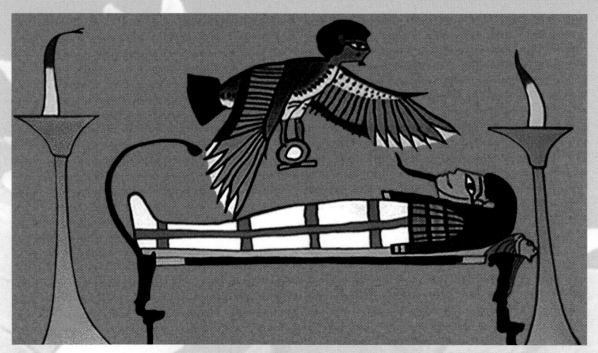

Plate 23. The "soul" of a mummified pharaoh revisits the body. (Exhibition panel from the Mysteries of Egypt exhibition, 1998–99, "Ba bird" © Canadian Museum of Civilization, 1998–99, PCD 2001-299-074.)

Plate 24. Genesis (28.11–19) tells the story of Jacob's dream of a ladder between earth ▶ and heaven, which the angels of God were ascending and descending. This has been interpreted allegorically by many scholars and theologians through the centuries, all culturally conditioned, some even willful, but the fundamental idea is cognate with Hindu and Neo-Platonist concepts of the ascent of the human to God, and the successes and failures of spiritual life in the physical world. (William Blake, watercolor, ca. 1800. The Art Archive/British Museum/Superstock.)

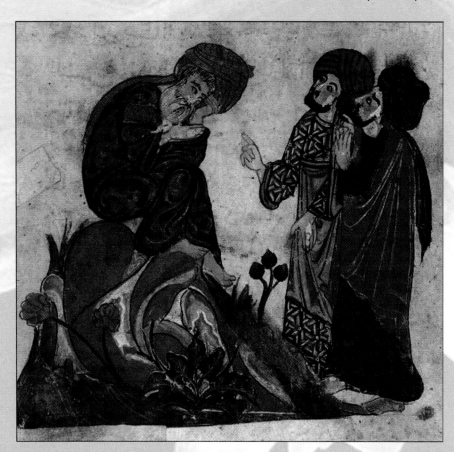

Plate 25. Abu Nasr al Farabi, the revered Islamic scholar who was the first to translate Plato into Arabic, is shown here (on the left) in debate with students of Aristotle. Among the scientific, medical, and philosophical texts translated were the earliest works ascribed to Hermes and Pythagoras. (Topkapi Palace Library, Istanbul.)

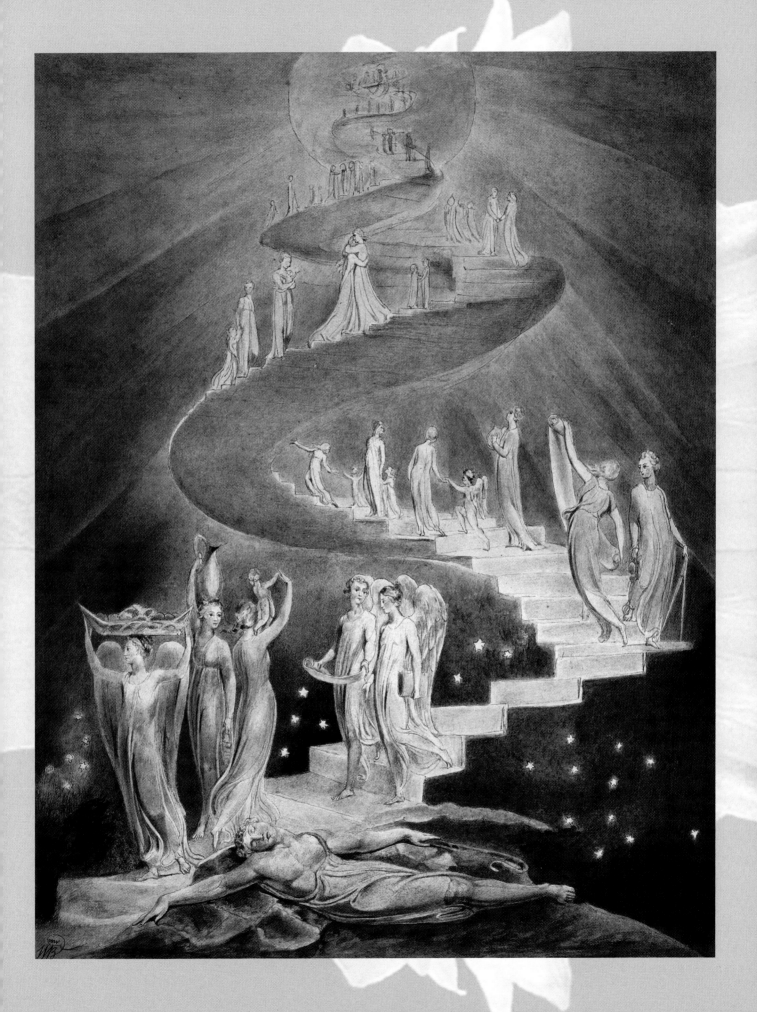

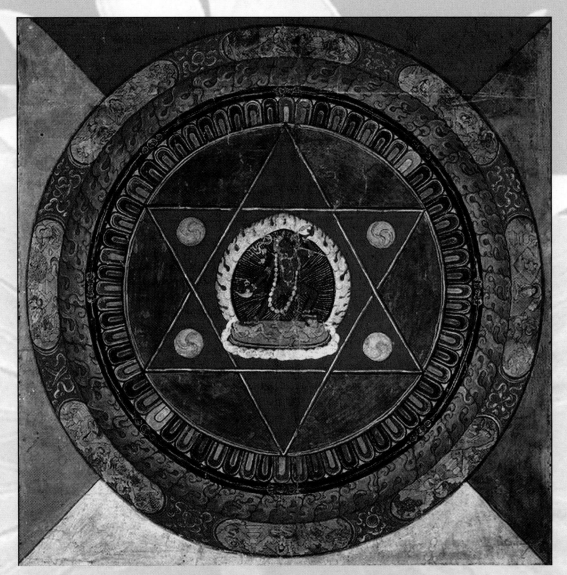

Plate 26. The mandala, humanity's oldest religious symbol, appears throughout the world and may even have existed in the Paleolithic period. The best-known forms of the mandala are used in Tibetan and Tantric yoga. Mandalas were noted by Jung in some four hundred of the accounts of dreams and visions given by his patients. They are of great significance because their centers contain the highest religious figures. In Jung's study of their spontaneous appearance in dreams he interpreted them to signify a psychic center of personality, not to be identified with the ego, but with the unconscious activities of the soul.

Plate 27. The circle as the symbol of completion can be found in many mandala-like forms in cultures ▶ from both East and West, from Native American medicine wheels to the formal gardens of medieval Europe. The rose window of Nôtre Dame Cathedral, Paris, pictured here, is typical, and one of the most impressive among the many such cathedral and church windows. The original idea is thought to have been brought back by Templar Knights returning from the Crusades in the twelfth century. Many windows depict God at the center surrounded by the days of creation, the order of the heavens represented by the zodiac, or Christ seated in the center "light" with his disciples around him. The rose window was first known by that description about the end of the seventeenth century, and is dedicated to Mary, mother of Jesus, as the "mystical rose," the feminine aspect of God.

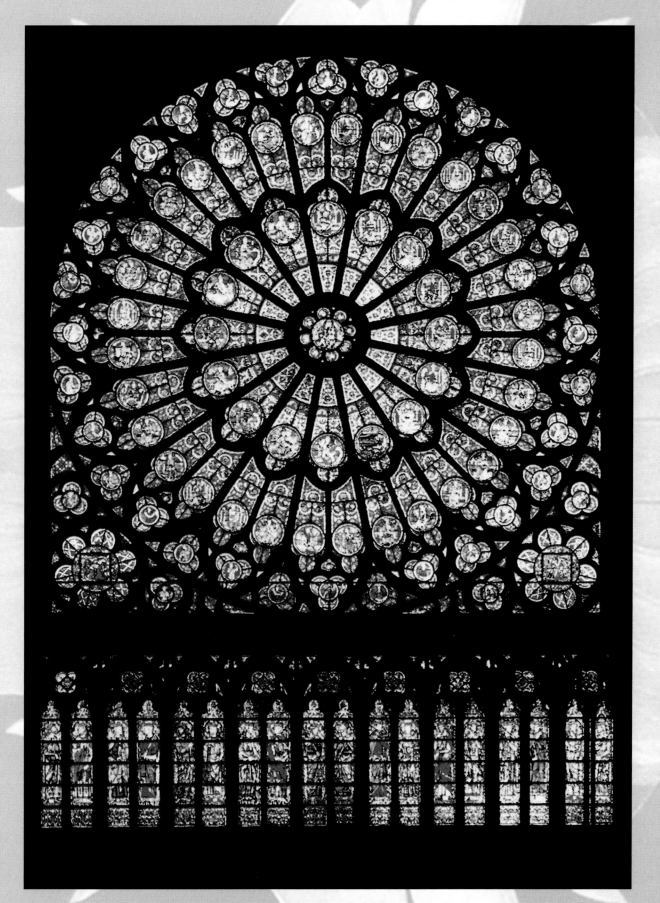

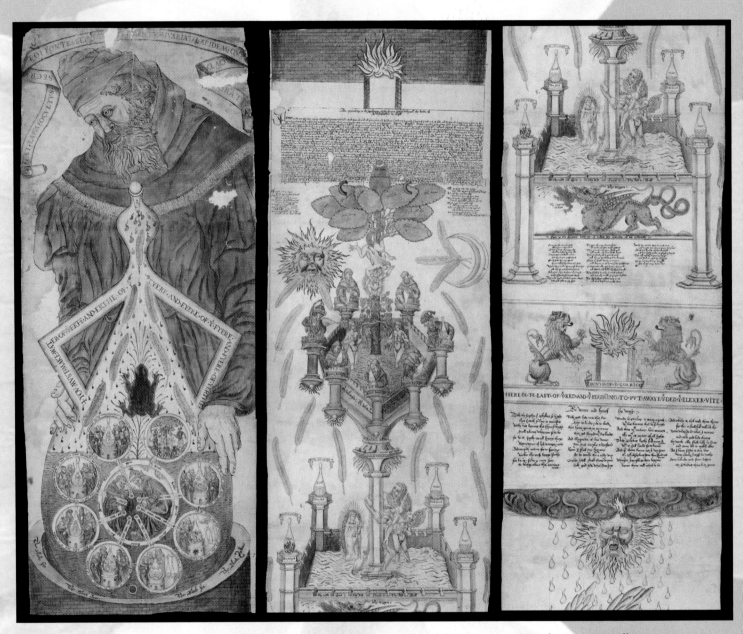

Plate 28. The Ripley Scroll, by the English alchemist, George Ripley, ca. 1470, illustrates the allegorical *Visio Mystica of Arnold of Villanova*, which relates the stages of alchemical transformation. Ripley's *The Twelve Gates Leading to the Discovery of the Philosopher's Stone* and his twenty-five volumes on alchemy earned him a reputation second only to that of Roger Bacon (ca. 1214–1294). Note how the Ripley Scroll evinces the concept of higher and lower levels that are similar, as asserted by the principle "As above, so below." (Beinecke Rare Book and Manuscript Library, Yale University.)

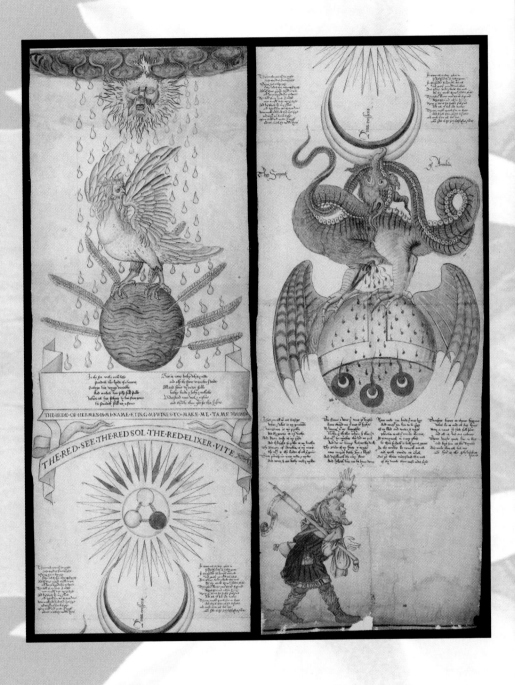
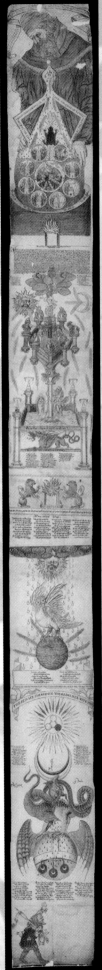

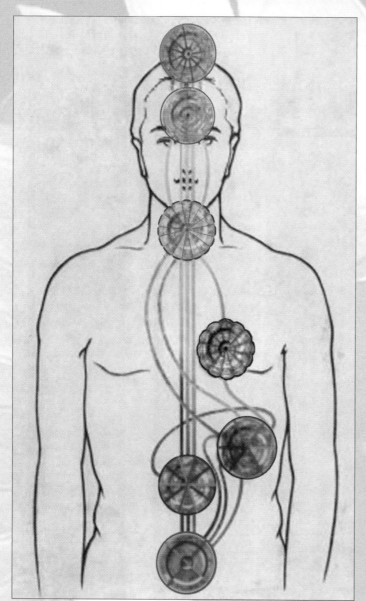

Plate 29. This is a depiction of C. W. Leadbeater's conception of the chakras, which the translator and scholar Sir John Woodroffe judged to be confusing and misleading, not least on account of Leadbeater's inclusion of a "spleen" chakra that does not appear in traditional Indian texts. Leadbeater was a clergyman, author, and clairvoyant, an early member of the Theosophical Society. He met Blavatsky in 1884 and followed her to India. Some of his ideas may have been influenced by Christian mysticism and he attempted to demonstrate in his book the analogies between his own theory of the chakras and the Christian theosophy of the German mystic Johann Georg Gichtel (1638–1710).

Plate 30. The cover of Leadbeater's book on the chakras published in 1927 shows the 1696 illustration by Johann Georg Gichtel, ardent follower of the German mystic Jakob Boehme, whose books he edited. Gichtel's illustration is based on Boehme's ideas of hermetic and alchemical correspondences, and has the sun at the heart center as the symbol of vital force and spiritual light. Some modern Western derivatives of the chakra system owe more to this medieval Judeo-Christian model of the subtle body than to the original Tantric conception.

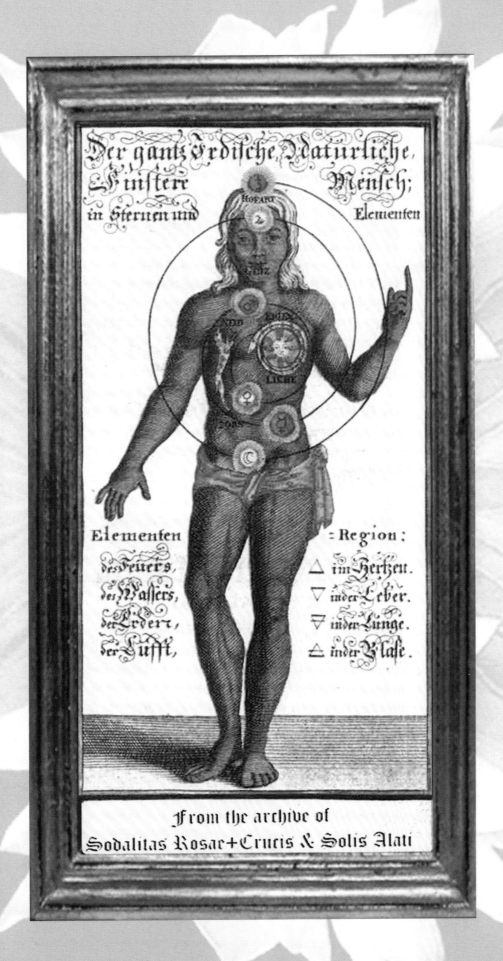

Der gantz Erdische Natürliche
Finstere Mensch;
in Sternen und Elementen

Elementen   : Region :

des Feuers,   △ im Hertzen.

des Wassers,   ▽ inder Leber.

der Erden,   ▽ inder Lunge.

der Lufft,   △ inder Blase.

From the archive of
Sodalitas Rosae+Crucis & Solis Alati

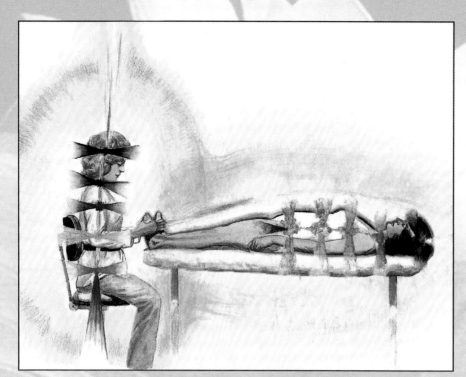

Plate 31. A healer at work balancing the auric field of the client, depicting the interconnections between client, healer, and the universal energy field. (Illustration by Jos. A. Smith from *Hands of Light* by Barbara Brennan.)

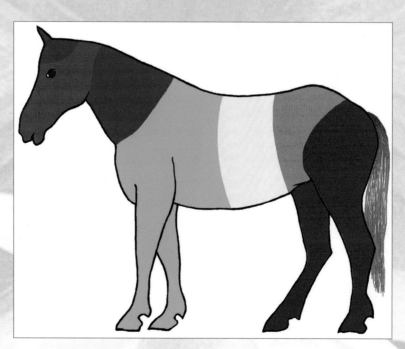

Plate 32. Here, the chakra areas of the horse are depicted in the same colors as are associated with the human chakra system, and healing is similarly performed on the animal from top to bottom. Healing is claimed to be as effective on animals as it is on humans, a fact often cited to prove that healing does not require faith in the one being healed. An analogous argument regarding treatment of animals suggests that homeopathy does not depend upon the placebo effect. Nonetheless, the animal's trust in the human healer may be effectual, but it seems unlikely that any animal would have any concept quite like our own notion of the placebo, and if the animal were unaware of a flavorless dose secreted in its food the placebo could hardly operate as it does in humans who are aware of being treated.

Plate 33. On the left of this diagram the mechanism of chemical combination of proteins and similar molecules, often referred to as "docking," is shown. The diagram is schematic and very much simplified. At *1* two molecules approach one another and oppositely charged points on the molecules attract each other. These points are, roughly speaking, the "docking" sites, points available for attachment by other molecules. The molecules then combine *chemically* by intimate *physical* contact, the opposed electric charges being shared, and so neutralized. This is a more or less stable state. The resulting combined state is shown at *2,* where the oppositely charged docking sites, now held in chemical combination, are indicated by arrows. However, recent research, theory, and calculation suggest that such chemical combination could not occur sufficiently often, or sufficiently quickly, for the body to function, which indicates that a faster, easier process must be at work. Field theory provides the explanation currently accepted, and this is shown, also simply and schematically, at *3.* The molecules do not have to approach closely, or physically "touch" each other, but interact, while still relatively distant, via their electromagnetic fields. James Oschman, in his book *Energy Medicine: The Scientific Basis*, gives a good introduction to all such matters, topically on pages 121 and following, where he also provides a more advanced diagram of an example of the field effect pictured very simply here.

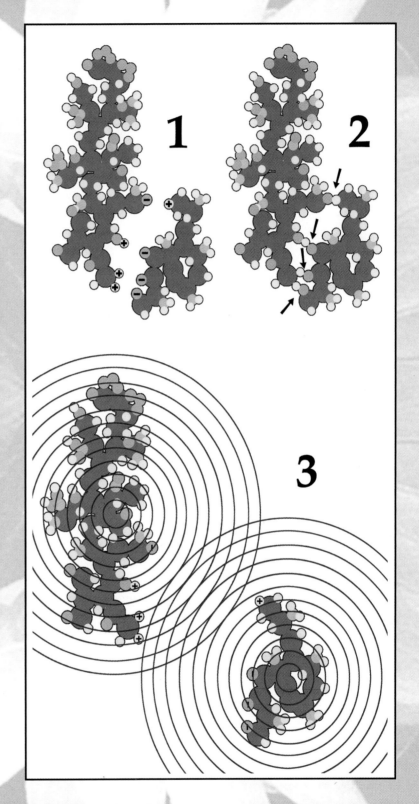

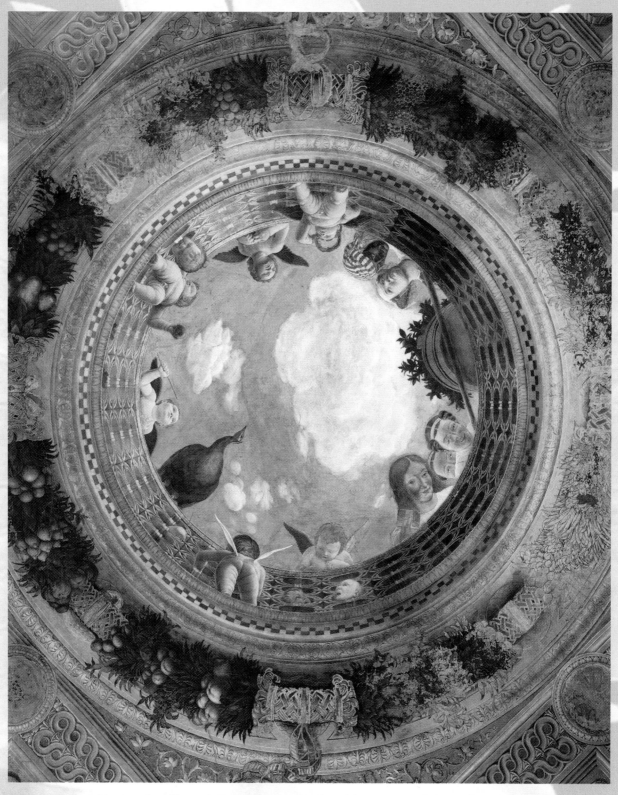

Plate 34. Andrea Mantegna's ceiling painting in the ducal palace, Mantua, one of the earliest such works, foreshadowed later attempts to depict the World-Above without human figures. Since all attempts to portray the invisible must fail, some much later artists turned instead to a new kind of spirituality, again entirely grounded in the human world-about, but attempting to convey spiritual awareness through the natural world itself, without emblematical figures of any kind. (Photograph © DeA Picture Library/Art Resource, New York.)

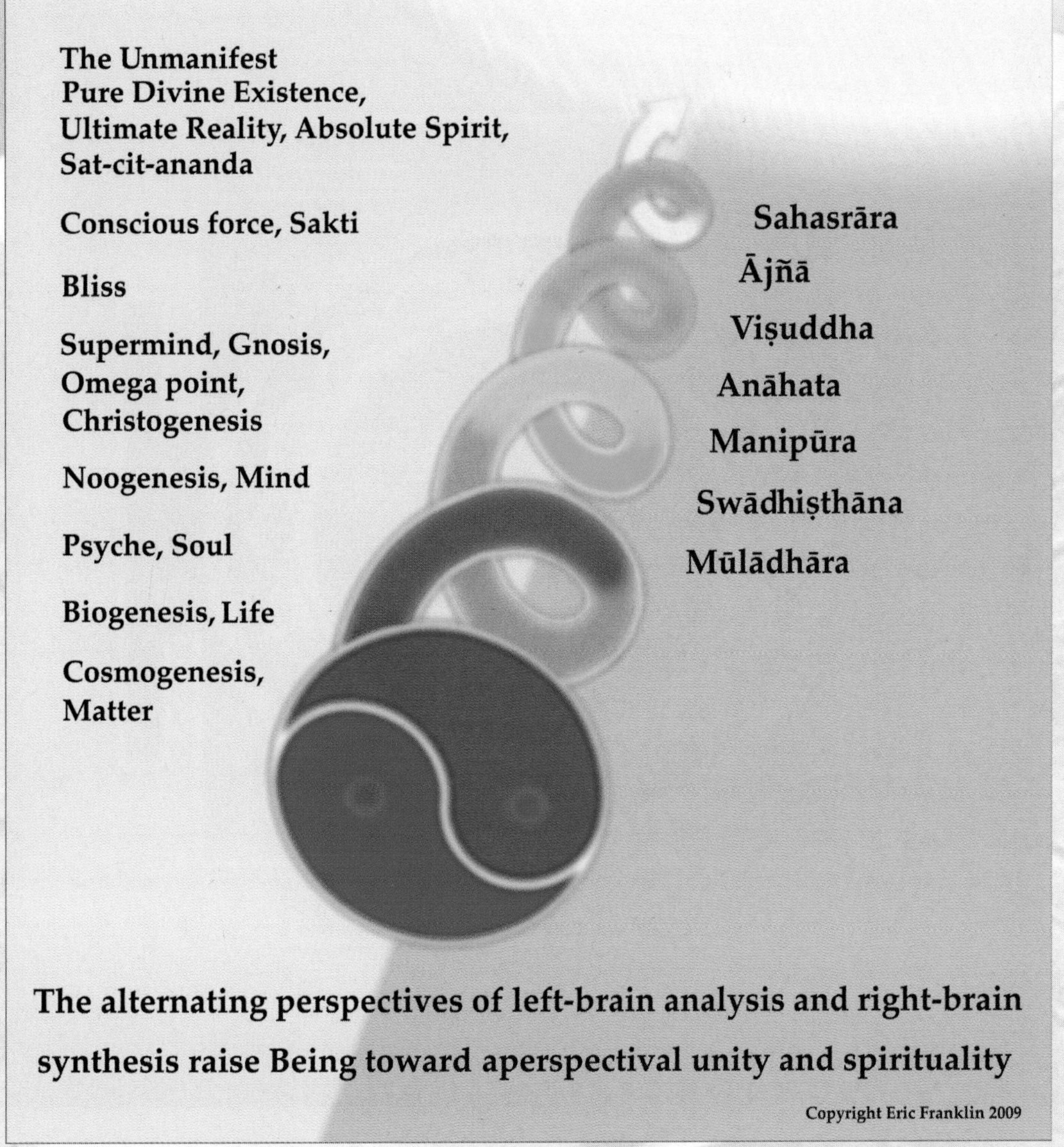
The Unmanifest
Pure Divine Existence,
Ultimate Reality, Absolute Spirit,
Sat-cit-ananda
Conscious force, Sakti
Bliss
Supermind, Gnosis,
Omega point,
Christogenesis
Noogenesis, Mind
Psyche, Soul
Biogenesis, Life
Cosmogenesis,
Matter
Sahasrāra
Ājñā
Viṣuddha
Anāhata
Manipūra
Swādhiṣthāna
Mūlādhāra
The alternating perspectives of left-brain analysis and right-brain synthesis raise Being toward aperspectival unity and spirituality
Copyright Eric Franklin 2009

Plate 35. Here in the world-about we live and think as we must, repeatedly analyzing and resynthesizing our understanding, and as we do so we progress, enlarging our consciousness from our initial limitedness toward the Oneness out-from which our very Being seems originally to have been born, to appear in this lower world into which, as Heidegger puts it, we have been "thrown." Spiritual growth is our way back, not, of course, a physical climb, but as if climbing the spiral path around a ziggurat, toward the Above.

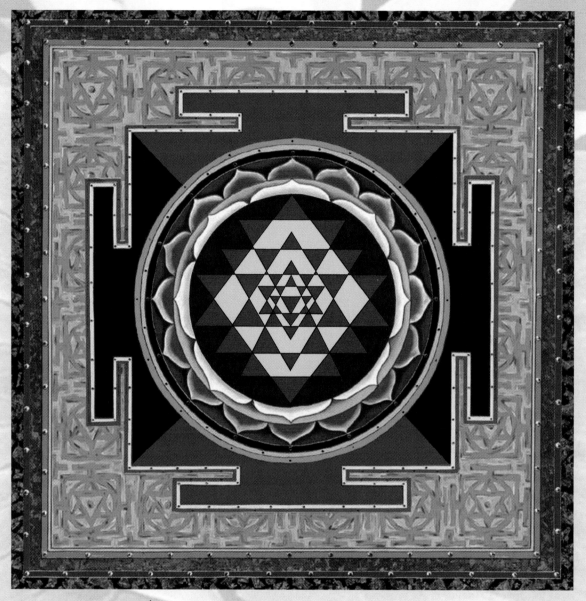

Plate 36. The Śri Yantra is the supreme sacred symbol, encapsulating the essence of Indian thought. At the center of this mystical construction, formed by the interpenetration of two sets of triangles, four with apex upward, representing the male principle, and five with apex downward, representing the female principle, is the *bindu,* the point of origin of the supreme consciousness from which everything issues and to which everything returns. The yantra is devised to give a vision of the totality of existence and hence has multiple layers of metaphysical meaning. Used both in rituals and in meditation, it activates the correspondences between the human as microcosm and the macrocosm through the internal yantras of the subtle body, revealing timeless truths that have inspired humans toward self-transcendence for thousands of years.

The recognition of a state of complete and balanced health that, in the present-day West, is beginning to be referred to as integral psychology is apparent. The Latin *Mens sana in corpore sano* (A sound mind in a sound body) is now coming to have deeper and fuller meaning than in any past era of the civilization that gave rise both to it and to modern Europe.

The American Buddhist teacher Sharon Salzberg, in her influential book *Loving Kindness,* offers the explanation that spiritual practice, by uprooting our personal mythologies of isolation, uncovers the radiant, joyful heart within each one of us and manifests this radiance to the world. We find, beneath the wounding concepts of separation, a connection both to ourselves and to all beings. She says that the Buddha described the spiritual path that leads to this freedom as "the liberation of the heart which is love" and he taught a systematic, integrated path that moves the heart out of isolating contraction into true connection.[25] The meditation practices that cultivate love, compassion, sympathetic joy, and equanimity are called, in Pali, the language spoken by the Buddha, the *brāhma-vihāras* (*brāhma* "heavenly," *vihara* "abode" or "home"). By practicing these meditations, we establish love (*metta*), compassion (*karuna*), sympathetic joy (*mudita*), and equanimity (*upekkha*) as our home.

Some Tantric practitioners believe that Buddhism, especially Vajrayana, better equips them to unravel the roots of suffering. Tantra embraces Yoga, with its postures (*āsanas*), breath control exercises (*prānāyāma*), and withdrawal of the senses from outer distractions (*pratyāhāra*), all of which make sitting still in meditation easier. The experience of mindfulness through the stillness of the gross body (*sthūla śarīra*) more readily facilitates awareness of the subtle body (*sūkṣma śarīra*), the mobilization and harmonization of energy, and the cultivation of the qualities that the Buddha regarded as the "skillful means" of bringing benefit and happiness. Buddhist Tantra places the heart at the center of all of them.

The Timeless Body

As will now be clear from the variety of traditions we have examined, the idea of a hierarchy of bodies, sheaths, or kośas is widely accepted as a "map" of human consciousness, though the bodies may vary in number, by means of which the aspirant may discover his or her own route to transcendence.

Historically, the model of the five kośas evolved during a period of self-discovery, of awareness of self, intellect (knowledge of a seemingly objective world), and individual willpower, which led to a dualist view. The Buddhist writer Roar Bjonnes suggests that this could be considered as the "adolescent stage" of humanity in terms of conscious understanding and intelligent evolution.[26] It could be related to our breaking away from the womb (mother nature), questioning and formulating our own inquiry, opinions, worldview, concepts, and beliefs, and then attempting an autonomous existence. As in adolescence, critical, rebellious, and creative thought dominate.

Bjonnes suggests that there are two stages of development in the first of which life is broken down into its constituent parts (*samkhya*) and in the second, as a result of yoga practice, the "map" itself is altered as an evolved, "timeless" body comes into being. Working on the "organs" of the subtle body through spiritual practice, he suggests, removes impurities from the gross body. Freeing the subtle pathways allows the mind and emotions to become disentangled from confusion and illusion. Through this "bright body" as he calls it, the dharma-kāya, or "adamantine body," the formless realm outside of time and space, becomes fully charged, inspired, and spiritualized.[27]

Thus the ānanda-maya-kośa is full of bliss and beauty when the gateway of the sahasrāra chakra has opened and becomes the sambhoga-kāya, the "bliss body" of Buddha. As the will and intellect no longer dominate, the subtle body is purified, activated, and refined and the gross body and the subtle body begin to act as one. "Here," Bjonnes says, "the end of ignorance is realised, hence [also] the end of suffering and bondage."[28]

He goes on to say that after all the karma has been cleaned up, there is only a seed potential, deep within the ānanda-maya-kośa. Here there is no sthūla (gross), sūkṣma (subtle), or even kārana (causal) śarīra. "This is *Śiva* in his absolute, formless, state (*nirguna*), timeless, but replete. . . . Here the mystery of absolute emptiness (*sunyata*), devoid of any constituent thing, and absolutely complete, is represented as the infinite buddha potential that permeates all of time and space, the *Tathagatagarbha,* the heart of hearts, the *hridayam,* the causal essence which itself has no cause."[29]

EIGHT

The Taoist Body of Inner Alchemy

Chinese terminology reflects subtle differences between states of a more or less ethereal quality, but of one and the same principle lying at the foundation of all the complex functions of man. The gross conditions of the body are as much included as are its finer essences and the higher mental states which make up holiness. This . . . is the reason why one can say that the Chinese do not make a clear-cut distinction between what we call body and mind. Their outlook is in general much more oriented towards life as an organic whole and ongoing process.

M. KALTENMARK, *LA MYSTIQUE TAOISTE*

In a contribution to *Esoterica,* the editor, religious studies professor Lee Irwin, tells us that the primary indigenous Chinese religion, Taoism, has a complex history. A highly esoteric tradition, it has many different strands, which evolved over thousands of years. It combines practices of meditation, spirit communication, conscious projection, physical movements, medicine, and "internal alchemy" within the theoretical frame of a profound transpersonal philosophy of nature and a metaphysics of human relationships, which is itself based on an ideal of spiritual transformation leading to immortality.[1]

In her introduction to *The Taoist Experience,* Livia Köhn, professor emerita of Chinese and Japanese religions, states that Taoism is an unknown and enigmatic, yet pervasive and ubiquitous, aspect of Chinese, even East Asian, religion and culture. She believes Taoism has greatly influenced Eastern thinking both as an organized religion and as a philosophy, as well as shaping the attitudes of individuals toward their lives and

the world. Taoism is not a religious system defined in terms of a founder, doctrines, pantheon of deities, scriptures, and practices. Its beliefs, doctrines, and deities appear in an incoherent jumble, mixing Buddhism and Confucianism, Chinese medicine and divination, alchemy and shamanism into a wondrous and multifaceted combination. Still, Köhn says that recent studies of Taoism in the West have helped to unravel its doctrinal intricacies and historical developments, making its complexity accessible, despite the obvious fact that no systematic *description* of the Taoist path can ever do justice to the actual *experience* of the religion.*

---

*This is true of all experience, an ubiquitous, unavoidable consequence of our being in the world. No description can be one and the same as what is described, but the descriptive "map" may be serviceable in the quest for the experience. A script and the play itself, as performed and attended, is an obvious example of this structure of referential relation (not identity) between our consciousness of it as a *reality* and of its mere *mapping.*

Lawrence Sullivan, professor of theology and anthropology, tells us that knowledge of the body is central to the history of religions in the form of physiologies that are religiously experienced and religiously expressed.[2] This being so, he asks "what kind of body should an individual attempt to acquire or cultivate, given his or her understanding of important powers attributed to the divine?" We saw in studying other traditions that *transformation* of the physical body is thought necessary if the embodied soul is to attain union with the universal soul, as in the jīvan-mukta. If this is so, the question next arising is whether a subtle body is necessary for this ascension to be accomplished.

Body and Cosmos

Kristofer Schipper, who is not only former professor emeritus of oriental studies at Leiden and religious studies at the Sorbonne but an initiated Taoist priest, suggests in his book *The Taoist Body* that the Taoist tradition has several ways of recognizing the relationship between the body and the cosmos. He classifies them as follows:

Theological: The cosmological system and the grand universal design that underlies it, with its elaborate system of correspondences, is linked to specific understandings of transcendental principles, including at least essential energies, souls, breaths, and notions of divinity associated with the composition of the body.

Symbolic: The body becomes an immense landscape during practices that heighten interior vision and reveal the laws and secrets of the universe through the exploration of this inner landscape.

Empirical: Instrumental therapies, such as acupuncture, based on a theory of elements and energy flows along meridians.[3]

Schipper argues that, of these three categories, only the specifically Taoist symbolic vision of the body is associated with a meaningful mythology. He explains that the heart of bodily vision is located deep within the interior world of the body and, in the most ancient descriptions, has no counterpart in the wider macrocosm. Only by turning the pupils of our eyes inward,

thereby channeling the astral luminescence of the outer sky down into the dark abyss of our inner physical mass, can we transform our eyes into the brilliant sun and moon of the interior universe. Through physical training, Schipper says, we can learn to illuminate the inner landscape and concentrate all light in its center in the middle of the forehead, between the brows,* a point identified with the Pole Star.† By this means, we create what he likens to a laser: the beams of light from the eyes are concentrated in the mirror-like center between the brows, which then reflects light into the depths of the body.[4] We cannot comment on how closely this might correspond with the findings of neuroscience, but note that the awareness of the outer sky and the Pole Star already marks a widening of the conscious view beyond its earlier limits, which recorded no parallel between inner and outer worlds. Since the earliest documents do not contain such references, this provides evidence of the increase of human consciousness of which Gebser wrote during the history of Taoism. It is also evidence of the syncretic thinking that produced the Vedic view of the universe, with the human a microcosm that is aligned with the polar axis of the macrocosm, the axis mundi.

Schipper describes the human inner landscape in some detail, from the highest chain of mountain peaks within the head, also the location of the "upper cinnabar field," to the lowest center, the "lower cinnabar field" (see plate 21).[5] The heart has an important position in Taoist meditation. Known as the "middle cinnabar field," its description and location show its resemblance to the hṛtpādma, the "secret heart" of the Tantric traditions. Each meditative position has a different inner landscape and inhabitants, which the initiate must come to know. Some are fierce and menacing and others helpful.

The key principles of structure and meaning in Taoist philosophy are change, mutation, transformation,

---

*In the Indian system this is the ājñā chakra.

†As we have seen elsewhere in Eastern belief, this is a recurrence of the symbol of the axis mundi. In this case it is the projection of the still center of the turning world upon the night sky, particularly to the more or less stationary star nearest to the envisioned extension of the axis through the poles, named for that reason the "Pole Star." Other connotations of the axis mundi were also present in the (later) Taoist mind, just as in the Hindu and Buddhist mind. (See the information in chapter 2.)

and flux. However, the flux takes place always within a wholeness, movement here being balanced by an opposite movement there. "The Dao, the most fundamental power of the Daoist universe . . . is always a totality."[6]* Known as the "Great One" in Taoist cosmology, it is the underlying principle, the primordial vital energy, the *yuangqi*.

Taoism, like most other religions, went through various phases of development. In one of its most significant phases, during the Han dynasty (206–6 BCE), it evolved various practices to attain immortality, physical longevity, and free spiritual access to the world of gods and spirits. "Crucial to the religious experience of Daoism," says Köhn, "the Dao is always there, yet has always to be attained, realized, perfected . . . to realise it one must go truly beyond."[7] Here Taoism parallels the Hindu traditions, with their quest for immortality even while in the physical body, the jīvan-mukta state, and so acknowledges a "spiritual" being living in or in some sense alongside the physical living body.

Mysticism and Meditation

Although the body plays a much more central role in Taoist mysticism than in any comparable Western model, Köhn says that descriptions of personal mystical experiences in the Taoist tradition are hard to find. She explains that this is because authors typically refrain by choice from becoming too personal, the overall tendency in the literature being, instead, to express the experiences of the mystic in generalized instructions and the listing of warning signs.[8] She compares this to Western religions where experience is pivotal and is described as overwhelming, ineffable, timeless, and yet full of knowing certainty[9] and where mystics have described its wonders time and again, as well as their agonies when it eluded them for a period in the so-called dark night of the soul.[10]

The challenge for the mystic, says Köhn, is not to overcome the body in favor of the spirit but to transform the entire body-spirit continuum to a higher level, in which the self is experienced as the divine replica of the cosmos in oneness with the Tao. This reminds us again of the jīvan-mukta and again shows Taoism's acknowledgement of a duality in our being. It is also an early realization of a truth now being perceived in the West, that earthly life must include acceptance of the body. We cannot live on earth, that is in the *physical* world, without the *physical* body, and life on earth is therefore maimed if we attempt to live it without the body's full complement of faculties in operation. This is obvious, a mere truism, yet we have lived for millennia as if it were not true, as if permitting the body fulfillment of its promptings were in all instances sin, yet our very being, as embodied humans, is being-*in-the-world,* all our perspectives depending upon the dipole of consciousness and world which would be meaningless, indeed, nonexistent, without both the body, with its perceptual apparatus, and a world perceivable thereby.

As if to confirm this, Köhn points out that the Chinese tradition sees the Tao as a divine force so strongly immanent and so much a part of the world that Oneness or union is the birthright of every being, not a rare instance of divine grace. She states that it is natural to begin with, and becomes more so as it is realized through practice. The Chinese mystical experience of oneness with the Tao, quite logically, is astounding only in the beginning. It represents a way of being in the world quite different from what is ordinarily perceived. The longer the Taoist lives with the experience and the deeper she integrates it into her life and being, the less relevant it is, or, it perhaps better phrased, the less obtrusive and surprising it is. Thus, Köhn concludes, "neither is the experience itself the central feature of the tradition, nor is there a pronounced "dark night of the soul," a desperate search for a glimpse of the transcendent divine."[11]

Taoist Meditation

The earliest document describing the form of Taoist meditation appeared in the Han dynasty. There are three basic "actions" in Taoist meditation: "concentration," "insight," and "ecstatic excursions," which are always linked together in practice and are all aimed toward the goal of immortality. The three actions are described as follows:

> *Concentration* is not only the foundation for meditation or higher spiritual exercises but the "rooting"

---

*The terms *Tao* (*Taoism*) and *Dao* (*Daoism*) are both correct. Authors quoted may use either in different works.

of the gods in the body, and leads to insight and ecstatic journeys to the other world.

Insight, borrowed from Buddhism and coupled with the concept of *sati,* "mindfulness," a state of active mental watchfulness or constant presence of mind, is a method of observing and evaluating the self and others, and attempting to apply the worldview of the Tao to our life and being.

Ecstatic excursions evolved from an earlier phase of shamanic journeying. When the physical body is left behind "the soul of the meditator surges up and beyond, meeting divine powers and spirits of the stars" and so becomes one with the Tao on its own plane.[12]

Concentration

While the three aspects are identifiable components of meditation, they are not seen as separate techniques, each guaranteeing a precisely determined different experience. Rather, they are seen as spontaneous results of meditation, particularly the second and third. In fact, one of the earliest techniques of Taoist meditation is based not on a wish to concentrate, or to gain insight, or to experience ecstatic travel, but on the more mundane matter of a medical analysis of the body. The visualization of different colored lights corresponding to different parts of the body was matched to the energies and their storage places within. This reminds us of Sufi beliefs and practices. The Taoist practice is known as the "ingestion of the five sprouts," and refers to the energy of "the five directions."[13]

The instructions from the *Taiping jing shengjun bizhi* (Secret Instructions of the Holy Lord on the Scripture of Great Peace) state that Great Peace can be attained by sitting quietly with eyes closed and "guarding the light of the One." Upon practicing this for a long time a brilliant light arises, in the radiance of which all five directions can be seen. By following it, the meditator can travel far, both beyond the body and deeply within the body. The scripture states that the host of spirits will assemble and that the physical body can be transformed into pure spirit.[14]

Although the Taoist concept of *dantiens* (energy centers, correlated with the zones) does not precisely parallel the Indian system of chakras, there is something closer to an exact mapping between the chakras and the colored lights in the Taoist practice of "guarding the light of the One," through which, the doctrine states, the meditator can "go beyond the world and ascend to heaven."[15] Thus we read:

> In guarding the light of the One, you may see a light as bright as the rising sun. This is a brilliance as strong as that of the sun at noon.
>
> In guarding the light of the One, you may see a light entirely green. When this light is green, it is the light of lesser yang.
>
> In guarding the light of the One, you may see a light entirely red, just like fire. This is a sign of transcendence.
>
> In guarding the light of the One, you may see a light entirely yellow. When this develops a greenish tinge, it is the light of central harmony. This is a potent remedy of the Tao.
>
> In guarding the light of the One, you may see a light entirely white. When this is as clear as flowing water, it is the light of lesser yin.
>
> In guarding the light of the One, you may see a light entirely black. When this shimmers like deep water, it is the light of greater yin.[16]

The meditator is then told that if he or she sees nothing but utter darkness without and blackness within, this is the light of human disease, and requires medicine. After medicine has been obtained, an attempt should be made to see any of the seven lights. There are further instructions in this text concerning meditations on emptiness and nonbeing, the regions of the body, the gods residing in the "five orbs" or the five elements, on foreign gods, and the ancestors.

Early meditations often combined practices, which included techniques aimed at achieving longevity and the health of parts of the body, rituals, alchemy, and visualizations of the gods, while later practices became simplified and focused upon keeping the thoughts from scattering, and on pulling energy together and harmonizing it, a process regarded as "the swiftest path to the Dao."[17]

Insight

The second of the three basic forms of meditation, described above, is "insight." Insight meditation is focused on a conscious inspection of the body-mind and its energies in relation to the constant movement of nature and the world. Taoists have to learn how to maintain a high awareness of their actions together with a strong sense of detachment and equanimity. Insight practice, Köhn explains, consists of two kinds of observations: observation of energy and observation of spirit. As body and spirit are not seen as distinct substances in Taoism, but as different aspects of a continuum, the human body is regarded as part of the same framework, as an accumulation of the cosmic, vital energy, known as *qi*.

The indeterminate essence of qi is *jing,* which is best understood in Western terms as "primal matter." It is the raw fuel that drives the pulsating rhythm of the body's moment-to-moment cellular division and reproduction of itself.[18] In its concrete form jing in the body appears as sexual energy and sexual fluids, so Taoist practices begin with control and reorientation of sexual energy, as practiced by some schools of Indian and Tibetan yoga. Some commentators see this as similar to the psychological "technique" of Freudian sublimation, others see it as kundalinī, and some claim that kundalinī itself is a "sublimated" or redirected orgasmic energy. Others vigorously repudiate this. Jing is purified through body movements, breathing exercises, meditations, visualizations, and rituals, which make it more subtle and transform it into qi. Moved consciously around the body in various cycles, it is eventually moved upward. In that movement it is further rarified and turned into shen (spirit).

Shen is understood to be the inherent higher vitality of life, as consciousness, the ability to think. Closely related to the individual's personality, it is said to reside in the heart, where it governs the emotions and has the most important impact on mystical transformation. Spirit, shen, the goal of mystical attainment, transformed from the baser form of qi, is understood as our true nature, as part of the Tao.

Ecstatic Excursion

The task, says Michael Winn, a longtime practitioner of both Indian and Chinese traditional techniques, is "to understand the unconscious communication patterns that are always flowing between one's microcosmic (personal) qi-field and the impersonal (macrocosmic)

qi-field."[19] Thus, insight meditation will give rise to the third and highest kind, the ecstatic excursion, in parallel with the process of the raising of the jing up through the body into the head, where it will become shen. This also, then, parallels kundalinī or may even be the same experience.

This threefold development of meditation practice parallels precisely the structural concept of the three dantiens. However, language does not allow us to communicate two matters at once, but only in linear or serial fashion, so it can be difficult to convey a complete picture by words, even when augmented by diagrams.

The Dantiens

The dantien concept itself is entirely Taoist in origin. Early Taoist sects believed that certain deities called the "Three Pure Ones" dwelt in these areas of the body. Later Taoist sects, focusing on internal alchemy, saw them as places in the body where the internal elixir was produced. Taoist internal alchemy is the art of bringing the qi (energy) into balance through gathering, storing, and circulating it for physical well-being and spiritual transformation. The word *dantien* (sometimes spelled *tan tien*) literally means "elixir-field" and a contemporary qigong* teacher has referred to them as "energy-incubators."

The three dantiens are arranged in a hierarchy. A variety of spiritual impressions is nurtured in them, including heightened emotion and consciousness. In its stationary or "condensed" state a dantien does not occupy the whole of its zone but is active in the center of it. When they are in their expanded state the dantiens act as relay stations for the transmission of the self into the universe and the universe into the self. This function is like that of the chakras of the Indian traditions, active in both immanence and transcendence. In this expanded mode dantiens coordinate the impressions of self and universe. From a larger perspective, the body or universe as a

---

Qigong, pronounced "chee gung," which is sometimes spelt *chi kung* and is often printed as two words, *qi gong,* comes from the words *qi* meaning "energy" and *gong* meaning "cultivation." Described in detail below, it is sometimes referred to as "energy work" or even "breath work." Qigong differs from *tai chi,* which is a martial art originally designed to maim and kill opponents but which now concentrates only on self-defense.

whole can be related as dantiens or even as two mutually interpenetrating dantiens. Further, any body part can be made into a dantien, but here we shall use the word simply to refer to any of the three main dantiens recognized by Taoism and shown in the diagrams.

The Lower Dantien

This dantien is in the lowest part of the torso. Imagine a down-pointing triangle linking the *qi-hai,* just below the navel, the point opposite this on the spine (*mingmen,* the Gate of Life) and the perineum (*huiyin,* the Gate of Death). Within it and slightly lower than its center is the lower dantien. It is often associated with the "Sperm Palace" in men and the ovaries in women.

The lower dantien is the furnace for prebirth and physical qi; earth generative and root energies have a close affinity with it. In Taoist internal alchemy the vital essence or jing is refined here. In qigong the attempt is made to nurture the prebirth and physical qi and unlock its potential for spiritual growth. By expanding into and condensing energies from earth as well as cosmos, a new center is formed. This center, as fine as air, having a fiery core and a periphery as large as the universe, motivates the energy of transformation. The energy can move outward for the skillful empowerment of everyday life, or inward and upward in subtle internal alchemy.

The Middle Dantien

This dantien is in the middle of the torso. Some texts indicate its position at the solar plexus, others in the heart region. Many qigong practitioners will find that it is in fact movable between these two sites. Emotion is generated here, along with post-birth qi, which is accumulated from the essence of air and food. In Taoist internal alchemy, qi, or vital energy, is refined here. Esoteric Buddhism focuses in this area to visualize an enlightened form of self that expands into the universe to achieve a "mutual empowerment of self and other."

The quality of consciousness and qi that accompanies the middle dantien is subtler than in the lower dantien. Being associated with emotional warmth, the middle dantien is often a locus for the development of enlightened self-care and the care of others. Its image should be beautiful, its feeling-sense warm and pure, its emotional tone loving and serenely happy. When working with this dantien we recollect these qualities from

the beginning, move out toward them in expansion, and collect them on condensation. Fully nurtured, we can then radiate them outward in self-expression, or turn them inward, descending to nurture the vital essence or ascending to even more subtle spiritual realms.

The Upper Dantien

This dantien is found by imagining a line running from the medulla, at the base of the skull, to the third eye, between the eyebrows. At roughly the midpoint on that line is the upper dantien. Perhaps owing to the brain's centrality in all we do, we make a general association between the upper dantien and perception. Also, four of the five senses are sited in the head. In qigong the quality and depth of perception is important. Deep perception is attained by focusing awareness on the spatial nature of consciousness; quality perception is attained by identifying the consciousness with spiritual light. These are coordinated through the upper dantien, where spiritual and mental qi reside. In Taoist internal alchemy the vital spirit is cultivated in the upper dantien and the essence of qigong practice with it is to harness and focus mental and spiritual qi to expand consciousness and perception. The image, when working with this dantien, is almost always of pure light. Its feeling-sense is spacious, detached, clear.

Earlier, colored lights seen in meditation and their meanings were described. Briefly, utter darkness shows illness, but light as bright as the rising sun may be seen. Entirely green light is that of lesser yang; entirely red, like fire, signifies transcendence; yellow light, if green-tinged, is of central harmony, a potent remedy; entirely white is of lesser yin; entirely black, shimmering like deep water, the light of greater yin.

Microcosmic Orbit

In the third stage of transformation of jing to shen, which may include ecstatic excursions in the third mode of meditation, long periods of intense concentration and stillness are required. After ten months of nurturing the primordial qi, the newly developed subtle body, the immortal embryo, is ready to be born. For this, it is moved gradually upward along the spine until it reaches the upper cinnabar field in the head. From there it can leave the body through the top of the head, undertaking excursions to the celestial spheres as it pleases. The birth of the embryo as a free-moving spirit power signifies the adept's rebirth on a new level and the gaining of a new *yin* body, an immortal being of softness, purity, and light.[20] This spiritual rebirth is not described in great detail in the texts, but, Köhn points out, the yin body is said to be transformed into a body of pure *yang* through deeper meditation. It eventually becomes pure, luminous spirit, and is then reintegrated into cosmic emptiness. Note the persistence of sexual and natal symbolism.

There is a certain similarity between Tantric kundalinī practices and the willed circulation of qi known as the "microcosmic orbit," in that both make interior energy flow backward up the spine. In Taoism the goal is to circulate qi throughout the body and gradually build a spiritual self within, while in laya yoga the energy is guided in a linear fashion through the chakras to achieve union with the Absolute, somewhere above the head.[21] Despite these differences, there is also a resemblance to hatha yoga in that yang is seen as "solar energy" while yin is "lunar," and both systems anticipate a merging of these two forces in the inner alchemical process.

Lu K'uan-yü (1898–1978), translator and interpreter of Chinese Buddhist texts from the Ch'an and Zen traditions, explains that once the circulation or orbit is established, the qi energy is guided inward to the center of the body, where it is progressively refined and transmuted through the three centers, the lower, middle, and upper "elixir fields" or dantiens; the goal being to create an immortal spirit body through which the person can function on a higher plane of existence than the ordinary physical body.[22]

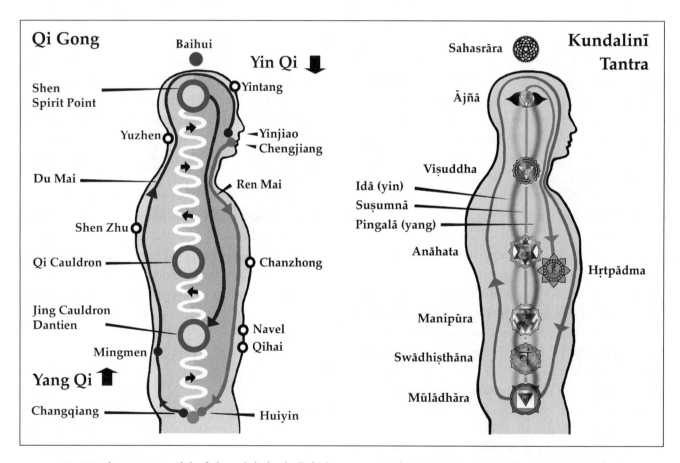

Fig. 8.1. The Taoist model of the subtle body (left) has some similarities to the Tantric model (right). The qi energy points and the dantiens, the main energy centers, are virtually parallel to the chakras. The circulation of energy in the Taoist practice is known as the "microcosmic orbit." Energy is guided up the spine, over the head from back to front, down the front, up in a spiral motion back to the head, and then focused in the dantien at the navel. This closely resembles certain kriya yoga practices in which the prāna (energy) is drawn up through the main spinal channel (suṣumnā nadi), down through the front (alambusa nadi), next up through and around each chakra, sending energy to the areas they govern, on upward to the crown, then ending in the "secret heart" (hṛtpādma) at the level of the diaphragm.

Since emphasis is on the dynamic flow and circulation of qi energy, very little importance is placed on the chakras themselves, these being, at most, points or stations of attention within the overall microcosmic orbit. One can, however, associate the three dantiens, located below the navel, behind the solar plexus, and in the center of the head, and the heart center (which is itself sometimes considered to be the middle dantien) with chakras.

We saw in chapter 1 that the Indian concept of energy is probably the earliest and most coherent hypothesis to the effect that there is a life force permeating all existence. By about 5000 BCE, a rudimentary model of prāna (energy) emerged, with polar opposite energies, the idā and pingalā, and a central channel, the suṣumnā, in which idā and pingalā combine to give the kundalinī experience. This is similar to the Chinese model of the qi, acting in its polar opposite modes, the yin and the yang, which appeared by about 3000 BCE. See the diagram on the previous page and compare it with the illustration of kundalinī printed alongside.

In the world of Taoism and Chinese medicine, qi is the material energy of the universe, the basic stuff of nature, as well as the life force in the human body, the basis of all physical vitality. There is only one qi, just as there is only one Tao, but it appears at different levels of subtlety and in different modes in inner, meditational experience. Primordial, prenatal, true, or perfect qi is contrasted with postnatal qi or earthly qi. There is *zheng qi* that flows harmoniously through the body and the world, creating health and harmony, in contrast to *xie qi,* which is deviant, wayward energy, causing upheaval and disease. There is the qi that is the root of, and stands between, the other key forms of body energy, the jing (essence) and shen (spirit), already mentioned. It is important to remember that these are seen as *modes of operation* of one kind of energy rather than as entirely independent energetic entities. There is qi that can be protective and nutritive; qi that is the yang counterpart to *xue* (blood); qi that transforms in the working of the "triple heater"* into various forms to nurture and energize the body.[23]

In the human imagination of the time of early Taoism, the concept of *qi* extended over a grand conflation denoting anything perceptible but intangible: atmosphere, smoke, aroma, vapor, a sense of intuition, foreboding, even ghosts. These were the more or less observable instances of an invisible essence, which human mindfulness had, by that date, evolved sufficiently to conceive. What would have been difficult for the mind of that era to grasp and hold was the notion that an "essence," a "being," might be totally imperceptible by the outward sense organs. Conflation was thus a natural process, a crutch for understanding, producing a hypothesis that was not seen until much later as being in need of testing. Such philosophy of science would have to wait some millennia of more or less blind investigation before human curiosity turned to examine the method of science itself. Meanwhile, the science of the time posited four (or five) elements, of which fire was perceptible, yet almost intangible, ethereal. It seemed obvious, at that period, that the nature or desire of fire was to rise toward the realm of the gods, for that was evidently its natural place or home. Such anthropomorphic notions remained acceptable explanations until at least the time of Aristotle.

In our attempt to produce a correct understanding of all the traditions, including the Western, we should note, before continuing, and in preparation for later chapters, that some contemporary writers on Taoist meditation and the subtle body have equated Chinese esotericism with specific Western esotericisms. Edwin Shendelman's *The Vision of the Body,* for example, compares the three body zones of qigong practice to the seventeenth-century Christian hermetic emblems of Robert Fludd. We shall begin to examine Western traditions in chapter 10, but now we must turn, in our necessarily linear treatment of the subject, to qigong itself, a *medico-energetic* theory, method, and practice.

Energy Cultivation: The Practice of Qigong

Qigong is a part of traditional Chinese medicine that became extremely popular in the West in the later twentieth century. It is both a preventative and a curative method of balancing and promoting energy flow for well-being and self-healing. It is based on the idea that qi is circulated in the bio-energetic system through the energy channels, the meridians, a similar notion to the concept of prāna circulating in the energy currents of the subtle body in the Indian traditions. Traditional Chinese medicine asserts that there are twelve main and

---

*The "triple heater" or "triple burner" is one of the meridians or energy channels of Chinese medicine.

eight secondary meridians carrying qi through the major organs and the whole body. In this system illness is regarded as the result of weak or blocked flow of qi. The blocks or weaknesses are corrected by exercises, which have the purpose of "massaging" the meridians so that the qi can flow freely.

The core of qigong practice employs a system of sophisticated body-mind interactions. For the sake of convenience we speak of distinct body and mind actions, but these converge in a vision of the body that is subtle in form. Mind-image and body-sense gravitate to a number of distinct zones. It is from these zones that the primary alignments (pathways of wholeness), activated in qigong, occur.[24]

While the purpose of qigong is mainly remedial, some practitioners and writers believe that it can also be a tool for experiencing spiritual states, and that it is, therefore, subtle and transformative *in the same way as meditation*. Thus it depends on the will, on conscious direction within the body. Qigong is energy medicine, healing by controlled supply of energy *itself*, rather than by administration of unnatural chemical or even natural herbal preparations as *carriers* of healing energy. Shendelman defines meditation by saying that it is a "gesture of total being" that encompasses and integrates body and mind.[25]

In qigong, the locus of activity of this gesture of total being is usually said to be the body-focus zones containing the dantiens. These are "the hub of the wheel of fundamental meditative intentions," according to Shendelman.[26] Qigong sees the body as having six zones, which are in spatio-*spiritual* relationship. These zones are not static, but interact, their effects being jointly produced. While perceptible as distinct entities, they constitute, above all, an organic, mobile, single wholeness. The six zones are: the Heaven-linking Zone, the Earth-linking Zone, the Lower Dantien, the Middle Dantien, the Upper Dantien, and the Hands, a movable zone.

We give a modified version of the earlier diagram, now showing the six zones, except that of the Hands, which is illustrated separately. It will be noted immediately that the three dantiens almost coincide with the Jing Cauldron, Qi Cauldron, and Shen or Spirit Point, respectively. In a personal situation where individual experience cannot be conveyed precisely to others, and a historical situation in which different systems of nomenclature arose, such confusions are inevitable. It is safe to conclude that the three dantiens are indeed very closely connected with or are even identical to the two Cauldrons and the Spirit Point. The similarity to the chakra system and to the Sufi understanding will also be seen. The three main zones also correlate with Western esoteric conceptions and especially with the works of the medieval alchemists John Dee (1527–1608) and Robert Fludd (1574–1637), and the Jesuit scholar Athanasius Kircher (1601–1680).

Shendelman presents a spiritual approach to qigong because he believes practitioners using this approach will consciously or unconsciously gravitate to the six zones. He states that while some schools of meditation focus on the zones with the intention that all objects of mind may disappear, qigong focuses on them so that the universe, heaven, and earth may appear, moving from the periphery of consciousness into its center. This "both-and" structure, reconnecting what had first been analyzed and understood as separate entities to give an overall vision, which is simultaneously the "bottom up" *and* the "top down" "map," is found in all holisms. Indeed, the very definition of *holism* requires it. Immanence, the "Above" revealed in the mundane sphere, and transcendence, spiritual growth upward from "below," transcending its low origins, thus meet and fuse into one global view.

The Heaven-Linking Zone

The crown of the head is the primary zone of interaction with heavenly energetic realities. "Heaven" means spiritual existence in its nonmaterial, transcendent forms. Within that understanding are many differentiations. We recognize realms of increasing subtlety and a variety of beings and energies existing in them. "Heaven" can also refer to general spiritual transcendence, whether the person becomes conscious of particular realms or not. The physical area of this zone encompasses the crown of the head and adjacent points. These points include the *baihui* (the Heaven Gate, posterior fontanelle area), *yintong* or *yintang* (the Seal Palace, the third eye area), and the *yuzhen* (the Jade Pillow, at the base of the skull). These cover a large area, but the crown itself is the most important part of the zone. The whole crown is a linking area and can become permeable to the energies of heaven. This is desirable, but it is most common for people to become aware of the area by the opening of its adjacent points.

The heaven-linking zone and its major point, the *baihui*, says Shendelman, is surrounded by a great deal of "spiritual lore." He has observed that many people start on a serious spiritual path after having a powerful spiritual experience. An energy-phenomenon on or through the crown of the head has sometimes been reported. This includes events and states such as baptism of the spirit, spiritual initiation, and empowerment. One qigong practitioner, upon simply hearing a holy book being chanted, felt, without any inward participation on his part, an incredibly powerful spiritual energy suffuse him through the crown of his head and pass down to his feet. The Tibetan Buddhist practice of consciousness-transference at the time of death (*phowa*) aims to eject consciousness through this point (via the central channel) rather than through any other point on the body, in order to obtain a high rebirth.

Three potential functions of the heaven-linking zone are:

1. Initiation into direct spiritual growth through an introduction to living spiritual energy.

2. To maintain the current of spiritual transformation by flexing this area through spiritual practices.

3. To open up the ability to ascend through spiritual spheres and, thereby, assist the transcendence of normal life.

The Earth-Linking Zone

The soles of the feet and the base of the spine are the primary zones of interaction with earth energies. One stands or sits on the earth. Important nearby points within this zone include a point a little below the navel (*qihai*) and the opposite point on the spine (*mingmen*, the Gate of Life). To understand the relation of qigong to earth energies it is helpful to review some religious and spiritual understandings of the earth:

1. *Anthropocentric:* this view sees humanity as the goal of God's creation. Earth, in this view, has value in relation to human beings and their fulfillment of God's plan.

2. *World-Denying:* some views of the mystical and

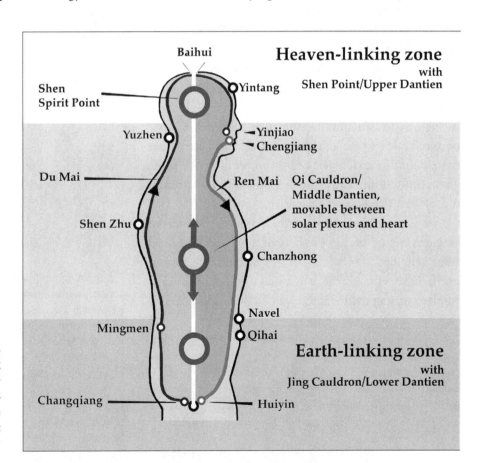

Fig. 8.2. The Heaven-linking zone, Middle Dantien, and Earth-linking zone of the Taoist system correspond approximately to the chakras and also to the three-part division of the body in Western esoteric traditions.

Gnostic type see the earth or earthly existence as a source of suffering, and therefore seek to transcend it. A corollary of this view is that the earth or earthly existence is essentially *unreal.* The spiritual is considered the only true reality (*acosmism*).

3. *Devotional:* in this view the earth is considered a divine being. She can become a source of spiritual meaning when approached in a worshipful way.

4. *Magical/alchemical:* positive spiritual magic sees humans as mediators between different planes of existence. This means that humans can function as "transformers," lowering the heavenly energies to earth level and raising earthly energies to heaven. In internal alchemy the energies of earth are brought within, for personal transformation.

Qigong most fully embodies the *magical/alchemical* point of view within Taoism. This implies that qigong is relational. The practice of qigong enables us to project subtle aspects of ourselves to embrace and harmonize with the earth. We then collect the subtle impression of the earth to act as a transforming agent within ourselves in all dimensions of our being. The Earth-linking zone is the first bodily area activated in this process. Transformation does often imply transcendence, but what we are transcending in qigong is not the earth *per se,* but an experience of reality that is entirely limited to the earth realm and has therefore remained disconnected from its true spiritual nature. The Taoist does not *relinquish* earth as she or he transcends it. She or he grows upward into the heavenly realm with feet remaining, always, firmly on the earth.

In Taoism, humanity's spiritual nature is considered as much a part of the earth as of anywhere else, and some religious antecedents of qigong, such as Taoism itself, have viewed the earth in a worshipful way.* Modern qigong retains the sense of cultivating harmony

---

*Reverence for the earth is important also for the North American "Indian" consciousness, though some other traditions have given it less respect. The account of man's creation in Genesis is not of this character, stressing rather an attitude of power and authority over the earth and its animate species, which has all too often allowed an exploitation of the earth, which ultimately harms the exploiter.

with, and by means of, the earth's own energies. The process is a transcendent one, but does not leave earth behind. Instead, the human self enlarges itself, extends itself upward to embrace heaven as well as earth. It is an *integral* way of being, accepting earth-nature, accepting our own essence as beings-in-the-world, but aspiring to become larger, and so to reach the "Above," to become, whether the term be used or not, a *jīvan-mukta,* to become liberated, immortal while embodied.

The Hands
The Movable Zone

The hands have special functions in qigong. For each of the other five zones the hands have the role of amplifying energies in and around them. They do this through "actions of picking up and pulling back," "expanding outward and condensing inward," in the region of the zones. They can also move energies up and down through the zones, along the *meridians,* either through a general "magnetizing" effect or by actual projection of energy into qi gates.

For the informed outside enquirer, a practitioner's hands are windows into the entire practice of qigong. The powers of giving and receiving, of initiating contact, and of expression, so important in qigong, are seen

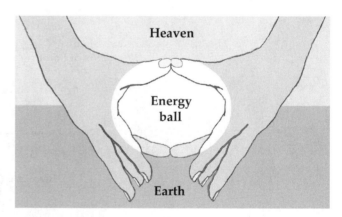

Fig. 8.3. Qigong (energy awareness) is a 5,000-year-old system of self-realization that emerged, in the words of Taoist master Lama Somananda Tantrapa, from "that vast pool of pre-historic Shamanic practices" that spread throughout Asia and Southeast Asia and encompasses Taoist, Buddhist, Tantric, and Confucian thought.[27] In the practices of energy work, such as the visualization of the energy ball depicted here, the hand positions, like the Indian mudras, magnify and expand the inner spiritual reality, "out-picturing" the unseen world and setting changes in motion to balance and heal the complete body-mind.

clearly in the actions of the hands, as though symbolic, analogic, but with real executive effect. Musicians will think immediately of the conductor of an orchestra, whose intentions are conveyed, not a little mysteriously, to the players. Of course, it is possible to doubt, when observing from outside, whether there is a real effect, but this example and others give an illustration of that same *executive intent* that is present in the hand-movements of qigong. Within themselves, the hands open and close, expanding and condensing around the center, the *laogong* (Labor Palace). As extensions to the organism, magnifying and amplifying spiritual realities as projections out from the other energy centers, they revolve and pivot in relation to the greater centers of the torso and the head.

Illumination of the Spiritual Mystery

Naturally, such verbal descriptions are difficult to frame and difficult to understand unless the listener or reader has actual experience or has observed a practitioner at work. Shendelman concludes that the vision of the body in qigong is evinced in the *practice* of qigong. In qigong, illumination of the spiritual mystery is gained in conjunction with, rather than in dissociation from, physical existence and embodiment. Physical and spiritual correlates are envisioned *together,* symbolized, "thrown together" as in the true meanings of the Greek roots of the word *symbol*. This "throwing together" in the mind is done because the visible world of the body is believed to picture the unseen world of the spirit and to have causal relations with it, which operate in both directions (though not necessarily with equal power in both directions).

The six primary body-focus zones in qigong coordinate the mind's impressions of the spiritual mystery so that the mind becomes conscious of them as sensation in these parts of the physical body. Pictured contemplatively by experienced meditators, they *become light;* they are sensed as interior light. The role of the conscious and subconscious mind in such a process is perhaps best seen with some knowledge of Western psychology, or, more particularly, parapsychology. Entities that the mind "throws together," or associates, appear to become *causally* connected; then the *complex* thus formed as a symbolic presence in the mind, the newly symbolized entity thus "thrown together," *itself* becomes causative.

The complex of *non*material will, or belief, becomes an active force in the *material* world. If the belief that the body precisely depicts or maps a world "Above" is paired with the belief that such a world is real, it sets synergies in motion between the *body* and *the belief concerning the higher world*. Belief becomes a tool of the will in the physical world. "As above, so below" *operates,* and is named intentionality.

Again, then, we have a link between Eastern and Western traditions. A number of Western concepts resonate, closely or loosely, with such a schema. Our words "psychosomatic," and "association," the Freudian use of the word "complex," and even the word "psychokinetic" may all have arisen from concepts that, while couched in modern scientific terms, are recognitions of the same truths about our way of being as conscious organisms that Taoists have long accepted. It has been habitual to regard Eastern and Western esotericisms as separate cultures, even as so different as to be antagonistic, but this is an entirely false impression, as we shall see in the following chapters. In discovering their own deep essence, human beings, wherever they happen to live on the globe, have always discovered the same self. Cultures and languages apart, why should East and West differ? Are we not one species, living under one sky? Only extreme racism could prompt a wish to claim that differences so fundamental could exist.

The Transsubstantiated Body

The attainment of the *Light Body,* the "Body of Enlightenment," or transformed body, of Taoism is the ultimate goal of many of the traditions and practices that we have reviewed so far. The *Body of Light* is the spiritual term for the nonphysical *subtle body* that is associated with the transubstantiated or enlightened state. In Taoism, those who have attained it are known as "the immortals" and "the cloudwalkers." We saw that the light body is known as the ānanda-maya-kośa, the "body of bliss," in Hinduism; it is known as the "divine body" in the modern *purna* (holistic) path of integral yoga. In Vedanta it is known as "the superconductive body," in Buddhism as the "diamond body," in Tantra as the "adamantine body," in Sufism as the "supracelestial body" (*jism asli haqiqi*), in early Christianity as the "heavenly" or "risen" or "ascended" body or, in the apostle Paul's words, the body that has "put on immortality."

We have seen that this universal expression of awakening to the presence of God, the Great Being, the All, takes many forms, and is not a single event but a process unfolding over months, years, or lifetimes. Some writers and teachers have referred to the process as the highest of all realizations of human potential. Enlightenment, it is claimed, is not solely psychological, for in the course of higher human development physical changes also occur, most dramatically in the later, and perhaps therefore most rarely seen, stages of the evolving enlightenment. In the final phase, according to various sacred traditions, the body is "alchemically" transformed into light. Enlightenment becomes literally a "light-making," through the transsubstantiation of flesh, blood, and bone into an immortal body of light. To what extent such a claim is to be taken as literally true (if we can define what that would mean), or to what extent it demonstrates the inability of language to describe to those who do not have the experience what something extremely unusual *is in itself* is uncertain. The claim is even made that through a combination of personal effort and divine grace, a human—a being of the earth, the soil—attains a deathless condition through the alchemical transmutation of his or her ordinary flesh body. Ultimately, it is claimed, the quest for enlightenment causes a person actually to become a "being of light." Ethics and goodness are then understood not as mere attainments of a human intellect lately become aware of the sufferings of others, apparently worthy but undeniably merely human value-judgments, but as a human reflection of the divine attributes. The practice of mysticism of all complexions is understood as a process of becoming, quite literally, more and more Godlike.

Conclusions are more difficult still to reach because, although the experience may be common to many traditions, they speak of the process in different ways. For that and other reasons, many questions remain for the seeker of truth. For example, some authorities, the apostle Paul among them, tell us that in at least some instances the change from mortal to immortal takes place "in the twinkling of an eye," not by a long process. So we must ask whether, in the case of one perfected during bodily life, the "immortal body" is newly created "inside" the mortal body? Or, was it already present as if in embryo, then simply manifested from within, as though the physical body were no longer able to withhold the effulgence of the developing light body? Was the light body earlier an "indwelling soul" sufficient only to keep the earth body alive, which has now grown to overcome its entropic degeneration, as if restoring it faster than it deteriorates? Is the light body preexistent within the individual and is the "gross matter" of the material body simply "burned" away, leaving a body that is not in the usual sense physical at all, but merely appears similar? Is the material body altered through a process not yet recognized by science, which changes the atoms of the flesh into something we cannot yet name that has no place in the periodic table of elements or in any catalog of organic compounds? But is that question merely one of semantics, of nomenclature? Alternatively again, is the use of the word *light* a reference to the very same light as the physical phenomenon we experience, or is it a metaphor for something seen as if it were akin to physical light but which in some manner transcends it?

As we have seen, there seem to be a number of routes to the ultimate state of the perfected body-mind, but we still do not know whether it is necessary to die biologically before we can attain it or whether we can reach it within ordinary space-time through the vehicle of altered consciousness. Is the perfected state, which is said to be composed of a finer, more ethereal form of energy-substance, and which mystics have long claimed to know by experience, an actuality or merely a delusion in their minds? If a delusion, why have so many individuals believed the claims and sought this most exalted state of development? And, if it is "real," are we, in the twenty-first-century West able to find it?

NINE

East Meets West

Development in Western thought usually involves destruction of the old to make room for the new, but development in Indian thought consists in retaining the insights of previous thought and building upon these insights.

TROY WILSON ORGAN, *WESTERN APPROACHES TO EASTERN PHILOSOPHY*

In his study of *Western Approaches to Eastern Philosophy,* Troy Wilson Organ points to a fundamental difference in attitude between East and West, particularly in philosophy. He points out the danger that the Western student might seek among Eastern cultures for a counterpart to the Western philosophical tradition, and, if successful in his search, identify this as "philosophy" without considering the possibility that in the East something vastly different might already exist which could and should be seen as an independent, "indigenously Eastern" philosophy. He points out that, ironically, we *did* believe that we could perceive differences between the two cultures and so *could* identify a distinct "West" and "East." The West, we thought, is scientific, empirical, rational, pragmatic, this-worldly; the East is poetic, intuitive, mystical, dreamy, other-worldly. We now realize this was somewhat simplistic, especially as in some senses it is the converse that is true.

What is often thought of as "the Eastern tradition" has shown itself to be in reality a complex web of variations upon the founding belief that we humans and our world are in some sense a small version of a greater world which is, ipso facto, like it, though believed to be more powerful and more permanent. As we shall discover when we explore the Western approaches to the subtle body, a complex of beliefs has existed for centuries in the Western world that is both profoundly similar and profoundly different.

If the word *philosophy* is used in the narrow sense of "argument for a position," the earliest philosophical writing in India did not appear, according to Organ, until 300 CE in the *Samkhya Karika* of Isvarakrishna, but if used in the broadest sense, as speculation, then philosophy can be said to have originated in India with the earliest *mantras* of the *Ṛg Veda,* about 4000 BCE.[1] Here we can illustrate the real difficulty of attempting to equate the two systems. We find differences of content on account of differences in mind-set. Since most Oriental philosophy is characterized by an intimacy between philosophy and religion, it may be impossible to, as Eliot Deutsch, philosopher, teacher, and writer, suggests, "avoid questions that lie in the fields of theology and mystical experience."[2] Note that this objection itself shows precisely the character predicated of Western philosophy, presuming without examination the appropriateness of that alleged Western analysis and categorization. Etymologically, the word *philosophy* derives from the Greek *philosophia,* and means "the love of wisdom." Wisdom is surely broad in scope rather than self-blindingly narrow. While "the love of wisdom" began "in wonder," Organ tells us that the mainstream of Western philosophy has been accented by the nonutilitarian pursuit of clarity and truth. He states that while he does not wish to affirm that the West is analytical and the East is existential, he does claim that the general tone of Western philosophy is primarily analytical and secondarily existential, whereas Eastern philosophy is primarily existential and secondarily analytical.[3]

Aurobindo confirms our thoughts when he states that, "In the West where the syncretic tendency of the consciousness was replaced by the analytic and separative, the spiritual urge and the intellectual reason parted company at the outset."[4] What is needed, then, if West is to meet East is for it to re-embrace esotericism even as the East embraces, indeed has already embraced, analysis and its offspring, science. As each restores its own balance, they will meet.

What Is Esotericism?

The word *esoteric* derives from the Greek *esoterikos,* and is a comparative form of *eso,* meaning "within." Its first known mention in Greek is in Lucian's statement that Aristotle taught both esoteric and exoteric doctrines. The word later came to designate the secret doctrines said to have been taught by Pythagoras to a select group of disciples, and, in general, to any teachings designed for or appropriate to an inner circle of disciples or initiates. In this sense, the word was brought into English in 1655 by Stanley in his *History of Philosophy.*

Esotericism, according to Versluis, describes the historical phenomena to be studied; *gnosis* describes that which is esoteric, hidden, protected, and transmitted within these historical phenomena.[5] Without hidden knowledge to be transmitted in one fashion or another, he states, one does not have esotericism. A whole range of disparate phenomena are included under the rubric of "Western esotericism": alchemy, astrology, various kinds of magical traditions, Hermeticism, Kabbalah, Jewish or Christian visionary or apophatic gnosis. They are connected primarily by one thing: that to enter into the particular arcane discipline is to come to realize for oneself secret knowledge about the cosmos and its transcendence. "This secret or hidden knowledge is not a product of reason alone, but of gnosis—according to esotericism, it derives from a supra-rational source."[6]

In every age and culture the vital questions have been about human beings and the universe: who we are, what we are, where we are going. For several decades we have looked to Oriental cultures for answers to these questions. In his article "Esoteric Wisdom East and West," Rensselaer gives what he believes to be the reason for this. Many in the West have been "turned off," he says, by their perception that the mainspring of the Western way of life is crass materialism, and by an apparent lack of moral or spiritual content in Western philosophy and religion. They see no improvement in the quality of life resulting from religious movements and institutions, nor in the individual or collective conduct of either leaders or ordinary members of society. Feeling their own tradition to be bankrupt, they very rationally look elsewhere for help, mainly to Buddhism, Hinduism, and the Chinese I Ching, although other less wholesome traditions have also received considerable attention.[7]

In his opinion, the quality of life in the contemporary Orient offers no more evidence of sound spiritual or religious practices or enlightenment than can be found in the West. Selfishness and a disregard for the sacredness of human life is as pervasive there as anywhere in the world. And among oriental religious authorities can be encountered as much useless dogmatism, ritual, and ignorance as our own tradition displays. The present-day East is experiencing a burst of material improvement and progress, he says, but "it still exhibits considerable degeneration from a once-lofty religious standard of life and offers little of enduring spiritual inspiration for us."[8]

What, then, Rensselaer asks, is the attraction of the East for the West? "In the first place," he states, "a long tradition of religious tolerance has allowed numbers of movements and sects to exist and flourish amicably side by side in the East." In an important sense, he explains, this represents the carrying out into the real world of central ideas in these religions in a way that our own religions have not seemed able to do. Then Eastern religions contain definite traditions of spiritual discipline by which a practitioner is said to be able to transcend his ignorance and achieve inner enlightenment. Because of their ideas on rebirth and karma, "Eastern religious traditions acknowledge the beautiful complexity of the total human nature, and offer a bright hope for man's future because time and scope are allowed for the full development of it through a long evolution of consciousness."[9] Those traditions, moreover, put the material world in its place and, by connecting thought and action with destiny, achieve great coherence and logic, which appeal to the questing mind.

By contrast, he believes that our tradition as given to us seems to constrict greatly the definition of what we are. It tends to disconnect us from the universe that surrounds us, and makes that universe a material shell having no true *raison d'être* and not much internal logic or philosophic cohesion. In fact, if—in accordance with Western scientific thought—we are only our bodies, which disappear forever after a short three score years and ten, that means *we* disappear forever. Then the concept of cosmic evolution and all of the mysterious and majestic experiences of our individual consciousnesses are meaningless and "without intrinsic value."[10]

Rensselaer thinks, as does Organ, that any attempt to compare Western and Eastern religious traditions must suffer because of our habit of separating knowledge of Reality into three distinct and often conflicting departments of thought: religion, science, and philosophy. Eastern traditions do not do this but rather seek to describe a total Reality, which has what we can term religious, scientific, and philosophical aspects, each a necessary part of the total vision. But he points out that while Oriental texts from the past cannot be surpassed for their "profundity of spiritual philosophy," and it is evident that their uniformity reflects the existence of an inner, or esoteric, wisdom that was much more a living reality during the time of their writing than it is today, that tradition has now become so enwrapped and encrusted with fable and allegory that the ancient reality and profundity are difficult to find.[11]

Western scholars began seriously to undertake the study of Eastern scriptures only at the end of the eighteenth century, eventually producing translations of original texts. It was not until near the end of the nineteenth century that Helena Blavatsky, in *The Secret Doctrine* and collateral writings, offered the first clear explanation of their esoteric content. Only then did we really begin to learn what the classical Oriental religious philosophy had to tell us.

Esotericism in the West

Blavatsky was, perhaps, the first to draw to the attention of nonspecialists the fact of an inner or spiritual tradition in the Western world corresponding to the traditions found in the East, and to show that Western traditions have always incorporated the same major ideas as are found in Eastern esotericism. These ideas are found in Platonic and Neo-Platonic thought and in the Gnosticism that formed a part of Christian doctrine until it was excised from canonical scripture by the Church Councils of the fifth and sixth centuries CE. These ideas can also be found in the teachings of scholars who flourished among the formal institutions of Christianity down to the Reformation and later, among them Giordano Bruno, Pico della Mirandola, Dante, the Meisters Eckhart and Wilhelm, Stephan Lochner, Cagliostro, the theosopher Jakob Boehme, Louis Claude de Saint-Martin, and the Reverend William Law.

This esoteric tradition in the West was also maintained by a series of apparently dissimilar movements and mystical brotherhoods, such as the Albigenses, the Masons and their Orders, the Rosicrucians, and the Illuminati. However, the deliberate excision of this inner body of ideas and its declaration as heresy was an important part of the early centralization of theological power in the official church hierarchy. As a result, those exponents of an esoteric tradition, notwithstanding that their tradition is truly worldwide in scope, had perforce to conceal themselves and their teachings to escape religious persecution.

The consequence of all this was, of course, that Western religion, as offered to the public, became steadily less able to address the perennial hunger of minds and hearts for satisfying explanations of ourselves and the universe, such as young people feel in our own time, says Rensselaer. However, he admits that "Paradoxically, the most useful interpretations of classical Oriental philosophy can today be found in the West" and suggests that what remains to be done is to "show Western seekers that the truth about ourselves and the cosmos can also be found in our own back yard, and perhaps more adequately stated for our real purposes than are some of the better-known Eastern expressions of the same."[12]

Esotericism in Academia

Esotericism, as an academic field in the West, is, pragmatically defined, the study of alternative or marginalized religious movements or philosophies whose proponents in general distinguish their beliefs, practices, and experiences from more public, institutionalized religious traditions. Among areas of investigation included in the field of esotericism are alchemy, astrology, Gnosticism, Hermeticism, Kabbalah, magic, mysticism, Neo-Platonism, new religious movements connected with these currents, nineteenth-, twentieth-, and twenty-first-century occult movements, Rosicrucianism, secret societies, and Theosophy.

The study of esotericism has at its central core the idea that the subtle body is a suitable subject to study the "several realities" that exist, and that as "nonbinary knowledge," that is, forms of knowledge that are not classical, not "logical" in a narrowly "rational" sense, it draws together a number of current discourses in contemporary Western thought: self and spirit, mind and body, reason and emotion, reductionism and wholeness.

On account of the erstwhile Western inadequacy regarding Eastern belief systems, the study of the subtle body in a Western academic context presents its students with an unfamiliar challenge. Traditionally, the subtle body has been understood by the intuitive modes of knowing that have been the very foundations of the East. What the Western academic must realize is that the evanescent, invisible, and fluid nature of the subtle body makes it a difficult subject to apprehend without an objective assessment of subjective knowledge, and such knowledge cannot exist without experience. However, research into the subtle body via an interdisciplinary, cross-cultural approach brings a unique opportunity to study the interrelations and correlations between distinctly separate Western traditions. It invokes "a radical renegotiation of the dualisms at the heart of dominant Western discourse."[13] According to author J. L. H. Johnston, Ph.D., such research necessarily includes a freeing of prejudices, which allows for new ways of seeing.

In the Indian tradition, yogis, mystics, and scholars have been preoccupied with the contrast between the materiality of the physical body and the nonmateriality of the subtle body, and have given the greater emphasis to the latter. We must show at least an equal breadth in the West. New studies in the West suggest that we need to extend our perception to include that space between bodies wherein our nonmateriality touches others. We must also include personal knowledge of the effects that meditation and what Johnston calls "everyday mystical" experience have on our perception of the "borders" between subject and object. It is in this arena

that the much celebrated but not always well-understood relevance of quantum physics resides, though even the conjunction itself is obscured by the difference in the language used in the relevant disciplines.[14] We shall attempt to unravel some of the confusion in chapter 15.

Johnston says that the subtle body is postulated to consist of a subtle form of matter-consciousness that "exceeds" the corporeal body. The postulate requires an understanding of embodiment that is not exclusively tied to materiality. The space between object and subject, or between subjects, becomes a space of mutual occupation, where an intersubjective relation is shared. This relation, she says, is simultaneously of and not of each of the subjects who are in relation. We would say that it contains each participant's personal perspective of I-thou relatedness. The apprehension and cultivation of the relation requires acknowledgment of our energetic and affective capacities, and an acceptance that self and other open to each other in ways that evade our grasp. The subtle subject, by its very ontological constitution, Johnston believes, is simultaneously in both an intimate and a detached relation with alterity. The subject is always innately *inter*subjective, creative, and open.[15] This re-expresses Heidegger's view that our being is, in its very nature, *Being-in-the-world,* and that that way of being is inherently and necessarily a *Being-with* with others. We are not Descartes' isolated and worldless thinking thing. We sense the "otherness" of those around us in the world, but our own personal being is essentially "in-the-world." Each of us is a Being, isolated to the degree that we are not conscious *of* another's consciousness, nor of the world's, but conscious *that* such consciousness is here alongside, while being one with others by virtue of being *here* in this same world as they also inhabit. We expound this idea in chapter 15, "Science, Philosophy, and the Subtle Body."

The study of the subtle body, then, is uniquely placed to bring together a range of understandings of the human condition, not only from Eastern and Western perspectives, but also from an integral viewpoint that expands our awareness and embraces many other attempts to explore and explain who and what we really are. Indeed, some of Rensselaer's remarks, like Johnston's, point directly toward the important matters of quantum (and other) interconnectedness and conscious intentionality, which will be introduced in chapter 15.

In part 2, we shall also consider what relevance and practical applications the subtle body has in a modern secular context, outside the religious framework, such as healing and psychology. Are these contemporary models equivalent to ancient religious views of the subtle body and do they allow us to produce in ourselves similar alterations in consciousness? Is spiritual awakening possible without faith or belief, or if our goals differ?

PART TWO

Western Perspectives

The study of the subtle body in Western traditions may require a different approach from that of the Eastern traditions. To begin with, study of the subtle body must use a corpus of material, under the general heading of "esotericism," which has only recently been recognized as a rich and coherent source of textual material for academic study *as a whole*. Until about the middle of the twentieth century the numerous and diverse strands of this huge field were each appropriated by specialist scholars. Although there are discernible threads, streams, or currents among the many teachings, indicating close connections between them, esoteric scholars Professor Emeritus Antoine Faivre and Karen-Claire Voss believe that a common vocabulary or language through which this field can be described as a dynamic, *living* tradition is only now emerging.[1] However, even the terms *tradition* and *traditional* are problematic when referring to Western esotericism or esoteric studies. It is therefore necessary to define these terms with some precision before we go further.

In this context, *tradition* usually refers to a set of metaphysical truths that were believed to have been imparted to humanity in primordial time and were thereafter forgotten, distorted, or for other reasons no longer accepted.[2] These truths can still be found embodied in the main tenets of most world religions, but more explicitly in the *philosophia perennis* ("eternal philosophy" or "perennial philosophy"), the term coined by the seventeenth-century German philosopher Gottfried Leibniz to refer collectively to certain universal, philosophical insights into the nature of reality, humanity, and consciousness that have recurred from epoch to epoch throughout history. According to Aldous Huxley, who used this term in 1945 as title for his book *The Perennial Philosophy,* it is: "the metaphysic that recognizes a divine Reality substantial to the world of things and lives and minds; the psychology that finds in the soul something similar to, or even identical with, divine Reality; the ethic that places man's final end in the knowledge of the immanent and transcendent Ground of all being; the thing is immemorial and universal. Rudiments of the perennial philosophy may be found among the traditional lore of primitive peoples in every region of the world, and in its fully developed forms it has a place in every one of the higher religions."[3]

The term *esoteric,* as we saw in dealing with the Eastern traditions, refers to the "secret knowledge" or "secret science," which has at its core the methods or techniques that lead to transcendence, and to the descriptions of the experience of transcendence itself. However, *esotericism* is a Western rather than an Eastern concept, with the particular feature that the *study* of esotericism in the West is separated from the *practice* of esotericism, ostensibly to prevent it from "being dissolved in a sea of incoherence," as Faivre and Voss put it, which some Western academics view as the inevitable result of mystical or ecstatic experience.[4] However, this viewpoint has been challenged by some writers, whom Latin scholar, editor, and translator Claire Fanger calls "pro-esotericists."[5] These would include Manly Hall and G. R. S. Mead, who regard intrinsic knowledge, that is, inner knowledge that changes the knower and is obtained in the esoteric experience, as essential to any understanding of the experience as a *whole*. Other writers, such as Pierre Riffard, attempt to find a balance between the esoterical position on the one hand and the extrinsic, scholarly stance on the other, by setting out a theory and methodology that allow for a study of the field from the broadest, deepest possible perspectives.[6]

The term *Western* refers to the medieval and modern Greco-Latin world in which various religious traditions, chiefly Judaism and Christianity, have coexisted for centuries and have periodically come into contact with other religions, philosophies, and ideas, identified by Faivre and Voss as forms of:

1. Hellenistic philosophy and religiosity (chiefly Stoicism, Gnosticism, Hermeticism, Neo-Pythagorism) linked at the beginning of the Common Era (CE).
2. Jewish Kabbalah and Neo-Alexandrian Hermeticism, containing ideas of analogy and universal harmonies, which appeared after 1471.
3. The *prisca theologia* (the doctrine that a single truth underpinned all religions), which became known as the *philosophia occulta* (occult or mystical philosophy) and, subsequently, as the philosophia perennis in the Middle Ages.[7]

Faivre and Voss state that "The historical or mythical representatives of the *philosophia perennis* were thought to constitute links in a chain. . . . The task of the scholar of esoteric studies is not to prove that such an invisible 'Tradition,' hidden behind the veil of the history of events, did or did not exist before the Renaissance; rather, the task consists of trying to grasp and describe the different facets of the emergence of this idea as it appears in the imaginary* and discourses of the last centuries." They point to the fact that much of this tradition emerged as a result of the separation between science and religion, leaving an "enormous abandoned field."[8]

Into this breach stepped the humanist scholars with esoteric leanings. Their contribution, Faivre and Voss believe, cannot be overemphasized. In particular, they dealt with the interface between metaphysics and cosmology, "thereby modelling a kind of *extra*-theological method for giving an account of the link between the universal and the particular and, in the light of these Renaissance influences, the field of esotericism developed over the next few centuries."[9] We shall be looking at some of these main trends in more detail in the next few chapters, but shall go further to include those that have appeared in the centuries following the Renaissance. That is not to say, however, that all the main strands from this vast tapestry have been included, but rather that a few, which are most obviously linked with our topic, the subtle body, have been selected for attention.

However, it would be appropriate to mention here some of the common strands in the study of esotericism, which have been identified by some writers as the *mesocosmos,* the realm *between* the human and the Divine, among which (in Pierre Riffard's model) the subtle body is listed. In his *L'Esotérisme,*[10] and in an anthology of essays edited by Faivre and Hanegraaff,[11] Riffard finds eight "universals," themes that provide a schema for the study of esotericism. Riffard's schema includes both internal and external modes of knowing and gives access to a broad range of cross-cultural religious, spiritual, and symbolic ideas. They are:

The anonymity of the authors
The opposition between the profane and the
    initiated
The subtle body
Correspondences
Numbers
Occult sciences
Occult arts
Initiations

It is unclear whether Riffard meant the order of this list to convey any particular significance, but for our purposes the universality of the subtle body provides an important key concept in this developing field of study. Of course, our contribution makes no claim to be exhaustive.

---

*The word *imaginary,* as used here, is a noun, not an adjective, a technical term of sociology, defined as follows: "An imaginary, or social imaginary is the set of values, institutions, laws, and symbols common to a particular social group and the corresponding society."

TEN

Symbolism and the Subtle Body in the Ancient World

The Mysteries taught that spirit, or life, was anterior to form and that what is anterior includes all that is posterior to itself. Spirit being anterior to form, form is therefore included within the realm of spirit . . . as the material nature of man is therefore within the sum of spirit, so the Universal Nature, including the entire system, is within the all-pervading essence of God, the Universal Spirit.

MANLY P. HALL, *THE SECRET TEACHINGS OF ALL AGES*

The word *symbol* is based on the Greek words for "throwing" and "together"; symbols are parallels, analogies, their components chosen because, when thus thrown together in the human mind, each illustrates the other. What Manly Hall here expounds is itself symbolic in this etymologically correct sense, and is often encountered as the principle "As above, so below." The fundamental notion is that the human being is a microworld living within a macroworld, and that each of those worlds reflects the other. Each might represent, or, in our habitual slight misusage of the word, symbolize, the other. We humans, in what came long afterward to be called "existential angst," have always been concerned about our own being, our own fate. As we have seen, early humans invented gods on this very account, and they looked to the gods for succor, for survival. It was natural, therefore, that the human body would become the most ubiquitous of all symbols. The Hindus, Egyptians, Persians, Greeks, and Hebrews all taught, though with characteristic variations, that the human constitution was a reflection of the universe, its laws, its elements, and its powers. While the universe is, for us, immeasurable in its immensity and inconceivable in its profundity, yet we may transcend briefly and by a small span the usual limitations of our natural being. In doing so, we trust that we will understand a little of that immense universe, and that, relying, since we have nothing else, upon our own intellectual and other powers, we shall not be entirely deceived by what we believe we find. But as the principle "As above, so below" itself predicts, in looking we see ourselves.

Accordingly, humans have proposed what in recent decades has been called the "anthropic principle," discovering a universe that allows us to exist, for, according to today's science, if the dynamic balance of its structure were to vary by a hair's breadth, we could not be present to see it, if, indeed, it could itself exist. Perhaps, then, the universe needs humankind as a part, just as we need it to be our home. Yet we do not feel at home until we see our own humanity writ larger still

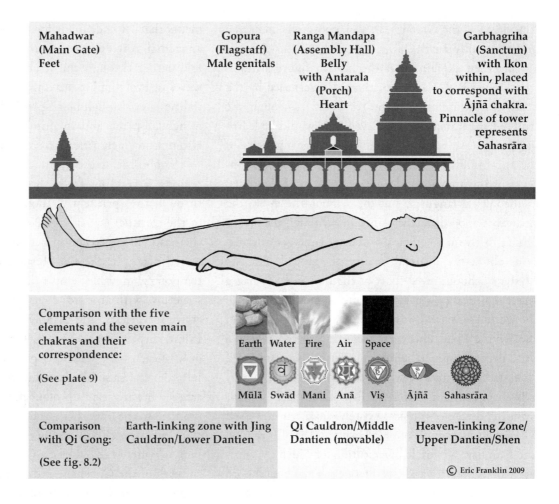

| Mahadwar (Main Gate) Feet | Gopura (Flagstaff) Male genitals | Ranga Mandapa (Assembly Hall) Belly with Antarala (Porch) Heart | Garbhagriha (Sanctum) with Ikon within, placed to correspond with Ājñā chakra. Pinnacle of tower represents Sahasrāra |

Comparison with the five elements and the seven main chakras and their correspondence:

(See plate 9)

Earth	Water	Fire	Air	Space		
Mūlā	Swād	Mani	Anā	Viṣ	Ājñā	Sahasrāra

| Comparison with Qi Gong: (See fig. 8.2) | Earth-linking zone with Jing Cauldron/Lower Dantien | Qi Cauldron/Middle Dantien (movable) | Heaven-linking Zone/ Upper Dantien/Shen |

© Eric Franklin 2009

in the great "above"; but to see that the better we must first enlarge ourselves. As a first step, and whether we question the logic or not, we appoint the human as the microcosmic symbol of the universe and reach out toward the gods, whom we have already made to be comfortingly like ourselves.

The Miniature Universe

Manly Hall explains that the early philosophers recognized the futility of attempting to cope intellectually with that which transcends the comprehension of the human rational faculty. Abandoning as hopeless any attempt to grasp the inconceivable Divine Being, they turned their attention inward, to what was familiar as the human experience of being a living Being in the everyday world, within which narrow confines they then asserted they would find manifested all the mysteries of those immensely greater external spheres. As the natural outgrowth of this practice, Hall tells us, "there was fabricated a secret theological system in which God was

Fig. 10.1. In ancient temples of the East, as well as in the churches and cathedrals of the West, the human form, within which the spirit lives, is taken as the microcosm and is surrounded by the building as a whole, which represents the world-enclosing macrocosm. On close inspection any such symbolism shows inconsistencies, of course, but, the impossibility of attaining it notwithstanding, the aim in sacred architecture was the creation of a building that would conform to both natural and spiritual laws. The vertical dimensions are associated with the connection between heaven and earth and the transcendent forces, and the layout in the horizontal plane expresses, and is believed to bring, change and transformation. Thus the building itself can inspire and elevate the spirits of all who enter its sacred enclosures. Many sacred structures are built on sites where energy lines were thought to meet or cross. Such lines are regarded as the meridians of the earth and are believed to bring revelation, healing, or transformation to those who meditate appropriately at the designated points.

considered as the Grand Man and, conversely, man as a miniature universe."[1]

He then explains that the human figure symbolized Divine Power and was, therefore, regarded by the priests of antiquity as their "textbook." Through the study of the human they believed they would be learning to understand the great and abstruse mysteries of the universe. Eliade observes that "the metaphysical concepts of the archaic world were not always formulated in theoretical language; but the symbol, the myth, the rite, express, on different planes and through the means proper to them, a complex system of coherent affirmations about the ultimate reality of things."[2] For the Mystery Schools,* every part of the human body had a secret significance, a parallel of some symbolic kind with the world above, and was, therefore, the living image of the Divine Plan. However, according to them only a third part of a human being temporarily dissociates itself from its own immortality and takes on physical, earthly existence, while at death this incarnated part awakens from the dream of physical existence and reunites itself with its eternal condition. Hall explains that "Both God and man have a twofold constitution, of which the superior part is invisible and the inferior part visible. In both there is an intermediary sphere, marking the point where these visible and invisible natures meet."[3] In chapter 15 we shall develop notions of a similar kind in modern scientific terms.

The idea that the body is the temple of the soul persists in many cultures and in some has been taken further. In the biblical New Testament the apostle Paul refers to the body as the temple of the Holy Spirit, superseding temples made in stone with the human being's own hands.

All the gods of the ancient world had their analogues in the human body, along with the four body centers of the elements, seven vital organs ascribed to the planets, and twelve principal constellations, the vehicles of the celestials. While the normally invisible parts of the human's "divine physicality" were assigned to various deities, the hidden God was believed to manifest through the marrow in the bones. Manly Hall com-

ments that "it is difficult for many to realise that they are actual universes; that their physical bodies are a visible nature through the structure of which countless waves of evolving life are unfolding their latent potentialities. Yet through man's physical body not only are a mineral, a plant, and an animal kingdom evolving, but also unknown classifications of invisible spiritual life."[4]

Symbolism arose from the human body's three regions, ascending from the embarrassingly "dirty," through the (penitently) thoughtful but still human, to the spiritual (considered either as in the heart or in the head. This perception became the template for the sacred place. In the Old Testament the tabernacle, a temporary, movable temple-in-a-tent, had a three-part structure, with an outer court for the people, an inner court for priests, and a Holy of Holies for the High Priest, in person and "not without blood," on one day only of each year. Solomon's permanent stone temple in Jerusalem had a similar layout in which a spatial progression led inward from a profane outer court, which corresponded to the lower body and the common people, first to a "holy place." Still further within was the "Holy of Holies" where the Shekhina Glory itself hovered above the Ark of the Covenant and only a select few humans might ever venture, on pain of death.

The Three Centers

It will be recalled that Taoists conceived the subtle body that underlies qigong to have a tripartite structure. The concept of unities-in-tripartite-division was widespread in the ancient world. In the Western world it appeared as a correspondence between three centers of the human and universal bodies, which, as we have seen, was itself represented in the three chambers of many designs of temple. In this way sacred architecture presented the understanding of the human body that was current at the time, itself conjectured, and believed, to be a close illustration at the mundane level of the inconceivable Great Being. It also appeared as the three degrees of the ancient Mysteries, a notion that persists in modern pagan traditions.

The first degree was the material mystery and its symbol was the generative system. It was seen as consisting of those parts of the body that had "animal" functions, known, further East, as the

---

*"Mystery schools" and "Mystery cults" refer to Eastern Mediterranean religious groups of late classical antiquity, c. 600–300 BCE, which practiced the "Mysteries," secret religious rites and rituals known only to initiates.

regions of the genital chakra, swādhiṣṭhāna, and the anal chakra, mūlādhāra. Progress began, as it must, at this level of low animality, and lifted the candidate through the various phases of concrete thought.

The second degree corresponded to the heart, in qigong the movable dantien, in the Indic traditions the heart chakra, anāhata, and it represented a middle-level power, that of the human mind, above the grossly animal genital and eliminative parts but beneath the god-like spiritual level, so forming the mental link that raised the initiate through mysteries of abstract thought to the highest attainments of the human mind. It will be recalled that the middle dantien of qigong is often seen as movable, as if carrying consciousness from below toward higher regions where it can transcend the physical body. The chakra system, a little more complex, is seen as providing the same ladder of upward transcendence.

The third degree occupied the highest position in the body, representative of the greatest dignity and, though given in the "brain chamber," was considered analogous to the heart, or to a spiritual level of the heart. Here we may note that the ancient Greeks were uncertain whether thought occurred in the brain or in the heart, and that the belief that there are two hearts, a mental and a spiritual, is characteristic of some schools of Sufism. Eastern ideas have always had parallels in the West, and the present-day Reiki schema conserves the concept of a multiplicity of hearts, with not only the physical heart and a sacred heart, but also an "ascending heart," which seems to parallel the movable dantien of qigong, and an "etheric heart" which is outside the physical body, and is itself triple in structure. See figure 14.6 on page 171.

Reunion with the Cosmos

Eliade points out that rituals and myths enacted in the ancient world reflected the cosmos and cosmic rhythms, and that we would understand these today as "primordial archetypes," creative repetitions of timeless, universal events.[5] He explains that the life of the archaic human,

like that of the mystic and the religious person today, evoked an eternal present outside of the consciousness of time. Through ritual and ceremony an ever-present state of union with the cosmos is regenerated. Many ritual and spiritual practices express nostalgia for a mythological "time" at the beginning of time itself. We see this, for instance, in the postulated correspondences between the human body and the celestial bodies whose cycles were said to be reflected in the parts of the human body to which they were believed to be linked (see plate 22).

Eliade gives as example the human's conceived relationship with the moon. "The moon is the first of creatures to die and also the first to live again."[6] He states that lunar myths are essential to the first coherent theories concerning death and resurrection, fertility and regeneration, initiation, and so on. The moon, varying its apparent form over a short enough cycle to have been noted, served to "measure time," and revealed the cyclical nature of the "eternal return." Lunar rhythm, he goes on to say, not only reveals short intervals (the week, by each quarter of the moon, and the month itself by the complete lunation), but also serves as the archetype for extended durations. In fact, he says, "the birth of a humanity, its growth, decrepitude . . . and disappearance are assimilated to the lunar cycle. And this assimilation is important not only because it shows us the 'lunar' structure of universal becoming but also because of its optimistic consequences for, just as the disappearance of the moon is never final, the disappearance of man is not final either."[7] The new moon, upon her return, was even holding the old moon in her arms. We can understand, then, the widespread belief in the eternal feminine principle, in the form of the moon goddess, which arose in most cultures.

Serpent Symbolism and the Subtle Body

As we have seen, the body as the locus of spiritual transformation has been a central idea in Eastern as well as Western traditions. Body-based mysticism evolved from the concept that the visible physical form is the container or vehicle not only for the postulated invisible subtle body but also for the knowledge of the mysteries of the universe. This knowledge, or "know-how," is represented using a variety of mythic symbols. In both Eastern and Western traditions the serpent is one of the oldest and most widespread of these. It is used to picture the rising, linear development toward spirituality, as in kundalinī, and in the related caduceus, representative of healing. When it forms a ring with its tail in its mouth it pictures the concept of the eternal cycle of birth and rebirth, giving a clear symbol of the "All-in-All." Recognized in this context throughout the ancient world, it symbolized the totality and completeness of existence—even of infinity, for the circle has no end—as well as the perpetually cyclic nature of the cosmos.

The best-known version of this is the Egypto-Greek Ouroboros. It has been important in mythological symbolism and religious traditions, particularly in alchemy, which we shall review in chapter 12. In some texts it is referred to as a serpent of light residing in the heavens and there is indeed a constellation so named. The much brighter Milky Way was also regarded as a continuous cyclical serpent, or, in Egypt, where the Milky Way, as viewed by earthlings, seemed to flow in heavenly parallel with the Nile, as a life-giving river. The whole of Egyptian life did indeed depend upon the Nile. In Gnosticism the Ouroboros symbolizes eternity and the soul of the world. The serpent in general was the symbol of the understanding granted by Sophia, Wisdom herself. Members of one of the Gnostic sects placed such importance upon

the symbol that they were referred to as the "Ophites" (Serpent People) by more conventional groups.

The symbol is also important in Christianity, though its prominence has been much reduced by the deep division of Christian history into gnostic (esoteric) and nongnostic (exoteric) traditions, and the highly oppressive political power gained by the latter. Manly Hall relates that the serpent always was, and is still, true to the principle of wisdom, for it tempts man to acquire knowledge of himself. In the Genesis account, humankind's earliest knowledge of self resulted not from obedience to Jehovah, or, to give the name more correctly, Yahweh, but from *dis*obedience to the Demiurgus, the jealous demigod who, according to some traditions, had created only this lower world in which humankind found themselves dwelling against their will. This account from the gnostic tradition, eventually proclaimed heretical, is nonetheless traceable even in the much-expurgated pages of the Bible as we have it today. While Genesis, as we have it, condemns the serpent as a deceiver of humankind, it admits that it was more subtle, that is, more wise and knowing, than any other beast. Another book of the Bible, Proverbs, particularly in its first four chapters, strongly advises humankind to pursue wisdom.[8] Indeed,

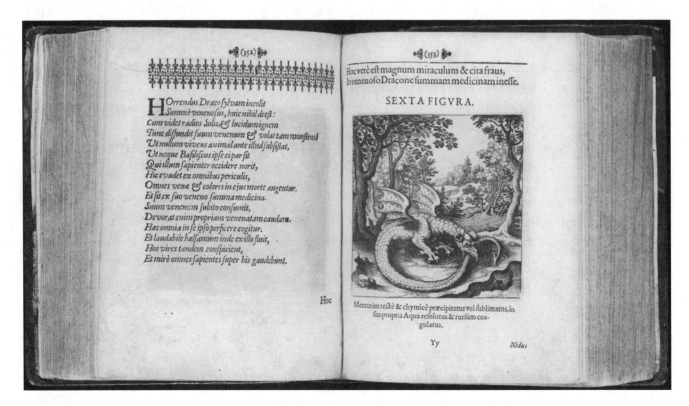

Fig. 10.2. The Ouroboros symbolizes totality and the eternal cycles of rebirth. From *Museum Hermeticum*, 1678. (Beinecke Rare Book and Manuscript Library, Yale University.)

the Genesis account itself cannot conceal the serpent's true significance as a symbol of wisdom, for how, if it were the evil beast it is normally conceived to have been, did it come to be in the garden of Eden when Yahweh declared "very good" all the creatures He had made? This question has never been satisfactorily answered by interpreters of scripture.

Furthermore, according to Hall and many other writers, the tree that, in the Genesis account, grows "in the midst of the garden" is in fact the gift not of the Demiurge but of the great serpent. Hall tells us that "The accepted view that the serpent is evil cannot be substantiated. It has been viewed as the emblem of immortality. It is the symbol of reincarnation, or metempsychosis, because it annually shed its skin, reappearing, as it were, in a new body."[9] Notwithstanding statements to the contrary, the serpent is the symbol and prototype of the universal savior, who redeems the worlds by granting to creation the knowledge of itself and the realization of good and evil. Jesus (Yahshua) himself acknowledged this by telling his hearers that he stood in relation to humankind as had the serpent in the wilderness. When, during their wilderness wanderings, the Hebrews were plagued by serpents, those who gazed upon a brass serpent specially erected by Moses were not cursed for idolatry, but recovered from the bite.[10] Referring to this, Jesus claimed to be the savior and healer to whom men would look, just as the serpent raised in the wilderness had been, over a millennium before.

"Parallels" were seen everywhere in those eras when science had scarcely begun and a kind of loose empirical observation-plus-imagination held sway. Thus, in the ancient Mystery schools, the seven coils of the snake corresponded to the simple or complex movements of the seven celestial bodies that continuously circled the earth, static at the center, and initiates were often referred to as "serpents," as their wisdom was regarded as analogous to the divinely conferred (if also imaginary) powers of the snake.

The Hebraic and Judeo-Christian tradition, while having unique features that were vigorously defended, and despite the eventual suppression of its own esoteric branches by its politicized exoteric establishment after Constantine, was not alone among Middle Eastern cultures in acknowledging the serpent. It was also recognized, indeed revered, in Egypt, Greece, and Rome. Thus,

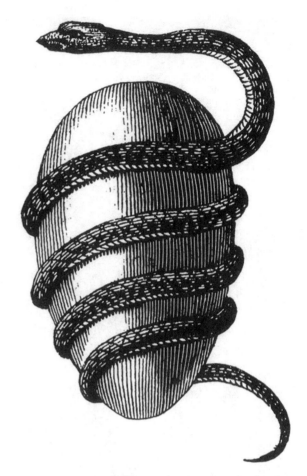

From Bryant's *An Analysis of Ancient Mythology.*

THE ORPHIC EGG.

The ancient symbol of the Orphic Mysteries was the serpent-entwined egg, which signified Cosmos as encircled by the fiery Creative Spirit. The egg also represents the soul of the philosopher; the serpent, the Mysteries. At the time of initiation the shell is broken and man emerges from the embryonic state of physical existence wherein he had remained through the fetal period of philosophic regeneration.

Fig. 10.3. The ancient symbol of the Orphic Mysteries, a Greek cult flourishing in the sixth to fifth centuries BCE, its founding myth that of Orpheus, was the serpent-entwined egg. The egg represents the cosmos and the soul of the philosopher, and the serpent is the creative spirit. During the initiation rite, the "shell" is broken and the person emerges from the state of physical existence, which, relative to the sought-for spiritual state, is merely embryonic. British scholar and philosopher G. R. S. Mead points out: "The 'egg of the universe,' besides having its analogy in the germ cell whence the human and every other kind of embryo develops, has its correspondence in the 'auric egg' of man."[11]

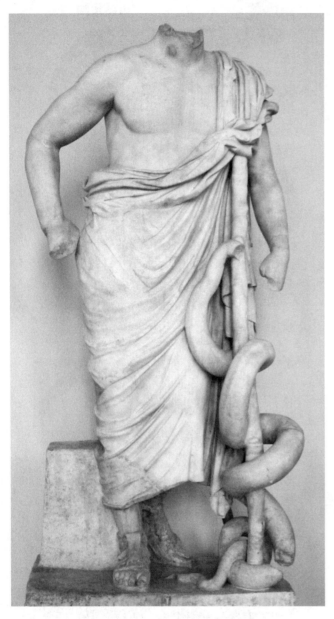

Fig. 10.4. Snakes appeared symbolically in the myths of many cultures. In the ancient world the serpent's role was to be wise mediator between this world and the next. The single snake shown here is the therapeutic symbol of Asklepios, the Greek god of healing. (Pergamon Museum, Berlin.)

in a curious parallel with the brass serpent displayed in the wilderness by Moses as a focus for faith-healing after snake bite, a single snake entwined the rough staff of Asklepios or Asclepius, the Greek god of healing.

The Hermetic Tradition

Greater even than Asklepios was Hermes. As his main concern is spiritual wisdom, wider and higher than heal-

ing, Hermes is usually shown holding a *caduceus,* consisting of not one but two snakes intertwined around a central staff. The snake was not duplicated merely for pleasing visual symmetry. Paired snakes had come to represent the union of paired or complementary opposites, forming a wholeness, a feature of any balanced wisdom, as the sages of the Taoist tradition, too, would claim. There are many such cross-cultural links, for this design also closely resembles the customary representation of the three most important subtle channels or energy streams of the Tantric system, in which the idā and pingalā spiral around the central suṣumnā, crossing over at each of the six main spinal chakras. But in what we now call the West, Hermes, the thrice-greatest, is head of a grand cult of his own. He has the role of psychopomp, escort of newly deceased souls to the afterlife, which explains the original choice of snake symbolism in the caduceus, for this was also the role of the much earlier snake-entwined Sumerian god Ningizzida, with whom Hermes has sometimes been identified. The symbol had probably first arisen from humankind's observation of the writhing, intertwining, *life-producing* copulation of snakes.

However, paired snakes were not the only distinguishing feature of Hermes' staff, for the wings at its head also identified it as his and his alone. He was the winged messenger, the Roman Mercury, recalling an earlier Egyptian incarnation of the ibis-headed god of wisdom, Thoth, embodiment of the universal mind. This bird-form represented the transcendent principle, the soul "taking flight," an idea that we saw in Hinduism. Hermes was also god of magic, diplomacy, and rhetoric, of inventions and discovery, the protector of both merchants and that allied occupation in the mythographers' view, the profession of thief.

While in all probability there actually lived a great sage and educator by the name Hermes, it is impossible, according to Manly Hall, to extricate the historical man (or men) from the legends. The system of philosophical and religious beliefs known as Hermeticism certainly had more than one root, and it has been speculated that there were three historical figures who contributed the teachings that came eventually to be attributed to Hermes Trismegistus. It is noteworthy that the name does mean *"Thrice* Greatest Hermes," suggestive, perhaps, of a trinity of sagacious authors whose teachings had been brought together in generating the cult.

Fig. 10.5. Hermes Trismegistus was believed to have revealed the truths of many systems of knowledge, but it is not easy to differentiate historical accounts of him from the mass of related myths and legends. He represents the awakening from sleep, a passing through earthly reality, and the eventual transcendence to the superconscious state of "living in the Light." *Museum Hermeticum*, 1678. (Beinecke Rare Book and Manuscript Library, Yale University.)

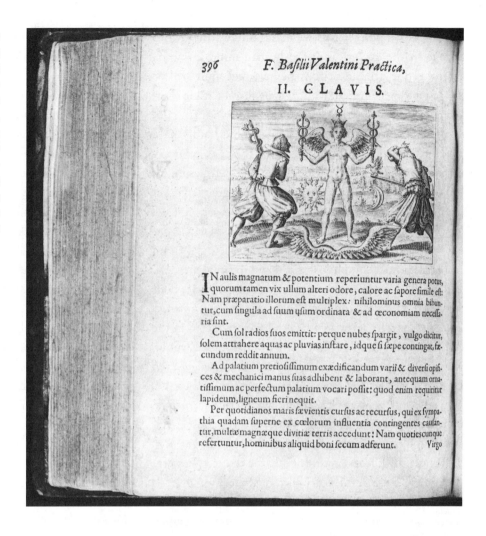

By whatever route, and with however many contributors, Hermeticism seems to have developed from long-standing direct influences from sources further East, augmented by relatively recent and geographically closer sources in Gnosticism and Neo-Platonism.

Hermes exemplifies, even personifies, a principle of thought about our relation with the cosmos that is reminiscent of Vedic notions of a vertical alignment from the gross material earth beneath our feet to the more subtly material sky above our heads.[12] In the four- or five-element science of the time all were considered to be material substances, for the modern notion of totally nonmaterial spirit had scarcely dawned. The earth was gross matter, water less gross, fire and air the subtlest, much nearer to the gods. Fire, especially, even seemed to float up to the gods. Clearly, its nature was close to theirs, for it sought them, rising into the sky. The invisibility of the gods was already a current notion, while the concept of mind as we construe it was only slowly developing. Still, a concept of universality, of a supreme,

overarching, creative influence within the cosmos, had already dawned. The notion of a greatest or highest of all gods was now required, and such a god could no longer be "likened unto wood or stone," or any material thing.

The instantly recognizable graphic symbol of Hermes was a flamboyant device of a kind that would surely have been eschewed by the modest Neo-Platonists and the secretive Gnostics, both of whom had influenced the cult. As mentioned, the insignia combined the entwined snakes, signifying wisdom and healing, with the wings of Mercury, the messenger of the gods, and a vertical staff reminiscent of the Vedic pole reaching from earth to sky, around which the snakes are coiled. Other facets of Hermes' complex character are not visible in the insignia, though (as befits the possible triple or even multiple authorship of the writings) he is believed to have revealed to humankind the truths of medicine, chemistry, law, astrology, music, rhetoric, magic, philosophy, geography, mathematics, anatomy, and oratory, rather too many achievements to find a place in just one symbol. If we ponder this we may gain an insight into a stage in the evolution of the human mind in which abstract concepts can scarcely be held, but must still be imaged and personified, while widely incompatible characteristics can be attributed to a single very human god-in-the-mind who, *qua* human being, could hardly have encompassed them all. What strikes the contemporary mind as puzzling is the curious ethic that Hermes might be conceived as a deity or at least as a very great sage, yet happily preside over both spirituality and theft.

The eighteen surviving books that form the *Corpus Hermeticum* date from the first centuries CE and contain texts with important philosophical and spiritual precepts, such as the concept of the unity in all things. The famous aphorism "As above, so below" comes from *The Emerald Tablet of Hermes,* a text reputed to have originated in the eighth century BCE, if not earlier. This source would, if the experts have correctly dated it, long antedate even Plato himself, let alone the Gnostics and Neo-Platonists who also influenced the full-blown Hermetic oeuvre. Hermeticism is probably the oldest and the most influential esoteric tradition that might, on account of its hold over much of Europe, meaningfully be termed Western, though the Eastern influences demonstrate, as so often, a multiplexity of historical threads that defies artificial categorizations, showing them to be merely useful, though potentially misleading, tools of thought.

The reader may wonder, on the basis of this chapter thus far, whether the Hermetic tradition relates closely to the subject of the subtle body, but one of the most important of the Hermetical texts, the *Poimandres* or *Pymander* (Shepherd of Men), shows the connection. It describes in allegorical language how spirit first descended into matter, fell in love with nature, and was trapped in space and time. This is clearly parallel to much else we have examined already, and shall yet examine. The initiate in the Hermetic tradition is enjoined to meditate in silence and so, by suppression of all the senses, which, of course, look out only upon the physical world-around, acquire the knowledge of God and salvation by an inward enlightenment. Upon achieving this he will ascend to Olympus through what is known as the "Vision of Light," the result being a rebirth, and a new sense of identity with the whole of creation and with God. "We must not be afraid to affirm," the text

says, "that a man on earth is a mortal god, and that a god in heaven is an immortal man."[13] In chapter 15 especially, but also elsewhere throughout this book, deeper understanding of our subtle being develops from contemplation of such passages.

Manly Hall describes an experience of Hermes in which, while wandering in a desolate place, he gave himself over to meditation. Following the instructions of the Temple, the school of priestly minds to which he belonged, he gradually freed his higher consciousness from the bondage of his bodily senses, whereupon "his divine nature revealed to him the mysteries of the transcendental spheres."[14] Hermes then narrates an awesome and sometimes terrifying encounter with the Great Dragon, Poimandres, the personification of universal life, "with wings stretching across the sky and light streaming in all directions." Poimandres teaches Hermes many things about the origin of life and being, then, "radiant with celestial light," vanishes, mingling with the celestial powers. "Raising his eyes unto the heavens, Hermes blessed the Father of All Things and consecrated his life to the service of the Great Light."[15]

Thereafter, Hermes preached, on the ground of his experience, that man should rise from his sleep and realize that his true home is not on earth but in the Light. He asks, "Why have you delivered yourselves unto death, having the power to partake of immortality? Prepare yourselves to climb through the Seven Rings and to blend your souls with eternal Light." In the "seven rings" we have a concept reminiscent of the seven coils of the serpent, of the seven planets, the sun being the greatest, and of the rising series of seven chakras of the Yogic and Tantric traditions, the highest bringing enlightenment. Thus the notion of the subtle body is not merely relevant but fundamental to Hermeticism, just as, in our own era, though to the surprise of many, it remains central to our understanding of ourselves and therefore to our understanding of what we call science. Science, more clearly than any other discipline, shows what is today called the anthropic principle, just as Hermeticism acknowledged the parallel principle "As above, so below," which, of course, included the physical body in its schema. Humankind is one with the world of its Being, yet, as Hermeticism affirmed, is also an alien wanderer in it. In chapter 15 we shall explore this matter in some depth.

ELEVEN

The Forgotten Philosophy

Neo-Platonism is a philosophic code which conceives every physical or concrete body of doctrine to be merely the shell of a spiritual verity which may be discovered through meditation and certain exercises of a mystic nature. In comparison to the esoteric spiritual truths which they contain, the corporeal bodies of religion and philosophy were considered of very little value. Likewise, no emphasis was placed upon the material sciences.

MANLY P. HALL, *THE SECRET TEACHINGS OF ALL AGES*

If we ponder these remarks of Manly Hall while holding in mind the ancient scientific concept of a scale of materiality from gross (earth) to fine (air), then allow ourselves the further notion of the fifth element, the empty but fecund "space" of the ākāśa, we shall begin to glimpse the change of direction in human thought that was already afoot as Vedic and Upaniṣadic texts reached first the Pythagoreans, then Plato himself, then, via his teachings, brought forth the Neo-Platonic worldview. Also within this shift of view was the Judaic realization, later expressed by the apostle Paul and others, that God should not be thought of as resembling wood or stone or any material thing, but as a Being of an entirely different essence. This new understanding thrust back into itself the earlier hylic pluralistic view that matter exists in four grades of fineness, placing them in one category, and positing instead that the essence of the great God must be quite different, and higher. This is the distinction we still make between matter and spirit. Chapter 9 of the New Testament Letter to the Hebrews is grounded in this then-new thinking. In our own chapter 15 this topic, this great uncertainty about material substances arising from humankind's increas-

ing consciousness of our own nonmaterial innerness, our thought, will be scrutinized in some detail, as it is central to what the word *subtle* might mean in regard to our nature as Beings-in-the-world.

This change of direction, having once begun and so produced in further process of time the perspective of our own day, distorts our view of all earlier philosophies, for all we have from any historical era are writings and works of art or craft. The human witnesses themselves are gone, and cannot be asked to explain. Artifacts need to be intuitively interpreted, with what the archeologist and the historian call "empathy" for the bygone age, yet that empathy is itself difficult to attain without *prior* knowledge of what is being investigated. Furthermore, investigation itself is obstructed by *our* preconditioned view. Writings are even more prone to misunderstanding than artifacts, for the meanings of words are never stable, changing even as they are being used. We saw an example of this in chapter 3, where we noticed the claim to derive both monistic and dualistic views from the same Vedic and Upaniṣadic texts, Feuerstein's interpretation of the resulting theories, and his demand that science now explain them. Insofar as history is the history of ideas it is also the history of the unreliability of words, and, in the absence of the author, written words from long ago are the most unreliable words of all. We must begin this chapter with all these cautions in mind.

As a starting point we have to attempt a deep empathy with the mind of the times. This requires a thoroughgoing logical grasp of a situation-of-thought that is entirely alien to most of us. We note Hall's remarks about the Neo-Platonists' very low valuation of corporeal bodies and the science of the material world of which bodies were a part. If, in sharp difference from earlier views, these came to be considered of little value, what was highly valued by the Neo-Platonists *must have been* entities postulated to be *non*material because *higher,* and also as *higher* because *non*material. This was not merely "new science," for a value judgment was also involved. Further, they must have been products of a new *imagination,* products of a mind now so developed that it had become capable of a process of *abstract conceptualization* never possible before. In confirmation of this we must also recognize that they were new postulates because *material* entities would be *things-in-experience,* taken by the mind of earlier eras to be *certainties,* the very opposite of postulates, which were *tentatively suggested* entities, or things *believed* rather than empirical *facts.*

The human mind was extending *in imagination* beyond the world of relationships with matter into an *inner* realm of its very own, and very recent, making. Perhaps *we* would use the word *spiritual* to describe the newly conceived entities, and, if that would be right, we must now expect a new form of dualism, postulating differences not of degree but of *kind-of-essence* to emerge. Earlier dualisms had had their grounds in what the Dutch writer J. J. Poortman terms "hylic pluralism," the belief that matter (Greek *hule,* meaning matter as differentiated from spirit or ether or any essence believed to be truly *non*material) occurred in different varieties, ranging from the finest—the fire that rose to the gods or the air that was inhaled and exhaled, and that brushed the cheek or blew down trees—to the grossest, the stony earth underfoot.[1] For long periods of history there had been little thought of what we would term the "logical possibility" of essences that *were not material in any sense at all.* Poortman's four-volume work *Vehicles of Consciousness* illuminates these often obscure topics. Here, we can allow them far less space, but alert the

reader to the need to be aware of them as the antecedents of the subject of this chapter, Neo-Platonism. In chapter 15 a new perspective on these topics will appear.

Despite the vagueness and ambiguity of earlier interpretations that may have lacked the present-day vernacular* sharp distinction between material and nonmaterial, G. R. S. Mead tells us in his introduction to *The Doctrine of the Subtle Body in Western Tradition* that the belief that the physical body is a manifestation and numinous expression of the soul is an extremely ancient one in the West. His study brings together ideas about the subtle body as they developed in Western traditions, from what he calls the "Alexandrian period" from around 300 CE to 642 CE, during which one branch of Neo-Platonism developed, to the scientific discoveries of his own day. The first published version of Mead's text appeared in 1919 and is still relevant today, highlighting, as it does, the dichotomies between matter and spirit and between mechanistic and holistic that still prevail in our society.

He makes the important point that "as a fact of history we find that innumerable thinkers in the past were persuaded of the existence of a subtle order of matter." This stage of hylic pluralism, to use Poortman's term, contained the seeds of its own transcendence for, as we saw, it led to the imaginative postulation of the utterly *non*material. Although they arrived at their hypothesis, as Mead puts it, by a simpler, or more naïve, procedure than that of present-day scientific method, he asserts that they "got at it" by the analysis of the whole of living experience, without prejudice, by speculating on the phenomena of dreams and visions as well as on the facts of purely objective sense-data, by reasoning about what happened to them without any arbitrary exclusion of everything not given in patent physical perception.[2] It was natural that in this wider, introspective, and meditative milieu the notion of spirit as something ethereal, yet quite different from atmospheric air, might develop. Of course, existing words, such as the Greek *pneuma,* would be used of this "new" entity, and, we wryly add, so increase the already great preexisting confusion.

This book is not an academic history of confused religious beliefs but a survey and discussion of ideas

---

*Present-day physics, as we shall see in chapter 15, no longer makes this sharp distinction.

about our essence from early and recent times, which turns to look forward to a more-than-holistic future of integral consciousness. A survey of some of Neo-Platonism's hinterland of beliefs about the nature and possible survival of the human being is appropriate here. Some of the Indic roots have already been revealed in earlier chapters. Ideas about the relationship between body, soul, and spirit had evolved, and continued to evolve, out of a common Indo-European culture. The Middle East mediated cultural contact between East and West. The process occupied many centuries, the westward movement during the later periods often impeded by the colossus of Christianity by then established in the north. Greek and Arabic texts on philosophy, natural science, and medicine began to appear in Europe only after the Christians reconquered Toledo in 1085, opening the way for access to material preserved by Islamic scholars. In this and succeeding chapters we shall follow, very approximately, this historical development, now dealing briefly with Egypt, where, during the late centuries of the pre-Christian era and into the first centuries of that era, Hermeticism was evolving side-by-side with the Alexandrian school of Neo-Platonism that was itself an influence upon it.

The early Egyptians had believed that the subtler parts of the human being included, among others, entities they named the *ka*, the *ba*, and the *akh*. The precise natures of these entities are, for the modern mind, very unclear, the categorizations implied being inconsistent with any present-day taxonomy. Poortman tells us that despite our having a great deal of information about the Egyptian beliefs, "there is very little rhyme or reason to be seen in the content of these ideas."[3] All that seems possible for us, therefore, is to make statements about each notion as if in isolation from the others, ignoring the overlaps and gaps that result, and the questions that arise.

The *ka* and the *ba* are, apparently, neither wholly material nor wholly spiritual, ba being sometimes described as if it were the raw material from which all souls are made, sometimes as a distinct entity having a shape of its own, just as any solid thing in the physical world (such as the visible body itself) has a unique identity and shape. This ambiguity is worsened when we find that the ka is described as the double of the visible, tangible living person, a copy of the physical body, but

made of finer or subtler matter. This apparent overlap of ka and ba is confusing to the modern mind, though it evidently confused the Egyptians too, for their own references to it are, the experts tell us, also confused and ambiguous.

The ba was believed to leave the body when a person dies, yet might revisit it later (see plate 23). This notion suggests the possibility that the concept of the ba came about as a result of introspection on the experience of dreaming, which seemed to be a traveling away from the sleeping body, followed by return to it. Despite the hawklike appearance of the entity hovering over the physical body in the illustration, the face of the ba was said to be the exact likeness of the face of the deceased person, which suggests deep confusion between ba and ka in the Egyptian mind. This is not the only confusion, for some writers interpret the sources as telling us that the akh, a third part of a sort of composite soul, was conceived to be the spirit of Ra, the sun god, without which, or whom, it was recognized there would be no life on Earth, but other writers, no less well informed, say that it is the ka that is an impersonal force, a "spiritual sun-matter," an undoubtedly very fine kind of matter that empowered not only the bodies of the primordial gods but also flowed into the body of the king, and even down into every living being. So, again, there is deep confusion, this time between the ka and the akh. However, this universality or ubiquity of akh seems to have ensured that it was also regarded not only as an *entity*, as *itself* a living being, but as a *quality* of living beings, lost at death, for in the Egyptian view it has an *opposite*. Independent substances may well be wholly distinct, but they can hardly have opposites, in the relevant sense. The negation of akh is *mut*, meaning "dead," as if the words are *adjectival* in function; akh was thus the *state* of a person who was alive, and mut the *state* of one who has died but has not been transfigured into light. We must turn away from such confusions and pursue this chapter's true theme of Neo-Platonism, which we shall find was wiser than its parent.

Plato's Three-Part Soul

To what extent Plato's thought derived from that of Indian and Egyptian precedents is debatable, but the idea of the body as external to a person's truest *self* had become quite common in Greek thought, the first known clear expression of it being Plato's own "human within," and for Plato himself the "true self" is the rational part of a soul that is immortal. According to R. M. Hare, who was Professor Emeritus of Moral Philosophy, Oxford University, and is recognized as a major authority on Plato in recent decades, "Both Plato and Pythagoras may have been influenced by ideas from the East and by the mystery religions, such as Orphism, which spread through Greece in this period. The early Pythagoreans seem (though this has been disputed) to have been mind-body dualists; that is to say, they thought, as Plato was to think, that the soul or mind (*psyché*) was an entity distinct and separable from the body."[4] As we have seen, Poortman makes more, and subtler, distinctions than the simple, even simplistic, contrast between a monism and a dualism that Hare is using here.

There is evidence that Plato derived some facets of his understanding from the Egyptian sources in the fact that in the *Republic* he speaks of three parts of the soul, *epithymia, thymos,* and *nous* or *logos,* which we shall very shortly define. These may have correlations with the ba, the ka and the akh, but the vagueness of the Egyptian concepts means that no firm statement here could be defended. More positive for us is that in the *Phaedrus* Plato makes a comparison between the soul and a chariot with a driver and two horses. This reminds us of the verse, cited in chapter 1, from the *Katha Upaniṣad,* which is worth quoting again here:

> *Know this:*
> *The self is the owner of the chariot*
> *The chariot is the body*
> *Soul (*buddhi*) is the body's charioteer—*
> *Mind the reins [that curb it].*

Like the ancient Hindus, the earliest thinkers in the West were interested in the cosmos (Greek, *kósmos*) and, in particular, its hierarchical structure and moral order. In Plato's *Timaeus,* where his primary purpose is to give a religious and teleological account of the world and the phenomena of nature, he not only refers to the three parts of the soul, just noted, but locates them in different parts of the body. This, too, is a schema we have noted elsewhere, for it is central to qigong. He locates the "divine and immortal part of the soul" in the head,

and the other two parts in the heart and the belly. He adds, "being mortal, they are closely connected with the physiological processes of the parts in which they are situated," and insists on "the close connection between mind and body."[5]

However, his tripartite schema also contains a psychological level, for he taught that the *psyche* or soul could be divided into: epithymia, desire, which is clearly not easy to conceive as a material thing, despite its corresponding with both the stomach and the masses of the people; thymos, which is spiritedness or righteous anger, and, despite its physiological *effects,* would seem in *essence* equally nonmaterial, corresponding to the chest and the soldier or warrior class; and, finally, nous or logos, which are mind or reason, also clearly not material substances, which correspond to the head and to the philosopher class.

While low desire was felt by all, and anger made the breast of the soldier heave, the philosopher calmly considered, in the highest part of his body, thoughts that (at least in his own estimation) were also *metaphorically* higher. Thus the notions of the *meta*phorical, the *non*material, the *non*physical, and even the *meta*physical were emerging; indeed, they were becoming *necessary postulates* as thinking left behind both the Egyptian confusedness and the Vedic simplicity (whether interpreted as dualistic or not). As such concepts as nous and logos emerged, enabling the human mind to think of what we would term abstractions, so the need to postulate different grades of matter from gross to fine began to recede. The chasm between an abstract concept such as "thought" and any everyday experience of "reality" was eventually seen to be greater than the difference between the solid, gross, matter of ice, and the water that resulted when the sun shone on it, yet was so obviously in some way the same matter.

This new capability of abstract thinking produced, in due course, a concept related to the Judaic realization that any God worthy of human worship would be *un*like a human, *not* an angry and vengeful Great Man, even if dwelling in the sky, as Yahweh had, by this epoch, begun to seem. However, human enlightenment proceeded by small steps, and anthropomorphic thinking could not be entirely expunged since humans cannot imagine the unimaginable. (We shall consider this human limitation further in chapter 15.) However, philosophers, while just as incapable as everyone else of imagining the unimaginable, *could* imagine that a realm might exist that contained *un*imaginable *things*. However, the overriding limitation could not be removed. Humans had always imagined the higher as *similar to* the lower, so, rather than fall entirely silent as to what a higher world might contain, as most earlier contemplatives had done, Plato conceived the further notion that in that highest realm there would exist things that, while *resembling* terrestrial things, all faulty in some way, would be the *ideal perfections* of those earthly things. The world of Forms, or Ideas, or Archetypes, was born in the Platonic mind.

Humankind's consciousness had, doubtless, been long developing at this time, but thinking brought new confusion, for this postulated higher realm of the Ideas must surely contain not only the perfect forms of *solid objects,* which would be patterns for the production of all earthly "thingnesses," all realities, all solid objects, even mundane things like tables and chairs, but consciousness now also conceived the notion that there would be perfect Forms of what *we* might term "things of the mind," *qualities* such as goodness and truth. The mind of Plato's time was not yet so conscious of its own consciousness that it could analyze what we see as a *categorial* distinction between "real being" and "abstract notion." Plato could go out into the street and find a stone, or a puddle, or a breath of air, or a fire, but he could not find a goodness or a truth. He surely saw this, but the categories could not yet be separated out. What he had conceived to be a world of the Ideas or Forms was itself not simple but complex, a place of confused categories, in reality nearer to what, more than two millennia later, the philosopher Karl Popper would call "World 2," thoughts, the content of mind, "World 1" being the physical world around us, full of material things, which include the fire, the breath of air, the puddle, and the stone. But Plato, with others of his and the immediately preceding eras, had nonetheless taken a great step forward, making possible belief in an invisible yet very real God, as well as the analysis of thoughts *about thinking.* Thinking about thinking spawned new concepts to complicate the already complex scheme. But only thought could think about thinking, and the new thinking was that there existed a category of things, or rather of *non*things, that must be distinguished. Not everyone knew this, so it was decided that nous alone is

able to contemplate the *spiritual* Forms or Archetypes, and the dignity of philosophers, who alone were capable of nous, remained intact.

However, Plato's understanding of physical anatomy was limited, for dissection of the human body was very little practiced in the ancient world. His understanding of the subtle anatomy was derived, according to Mead, from the astral or sidereal* religion of antiquity. The ancients' belief had long been that the creation of man in the image of God was to be understood literally. Everything was what *we* call "physical," though water, fire, and air were progressively more subtly physical than earth. They maintained that the universe was a great organism much like the human body, and that every phase and function of the universal body had a correspondence in the human. They termed this "the law of analogy." The restraints upon dissection of the body notwithstanding, any content regarding God's own form depended entirely upon such scant knowledge of the human physical body as humankind allowed itself to learn. No doubt what was effectively a proscription of dissection was, by a circularity of reasoning, itself partly grounded in the belief that the body, being formed in the image of God, was too holy to be cut up (except, of course, in battle, which did allow humans to learn that it contained the entrails).†

A Greek System of Chakras?

Many of the ideas about the soul, its functions, and its parts, which form the basis of the Western esoteric

---

Sidereal (from the Latin *sider,* meaning "star") relates to the distant stars and constellations of fixed stars, but not to the planets (from the Latin *planetes,* meaning "wanderer"). In *The Doctrine of the Subtle Body in Western Tradition,* Mead explains that "The astral or sidereal religion of antiquity revolved around the central notion of an intimate correspondence between man's sensible and psychical apparatus, or his inner embodiment, and the subtle nature of the universe. The relative positions of the celestial bodies in the aether at any moment were regarded by the most advanced thinkers solely as indices of the harmonious interaction of invisible spheres, with appropriate fields of vital energy."
†We wonder whether battle was seen as a Godlike activity, and the Old Testament assures us that it was, God himself doing battle, not least (we now think) because his people practiced the same, and he, being their leader, must follow them, having been created by them in their image.

traditions, came from the works of the Greek philosophers. Although correspondences between Eastern and Western perceptions of the soul and the subtle body are not exact, we find a certain similarity in ideas across the Eurasian continent. Plato's account of the parts of the soul described in the *Timaeus,* for example, bear some relation to accounts of the chakras. Herbalist and holistic practitioner David Osborn cites a conceptual model of an equivalent system (see fig. 11.1) from an original idea by former professor of Greek and Latin John Opsopaus,[6] which Osborn believes underpins Greek medicine and many of the holistic therapies practiced today.[7]

Opsopaus studied the *Timaeus,* which would seem to be the ideal starting place to find a Greek system of energy centers since, as H. P. D. Lee describes it in his translation, the *Timaeus* was "the first Greek account of a divine creation," which "remained influential throughout the period of the Ancient World, not least towards its end, when it influenced the Neo-Platonists."[8] Lee also states that it was one of the few works of classical antiquity to survive in its Latin translation into the Dark and Middle Ages, and that it achieved an immense importance in European thought that continues even at the present day. The model illustrated by figure 11.1 is based on three basic principles that, Opsopaus suggested, a Greek model of energy centers might embody:

1. Seven energy centers (the average number, as we saw in the Hindu traditions).
2. The centers should be located in the same places as the chakras.
3. They should have similar functions.

However, there are inherent difficulties in the search for a Greek system of chakras or energy centers of the subtle body to parallel the Indian. As Oxford professor of ancient philosophy Richard Sorabji observes, there is no uniformity of ideas in Greek philosophy about what constitutes that immaterial part of our being to which we variously refer as "spirit," "self," or "soul." "The Greeks did not at first find it easy to articulate the idea of things being immaterial," he says.[9] This, too, we noted earlier, along with the similar confusion between the Egyptian notions of ka, ba, and akh. Sorabji also points out that feature of what Poortman calls hylic pluralism

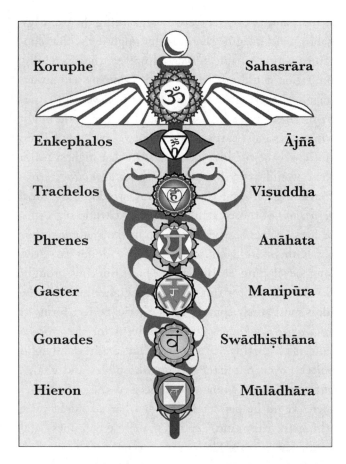

Fig. 11.1. This figure illustrates the correspondences between a Greco-Roman conception of chakras (left) and the Indian system (right), arranged around the Hermetic insignia with its wings and entwined snakes.

that produced inconsistency of belief as to whether or not the soul is a body and whether or not it is mortal. The first extensive discussion of the soul's immortality appears in Plato's *Phaedo,* in which he claims that the soul is like the *universals,* such as equality, or the goodness or truth we mentioned earlier, which are different from *particulars,* such as physical objects, since the universals cannot be perceived by the senses.* While Homer, Pythagoras, and Empedocles had, much earlier, all emphasized the soul's immortality, Aristotle and Epicurus, about a generation after Plato, made it mortal, despite denying it had a body. The earlier philosophers had described it *as* a body, while later philosophers thought that the soul is not a body but is dependent on a body. The Stoics consciously made the soul a body, and

---

*We notice here a pointer to the true nature of the physical sciences, whether ancient or modern.

not immortal, yet allowed it to persist a long time after death. Whole chapters could be written around these uncertainties, with no firm conclusions resulting. At the end of chapter 15 we shall suggest an understanding that present science can support.

Another problem is that some of the terms for these concepts have been transferred unchanged from their original languages and are now in common English usage, while others have been translated with preexisting English words. In neither case can we be certain that the precise *meaning* of any of them has been accurately preserved, or that any word now in use truly describes to us what was understood by the originators of the term. The word *psyche* serves as an example. In present-day English it is used interchangeably with both "spirit" and "mind," as in psychology, which is "the study of the mind and its functions," and psychiatry, "the study and treatment of mental (i.e. mind) illness." The words *soul* and *spirit* are vague and interchangeable in colloquial speech. Adding to the confusion, present English usage also has the phrase "body, mind, and spirit," used as if these were distinguishable entities, each with a well-defined, mutually exclusive meaning. In fact, we are not much less confused today than the ancient Egyptians and Greeks, despite our diligent pursuit of understanding. Discerning our own nature, and finding the right words for it, is difficult indeed.

Even during the ancient Greek period itself, before any translation took place, the word *psyche* was given different meanings at different times. As Opsopaus points out, in the Homeric age (eighth century BCE) it referred to the "vital spirit" or "life principle" or "life soul," the immortal part of the soul, which was represented as a snake and had its physical counterpart in the cerebrospinal fluid. Here we may have a correspondence with the Indian kundalinī, the serpent power that also rose around, or within, the spine. Both Homer and, some three centuries later, Plato believed that the psyche, the rational soul, was lodged in the brain at the level of the ājñā chakra (literally the "command wheel") in the middle of the head. Here, according to Tantra, when the serpent power is aroused, the left-channeled and right-channeled energies, idā and pingalā, having crossed over and over, meet again at the crown center. Qigong shows a similar notion, though without the heavy emphasis upon the spinal column that Tantra inherited from the

Vedic seers. We might note also that the concept of a wheel within the head, the ājñā chakra, must have been a metaphor of great resonance and scientific significance for the ancients, for whom the wheel was the highest, most magical technology, as momentous and as prominent in the cultural awareness of the era as the computer is in ours.

As we have seen, Plato considered the human being as having a soul that was tripartite. This analysis was based on the fact that the physical body seemed to have three diverse main functions, ranging from animal, at the base, to what we might term spiritual, in the heart or head. However, he also espoused notions of a triple division of the nonphysical, mental capacities mentioned earlier, of which he used terms such as "forms," "kinds," "characters," and even "souls." We note the confusion (which bedevils philosophy to this day) about the question of whether a *quality* of a thing (something rather adjectival) could *itself* be a thing (something substantive, requiring use of a noun). Today's psychologists explain this triple constitution of the Platonic soul as "having three elements of consciousness." However, a number of scholars have pointed out that this should be seen in the context not of psychology but of ethics since, they believe, it evinces three types of ethical problem, or moral quality, with regard to three types of life, namely the ideal contemplative life and two alternatives to it, the search for honor and the search for profit, each style of living being grounded in one of three corresponding modes of cognition or cognitive style.[10] Here we see a close parallel with the Indian system, which also has three paths, the "verticalist, horizontalist, and integral approaches" as Feuerstein describes them, denoted by the Sanskrit terms nivṛtti-marga (the path of cessation), pravṛtti-marga (the path of activity), and pūrna-marga (the path of wholeness),[11] in each of which one of the three cognitive styles dominates.[12] Interestingly, Heidegger, a recent philosopher who grounded his reexamination of the question of our Being in ancient Greek belief, found a number of trinities-in-indissoluble-unities as he built an ontologically fundamental psychology of our nature and of our modes of living as Beings-in-the-world.

We can compare what Plato referred to as the nous, the divine, immortal part of the soul that has the qualities of spiritual insight, wisdom, and intellect, to the Indic sattva guna, the disposition of "divine character," expressed through the sahasrāra (crown) and ājñā (brow) chakras.

The thymos, the seat of the emotions, identified as "the breath" or, in Plato, as the "breath-soul," is similar to the raja guna, the source of stimulating, dynamic energy expressed through the viṣuddha (throat), anāhata (heart), and manipūra (solar plexus) chakras.[13] Osborn comments that the thymos is also the essence of the vital faculty, the heart and lungs, related to pneuma, the breath or spirit.[14] In Homer's time it had been considered to be the seat of all thought, feeling, and consciousness. By Plato's time the heart center had become the seat of the passions, the emotions, the feeling mind, whereas the brow center was the seat of the rational mind and soul. In Plato's system, a midriff partition, which manifests physically as the diaphragm, exists between the heart center and the lower center, which is primarily concerned with the body and its needs. Being the first of the centers that is truly concerned with spirit and that higher life, which gave scant attention to the needs of the body, a kind of spiritual rebirth takes place in the heart center, and so allows spiritual progress toward the highest center to continue. We are reminded yet again of Sufism and qigong.

The epithymia, the level of desire and instinct, would appear to correspond with the tamas guna (inertia and dark, heavy energy) expressed through the swādhiṣṭhāna (sacral) and mūlādhāra (root support) chakras. In Sanskrit the word *swādhiṣṭhāna* means "one's own place," and parallels the Greek *gonades,* the generative and procreative function that Plato believed was the place where "the bonds of life unite the soul with the body," the seat of the desire for life which draws new souls into physical embodiment. The ancient Greeks, like the Tantrics, considered semen and female sexual fluid to be the physical manifestation of the life force. The female must, it was thought, contribute something of herself to the child to be gestated, but both the taboo on dissection and the inconspicuousness of the ovum had prevented its discovery. "Female fluids," therefore, were seen as the necessary counterpart to male semen, and the Gnostics concurred.

The Tantric belief was that a postulated substance named, in Sanskrit, the *ojas* (spiritual essence), a kind of numinous energy that illumined the entire body-mind, was drawn down the cerebrospinal channel into the womb, and there produced new life (rather than return-

ing upward as the kundalinī). Based on scant and, we now know, highly unreliable empirical "evidence," this produced obvious confusions, for the ojas was held to be so potent that, when sublimated by a celibate meditator (particularly males), it would enable an ascetic to influence his or her destiny and the destiny of others.[15]

The West is not without equally ill-conceived notions, for in Descartes' time the sperm was often thought to contain a human being, already complete, but tiny, which the woman's body merely fed until it became of sufficient size to be born. Even within the past fifty years, some reasonably well-educated people without physiological knowledge have thought the sperm the only ingredient involved in procreation, because it is the "seed"—a naïve misunderstanding having a merely verbal basis.

There appears to be no concept expressed in Greek language to parallel kundalinī as such, but its sublimation of sexual energy into the rising serpent power finds at least a faint resonance in that the Greek term for the lowest of the psychoenergetic centers, *hieron osteon,* means "sacred bone," "holy reed" (Greek *hiera sphinx*), or "holy bone" and was believed by the early Greeks to generate all life and to distribute spiritual energy.[16] It bears some resemblance to the *kanda* (bulb), the root of all the nadis, from which the primal spiritual energy emerges through the "hollow tube" of the innermost spinal channel, the *citrini,* the "radiance of Consciousness itself."[17] Perhaps this faintness of resonance should not surprise us, for Tantra itself was not the main stream of Indic influence on the Greeks.

Plato and Reincarnation

Plato, believing the one soul to be in fact tripartite, argues that if the soul is embodied, then all its parts must be necessary to existence, for without all three, embodied as a group, nothing at all would be embodied and the human race would perish. It has been assumed by some Greek scholars that since nous is the only part of the soul that is immortal, it will escape rebirth. However, the author James Robinson offers an alternative interpretation, contending that the tripartite soul is "everlasting" but *not* immortal, a view with which Plato himself evidently concurred; but, Robinson adds, if his interpretation is correct the soul *has no escape*.[18] He comments that Plato seemed to believe that the soul's escape from rebirth was only temporary.[19] In Plato's conception, the best souls are reincarnated in heavenly bodies, the worst in the bodies of snakes or fish. This raises the questions of what "heavenly" would mean, and by what ethical standard the soul would be judged, and also suggests a developing ambivalence in humankind's attitude to the snake, presaging its latter-day characterization not as wise but as evil. Robinson notes that the destiny of the soul is best expressed in the metaphor of a ladder—an idea that we also see in the Indic traditions (and a relic thereof in the board game Snakes and Ladders)—which the soul ascends and descends.[20] Clearly, if a ladder allows ascent to heaven, as Jacob's and other ladders do, the snake has now become the enemy of such progress, its former high reputation suffering in consequence. Here is a concept similar to that of *karma,* in which the body serves as the vehicle through which the soul experiences the trials and tribulations of the world. It also illustrates the way in which arguments over religious understanding gave rise to zealous persecution of gentle thinkers who happened to have thought rather more than those who perceived it their duty to destroy fellow humans on behalf of an angry God. The power of ideas is immense.

St. John of the Ladder

The ladder of ascension was a recurring theme in both Eastern and Western societies of the ancient world. One of the most revered saints of the Eastern Church is St. John Klimatos, "St. John of the Ladder," born in Constantinople in 570 CE. A great ascetic and author of a spiritual work called "The Ladder," he describes the steps to spiritual perfection attainable by the ascent of a "fixed ladder leading from earthly things to the Holy of Holies," starting with renunciation of worldliness and ending with "God who is love." Although written for monks, the book is still recommended as an unerring guide and support in the spiritual life for any Christian living in the world.

That the nous cannot, by its very nature, escape is a very different idea from the Indian concept of the jīvan-mukta (the "liberated while living") who can tran-

scend the human condition by perfecting himself or herself through spiritual practice. Yet, as mentioned, Plato seems to have believed that something can last forever *without becoming immortal* and that, since the human soul contains something divine fashioned by the gods, it does have the opportunity to become "virtuous," that is, ordered, and, by doing so, improve itself. The description "ordered" brings to mind the modern physicist's concept of entropy, and the thought that so long as energy is continually injected into a system to restore the "order" lost from it there is no reason why that orderedness should not persist indefinitely. Such a Being would not be inherently immortal but a system that was everlasting because it was under perpetual repair and maintenance. Many spiritual paths have considered the maintenance of the physical body important, and perhaps equally many have believed the reverse, looking instead for ultimate salvation by leaving the physical world behind. Each is based upon a view of our being that is directly opposed to the other, the one being hylic pluralistic, the other dualistic.

Although it would seem that Plato's schema dooms the soul to reincarnate perpetually, we see an interesting development in his *Timaeus,* which postulates a parallel to the Buddhist concept of spiritual rebirth as a bodhisattva, an evolved soul who remains behind on, or revisits, earth to help other souls and to aid the world soul to maintain order and harmony in a realm of becoming.

The Radiant Body

Mead states that while the idea of the subtle body perhaps reached its most mature expression in Indian thought, the parallel notion that evolved in the West also asserted that the perfection of a person is achieved by following the path of ascension, which, in the semispiritual but still largely physicalistic mode of the times, was usually conceived as an ascent toward the stars. He writes:

> The speculation of sidereal faith rose to ever more sublime heights, and brought such minds as could struggle to the topmost peaks of the mount of contemplation into communion with the ever-living ideas or realities of the spiritual

state which energized in the second degree as the formative principles of the world of becoming. He who could reach to such communion, we are told, had firmly planted his feet on what Plato calls the plain of truth.[21]

Amid the confusing plethora of incompatible and shifting notions, the terms *pneûma* (spirit or breath) and *sôma pneumatikôn* (spiritual or breath body) were, according to Mead, the most commonly used by the Greeks in referring to the soul vehicle.

The spirit body, or spiritous embodiment, was often called the aëry or ethereal body. But, as a distinction was usually drawn between the lower air (*aēr*) and the upper air (*aithēr*), ethereal should perhaps be reserved for the celestial state of this psychical vehicle . . . and after death it was known as the image (*eidōlon, imago, simulacrum*) or shade (*skia, umbra*).[22]

Sometimes it was referred to as the subtle or "light" vehicle of the soul, to distinguish it from the gross, dense, solid, or earthy body, which was often called the "shell," or shell-like body or "surround," reminiscent of the famous phrase of Plato in the *Phaedrus* (250c): "We are imprisoned in the body like an oyster in its shell," a sentiment that echoes that of the Hindus for whom the human condition is "bondage," and underpins the whole spiritual enterprise, as we saw in chapter 1.

Mead emphasizes that it must be clearly understood that, for the Hellenic philosophers, *spirit* in this sense is subtle *body,* an embodiment of a finer order of matter than that known to physical sense, and not soul proper. This is also one of Poortman's main contentions. By *body,* moreover, is not meant a developed and organized form, but rather an "essence" or "plasm" that may be graded, or "woven into various textures." In itself unshaped, it is capable of receiving the impression or pattern of any organized form. The soul proper, Mead says, is thought of as utterly incorporeal. Psychic life is classified according to its manifestations in body, but is not itself body.[23]

According to Mead, the fundamental notion that was absorbed into Greek philosophy from the influence of the mystical doctrines of Asia Minor was of a

"star body" or "radiant body." This was known in classical Greek as the *augoeidēs,* that is, possessed of *augē,* a form of splendor, brightness, radiance, or glory. It was regarded as the prime essence or substance of all bodies and all embodiment and the vehicle of purity and truth. The apostle Paul refers explicitly to the necessity for believers to "put on immortality" in order to resemble Yahshua, who has a "glorious body."[24] Damacius, the last of the Academics* of the old school,† writes of the radiant body:

> In heaven, indeed, our radiant (*augoeidēs*) [portion] is full filled with heavenly radiance (*augē*)—glory that streams through its depths, and lends it a divine strength. But in lower states, losing this [radiance], it is dirtied, as it were, and becomes darker and darker and more material. Heedless it grows, and sinks down towards earth; yet in its essence it is still the same in number [i.e. a unity]. So also with our soul itself, when it strikes upwards unto Mind and God, then is its essence [that is the *augoeidēs*] full filled with gnostic light divine, of which it previously [that is in incarnation] was not possessed, else had it always been divine.[25]

Although Plato's philosophy was soon rivaled by that of his more scientific, materialistically oriented student and successor, Aristotle, the seeds of an esoteric psychology were carried on by the Middle- and Neo-Platonists, particularly Plotinus. Manly Hall points out that, to the ancients, "the study of the stars was a sacred science, for they saw in the movements of the celestial bodies the ever-present activity of the Infinite Father."[26] This is clearly evidenced in the following reference to the nature of the radiant body and its relationship to the stars made by Proclus, the last major classical Greek philosopher. He states in his commentaries on Plato's *Timaeus:*

> Man is a little world (*mikrós kósmos*). For just like the universe (*tò pân*), he possesses both mind

---

*The Academics were members of the Academy of Athens founded by Plato ca. 387 BCE.

†Despite the similarity between Damacius' belief and that of Christ's apostle, the Christian emperor Justinian drove him from his post in 529 CE.

and reason (*nous* and *lógos*), both a divine and a mortal body. He is also divided up according to the universe. It is for this reason, you know, that some are accustomed to say that his gnostic [principle] (*tò noeròn*) corresponds with the nature of the fixed stars. His reason [corresponds] in its contemplative aspect with Saturn, and in its social aspect with Jupiter. As to his irrational [part]—the passional [nature corresponds] with Mars, the eloquent with Mercury, the appetitive with Venus, the sensitive with Sol [sun], and the vegetative with Luna [moon]. Moreover, the radiant vehicle (*augoeidḗs óchēma*) [corresponds] with heaven, and this mortal [frame] with the sublunary [region].[27]

Through the Neo-Platonists the ancient philosophers' musings about the subtle body had an impact on Western thought well into the Middle Ages. In Jean Fernel's *De Naturali Parte Medicinae* published in 1542, for example, we find the following passage:

In order that the necessity and the substance of the spirit may be more fully shown, we must revisit and recall the doctrines of the ancient philosophers. The Academics were the first to suppose, when they realized that two entirely dissimilar natures cannot be associated together without the interposition of a suitable mean, that our soul, created by the supreme maker of all things, before its emanation and immigration into this thick and solid body, put on as a simple garment a certain shining, pure body like a star, which, being immortal and eternal, could never be detached nor torn away from the soul, and without which the soul could not become an inhabitant of this world.

Then they surrounded the soul with another body, also fine and simple, but less pure, less shining and splendid than the first, not created by the supreme maker, but compounded of a mixture of the finer elements, whence it is named aerial and aethereal. Clothed with these two bodies, the soul, entering this frail and mortal body, or rather thrown like an exile into a loathsome and shadowy prison, becomes a guest of the earth until, having broken from this prison and having returned, joyful and free, to its home, it is made a fellow-citizen of the gods.[28]

As late as the Renaissance,* books on medicine still contained theories about the relationship between illness and the astral body, even though the concept of the astral body, as a subtle body intermediate between the soul and the physical body, was by then considered "unsafe," that is, unscientific.

The Neo-Platonist Philosophers

The first successors of Plato sought to preserve his teachings, and therefore did not consider or describe themselves as *Neo*-Platonists. The *Enneads* of Plotinus is the foundational document of Neo-Platonism, and contains a theoretical part dealing with the origin of the human soul, and a second, practical part showing by what way the soul may return to the One.

Name/Dates (all CE)	Description
Ammonius Saccas (death ca. 265)	Teacher of Plotinus
Plotinus (ca. 204–270)	Greco-Egyptian philosopher, widely regarded as the father of Neo-Platonism
Porphyry (ca. 232–305)	Syrian polymath, disciple and editor of Plotinus, also wrote commentaries on Plato and Aristotle
Iamblichus (ca. 245–325)	Syrian Neo-Platonist, best known for his compendium on Pythagorean philosophy
Proclus (ca. 410–485 CE)	The last major classical Greek philosopher; a systematic Neo-Platonist, he influenced subsequent Christian philosophers

---

*The Renaissance (rebirth) was a cultural movement that began in Italy in the late Middle Ages and later spread to the rest of Europe, spanning the fourteenth to the seventeenth centuries.

Climbing the Neo-Platonist Ladder of Being

From the sixth century BCE onward, the urge to reconcile the many with the One, an incomprehensible, all-sufficient unity, had been a recurring theme throughout Greek philosophy, and particularly in Plato. The theme remained central, and in the school of mystical philosophy known as Neo-Platonism was elaborated into a scale of graded levels of consciousness descending from the perfection of the One to the lowest levels shown by beings on earth. By the process of emanation the One had given rise to the Divine Mind or *Logos* (Word), which contained all the forms or intelligences of individuals. In the third century CE Plotinus expressed the central concerns of the new Platonism as arising from aspirations for a life in which the individual soul would rise through contemplation to the level of intelligence (the Divine Mind) and then, through mystic union, be absorbed into the One itself. Conversely, a privation of being or lack of desire toward the One was the cause of sin, which Plotinus held to be a negative quality, not so much the deliberate commission of evil, but, rather, a failure to do good, and thus a *nonparticipation in the perfection of the One.*

There are thus two reciprocal movements in Neo-Platonism:

- The metaphysical movement of emanation from the One
- The ethical or religious movement of reflective return to the One through contemplation of the forms of the Divine Mind

While the thinking of Plotinus was mystical, concerned with the infinite and invisible within the finite and visible world, his method was thoroughly rational, stemming from the logical and humanistic traditions of Greece. Many elements of his philosophy came from earlier philosophers. R. T. Wallis, formerly associate professor of classics at Oklahoma University, observes that "Until the dating of the *Hermetica* in 1614, the Platonic tradition was regarded as a later development of the pristine Egyptian wisdom of Hermes Trismegistus, the supposed original source of the *philosophia perennis*."[29] The existence of the One and the attendant theory of ideas or forms were aspects of the later writings of Plato, particularly in the *Timaeus,* and Stoicism had identified the World Soul with transcendent universal reason. What was distinctive in Plotinus's system was the unified, hierarchical structuring of these elements and the theory of emanation, as we see in the chart below.

Wallis observes that between the human soul (or consciousness) and the One there is a "ladder of being," which reminds us of the chakras of the Indian system. We have also seen that similar models are found in the three zones and three dantiens of the Chinese (qigong) system, in the Sufi system, and in Western descriptions of the subtle body such as those of the English alchemist Robert Fludd. Wallis specifically notes:

> The later Neo-Platonists have various terms, their favorite being the "summit" or "flower" (*anthos*) of Intelligence (*nous*); elsewhere a yet higher principle, "the flower of the whole soul," is distinguished. It is this principle, at the core of our being, that we attain by unifying our mind, and through it that we contact the divine.[30]

The methods employed to contact the Divine came from different sources. One strand of belief came from

THE NEO-PLATONIST LADDER OF BEING

The One	Intelligible Henads	Intellectual Henads	Supercosmic Henads	Intracosmic Henads
	Unparticipated Being	Participated Being	Participated Being	Participated Being
		Unparticipated Divine Intelligence	Participated Divine Intelligence	Participated Divine Intelligence
			Unparticipated Divine Soul	Participated Divine Soul
				Divine Soul

the "sympathetic magic" of pre-Neo-Platonic thought, in which *theurgy,* human ritualistic action taken in the hope of procuring supernatural or divine intervention, seeks to call down and use divine power to achieve a humanly intended result, and is essentially the same as ritual magic. The magician invokes divine force within a sacred object or in him- or herself, resulting in prophetic trance. Wallis says that this ancient idea of the principles of correspondence—"that each part of the universe mirrors every other part of the universe" and that "the whole material world is the mirror of invisible divine powers"—rests on the principle that "everything is in everything, but in each appropriately to its nature." It was "common ground for all Neo-Platonists that the sympathy linking all parts of the sensible cosmos enabled the magician to draw power from the celestial spheres."[31]

The idea of the interconnectedness of all things is common to many cultures, and there are many related myths. One version, from the sixth century *Avatamsaka Sutra,* tells the story of Indra's Net. Indra was a king in ancient India who, as kings are wont to do, thought a great deal of himself. One day he summoned the royal architect and said that he wanted to leave a monument to himself, something that all the world's people would appreciate. The king's architect seems not only to have perceived the king's pride but also to have been something of a mystic. He created an immense net, which extended throughout all space and time. The king's treasurer then placed a bright, shining pearl at each node of the net so that *every pearl was reflected in every other pearl.* No pearl, not even the king's, took precedence over any other, yet each single pearl, each person, each event, reflected, and so contained, the whole of Indra's Net, which included all of space and time, everything that is or ever was or will be. Despite the acknowledgment of terrestrial time inherent in this description, Indra's Net did *all* this *simultaneously.* The idea also points clearly toward the modern physicists' notion of an underlying field of all potentials, of which we shall say more.

These two illustrations, from Neo-Platonism and from India, afford a neat demonstration of the similarity, indeed, the *fundamentally human* natural identity of Eastern and Western concepts. Human thought is *necessarily* limited by our nature, regardless of history and geography, and our nature is *necessarily* compatible with the cosmos in which we live. Our view of that cosmos is

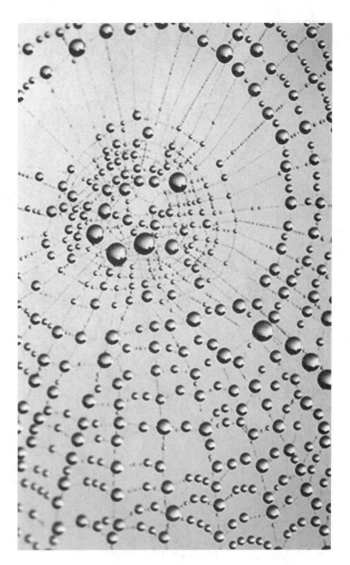

Fig. 11.2. Indra's Net. The symbolism of this allegorical tale helps us to understand the idea of an interconnectedness between all things, suggested here by droplets of dew on a spider's web, each reflecting all the others.

necessarily limited to what is within our power to imagine. For this reason, science can never expand beyond the range of human sense and imagination, though it can continue without obvious limit to discover facts within that realm, and to make better correlations with all other human knowledge.

Wallis notes that the increasing importance attached to theurgy in later Neo-Platonism corresponds to the great stress laid on ritual in the later, Tantric, forms of Indian religion. In both cases the contempt with which modern scholars formerly spoke of the later developments is now giving way to a more respectful interest.[32] This development is welcome and very long overdue. As always,

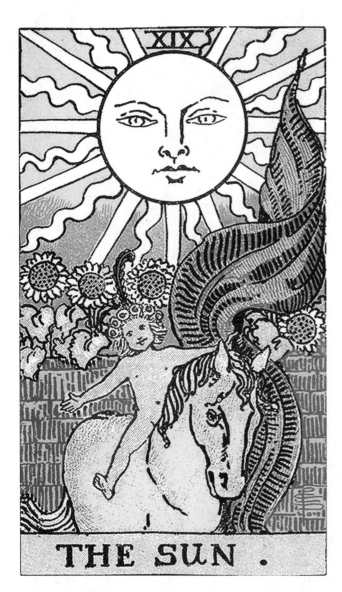

Fig. 11.3. Neo-Platonists believed that power could be drawn from the cosmos. Sol, the sun, represented generative and transforming power within the human and the cosmos, a source of universal power of growth, healing, and magic, and expression of the physiological and psychological urge to return to an incorruptible paradise, the uncursed world existing before the fall.

the concepts are human, the underlying forms already familiar, but the same intuited truths have new clothes. As we shall see in chapter 15, "Science, Philosophy, and the Subtle Body," Neo-Platonism now finds expression in postulates of interconnecting cosmic and human energy fields, and even in the concept of "three worlds": the Platonic "world above" of Ideas or Forms (including the eternal truths of mathematics) or something resembling it, the physical or material world in which we live, and the mental world, in which we also live.

Confusions and Uncertainties
What Parts of Our Being Are Immortal, What Parts Perishable?

While most Neo-Platonists agreed that what they termed the *soul* is immortal, some disagreed about whether the astral body dissolved after death or was immortal and celestial (hence *astral,* "starry"). Here we have one of our main questions: What is it that the subtle body is? Where should we draw a distinction between physical and nonphysical? Should we discard the terms *physical* and *metaphysical* as prejudicial to our attempt to answer the question? Does the subtle body have layers, as the Neo-Platonists all agree, while disagreeing about what, and how many, layers there are? If there are indeed layers, as the Upaniṣadic notion of kośas also attests, in which "worlds" do the layers exist? Or, if that question is wrongly put—for it may be based on a faulty prior hypothesis concerning the matters we seek to elucidate, and we must not assume what we seek to prove—should we see the question as if from above, as well as from below, and ask instead what unitary complex is the subtle body? Recall the image of a part beholding the whole, and the reverse, which is the central feature of Indra's Net, and the column of chakras that, along with the spinal column, places the human being in vertical relationship with the cosmos. What is the worth of holism if it is not big enough to embrace this mutuality of two-way, opposed-direction gaze?

This is really all one question, of course, but we need to analyze it into its subsidiaries if we are ever to be able to answer it. And however we finally answer it, we shall certainly have to modify it as we proceed, in the light of what we find at each step. Karl Popper, the highly regarded philosopher of science, would approve, for this testing and correction of hypotheses, he contends, is the best and safest procedure for science.

After this utterly central "aside" (we ask the reader to ponder the *merely apparent* contradiction in terms) let us return to Neo-Platonism itself. Porphyry, the immediate disciple and editor of Plotinus, believed that the soul's "pneumatic envelope," the subtle, astral body acquired during the descent from the celestial realm, needed to be, and could only be, purified by theurgy. "By this means, in virtue of the interconnections of body and lower soul, the latter could be purified sufficiently to enable man's higher soul to pursue contemplation without distraction."[33] This picture contains strong traces of the three-part division of the body accepted by Plato himself and by the Hermeticists. The notion of the soul was particularly complex, confused, and problematical, so much so that even rational discussion, let alone reliable definition, of the terms and their significances is almost impossible. The ancient Egyptian confusions over the ba, the ka, and the akh were still unresolved. While the Neo-Platonic soul was considered to be an "intelligible cosmos," as if an inherent part of the Great Being, or the One, and therefore greater and higher than an individual person, greater or higher than what we might term an "instance of incarnation," the soul embodied in the human being was nonetheless capable of choosing either a "rational" level of life or the "irrational" lower level of a subhuman animal. Such a proclivity seems to us, unless the soul is an impersonal pervasive essence, inconsistent with the exalted ethical nature of that higher realm from which it came, for it suggests that an emanation of the Great Being could choose to live in a much-inferior way. But if "soul" were an *impersonal* essence of this type, a kind of soul-*substance,* a raw material for soulness, profligately spread throughout the created world, how could it be in any real way a *central* essence of an *individual* human being? Perhaps there were indeed several souls, at different levels of being, whether so named or distinguished by other names.

According to Porphyry, theurgy could not confer immortality either on the irrational soul or on her vehicle, which, on a person's return to the intelligible world—that higher world that the human *intellect* could *grasp or envision* but that could not be *observed* by any of the body's *senses*—would therefore be dissolved into the spheres from which they had originated.[34] Beliefs were, as ever, confused and in still-ongoing flux. The fifth century Neo-Platonist, Proclus, the last notable philosopher of premodern Greece, who tackled the same long-standing questions concerning the permanence or otherwise of the postulated parts of Being, posited two subtle bodies or "vehicles" (*okhema*) connecting the soul with the physical body: the *pneuma* ("breathing" or "spiritual") vehicle, which he considered mortal, and the astral vehicle, which he believed was not the soul itself but the *immortal* vehicle of the soul. We have to invite those who are willing to tackle the uncertainties to consult writers such as R. T. Wallis.

Wallis points to an ambivalence in Porphyry's writings that may have come from a dilemma in Plato's thinking about whether or not body and soul constitute two distinct orders of reality, and whether a union between the two bodies would destroy the soul's separate existence. He also points to another fundamental question, whether or not incorporeal entities are subject to the spatial restrictions that are all too obvious in our lives in the physical world. How many angels can stand on the head of a pin? With reference to this question, Wallis tells us that

For Porphyry, as for Plotinus, they [incorporeal entities] are "everywhere and nowhere." The

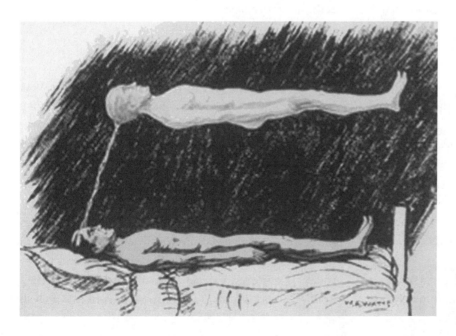

Fig. 11.4. The astral body was believed to travel out of the body during sleep, remaining linked to the body by a silver cord, which it could not sever because of the soul's emotional attachment to the body. Out-of-body experiences, the term introduced by G. N. M. Tyrrell in 1943, are experienced by around one in ten people today and are often part of the near-death experience. Little is known about the phenomenon as yet because Western researchers have been reluctant to explore it on account of its association with beliefs in the immortal soul that offend recent philosophical fashion.

soul's "presence" in the body is therefore not a matter of spatial location, but consists in a "relation" (*schesis*) towards that body. . . . The soul is therefore present "in" Intelligence when she exercises intuitive thought and "in" her own sphere when she reasons discursively; conversely she "descends to Hades" if the pneumatic vehicle to which she has grown attached becomes so coarsened that after the death of the physical body it sinks to the subterranean regions. For it is the soul's emotional attachment to the body that binds her there . . . and physical death, while separating body from soul, does not necessarily free the latter from the body's influence.[35]

Like so much else, this reminds us of the Egyptian confusions, in this instance the belief that the ba might revisit the dead body.

Wallis and other writers consider Neo-Platonism to be the last of the pagan philosophies that has had enduring influence on Western metaphysics and mysticism. "The notion of a subtle embodiment . . . may indeed prove to be that mediating ground in concrete reality which is so badly needed to provide a basis of reconciliation between the two dominant modes of opposed and contradictory abstractionising that characterise the spiritualistic and materialistic philosophy of the present day."[36] In considering whether Neo-Platonism has anything to offer us today, Wallis concludes that if we confine ourselves to the school's main trends, its religious and experiential side seems to offer more than its deductive metaphysics, but this by no means destroys Neo-Platonism's philosophical importance.

However, he also points out that "not all the Neo-Platonists' religious attitudes can still be accepted; in particular, even at their best they give too little importance to the body and the material world. Yet . . . our reaction to such excesses must be a *purification* of the spiritual life, not the wholesale abolition of an important part of human experience."[37] This goal will be achieved only by those who acknowledge both the necessity for discrimination and self-discipline as well as the necessity for acceptance of the body and ethical satisfaction of its needs and desires.

Although Wallis states that the dilemma of reason's place in the spiritual life is an acute and ultimately insol-

uble one (since too rigid a system leads to ossification but too little rationality leads to chaos), both in theology and in the individual mind, the Neo-Platonists' successes and failures have much to teach us in our own spiritual search, "for it is on our own success or failure in attaining a due balance that the future of our civilization depends."[38] We would add that the concept of the *integral* body, with its healthy (that is, whole) acceptance of *all* it contains, must be the best way to solve the dilemma. Perhaps, if the "liver" of the "lived body" is simply allowed to be him or her self, the "insoluble" problem will solve itself because it will shun the realm of left-brained intellect and turn to that of spontaneous but fully self-aware living.

Some problems are problems only because we have forced them to become so, and then, believing them to be problems, we have blocked their natural, unproblematic self-resolving flow. Perhaps the real problem has always been the human proclivity to raise so-called moral barriers against the happy embrace of a natural wholeness of life. Law has always been at loggerheads with the spirit, as the apostle Paul pointed out, though he may himself have failed to resolve the problem, for this opposition raised for him, and still raises for us in a civilization much influenced by his teaching, the important question of what we should *do* with our bodies, both subtle and physical. If we seek wholeness we must surely *allow the body*. The liver within the lived body is its own moral agent, as well as a vivifying force or personal, individual will. We leave these thoughts for readers to ponder and act upon for themselves.

Two Worldviews

Some contemporary thinkers believe that in the West (and here there is a strong contrast with the East) our being has been divided between, and therefore paralyzed by, two worldviews: fundamentalist Christianity and scientific materialism. According to author and broadcaster E. A. Meece, "A greater view of life than what is provided us by the two dominant, warring and extremely limited cultures is being created on the fringes of society. The revival of mystical vision, updated where necessary to better fit with our own reality and values today, is our eventual hope for renewal."[39] In Meece's opinion, a renewed Neo-Platonism is part of this revival,

Fig. 11.5. The Neo-Platonic ladder of the seven planets, an idea that parallels the Eastern idea of a correspondence between human embodiment and the cosmos.

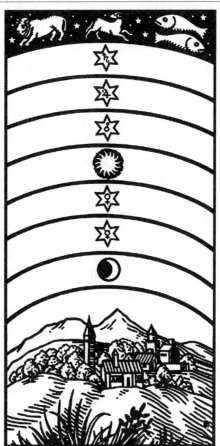

The 'crystal sphere' of 'fixed stars', three Zodiac signs, Taurus, Aries and Pisces, shown in the night sky

Saturn, the planet, or 'wanderer', with the longest period, bringer of taciturn old age

Jupiter, supreme Father, the thunderbolt his symbol, yet also 'jovial', escaped being devoured by Saturn, correlated with tin

Mars, the red planet, bringer of war, cabalistically correlated with iron

Sol, the sun, rational basis of the solar calendar of northern peoples dependent on the sun's return

Venus, the peaceful 'morning star' and 'evening star', always seen near the sun

Mercury, the fleet-footed winged messenger, the closest of all to the sun

The Moon, empirical basis of the lunar calendar of southern peoples who experienced less seasonal variation

Earth, the sublunary world, the realm of the 'Below' of the Hermetic system, reflecting, imperfectly, the 'Above'

though it is seldom known by this name today. This forgotten philosophy is one of the keys to unlock the shackles of current dogmas so that we can become a more creative and enlightened people. Whenever such things as sacred geometry, an organic cosmos, the Tree of Life, holography, or the soul centers within our bodies are discussed, Meece says, we are witnessing a revival of Neo-Platonism. The change has not been unheralded, but has merely taken a century to arrive, for one writer of the early twentieth century, the British theologian William Ralph Inge, though reviled by conservative religionists in his own day, claimed that "Neo-Platonic thought is, metaphysically, the maturest thought that the European world has seen." He admitted that our science is more developed with regard to some special problems, but still felt that "the modern time has nothing to show comparable to a continuous quest of truth about reality during a period of intellectual liberty that lasted for a thousand years."[40]

The central notion of an intimate correspondence between the subtle body of the human and the subtle

nature of the universe has persisted as a map of reality in Western traditions, as it did in Eastern traditions, until relatively recent times (see plate 24). In Neo-Platonic philosophy, the "world axis" along which the sun appeared to ascend and descend each year in a continual cycle seemed to present a symbol of the living, yet immutable, divine essence of the world. This axis mundi corresponds, in the *mikrós kósmos,* to our backbones, the stabilizing spiritual axis within our own bodies. This concept, as we have seen, is as old as the Vedas. Furthermore, there are seven "soul centers" or chakras along this axis corresponding to the seven planets and metals, an idea that author Robert Place believes was not merely imported from India. He believes that there is evidence that the seven soul centers were already known to the ancient Pythagoreans, and had in their time been already a part of Western culture for centuries. As trade and other contact between the Mediterranean and the Indus Valley people was well established by 1000 BCE, *mutual* influence of philosophical thought was at least possible, and there is little doubt it took place. "In the ancient world, the seven soul centers were related to the Neoplatonic ladder of the planets. . . . The soul centers or *chakras* are thought of as seven energy centers located in ascending order from the base of the spine to the top of the cranium."[41]

The Perennial Philosophy Returns

Much has changed since Inge's and Mead's writings were first published about a century ago. Although what Mead says about the schism between philosophy and spirituality is still relevant, there is a growing understanding of the nature of reality, and of our potential for transcendence and the evolution of consciousness, which is at the core of all belief systems. The spiritual context in the West today is a rediscovery of the philosophia perennis. In *The Return of the Perennial Philosophy*, John Holman, who describes himself as "an independent scholar," explains that "perennial philosophy" is a universal set of truths, common to all cultures and religions, found in the writings of philosophers, no matter how diverse their presentation of truth.[42] He says that views among philosophers since Leibniz (1646–1716) have differed on the question of whether a "final" philosophy had already been achieved before their time, and even as to whether it is achievable at all. Now, as the twenty-first century gets into its stride, we can certainly speak of the perennial nature of philosophy and the universality of certain of its questions and concerns. In 1944 Aldous Huxley articulated the chief among these matters as the main principles of a perennial philosophy:

> The immanence and transcendence of God as a pure consciousness that lives the human self as an actor lives his part, making the manifold world of our everyday experience "real with a relative reality . . . but this relative reality has its being within and because of the absolute Reality."
>
> The principle that the work to be achieved by human beings is union in consciousness with God and that this requires us in some measure to "die to self" in order to "make room" for God.
>
> The principle that in no period has God or Divine Reality left Himself (or Itself) without representation through prophets, mystics, and their teachings.[43]

Perhaps, John Holman believes, the most important principle in understanding this esoteric field devolves from the scholastic debate on *how to study* the perennial philosophy itself. Specifically, this relates to questions regarding what should be included in it and what excluded, not only in terms of subject matter, that is, the philosophical systems themselves, but the approaches to knowledge employed by the student. As we have pointed out elsewhere, some researchers take the view that the approach commonly promoted, if not prescribed, is the "agnostic empirical," but this is inadequate for it leaves out the rational view of subjective experience.

Holman rightly says that what we can all observe, with some effort and with the ordinary human mind, are the *conceptions per se* of the esotericists rather than the *realities about which* these conceptions may be held, namely Divine Reality. Current academic fashion requires these conceptions to be presented "neutrally" (that is, without expressing an opinion on their veracity), and, as Holman puts it, the "student of Western esotericism is, to be clear, *operationally* not an esotericist but, as Faivre proposes to differentiate them, an 'esoterologist'."[44] As Arthur Versluis, religious studies professor and founding president of the Association for the Study of Esotericism, has also pointed out, the problem with the approach of detached observation and report is that if we want an esotericist's view to be conveyed accurately and adequately "It is essential for scholars to engage at minimum in a process of imaginative participation. . . . I am suggesting that in order to fully understand what we are studying, there is a point in this field . . . at which the practitioner's expertise takes on more importance than purely academic knowledge."[45]

This is increasingly the view expressed by researchers in this field, and one that I, a meditator of many decades standing, have expressed several times in these pages. We cited music as an example comprehensible by all, including those with no experience of the esoteric, noting that "mappings" such as the printed score or the program note accompanying a public performance are far divorced from *the music itself as experience,* having *nothing, absolutely nothing,* in common *except* to a person who is already totally familiar with music *itself.* But what is the relevance of this? It is greater than one might think, which is why we stress it yet again, for Huxley presses the still stronger view that if we are to understand the essential content of the philosophia perennis—in other words, Divine Reality and our relation to it, via our subtle selfhood—we must recognize first that it cannot be directly apprehended unless we submit ourselves to the same spiritual discipline as those who have "trod the Path" before us.[46] Few could argue convincingly against him. The truth of what he says is obvious, and yet there is in this situation a difficulty, possibly unsuspected by observers from outside, which it may be *impossible* to overcome. A series of questions will point to it.

Can we be whole without becoming active esotericists?

How can one become an active esotericist without ascetically cutting off part of our natural selfhood?

If we cut off any part of our natural selfhood how can we be whole?

But perhaps there is a way to save the situation, so we ask a further question:

Does the concept of and the aim to become integral Beings help, or is it a forlorn endeavor, doomed by what some might still see as inherent internal contradictions to fail?

The questions to answer before attempting to diagnose our situation and our future prospects are:

What has the history of human consciousness achieved thus far?

Does our current standing promise us the ability to go further and to synthesize a greater wholeness than humans have ever experienced before?

Can we, now, become complete: completely natural, and spiritually complete too?

Perhaps we can achieve all possible objectives, but *successively,* pursuing one for a time, then another, as does Katavul, of whom we read in chapter 2. He meditates, he pursues the demons, and he pursues and enjoys Sakti. There is no prudery in him, no abnegation, no amputation, and no entering life maimed; over time he achieves a balance, and he fears no Gehenna of fire. If we attempt to become complete, memory will be crucial, retaining the result of the experience of one mode of living while, for a time, we pursue another. Over a lifetime a human would aim to build a balanced whole. Over many lifetimes, some male, some female, why should full perfection, at least full *human* perfection, evade us?

Has the rejection of sex not been the extreme and persistent vice and disease of many religious traditions, not least the Christian? Perhaps there is an alternative to the ascetic path: not the gradual relinquishment of the so-called lower parts of our being, but rather the integration of *all* we are into a healthy whole. If we are sufficiently aware of the meanings of these two words, *healthy* and *whole,* their juxtaposition will jar, of course, because it is a repetition, a tautology, which we allow ourselves for emphasis. To be healthy *is* to be whole. To be whole *is* to be healthy. Shall we be right if we take *this* aim as a guiding principle for our development? Is the era of ascetic spirituality over, about to give place to integrated Being, the being of an entity who is "very man and very god"?

Aldous Huxley himself advocated ascetic development, pointing to its long tradition; he claimed that it had always been found necessary, and that it surely remained so now. However, we might rationally consider whether, in a world in which more people are awakening, he might seem to have been unnecessarily ascetic. Would we be right to think this, and to act accordingly? Living, as we do, as biological organisms on a planet ruled by entropy and cyclical processes, would we be right to live as the animals we are but also to "sanctify" our so-called lower, but absolutely necessary, characteristics, not by leaving them behind (whether by asceticism or suicide), but by cherishing them even as we also seek a "higher" spiritual growth? Instead of entering life maimed, if our everyday desires "offend" us, as Yahshua advised, is it not now possible to enter life whole, those desires remaining but harming none because balanced both within the person and in the person's relationships with others in the world? The Hindus who conceived Katavul as a god in their own image evidently thought a "cyclical integrity," that is, "integration over time," necessary to his and our wellbeing in the world of time. "To be or to be whole?" is now the question, and if to be whole is the better way, is not an understanding of the newly returned philosophia perennis a good place to start a new cycle of discovery of the truth of its perennial principle, "As above, so below"?

TWELVE

The Alchemical Body

> *One of the most important tasks of alchemy was the transformation or transmutation of the unrefined into the refined. The unrefined was the so-called prima materia, the refined, the lapis, the philosopher's stone, the philosophical gold or the corpus subtile (subtle body) which in far-eastern alchemy is the Diamond Body. . . . [T]he alchemist's work prefigured the task we have at the start of the 21st century: to consciously realise the importance of the body, the feminine principle, or Eros functioning, for it is pure gold. Such a conscious realisation of the feminine principle will provide a much-needed balancing of the human psyche and thus [of] how it relates not only to others but also in how it values and honors the earth and its resources.*
>
> R. F. ROTH, *THE ARCHETYPE OF THE HOLY WEDDING IN ALCHEMY AND IN THE UNCONSCIOUS OF MAN*

In surveying the alchemical art G. R. S. Mead discovered that "never in the history of human culture has there been evidence of so long-continued a conspiracy to disguise the subject-matter and operative processes of an art" but that, in spite of the obscurity, which provides stumbling blocks to the sincere seeker and deliberately misleads the honest inquirer, there is no doubt that the alchemists possessed knowledge of the subtle forces of matter and of the activities of life and mind.[1] Jungian analyst and yoga practitioner Iona Miller concurs in her *Introduction to Alchemy in Jungian Psychology:*

Alchemy is much more than the historical predecessor of metallurgy, chemistry and medicine—it is a living form of sacred psychology. Alchemy is a projection of a cosmic and spiritual drama in laboratory terms. It is an art, both experiential and experimental. It is a worldview which uni-

fies spirit and matter, Sun and Moon, Yang and Yin.[2]

Mead was not interested in whether in the lowest phase of the art any of its practitioners really succeeded in making gold or in discovering an elixir of life. While it was clear to him that modern chemistry dethroned alchemy and that astronomy superseded astrology and exiled it from the realm of science, there was "a deeper, more vital side . . . a subtler phase intimately bound up with the highest themes of sidereal religion, a supra-physical, vital and psychical side to alchemy—a scale of ascent leading finally to man's perfection in spiritual reality."[3]

He goes on to say that a subtle embodiment of the life of the mind was a fundamental dogma for the alchemists, and that the prime secret of alchemical transmutation was an inner mystery, the purgation and perfecting of this subtle embodiment. "For their grand secret was the soul-freeing doctrine of regeneration, which, as a demonstrable fact of history, was undisguisedly the chief end not only of the higher mystery-institutions but of many an open philosophic school and saving cult of later antiquity."[4]

The history of alchemy is a long one. It spans several thousand years in both Eastern and Western traditions. Although it is thought to have its roots in ancient Egypt, where metallurgy and mysticism were inseparable, it is known to us through the writings of the Greek philosophers of the Hellenic period. Professor Hamed Abdel-reheem Ead, from the University of Cairo, tells us that when Alexander the Great conquered Egypt in 333 BCE and his general, Ptolemy, became King of Egypt, Alexandria became the most important city in Egypt and the acknowledged center of the intellectual world. A library of some 400,000 to 500,000 manuscripts attracted teachers and scholars from all parts of the then civilized world. A unique culture, blending Egyptian arts, Greek philosophy, Persian, Hebrew, and Chaldean sciences and mysticism, evolved and flourished (see plate 25). However, Alexandria became a Roman province in 80 BCE and an important part of the Alexandria libraries was burned. Ultimately, in the third century CE, the Roman Empire itself began to collapse.

However, certain ideas survived, preserved as secret doctrines by the mystical cults of the period. Through their transmission by Arab scholars they found their way to Europe by the twelfth and thirteenth centuries CE. According to Professor Ead, "Arabian mathematicians, physicians, alchemists, were held in high esteem as scientific experts. Arabian translations, elaborations and commentaries from ancient Greek and Greek-Egyptian authors received from Syrian versions and finally translated into Latin in the twelfth and thirteenth centuries became the great authorities in natural science."[5]

The earliest alchemical writings, Professor Ead goes on to say, date from about the beginning of the Common Era. They not only contain references to the devices and methods of experimental chemistry but also obscure allegorical narratives and descriptions analogous to the ideas of the later Alexandrian Neo-Platonic philosophers involved in the mystical cults of the period. He states that there is evidence this knowledge spread as far as India*

and China, where it acquired its own character through local cultural influences, though it was largely based on theories of matter and transubstantiation developed by Plato. Among these surviving doctrines, the forty-two books of Hermes Trismegistus, who was mentioned in the previous chapter, form the basis of early alchemical philosophy and practice.

Titus Burckhardt (1908–1984), scholar of wisdom traditions and major proponent of the perennialist school of thought, states that by the thirteenth century CE alchemy had developed into a fairly structured system of belief.[6] This belief system was based on an integrated body of ideas derived from a number of sources, including Christianity, which viewed alchemy as a useful system to explore theological ideas such as the fate of the human soul after the fall of Adam and the reunification with God, as well as an understanding of how the universe operated, gained from chemical experimentation.

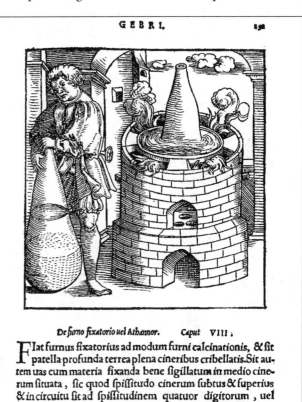

Fig. 12.1. Chemistry as we know it was unknown to the early Islamic world, but experiments by Jabir ibn Hayyan (also known as Geber) in the ninth century were a crucial step toward it. After Geber's time, alchemists' belief in transmutation dwindled. The more fundamental physics of today confirms its possibility, but shows why it does not normally occur. (Beinecke Rare Book and Manuscript Library, Yale University.)

---

*The poet-philosopher-yogis, the Siddhas of South India, evolved alchemical practices called *Rasayana* that continue to be integrated with their medical system even today.

The Philosopher's Stone

The idea of the *lapis philosophorum,* the philosopher's stone, was fundamental to alchemy, especially during the troubled fourteenth century, when it was kept alive, according to Burckhardt, by men such as Nicolas Flamel, who lived from 1330 to 1417. Unlike many of his predecessors he was not a religious scholar, nor a scientist in any manner we could recognize today. Most of his work was aimed at gathering alchemical knowledge that had existed before him, especially regarding the philosopher's stone, which he is reputed to have found. His work gives a great deal of space to describing the processes and reactions, but never actually gives the formula for carrying out the transmutations.[7]

The conflation of concepts of which the philosopher's stone is a central part shows strong links with the Hermetic tradition. The stone is the legendary substance believed capable of turning "base" metal into gold, and also of prolonging life. Hence, we also have the term "elixir of life." In Arabic this is *al-'iksīr,* derived from the Greek *xērion* (from *xēros* "dry"), a "powder for dry-

ing wounds." The elixir was said to be a blood-red powder (for drying wounds and for prolonging life) obtained from mercury. At the time blood (and therefore life) was associated by color with a red chemical substance obtained from "quick," that is "living," silver, known as mercury, one of only two elements (using that word in its modern scientific sense) that are liquid (quick) at terrestrial temperatures. Mercury is, as we saw, also the name of the Roman god of trading (from the Latin *merx,* "merchandise"), thieving, eloquence, and skill. He is also Hermes, the herald and messenger of the gods. Note in this confusing mêlée of ideas the naïve conflation of verbal labels with the entities that the words signified, along with associations with shallow characteristics such as color.

The red substance is also known as *cinnabar,* which is an ore of mercury consisting, in modern terminology, of a mixture of its two sulphides. Like most mercury compounds this purported extender of life is in fact highly poisonous, but we know from the writings of the period, such as those of the traveler Marco Polo, and from modern studies, such as David Gordon

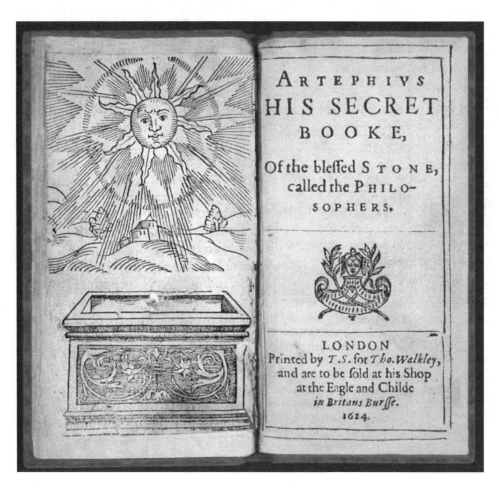

Fig. 12.2. Flamel's book, based on an alchemical work of 1357, stresses moral, philosophical, and spiritual transmutation rather than the "protochemistry" already suspect in his day. (Beinecke Rare Book and Manuscript Library, Yale University.)

White's *The Alchemical Body,* that cinnabar was commonly used in China, India, and Europe because it was believed to prolong life and promote well-being. As late as the sixteenth century, the Swiss alchemist and physician Paracelsus (1493–1541) used it in treatments alongside other chemicals and minerals, though evidently in tiny doses, which had a homeopathic effect and did no harm.

Paracelsus wrote, "Many have said of Alchemy that it is for the making of gold and silver. For me such is not the aim, but to consider only what virtue and power may lie in medicines."[8] His Hermetical views entailed the idea that sickness and health in the body relied on the harmony of man the microcosm and nature the macrocosm. Despite this awareness of and respect for the Hermetic principle "As above, so below," he nonetheless took an approach to healing that differed from that of his predecessors, using this analogy not in the cause of soul-purification but with reference only to the physical realm, believing that humans must have certain balances of minerals in their bodies, and that certain illnesses of the body could be cured by chemical remedies, an idea that persists to the present day.[9] While his attempts to treat diseases with such remedies as mercury might seem ill-advised from a biomedical point of view, he found that they could have beneficial results when given in minute doses. Hence he is not only known as "The Father of Drug Therapy" because of his ideas about chemical medicines, but also as "The Father of Homeopathy" on account of his belief in the principle *similibus similimum curantur* (like cures like) and the use of very small dosages.

Spiritual Alchemy

The art of alchemy rose and fell in popularity during the Middle Ages. By the eighteenth century it was reduced to the status of an arcane philosophy by scientific materialism and the beginnings of modern chemistry. Still, the esoteric idea of "spiritual alchemy" survived. In his article on spiritual alchemies of seventeenth century England, Dr. Robert Schuler from the University of Columbia states that recent studies have begun to answer the "vexed questions" of the "enigmatic subject of alchemy" such as "to what extent its suggestive allegorical language [could] be seen as a vehicle for 'spiri-

tual' or 'religious' significance" and "when and where did the practice of alchemy have specific religious significance?"[10] Schuler points out that, in spite of claims that alchemy is a homogeneous tradition of mystical beliefs going back to Hermes Trismegistus, it was subject to variations of religious interpretation according to context even within the brief period of English history discussed in his article. Between 1600 and 1650, he points out, moderate Anglicans, orthodox Calvinists, and radical Puritans all found in alchemy something to harmonize with their very different beliefs and experiences.

Among the documents that Schuler studied is the *Enchyridion,* written in the seventeenth century by d'Espagnet, which became the chief nonscriptural handbook of the Royal Society (a learned society for science founded in England in 1660), after it had been translated from the French by Elias Ashmole, one of the Society's founder members. Schuler states that according to Ashmole "the chief task of the spiritual alchemist is to tap the Universal Spirit, which is in all things." "With the help of Hermetic and other Neoplatonic ideas supplied by d'Espagnet," says Schuler himself, "members of the Society of the Sun in Aries [a secret Hermetic society that may have been a precursor of Rosicrucianism, some of whose members were founders of the present Royal Society of Great Britain] appear to have been seeking a spiritual enlightenment, chiefly through prayer and meditation."[11] One paragraph of Ashmole's translation is of special interest to us. It reads:

> Hence it is that the *Power* and *Vertue* is not in *Plants, Stones, Mineralls, etc* (though we sensibly perceive the *Effects* from them) but tis that *Universall* and *All-piercing Spirit,* that *One operative Vertue and immortall Seede of worldly things,* that *God* in the beginning infused into the *Chaos,* which is every where *Active* and still flowes through the *world* in all kindes of things by *Universall extension,* and manifests it selfe by the aforesaid *Productions.* Which *Spirit* a true *Artist* knows how-so to handle (though its *activity* be as it were *dul'd* and streightly *bound up,* in the close *Prison of Grosse* and *Earthe Bodies*) as to take it from *Corporiety,* free it from *Captivity,* and let it loose that it may freely *worke* as it doth in the *Aetheriall Bodies.*[12]

An anonymous text written about 1655 documents "a characteristic habit of mind which enabled even those Puritans who were not members of radical sects to embrace alchemy: that is, they identified the Calvinist *electus* with the alchemical *adeptus*. Just as they were chosen by God for salvation, so the *adepti* were not merely initiated by other *adepti*, but were granted a spiritual perfection (sometimes through a direct revelation) which in turn made them worthy of the philosopher's stone."[13]

A volume of materials collected by Sir Hugh Platt (1552–1611) has a section ruled into two vertical boxes, on the back of which is written: "It is possible to make a Body of the nature of a spirit, which then hath power ouer all inferior bodies." The two boxes contain parallel columns with the heading: "That the Regeneration of Man and the Purification of Metall haue like degree of Preparation and Operation to their highest perfection" followed by a comparison of the two processes, material and spiritual.[14] While accurate interpretations of both d'Espagnet and Platt might escape us, it is clear that the spiritual aspect of alchemy had survived, and that neither the jīvan-mukta nor the ritual magician would fail to understand this worldview.

Medical Spirits and the Astral Body

The nature of the relationship between body and spirit was a main concern of sixteenth and seventeenth century alchemists, a concern that was reflected in medical ideas of the period. "In spite of certain inherent weaknesses and vaguenesses, the theory of medical spirits maintained itself throughout the Middle Ages in a fairly constant and coherent form," states D. P. Walker in an article on Renaissance Medicine.[15] These ideas, he says, were based on Aristotle and Galen and were systematized by the Arabs. He is referring here to an Arabic treatise attributed to the great Islamic scholar, philosopher, scientist, and physician Avicenna (Abu 'Ali al-Husayn ibn Abd Allah ibn Sina, 980–1037 CE), who is known to have written some 450 works, of which about 240 survive. These include the *Book of Healing* and the *Canon of Medicine,* which had widespread influence on later medical practice. Despite predating Paracelsus by three centuries Avicenna already held prototypically modern physicalistic notions regarding chemistry. He wrote a number of treatises against alchemy, discrediting the theory of transubstantiation of physical substances. At the same time, his metaphysical theories and doctrines on the nature of the soul, his distinction between

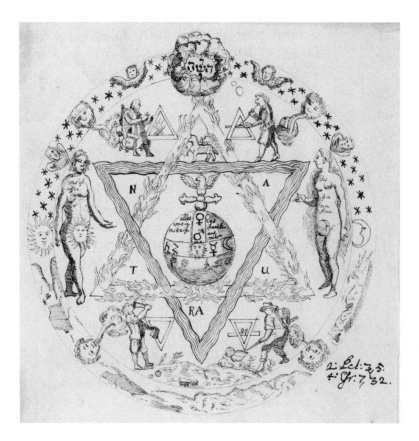

Fig. 12.3. The circle was perceived from earliest times as the perfect form. (See plates 26 and 27 for other circular representations of spiritual ideals.) Alchemists regarded the circle as a hermetically sealed space in which transformation could take place. Hence it appears frequently in alchemical images as a symbol of wholeness and, therefore, of God. Pen and ink sketch, *Alchemical and Rosicrucian Compendium,* German ca. 1760. (Beinecke Rare Book and Manuscript Library, Yale University.)

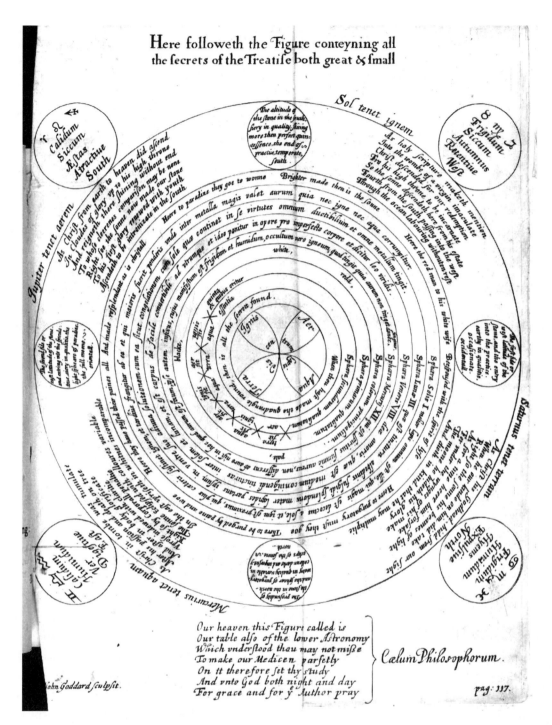

Fig. 12.4. "The Secrets of the Treatise" from the *Theatrum Chemicum Britannicum,* is taken from Elias Ashmole's 1652 collection of alchemical writing in poetical form. Such texts combined arcane knowledge from many sources, from magic to Pythagorean mathematics. Contributions from several famous English philosopher-alchemists including George Ripley, Geoffrey Chaucer, Thomas Norton, and Sir Edward Kelle expound various aspects of the alchemical process. The process described seeks to break down the original chaotic unity into the four elements, then recombines them in a higher unity so that the soul or spirit can be "extracted in the purest state." Here the alchemical process is presented in a diagrammatic but verbal manner, while in the Ripley Scroll (see plate 28) it is illustrated graphically. Both expositions raise many questions for today's mind, and show two things that neither intends, the insuperable difficulty of presenting in graphic or verbal mode the ideas themselves, and, an even more fundamental problem, the impossibility of depicting spiritual "things" in any physical form or medium whatsoever. Painters of the "sublime," such as Friedrich, made heroic attempts to depict spirituality, but inevitably failed for the same inherent reason: the transcendent is not the physical, and cannot be depicted for physical viewing. (Beinecke Rare Book and Manuscript Library, Yale University.)

essence and being, and, especially, his "floating man" thought experiment, imply an understanding acceptance of *spiritual* alchemy. However, the main relevance of the "floating man" for us is that it concerns the question of what we are as Beings.

We shall present a view of the matter in chapter 15, but Avicenna used essentially the same reasoning more than a millennium ago. He imagined the experience of a human being floating freely without sensory inputs from the world around, who has entered a state of awareness of him- or herself alone. The lack of sensations notwithstanding, the experience would not be void. The person would not cease to be, nor even lose consciousness upon losing all sense of the world, for the "floating human" would still be conscious, not least conscious *of being conscious*. Such a self, Avicenna argues, does not depend for its reality on external objects, but remains present and real when all else has left its consciousness, and its being real is thereby self-proving, at least to itself. The self is therefore a *real* substance, whatever that "real substance" *itself* might consist of. Whatever its nature, whether fine matter, or "spirit," or even mere *mathematical pattern in a nonmaterial "aether,"* it must be granted the reality by which we can justify using the word "substance," and must be acknowledged to be a living entity, which we honor by using the word Being, with the capital B.

Heidegger, centuries later, called this consciousness "a genuine pre-phenomenological experience" of the "I," and might have agreed, at least partially, with Avicenna. Of course, the fact of a state of consciousness that is aware *only* of being-the-Being-who-is-aware does not entail denial of the reality of our external world, as Descartes might have wondered, but simply acknowledges what Heidegger called (in translation, of course) a "bare consciousness's" perception of itself. The world had not ceased to exist, but was simply not, for the present, the object of the floating human's consciousness. Even the body becomes external to the Being in this context of meditative consciousness. Today's meditators do experience such a state, and Avicenna himself may well have based his view on his own identical personal experience.

The great spiritual-physical divide that would modify hylic pluralism, postulating a "spirit" that was *entirely* nonmaterial, was now beginning to open. Avicenna's ambivalence is unsurprising, despite his early date, for

Walker points also to the great confusion of those who attempted to define the physical and the spiritual, which we have already noticed many times. What we would class as *physical* difficulties were often attributed to the *astral* body, on the nature of which also there were conflicting opinions. As we have seen, Porphyry, centuries earlier still, had held that the *nonmaterial* part of us was but one subtle body, while Proclus had claimed that it was a multiplex. This reminds us of the three, or even seven, but usually five kośas of Indic belief and the confusion of material and spiritual within that system.

Whatever the confusions, which were legion, the presiding metaphor of the medieval age was one of "spirits" that carried out the body's functions. No wonder, then, that the notion of a completely nonphysical spirit produced yet more confusion. A 1556 monograph on medical spirits states:

> The central ventricles must contain something, which must be airy, since they are empty in dead bodies; the spurting forth of arterial blood shows that these heavy liquids must be mixed with something light and mobile; the fact that if one eye is shut the pupil of the other dilates must be due to some kind of spirit being constantly transmitted to both; the instantaneous transmission of heat and cold which produces blushing and pallor from fear must be due to a *subtle body*.[16]

Even Descartes, the advocate of a strong dualism, refers, in a letter of 1643, to some kind of *matière subtile* contained in the cerebral ventricles and other cavities. While a little of this could be translated into terms that modern science could encompass within its paradigms, more could not, and the superiority in explanatory power of today's science over the ancient four- or five-element science that was still fundamental to Descartes' view is undeniable. Nonetheless, as we shall see, today's physics is as "humanoid" as alchemy was, and some startlingly similar broad paradigms remain.

Commenting, in his article *The Astral Body in Renaissance Medicine,* on the difficulty thinkers of the period found in reconciling a thoroughgoing astro-spiritual cosmology with the Christian doctrine of the soul (which doctrine Gilbert Ryle, centuries later, took to be an example of that concept of mind that he disparaged as the erroneous "official theory," "the dogma of the Ghost in the Machine"), D. P. Walker concludes that philosophies dominated by the concept of the spirit tend to be immanentist, and so leave little or no room for a transcendent incorporeal soul that must be injected into a half-formed body that has been elaborated by its own spirit.[17]

Using Fernel as an example, confusion seems to stem from the term *spirit* and from the various groups of ideas that are distinct from, but intimately related to, it. Firstly, he believed that medical spirits are a very fine, hot vapor, deriving from the blood and breathed air. They are corporeal and of three kinds: natural, vital, and animal, of which the vital spirits are of most concern to the human body. Fernel believed that these vital spirits are manufactured in the heart and conveyed to the arteries, and that their main function is to distribute innate, vital heat to all parts of the body. Secondly, he believed the animal spirits to be derived from vital heat and to be contained in the ventricles of the brain and transmitted through the nervous system to the sense organs and muscles for motor activity, sense perception, and what he called "lower psychological activities," such as appetite and imagination. Fernel believed that these medical spirits were the first, direct instrument of the soul. The only thought that seems clear is that, as science began to develop and demand explanations of human life that could not but differ from earlier religious doctrines, the earlier confusions were, if anything, compounded.

Today, we would surely reject almost everything from bygone eras of ignorance and devise explanatory concepts of our own. One of Ryle's most serious errors was to try to define a standard doctrine to criticize when no such clarity was available, for, as we shall see in chapter 15, he misrepresents even the so-called official doctrine itself. Philosophical discussion of confusion is liable to lead only to further confusion. What is needed is science, not a kind of abstruse etymology of the habitually abused competing preexisting terminologies of ecclesiasticism on the one hand and a very juvenile science on the other. But, useful though such pointers are, this is to look a chapter or two ahead, so for the present we return to the late medieval and early modern world and its views.

When the already confused concept of spirit was combined with astrology, as in Fernel, the difficulties became even greater; what transcendence there was in the system, Walker explains, was put into the stars and, therefore, since the spirit must then derive from these, it became almost a double of the soul (or vice versa), for "both have a celestial or divine origin . . . both are the total form of the body, both perform psychological activities." Walker comments that it is impossible to assemble any coherent system using Fernel's juggling with the notions of spirit and soul; and it is not therefore surprising that his immediate successors, themselves often unclear in their views, criticized this aspect of his medical philosophy. Fernel is often cited as chief of those who abused the concept of spirit. The English physician William Harvey (1578–1657), first to describe accurately the systemic circulation of blood to the heart, criticizes Fernel for resorting to a *deus ex machina* to resolve all difficult problems.[18]

Gebser, the reader will recall, sees the period of Fernel, Harvey, and more recent researchers as that in which mental consciousness, rare at earlier times, became the prevailing mode of (educated) human mindfulness. Once established, it proceeded to undermine many long-established beliefs, and to build others. In doing so, far from expanding knowledge, it narrowed science to what it could, at the time, explain by paradigms acceptable to itself, a self-centered way of proceeding, and threw away all it could not. The method proved very serviceable, but we should note this description of its modus operandi, for we shall begin chapter 15, "Science, Philosophy, and the Subtle Body," from this realization, and show that while it seems, here, to represent final and authoritative rationality, in fact it does not.

But we must return once more to Fernel and his critics. "These criticisms," Walker says "are directed with special vehemence against Fernel's astrological spirit, against his assertion that the spirit, or the innate heat in it, is celestial, *aethereal;* and . . . his use of the astral body is quite often attacked as well," especially by Argenterius, a "revolutionary" medical writer who attempts to make medicine more rational than it had earlier been. He condemns Fernel's astral bodies and asks "for who could believe, let alone prove, that the soul is wrapped up in these garments and spirits?" implying that there is no authority for belief in an astral body, an assumption later corrected by Domenico Bertacchi, who reproved Argenterius for ignorance of Neo-Platonic accounts of the astral body in his 1584 monograph, which *had* been accorded authority (whatever their standing would shortly become).[19]

Harvey denies that there can be "a body most simple, most subtle, most fine . . . aethereal and participating in the quintessence." "Nowhere," he continues, "have they demonstrated that there is such a spirit, or that it acts beyond the powers of the elements, or that it performs greater work than blood alone could do. We indeed, who in our investigations use sense as our guide, have not been able to find any such spirit anywhere."[20] However, today's more open-minded scientists and philosophers would point out to Harvey his failure to see that a spirit body *could,* as at least a logical possibility, cohabit with or even control the physical body. It could even be logically *necessary* to postulate its existence, as a step toward explaining the as-yet inexplicable, or to correct explanations that are evidently false yet which, without the new postulate, would remain unexplained.

If you declare something impossible, as Harvey did, you can be sure you will never find it, even if it is staring you in the face. Considerable scientist though he was, in this matter he seems to have assumed what he thought he was proving, for we would ask him why a *nonphysical* body such as a "spirit" should ever be *expected* to be the *direct* cause of circulation of *physical* blood? So if it were *not* the cause, that fact would, in itself, provide neither proof nor disproof of the spirit's existence, and would have to be seen as irrelevant to the physical question. Christ, in whom most believed and whose words Harvey surely knew, had averred that "flesh and blood cannot inherit the kingdom of God." He thereby asserted the reality of something fleshless and bloodless that *could* inherit the kingdom. Sure enough, even *within* what we now consider the physical world, an entity lurked utterly unknown to Harvey, which was indeed a "prime mover" in circulating the blood, and in everything else in the physical world-about, namely electricity. Denial of entities by an overzealous application of the principle of preferring the simplest explanation, and simplistic confusions of levels were both easy errors, are just as common today.

In this world of burgeoning scientific reason, with its criticism and countercriticism of long-held philosophies, we see the beginning of the schism that later separated the mechanists from the vitalists in medical theory, but

what then happened to the alchemists and, in particular, what happened to the spiritual alchemists? Although, as Mead tells us, physical alchemy virtually disappeared from the public world over the following centuries, it has persisted in various forms, preserved in the rituals of secret societies such as the Rosicrucians and the Masons, in the unitive spiritual philosophies of the Theosophists and the followers of Steiner, in holistic healing practices, and in the resurgence of interest in oriental systems such as Yoga and Taoism.

The Subtle Body, Alchemy, and Individuation

A revival of interest in medieval alchemy has been created through the work of the Swiss analytical psychologist, C. G. Jung (1875–1961). He found in the symbolism of the medieval texts a parallel to his concepts of archetypes and the individuation process, and in the "secret art of alchemy" a practical guide to the "laboratory of the unconscious" and the process of transformation of the personality (see plate 28).[21] Thus, he perceived symbols and levels of reality that had eluded so many before him, and too often still elude thinkers today.

Jung's interest in alchemy grew from a vivid dream of an ancient library full of books on arcane subjects. During the following fifteen years, which he spent collecting his own library of works on alchemy, he recognized certain major symbols used in the alchemical literature cropping up in his patients' accounts of their dreams and fantasies.* They recounted dreams of such entities as a sealed vessel, or the conflict and final unification of opposites, an inner quest, a philosophical tree, a golden flower, a fountain of eternity, a stone, a sacred wedding. This last was known to alchemists as the *coniunctio,* which sought to unite spirit, seen as male, with matter, seen as female, so creating the "homunculus," a fully formed microscopic human being from which an embryo was supposed to develop.

Jung believed that the psyche cannot be understood in "conceptual terms," but only through "living images or symbols," which are able to include ambiguities and

---

*Jung's works on alchemy include *Alchemical Studies, Psychology and Alchemy,* and *Mysterium Coniunctionis.*

paradoxes without the intellect protesting at such "illogicalities." The truths of which the symbols spoke were directly and intuitively seen in the symbolic pictures themselves. He saw in alchemy a metaphorical representation of the process of personal individuation that he himself had discerned. Alchemy, he concluded, was therefore a system of self-initiation. Whether it was *only* a system of self-initiation remained, logically, an open question, but following his espousal of this belief he often turned to the images of alchemy, mythology, and religion to help describe psychic life. But what should we take the phrases "conceptual terms" and "living images or symbols" (or any alternatives and equivalents) to mean? They are not defined for us, either in terms of or in distinction from each other. Iona Miller, writing about Jung and alchemy, says his view was that for an image to be a "living symbol" it must refer to something that otherwise cannot be known.[22] But this, too, does not logically follow; nor does it seem to help us, for, while it may be true, it is not immediately clear why it has to be true, nor even what is meant.

In any case there is a danger in interpreting the arcane literature of an arcane subject in terms of the equally arcane contents of the mind of the patient "on the couch." The danger is that of tumbling too quickly, perhaps even wrongly, toward the view that both alchemy and the dreams and fantasies of patients might be rationally assumed to have a common provenance in the psyche. This was unlikely to be untrue, of course, but for reasons of which Jung might not have been fully aware, for the psychoanalyst's own mind was itself in that very same category, and was steeped in predisposing lore, predetermining what might be (even rationally) concluded about what were acknowledged to be rather nonrational matters. The thinker was embroiled in the very content of the thoughts being examined. This, like the alchemy that itself had given rise to some aspects of Jungian psychology, was hardly science in anything approaching the Popperian manner, in which the researcher devises explanatory hypotheses, the content of which will allow the design of experiments to test the hypotheses, and so lift the whole process out of the realm of unprovable imaginative constructs. That ideal might be impossible to satisfy in such a matter as psychology, as Popper himself knew.

Still, the discoveries were nonetheless probably

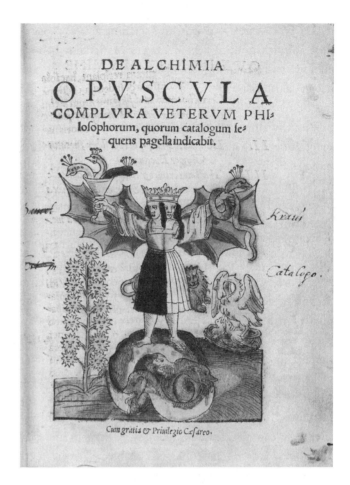

Fig. 12.5. The coniunctio, or alchemical marriage, depicted here is one of many symbols Jung studied. In *Alchemical Studies* (CW Vol. 13), he concluded that the purpose of alchemy was to separate the prima materia, so-called chaos, into the active principle, the soul, and the passive principle, the body, which would then reunite in personified form in the "chymical marriage." ca. 1550. (Beinecke Rare Book and Manuscript Library, Yale University.)

veridical, not for an understanding of alchemy per se, nor of patients' neuroses per se, but rather regarding the constitution, capability, and scope, but also the opposing constrainedness, of all human thought. We shall have more to say about this when we attempt the difficult task of placing humankind's study of humankind into the mold of humankind's more recent science of humankind. Our repetitions may help readers unfamiliar with philosophical thinking see our point. The science of other animals and the science of angels must necessarily differ from our own.

Any conclusion that in both alchemy and psychoanalysis everything was "all in the mind" was, in fact, less a great revelation than merely an easy assumption to make. True or not, and alchemy's seeming arcane profundity notwithstanding, the discovery of alchemy in psychology and psychology in alchemy does not really take us very far, for in itself it contains no key to what Jung meant or what the alchemists themselves had meant, nor to any final truth, but only to man's own view of man. Indeed, it might be even less than that, nothing more than an empty truism, a contentless analytical fact of language: the mere truism that "humankind is as humankind is," and that all our theorizing tells us only about ourselves.

However, all is not lost in an ocean without landfall, for if real self-examination is taking place, the fruits of the process are not useless, and meditators do claim to find understanding of our relation to a greater Being and a sense of safety within that greater Being. Today, those who have near-death experiences and afterward remain in this world often speak of their great joy at what they find. "Know thyself" has always been recognized as good advice. And this is the aim we have set ourselves, to know ourselves a little better by discovering, if we can, what the subtle body is. Perhaps alchemy and some recurring psychological problems are products of the right brain, rather than the left (which assuredly makes many problems of its own), but this matter was unknown territory until the very last years of Carl Jung's life. Nor can neurophysiology itself answer all our questions. Here and there Jung's studies of alchemy throw up matters relevant to the subtle body, so reference to some further material will not be out of place.

Jung spent most of the last years of his life studying alchemy, the symbolism of which, according to psychologist Marvin Spiegelman, was "the attempt to both produce and explain the experience of a Self which is non-producible and unexplainable."[23] Although he was interested in Eastern thought, and particularly admired the idea that we each have the potential for self-liberation, Jung found the historical grounding for his experiences in Western alchemical and Gnostic tradition.[24] Many Gnostic texts had been destroyed by the Church and he feared he might never make the link between Gnosticism and contemporary experience. Nonetheless, he found in alchemy a close resemblance to the teachings in Gnosticism's surviving documents, in which "man's unconscious psychology [is] in full flower."[25] He found there a contemplative "knowing,"

a seeking of direct, personal revelation of the Divine, mediated through dreams and visions, and a recognition that things are as they are, which was not the product of rational intellect, and might, therefore, not be amenable to logical explication. In Gnosticism he also saw "an anticipation of the intuitions of German mysticism, so important psychologically," whose greatest exponent was Meister Eckhart.[26]

In 1929, Jung wrote that "the alchemical operation consisted essentially in separating the prima materia, the so-called chaos, into the active principle, the soul, and the passive principle, the body, which are then reunited in personified form in the *coniunctio* or 'chymical marriage.'"[27] Many of the terms used by the alchemists—who regarded the soul as the "active principle," which combines with the spirit to animate and vitalize the body—are related to terms for the breath. The concept of an "inspirational" function had evolved from the earlier meaning of "breath-soul" (pneuma or spirit) (which we also saw in the prāna of Indian traditions and the shen of Taoism) and developed further, via the concept of the *corpus subtile* (subtle body) and the *anima* (Jung's term for the feminine part of a man's personality), into the *ligamentum corporis et spiritus,* meaning, literally, "the soul as that which ties body and spirit together."[28]

This seems, semantically, and despite centuries of thinking, to resemble the ancient notion of the tripartite soul. Jung explains that the ancient view was that the soul was essentially the life of the body, the life breath, or a kind of life force, which assumed spatial and corporeal form at the moment of conception, or during pregnancy, or at birth, and left the dying body again after the final breath.[29] The soul in itself was a being without extension, that is without spatial size, a point, in Leibnizian terms a "monad," a single indivisible entity, an organizing principle (a term later adopted by Blavatsky and the Theosophical movement to describe Ultimate Reality, similar to the Hindu *Narayana,* the "Divine Flame" or "Flame of Truth," from which the whole cosmos has sprung); because it existed before taking corporeal form and afterward as well, it was considered timeless and therefore immortal. The conflations encountered in earlier chapters at both terminological and conceptual levels, and the resulting uncertainty as to the reality of postulated entities, remain with us.

Jung's theory of individuation, a construct of his

Fig. 12.6. This is the fifteenth-century Benedictine monk Basil Valentine's depiction of the seven stages of alchemical transformation, which parallels the seven planes of consciousness in the Hindu chakra system and Jung's seven stages of individuation.

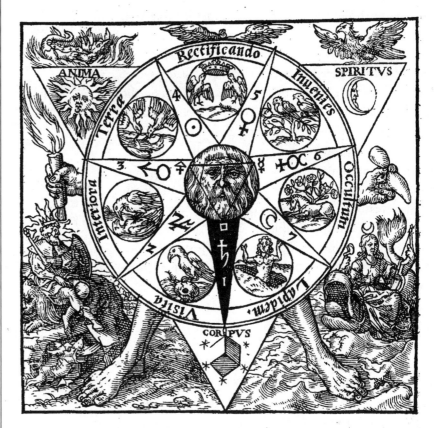

mature years, is generally believed to have evolved as an element of his alchemical model, although some writers disagree. Spiegelman claims that Jung discovered psychological types independently of alchemy.[30] Nevertheless, it appears to be generally acknowledged among Jungian analysts that he conceived of individuation as a process of personal transformation emerging from the depths of the psyche and leading to a development of the individual's own values, independent of, but cognizant of, those of the collective culture, a movement toward wholeness that involves a rounding out of the personality and employs all the psychological functions, including the religious impulse. This is not unlike the ultimate aim of alchemy, which he said, was to produce a "corpus

subtile [*sic*]," a transfigured and resurrected body, a body that was at the same time spirit.[31] This reminds us of the Indic concept of the jīvan-mukta.

In *Psychology and Alchemy,* when discussing the role of the alchemist, Jung states that "it always remains an obscure point whether the ultimate transformations in the alchemical process are to be sought more in the material or more in the spiritual realm."[32] We immediately ask whether these realms are correctly understood and defined, and Jung himself continues, "Actually, however, the question is wrongly put: there was no either-or for that age, but there did exist an intermediate realm between mind and matter, i.e., a psychic realm of subtle bodies whose characteristic it is to manifest themselves in a mental as well as a material form. This is the only view that makes sense of alchemical ways of thought, which otherwise must appear nonsensical." He goes on to say that, obviously, the existence of this intermediate realm comes to a sudden stop the moment we try to investigate matter in and for itself, apart from all projection (which is what science has done for some three centuries) and it remains nonexistent so long as we believe we know anything conclusive about matter or the psyche. But, he states, the moment when physics touches on the "untrodden, untreadable regions" and when psychology has at the same time to admit that there are other forms of psychic life besides the acquisitions of personal consciousness—in other words, when psychology, too, touches on an impenetrable darkness—then the intermediate realm of subtle bodies comes to life again, and the psychical and the psychic are once more blended in an indissoluble unity.[33] We agree wholeheartedly with this, and note that today we are very near this turning point.

Jungian Archetypes and Seven Stages of Individuation

There are references throughout Jung's writings to the sequence of archetypes associated with seven stages of individuation. Professor James Whitlark explains that these archetypes are the configurations of the unconscious at various points in human development and that the following list was charted by the American psychologist and professor of human development Clare Graves (1914–1986):

Stage 1. Survivor/Transitional-Object
Stage 2. Truster/Trickster
Stage 3. Unscrupulous Competitor/Hero
Stage 4. The Virtuous/the Shadow
Stage 5. Materialistic Analyst of Things/Anim(a/us)
Stage 6. Empathizer with Every Person/Wise One
Stage 7. Distancer/Self

Although he had no clinical evidence for further stages, Graves speculated that there may be further stages of numinous experience that psychology has not yet charted.

Post-Jungian Interpretations

Meanwhile, some commentators, such as Remo Roth, a student of Marie-Louise von Franz, Jung's closest collaborator and friend, continue the attempt to present alchemical interpretations as rational and scientific. Roth himself admits that "a breakthrough to the conscious observation of the creation of the *subtle body* in the Hermetic alchemical meaning was yet impossible for Carl Jung. This task remains, therefore, the challenge for the beginning of the 21st century."[34] With this we strongly disagree if his claim implies that the breakthrough could be based in any way upon the alchemical writings. As we hope to show in chapter 15, it will be far better to start again, with today's science speaking simply for itself, without regard to any historical precedents. (But this new science will, as we said earlier, still be the human mind speaking about its study of the human mind's own imaginings.)

In Jung's defense von Franz points out that, although his interpretation of the alchemical texts may seem impossible to understand, he has, in fact, simplified enormously, which gives us some impression of how obscure the medieval writings must be.[35] This reminds us of Mead's observation that at least some of the opacity was deliberate, but we have to say also that much of it resulted from the simple but catastrophic confusion of levels and misunderstanding of the different natures of physical and nonphysical entities. If the mind sets itself impossible premises it must not be surprised if no logical solution appears. What was needed was good science, so should confused prescientific alchemical writing now be set aside?

Von Franz gives an example of how the subtle body *might* be interpreted *now* by borrowing the ancient Egyptian idea that if a person did not go through the proper funerary rites and so attain a resurrection, his or her spirit would be trapped in the coffin chamber. She illustrates her example with a story of a patient in a modern hospital who, after undergoing an operation, "wakes up from the anesthetic" and walks out of the hospital through its closed doors. Although that does not make much of an impression on him, he is, finally, a little shocked when he hears a voice saying "If you want to return, this is the last moment—quick!" At that moment, he "really does wake up" to find that the doctor is massaging his heart, which has failed, and he hears someone say "My God, we nearly didn't bring him back!"* With her remarkable gift for translating esoteric symbolic material into everyday experience, Dr. von Franz explains that the patient had just had the *subjective* experience of walking out through a closed door. "So you see," she says, "that is the *subtle body* in a parapsychological form, the ghost of the dead already capable of walking through shut doors . . . the surviving soul can walk through material objects" and this universal belief "is looked on as proof of the immaterial, immortal aspects of the psyche."[36]

But how should we interpret this? The patient certainly knows what *he* thinks, for *he* has the experience, but what Dr. von Franz means by the words *subjective* and *proof* is unclear to us. As if to show our uneasiness justified, she *reverses* her "remarkable gift" by translating what has now become everyday hospital ward experience into esoteric symbolic material, like that of the alchemists, by embarking upon a symbolistic interpretation, and almost admits the disingenuousness of doing so:

If we take this [my emphasis] not as an experience of the death process, but as the experience of a living being, it *could be* [my emphasis] the influence of the unconscious on the surroundings—not an intentional one, but because one is in connection with the Self . . . if one is connected with the Self inwardly, then one can penetrate all life situations. Inasmuch as one is not caught in them, one walks through them; that means there is an innermost nucleus of the personality which remains detached, so that even if the most horrible things happen to one, the first reaction is not a thought, or a physical reaction, but rather an interest in the meaning.[37]

No doubt this is one facet of truth, but the victim of torture will probably confirm that in the immediate experience it is *not* the immediate preoccupation von Franz pretends. Instead, the simple-hearted view, without tendentiousness, may be *objectively correct* and *subjectively verifiable*. The soul may be shown, to any

reasonable mind (and certainly to the experiencer), to be a *real* non*physical* entity, which *really* "walks" through *physical* matter such as hospital doors. Von Franz goes on to say, and again we think disingenuously, that "if one has an awareness of and a constant alertness to the Self, one is no longer caught in anything; there is an innermost part of the personality which remains free . . . the state of helplessness in which one is caught by one's own inner processes stops, which amounts to a tremendous steadying* of the inner core of the personality."[38] This is, she believes, comparable to possession of the philosopher's stone, which symbolizes what the steadying of inner experience produces, and the real purpose behind spiritual alchemy, what the alchemists were *really* looking for: emotional balance and wholeness.[39]

This seems, again, a trite substitute for the kind of assurance about our eternal being that virtually all of us long for. Emotions come and go in our daily lives, but we would surely all agree that the far future matters, and our life therein, and the quality of that life. Von Franz, in this passage at least, sets all this aside, replacing it with parochial theorizing of her own. She is right that within the tiny limits of our personal lives emotional balance and wholeness are pleasant, but one suspects special pleading on behalf of her profession in so casuistic and so paltry an explanation. A problem with psychoanalysts is not that they are too scientific but that they are not scientific enough.

Jung's Problem with Kundalinī

Von Franz, as we have just seen, attempted to explain empirical observations and authentic personal experiences by imposing upon them an alien psychoanalytic theoretical structure grounded in a psychology, not in real-world entities. Decades earlier, Jung had taken an interest in Indian psychology and spirituality, especially kundalinī, and had, to a degree, done something similar. In 1932 he and the German Indologist J. W. Hauer jointly presented a seminar in which Jung's students heard an exposition of kundalinī by Hauer, an acknowledged expert, and found it exciting but deeply puzzling. Jung then delivered four lectures in which he gave his

* This not uncommon event, now that resuscitation is so often successful, serves to demonstrate the distinct natures of the physical and the nonphysical, so important, and so often unperceived or denied.

* One wonders what a "tremendous steadying" could be. Steadiness does *not* tremble. Accurate verbal usage is more important than von Franz appears to realize.

students an understanding in terms of his own psychology, which was criticized by kundalinī practitioners who considered that he had misrepresented their position.

Ironically, in view of his other interests, rather than produce an interpretation of kundalinī that distilled and continued the alchemical precedents he had already at that date been studying for many years, he set aside the understanding, common to Western and Eastern conceptions, that the lowest three chakras are earthly, animal, even profane. He claimed instead that the mūlādhāra, since it was the everyday mode of consciousness of the "average man," in fact contained the *un*conscious, which it was the objective of his psychology to bring into union with the conscious mind.[40]

This turned at least some aspects of the Tantric system on its head, for a part of the very essence of all Indic spirituality is to *transcend* that everyday consciousness *by quiet withdrawal from it*. The Tantric did not see his highest objective as hidden in the quasi-unconscious, *everyday sleeplike* consciousness of the mūlādhāra, but in the spiritual world six chakras higher, above his head. That Jung did somewhat misinterpret the Tantric quest seems confirmed by his dismissal of the two highest chakras, the ājñā and the sahasrāra, not only as irrelevant and dangerous to Western seekers, but because he himself, despite his spiritual aspirations, failed to see the reality and worth of what the Tantric meditator experienced at those levels. By the tragic irony of being true (for most Westerners did indeed fail to aspire so high), this merely confirmed that the Western mūlādhāra consciousness failed utterly to envisage higher possibilities than its own mundane and animal concerns. The higher spirituality found by meditators in and only in meditation, that is in *withdrawal from* the mūlādhāra world, is precisely what that everyday mūlādhāra *sleeping* consciousness fails to see, let alone encompass, and is precisely what Jung denied had value. He discouraged his hearers from seeking the very thing, the *kundalinī experience*, which he had himself purported to search out.

We do not have space for a full account of Jung's conflict with the Tantrics, and must be content to sketch his interpretations of the chakras and pass on. We do this largely so that readers can make a comparison with Plato's view of the chakras. However, this brevity is also indicated by our subject, which is not Jung's psychology per se, nor Tantra per se, nor yet the chakras

as understood by Plato per se, but the subtle body and its reality.

Jung's "Journey" through the Chakras

Harold Coward suggests, in his study *Jung and Eastern Thought,* that "in the development of Jung's thinking Yoga led him on from his early fascination with Western gnosticism and then back to Western alchemy, which then remained the keystone for the rest of his life."[41] Coward explains that rather than focusing on the kundalinī theory of the process of spiritual unfolding (concerning which he disagreed with Tantric practitioners over important details) and on the obvious parallels with the individuation process, Jung stressed instead the symbolic meanings of each of the chakras (though even so devaluing the ājñā and sahasrāra, the highest chakras within the body). Jung regarded the chakras, he says, as a complex manifold of ideas, which can be understood from three aspects, each of which is evoked and incorporated in the symbolism of each chakra:

> *Sthūla:* things as we ordinarily see them (the observations of the mūlādhāra mind)
> *Sūkṣma:* the level of theoretical understanding, abstraction, or wisdom
> *Para:* the transcendent level beyond sense experience and mental theory (the Eastern goal about which Jung had grave doubts)[42]

In his doctoral thesis, *Individuation and Subtle Body,* psychologist Gary Seeman explains how Jung perceives the journey through the chakras in a way that shows an interesting parallel with Gebser's consciousness structures discussed in chapter 1. Seeman says that, as in kundalinī yoga, the journey of individuation begins in the mūlādhāra, the root chakra, whose element is earth and whose consciousness is one "where the ego is awake and the self is asleep."[43]

The next station in this journey is the second chakra, the swādhiṣṭhāna, where, according to Jung, a person is baptized in the unconscious, which ritual is represented by the swādhiṣṭhāna's association with water. Jung interprets immersion in the swādhiṣṭhāna through the universal imagery of the sun myth, in which the sun disappears into the unconscious on a night sea journey, a journey into the underworld. On this journey, the hero confronts the Leviathan, or Great Mother, represented by the *makara,* an alligator-like animal in the lotus symbol of that chakra. However, Jung sees the swādhiṣṭhāna as inferior to the mūlādhāra, an assessment with which Tantric experts have always vigorously disagreed.

Like the sun, the hero emerges from the depths of the sea at the next center, the manipūra, a fiery realm of jewels. After surviving the perilous descent, as Jung sees it (though all the Indian traditions see it as an ascent), the person is initiated into the light and heat of the passions. She or he identifies with God and is possessed by the passions and their oppositional tendencies, symbolized by the fire element in the manipūra. If the aspirant begins already, by thought, to differentiate self from passions at the manipūra, the individuation process proper begins when she enters the world of the heart center, the anāhata. As the passions are tamed, she becomes, perhaps dimly at first, but increasingly, aware of the self, the puruṣa, at the center of anāhata, and learns objective love or empathy.

As the influence of the self increases, the person enters viṣuddha, the center at the throat. Viṣuddha is a realm of abstraction and psychical reality. It is the mode of consciousness in which the individuating person makes meaning of synchronicity and dream symbolism. Through the transcendent function, the ego's conflict is mediated by the self, which transcends apparent opposites to enable it to choose between alternatives.[44]

Beyond viṣuddha, one encounters the consciousness of ājñā, the center between the eyebrows. Jung interprets this as the level of consciousness at which a person begins to experience unity with God because it is where, in kundalinī yoga, the divine masculine and feminine, Siva and Sakti, unite, and the animal symbolism disappears, suggesting that instinct is subsumed or transcended. But, as we have said, Jung sees the unitary consciousness, said to center in both the ājñā and the sahasrāra at the top of the head, either as beyond his reach and that of his Western audience, or even as a figment of the Eastern imagination, a metaphysical speculation on the part of Yoga philosophers. His brief, dismissive treatment of the ājñā and the sahasrāra is, unsurprisingly, somewhat controversial. Since he did not himself experience what the Tantric meditators claim to experience through them we have to suspect a certain arrogance on his part.

We venture, before continuing, a contribution to the understanding of the rift between Jung and the practitioners of Tantra. The reader will recall that the developing Christian church had driven out its more esoteric parties, chief among them the Gnostics, and destroyed much of their literature. Continuity with later study of such ideas was lost from the Christian heritage (though it continued via Arabic and, eventually, Muslim thinkers, who also began the development toward modern mathematics and science). This hiatus may well have been a major cause of the babble of alchemical multiple entities and overlapping terminologies, which then developed in Christian Europe and which Jung and others failed to unravel. Such writings as we still have are even more divorced from their experiential origins than they might have been had not the Constantinian political Church been so antagonistic toward the Gnostics, whose spirituality it surely feared.

Furthermore, alchemy, necessary as forerunner of the vastly better scientific hypotheses we have now, was enabled by the church's banishment of it to stumble forward in the darkness of both ignorance and secrecy toward the schematic insights of our day. If alchemy lost its way (later to find it again in chemistry) because its antecedents had been suppressed, it is not to be wondered at that the experiential meanings—the only *reliable* meanings—of its terms had, long before Jung's day, become not merely complex and speculative but also inaccessibly arcane. Separated from its earlier roots in the East, religion, in all its aspects, had, in the West, taken a new route. There was, of course, a compensation, the unexpected but utterly indispensable development of rational, empirical science. But the Western science of psychology had lost touch with its Eastern antecedents, and had not only to begin again, but to begin again under the cloud of both scientific ignorance and a God-versus-Devil dualism, which a priori set empirical neutrality beyond all possibility of attainment. No wonder Jung on the one side, and Hauer and Tantric practitioners on the other, when they met some centuries later, found they did not totally agree.

Is Alchemy Relevant Today?

We have already hinted at the answer to this question, for alchemy was, or still is, necessarily a part of human study of the human, which can be carried out only along the lines of human modes of observation and thought. In the broad perspective, then, alchemy will be relevant, though in what sense remains a question, for it is undeniable, now, that its understandings of chemistry itself were almost totally incorrect. Today's understanding, grounded in atomic structure and interatomic forces, has so hugely outperformed alchemical correspondences and the like that it has removed alchemy, in its narrow, chemical sense, from serious discussion. The sheer size and success of the organic chemistry industry proves the reliable predictive power of current theories of chemical reaction and combination.

Alchemy's longevity, if indeed a fact, will lie elsewhere, in our interior, psychospiritual world, related in some way to that fundamental fact to which we have drawn attention, the human mode and limitation of human thinking, and it is this that is worthy of further space. On the basis of what we have already said we shall look for patterns of alchemical thought that might provide a perspective on current scientific thinking. We could ask, then, whether there is a place, today, for a hermeneutic of alchemy. On this topic Seeman offers the view that Jung's profound interpretation of Western alchemical texts may not be the final word in understanding the symbolism, since some of the practices may have disappeared with the oral tradition, and a comparative study between the advanced spiritual practices of Tantra and Western alchemy might recover lost answers and provide new knowledge.[45]

As Iona Miller has already found, there are indeed parallels between Western alchemy and Indian Yoga and common symbols for the process of transformation.[46] This is not greatly surprising, for India also has an alchemical tradition called *Rasayana,* which in the first centuries of the common era was practiced by the Siddhas, the poet-philosopher-yogis of South India, as part of their Siddha medicine system. By the twelfth to fourteenth centuries CE, this system, probably the world's oldest medical discipline, had become part of the less ancient Ayurveda, which remains India's mainstream medical practice to the present day, although Siddha medicine persists in the South Indian state of Tamil Nadu and other places in the world to which the Tamils have migrated.[47] In her book on alchemical and therapeutic methods of healing, Miller compares the two systems, noting that Yoga, like alchemy, is also experimental in nature, though with the

difference that the experiment is performed on oneself, in the "inner laboratory."*

It is possible to draw metaphysical or symbolic correspondences between the planetary and metallurgical attributions of alchemy and the chakras, the energy centers of the subtle body, an idea that appears also in Indian astrology and gem therapy, as follows:

Metal	Planet	Chakra
Gold	Sun	Heart chakra
Silver	Moon	Brow chakra
Copper	Venus	Throat chakra
Tin	Jupiter	Solar Plexus chakra
Lead	Saturn	Root chakra
Iron	Mars	Sacral chakra
Quicksilver	Mercury	Crown chakra

We have arranged the planets in their sequence of lessening brightness in the sky, which presents the chakras in incorrect sequence. We do this to show that various systems of "correspondences" threw up anomalies that the human mind failed to see, or glossed, or even ignored. Often, the observed characteristics could have given wholly different hierarchies and correspondences from those actually chosen. It took many centuries for the human mind to discern that more rational systems could be based on the observations if exclusions from and narrowings of the subject matter had first been made, and earlier alleged parallels had thereby been excluded from the hypothesis-making process. It was only by such processes of exclusion that the modern systematic sciences could come into being. Now, in the twenty-first century, with these successful narrowly defined systems

---

*In the application of the word *laboratory* to both the self and the alchemist's workplace, we see the mind's tendency to conceive parallels, and also the tendency of repeated verbal usage to confirm such notions, as if usage provided objective proof of their validity. Of course, in the majority of scientific situations this would today be considered invalid, but in the past it was not thought so, nor may it be in the future, since the ubiquitous presence of the human mind raises questions concerning the power of intentionality, which are certainly within the proper realm of today's science.

(especially, of course, physics and mathematics) as foundation, we seek a reexpansion of them that will include the whole of human-beingness without anomalies. We shall have more to say, but now continue our description of the parallels between Eastern and Western alchemies.

Alchemy is not concerned only with consciousness, but also seeks the subtle transformation of the body, so that the physical level also is brought into perfect equilibrium. Another parallel can be drawn between the three major principles, or qualities of energy, which, as we have seen, are known to Indic culture as the gunas: sattva, rajas, and tamas. We display them alongside their alchemical and other correlatives at the bottom of the page.

In Indic thought, other correlates of the gunas concern foods: sattvic foods, such as fruits, vegetables, nuts, and grains, incline one toward meditation and the spiritual life; rajasic foods are spicy, and therefore stimulating; tamasic foods, such as animal flesh, incite the so-called "baser" instincts. That physiological correlations of such kinds exist is surely beyond doubt, but whether the Eastern and Western alchemical analyses are correct need not concern us. Our point is, rather, that there were parallel developments in both camps over historical time and, while some contacts were stretched or even destroyed, many similarities survived the separation. Today's rapprochement between the cultures under a new scientific aegis rediscovers these and builds upon them, but with the advantage of new insights from the rational, empirical, mathematical, and analytical (left-brained!) science, which, if historical and geographical discontinuities had not intervened, might not yet have developed.

Furthermore, preparation for the practice of either alchemy or Yoga requires a moral or ethical self-examination. Both stress that "negative" tendencies should be overcome while "positive" virtues are to be developed. This requirement applies to both behavior and the "purification" of various body centers. The objective is not wealth, the transmutation of base metal into gold, but

health or wholeness. What many today would demand, the "objectivity" of science, is here prevented by value judgments about what is to be regarded as "negative" and "positive," "base" and "higher," "pure" and "impure," and also by a lack of detail not only about what the practices should consist in but also *why* they should be as recommended. The consideration of this question of independent support for ethical valuations and judgments is in itself a productive introspective process, regardless of what is found, since it is a process of *self*-examination by the investigator of the modes of *his or her own* living, and of the factual, ethical, and other consequences. It is as if an undeniably valuable personal inwardness can only ratify itself, there being no possibility of scrutiny by others. Hence the warnings by the experienced that embarking recklessly upon spiritual practice can damage both the naïvely unwary and the arrogant novice.

Many questions arise, all difficult to address. Science is wary of a priori views, for example, upon what is "pure" and what is to be purged as "impure," unless some independent substantiation has been found for the judgments imposed. The word *pure* itself provides a notable example, for it is often applied, with connotations of condemnation, to matters of sexual conduct, yet often the matter is not one for purgation, not a matter of "whether," but rather of how and when and with whom. The conflation of taste with morals is no new error, for all cultures have given instances. Most thinking people today recoil with horror from the ethics of the Old Testament patriarchs, for instance. But we must return to alchemy and Yoga per se.

Alchemy speaks of a "secret fire," which is often compared to a serpent or dragon. Here again, we find correspondence with the Tantric kundalinī, the serpent-power. Alchemy is performed by the aid of Mercury, the illuminative principle, and the powers of the sun and moon. Both alchemists and Tantrics practice with the essential aid, sometimes sexual, of a mystical sister, the alchemist's *soror mystica* or the yogi's yogini, so making the complementarity

Guna	Character	Alchemical Character	Correlate of Guna	Substance	Correlate of substance
Sattva	*illuminative*	Mercury	*vital, reflective*	Spirit	*spiritual, good, intelligent*
Rajas	*desirous, attached*	Sulphur	*fiery, passionate*	Soul	*active*
Tamas	*arrestive, binding*	Salt	*gross, material*	Body	

of king and queen, Siva and Sakti, god and goddess, yin and yang, joined in the miracle marriage. Where extremes of character, in all the senses of that word, found alone and unbalanced, cause only harm, the union and harmony of *complementary* "opposites" brings only good.

The Yogic system works in three channels in the subtle body, as we have seen before. Pingalā is conceived to be correlated with the sun, idā with the moon. Suṣumnā, the combining and harmonizing channel, is associated with illumination. As we have also seen, in the caduceus twin serpents twine together and open up into the third way. The yogi seeks to arouse the latent power of the kundalinī serpent so that it rises through the chakra centers until it opens the third eye of mystical vision and illumination. Alchemists perform the process in outward symbol, reminiscent of the fire rituals surveyed in chapter 5, "The Yoga of the Subtle Body," and also reminiscent of Rasayana. Slow heat is applied to the alchemical vessel to sublimate and refine the contents. The yogi uses breath control, the alchemists use bellows to control the fire. Interestingly, yogis employ breathing exercises called "breath of fire" and "the bellows," as we also noted in chapter 5.

The human mind has long been an inventor of symbolisms and a seer of correspondences, and there are also parallels in the respective histories of alchemy and Yoga. Iona Miller draws attention to some of these, pointing to correspondences resulting in the alchemical production of a new kind of human being, one made "hale" or whole. We reproduce information from her article with small changes of our own:

1. Both the Yogic and the Tantric alchemical systems agree that all things are expressions of one fundamental energy.
2. Both affirm that all things combine three qualities:
Wisdom, sattva, superconsciousness, or Mercury
Desire, rajas, compulsion, or Sulphur
Inertia, tamas, darkness, or Salt
3. Both recognize five modes of expression:
Ākāśa: spirit, or the quintessence
Tejas or Agni: fire
Apas: water
Vāyu: air
Pṛithvī: earth*

4. Both systems mention seven principal vehicles of activity, yogis referring to seven chakras, alchemists to seven metals.
5. Both say there is a secret force, fiery in quality, which is to be raised from one chakra or metal to another, until the power of all seven is sublimated to the highest.
6. Yoga says sun (*surya*) or prāna, moon (*chandra*), and wisdom (sattva) are the three agencies of the work (or idā, pingalā, and suṣumnā). Alchemy says the whole operation is a work of the sun and moon, aided by Mercury.
7. Both systems stress the need of preparation by establishing physical purity and ethical freedom from lust, avarice, vanity, attachment, anger, and other antisocial tendencies.
8. Both allege that success enables the adept to exercise extraordinary powers, to heal all diseases, and to control all the forces of nature so as to exert a determining influence on circumstances.[48]

Miller ends the above comparison by saying "What both alchemist and yogi do is to recognize what goes on in the body and to use this knowledge of the control exerted over subconscious processes by self-consciousness to form a definite intention that this body-building function shall act with maximum efficiency, [so] creating increased vitality." This "supercharge of libido," she explains, then awakens the spiritual vision of the pineal gland to full activity. In some modern interpretations this is said to override biophysical mechanisms that normally inhibit the production of endogenous DMT, or, in other words, it allows the production of endorphins.* "The 'Great Work' of alchemy consists of stabilising this *vision* of Light into a full *realisation* [my emphases]. The by-product is that the body-building power of the subconscious changes the alchemist him- or herself into a new creature."[49]

---

*This is the order in which Miller gives the five elements. More often they would be presented in the following hierarchy: ākāśa/tejas or agni/vāyu/apas/pṛithvī.

---

*Regarding endorphins, the reader should consult the work of Candace Pert, mentioned in chapter 16, and listed in the bibliography.

THIRTEEN

Theosophy, Anthroposophy, and the Subtle Bodies

Each of the centres can, when fully awakened and consciously and scientifically employed, serve as a door through which awareness of that which lies beyond the individual human life can enter. The etheric body is fundamentally the most important response apparatus which man possesses, producing not only the right functioning of the five senses and consequently providing five major points of contact with the tangible world, but it also enables a man to register sensitively the subtler worlds, and when energised and controlled by the soul, the spiritual realms stand wide open also.

ALICE BAILEY, *ESOTERIC HEALING*

"Knowledge of the constitution of man and the nature of the various bodies, both dense and subtle" is the fundamental subject matter of Alice Bailey's influential book, *Esoteric Healing*. First published in 1934, it has gone through numerous reprints as each succeeding generation of healers has discovered it, and it is now regarded by some as the "bible" of the "New Age." Alice Bailey (1880–1949) was a prolific writer on healing, spiritual psychology, esoteric thought, Christianity, and other religious themes. Her works were influenced by those of Helena Blavatsky, the founder of the Theosophical Society, which Bailey joined in 1917. Although her teachings eventually differed from Blavatsky's—she split from the Theosophical Society in 1923 and founded her own esoteric school with her husband, Foster Bailey—she continued to promote and develop Blavatsky's theories.

Since its founding in New York in 1875, the

Theosophical Society has spread throughout America, Europe, and the Near and Far East, with over a hundred branches in India alone. In an article assessing its relationship to Hinduism and Buddhism, written twenty years later, Merwin-Marie Snell notes that "the word *theosophy* properly means the theory or practice of the acquisition of knowledge or wisdom from a divine source as opposed to a human source; it is thus the correlative of *theopathy,* the perception of the divine by feeling, and of *theurgy,* action through divine power."[1] She points out that the word *theosophy* has long been in use to designate Neo-Platonism and the philosophies of Paracelsus and Jacob Boehme. She continues:

The Theosophical Society professes to have as its object not the propagation of a special creed but the promotion of human brotherhood, the investigation of the occult powers and forces of nature, and the study of Oriental literatures. Nevertheless, it has taught from the beginning a distinct system which has crystallized more and more into an accepted orthodoxy. . . .This system is in theory a true theosophy, as it holds that the fundamental source of religious knowledge is not reason, objective revelation, or historic tradition, but an interior illumination, or, rather, direct spiritual vision resulting from oneness with the divine universal Spirit.[2]

However, she points out that it surrenders this principle by its implicit acceptance of the authority of the "Mahatmas," claimed to be the highest spiritual adepts, who have exerted continuous influence on the human race. The disciples of the new theosophy are, therefore, not left to construct their own worldview through study and intuition but are expected to accept implicitly the body of teaching, believed to be part of a secret tradition of absolute religious, philosophical, historical, and scientific truth, handed down from the earliest progeni-

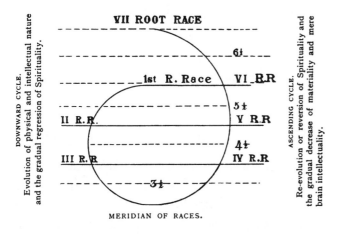

MERIDIAN OF RACES.

Fig. 13.1. Blavatsky believed that humanity is currently passing through its fifth cycle of evolution. In her magnum opus, *The Secret Doctrine*, she states that while the first of the "root races," the "First Spiritual ethero-astral race" was "devoid of the intellectual brain element" because it was on its descending line from the Universal Mahat (Great Being), we are on the ascending line and therefore lacking the spiritual element "which is now replaced by the intellectual," an idea related to Gebser's view that we have in recent centuries been dominated by the mental aspect of our development. Blavatsky, like Gebser, believed that we are now passing through a transition period and are again turning toward spirituality.

tors of the race, their predecessors of other worlds and races, constantly confirmed and corrected by seers and sages, which was communicated to Madame Blavatsky and her inner circle.[3]

Theosophy was, in its earliest days, called "Esoteric Buddhism" and "Pre-Vedic Brahmanism." Thus, the next part of Snell's article is devoted to a comparison of Theosophy, with its claims to esoteric truth, and the "outward material form," which the Buddha taught, the true esoteric knowledge being taught only to his elect. Most of Blavatsky's teaching, thus referred to by Snell, is found in two particular works, *Isis Unveiled* and *The Secret Doctrine*. The latter is a prodigious work containing the cosmogony, theology, and history of the long spiritual evolution of the human race as it first descends into matter and attempts the long climb back to Godhead, an unfoldment directed by the divine powers (the *dhyan chohans*) and the seven great hierarchies, which include the dhyāni buddhas, the devas and *prajapatis* (creators) of the Hindus, the *elohim* (gods) of the Jews, and the angels and gods of other religions. "Although consisting of vast hosts of individual beings, their consciousness is to such a degree fused that as a whole or in any of their subdivisions they may be spoken of either as one or as many."[4]

The Bodies in Theosophy

Central to Blavatsky's cosmogony is the theory that a sevenfold constitution of the universe is reflected in a sevenfold human constitution. These seven parts of the human are:

> spirit (the spark of the Absolute Being within us)
> spiritual soul or god within (buddhi)
> human soul (manas), which is cast off with the lower bodies at death
> animal body (*kama-rupa*)
> subtle body (linga or sūkṣma śarīra)
> vitality (jīva)
> gross body (sthūla śarīra)

However, Bailey also taught that the human being consists of a *soul* of abstract mental material, working through a *personality*, a technical term used to describe the physical, emotional, and less-abstract mental *bodies*, considered holistically. She uses traditional terms for these lower three "vehicles" or "sheaths": *etheric* body, *astral* body, and *mental* body. These auric aspects of the human being are defined as partial emanations or expressions of the soul, which is itself identical with the evolving human consciousness. The mind is not conceived to be simply an ephemeral brain effect,* but as the motivating energy responsible for the inner constitution of individuals, which also manifests as the aura, the energy field that surrounds all matter. It is not a flaccid effect but a preexisting executive force. This "explanatory description" raises as many questions as it sets out to settle, not least the overriding question whether Bailey's description is of the same entities as Blavatsky's or reflects divergent beliefs as to our nature and constitution. As related, Bailey parted company from Theosophy, though without relinquishing all its doctrines, so the question arises whether her later views on the structure of the human remained compatible with the seven levels of being posited by Blavatsky. The perpetual problems of language not only exacerbate the difficulty but also prevent the reader reaching certainty on the point.

In introducing *Esoteric Healing,* Bailey explains her interest in healing, writing:

All initiates of the Ageless Wisdom are necessarily healers, though all may not heal the physical body. The reason for this is that all souls that have achieved any measure of true liberation are transmitters of spiritual energy. This automatically affects some aspect of the mechanism of the souls they contact. When I employ the word "mechanism" in these instructions I refer to different aspects of the instrument, the body or form nature, through which all souls seek manifestation.[5]

The book is divided into sections, the first of which deals with the causes of disease (which, interestingly, include discussion of the illnesses suffered by disciples, mystics, and occultists). It is followed by a section on the

seven methods of healing "as practiced by the initiates of the world." Then follow sections on the training of healers, the "Psychological Causes of Disease" and "Causes Arising in the Emotional-Desire Nature," in which she discusses the "subtler bodies." She writes a passage that hints at some of the difficulties we have mentioned, observing:

First, the phrase "subtler bodies" is somewhat meaningless, is it not? They are not bodies like the physical body. They can be regarded as centres or reservoirs of particular types of force, attached to each individual, and possessing their proper inlets and outlets. They are collections of atoms, vibrating at high speed and colored (according to some schools of occultism) by certain definite hues; they emit a certain tone, and are at varying points of evolution. According to others they are states of consciousness, and some regard them as made in the likeness of a man.[6]

We wonder whether, upon reading such a passage, a scientist of today, even one with the deep interest in matters spiritual that many of them evince, would attempt to clarify her meaning, or pass by.

Bailey then suggests that for the majority of humankind, the astral body is the most important, as it is an outstanding cause of ill health. The reason for this, she says, is that it has a potent and predisposing effect upon the vital and etheric body. The physical body is an automaton of whichever inner body is the strongest. She states that when you remember that the vital body is the recipient of the streams of energy and is in fact composed of such streams, which drive the physical body into activity, it is apparent that the stream that is the most potent is the one that will control the action of the physical body upon the physical plane. She then refers to two other streams that are predisposed to disease:

1. The stream of life itself, anchored in the heart, which determines the vitality of the man, his capacity for work, and the term of his existence.
2. The predominating stream of energy coming from the astral, mental, or soul bodies, which control his expression upon the physical plane.

---

*This vague phrase may express an equivalent to the claim that consciousness is merely an epiphenomenon of the brain's working, an incidental accompaniment having no causative power or function. Sources such as Popper and Eccles' *The Self and Its Brain* contain references to this hypothesis, which these writers reject.

(Perhaps a little clarity results from realizing that this amounts to a description of the ancient notion of karma.)

Bailey states that these energy streams differ in different people, whom she classifies into four groups:

The masses of people throughout the world
The thinking public
The intelligentsia and spiritual aspirants
The mystics and creative workers[7]

Here, again, are the temperaments we discussed earlier in writing about the Hindu system and Neo-Platonism, though we also see categories that, if they are accurately described, cannot but overlap, preventing valid definition. The healer, Bailey states, must understand these different types of energy in order to work constructively, and she sums up these "occult facts" about the subtle bodies and the seven energy centers in the following description of their forms, colors, locations, and behaviors. We shall allow her to speak at some length for herself:

1 First of all, there is nothing but energy, and this energy manifests itself as many differing and varying energies. Of these many energies, the universe is composed. Likewise man's bodies or vehicles of manifestation are without exception constituted of energy units. These we call atoms, and these atomic units are held together in body form by the coherent force of more potent energies.

2 The major focal point of energy to be found in human beings is that of the soul, but its potency as an agent of cohesion and of integration is as yet greater than its quality potency. In the earlier stages of human evolution it is the *coherence* aspect that demonstrates. Later as man's response apparatus, his bodies, becomes more developed, the *quality* aspect of the soul begins to demonstrate increasingly.

3 Seen from the inner side where time is not, the human creature demonstrates as an amazing kaleidoscopic mutable phenomenon. Bodies, so called, or rather aggregates of atomic units, fade out and disappear, or flash again into manifestation. Streams of colours pass and repass; they twine or intertwine. Certain areas will suddenly intensify their brightness and blaze forth with brilliance; or again they can be seen dying out and the phenomenon in certain areas will be colourless and apparently nonexistent. But always there is a persistent over-shadowing of light, from which a stream of light pours down into the phenomenal man; this can be seen attaching itself in two major localities to the dense inner core of the physical man. These two points of attachment are to be found in the head and in the heart. There can also be seen, dimly at first but with increasing brightness, seven other pale disks of light which are the early evidence of the seven centres.

4 These centres, which constitute the quality aspects and the consciousness aspects, and whose function it is to colour the appearance or outer expression of man and use it as a response apparatus are (during the evolutionary process) subject to three types of unfoldment:
    a) That unfoldment which takes place as a physical-plane child grows from an infant to a man. By the time he is twenty-one, the centres should normally have reached the same quality of expression as they had attained when he passed out of life in a previous incarnation. The man then takes up life where he had previously left off.
    b) The awakening of the centres through life experience. Occasionally only one centre may be dealt with in any one life; sometimes several are brought into greater functioning consciousness.
    c) There is, finally, the awakening of these centres through the process of initiation. This, of course, only happens when the man is consciously upon the Path.

5 The centres determine the man's point of evolution *as far as his phenomenal expression is concerned;* they work directly upon the physical body through the medium of the endocrine system. This point should be borne in mind, for the future occult healer will approach his

patient with this knowledge. He will then work through those centres and glands which govern the particular area of the body wherein the disease or discomfort is located. The time, however, for this has not yet come, for man's ignorance is great. Over-stimulation of the centres, and consequently of the glands, could easily be brought about, and the diseased condition might be stimulated also and increased, instead of dissipated or healed.[8]

Several points of interest in Bailey's text draw our attention. How far she adheres to "orthodox" Theosophical teachings is difficult to say, not least on account of her use of vague allusions, which seem to risk meaninglessness for most readers. However, she is certainly speaking from experience rather than merely stating received teachings. This is evidenced by her comment in paragraph 3 where she uses the phrase "Seen from the inner side where time is not . . ." Clearly she is referring to her own experience of meditation, when psychological time seems to fade away and the physical-world clock is not heard to tick. She did, indeed, advocate meditation as an important tool in the development of healers. It would also be interesting to know whether she had heard of, and had attempted to understand, what were at the time very recent developments in physics, as she seems to refer, though very vaguely, to certain newly discovered phenomena, such as the strange behavior of particles at the "quantum level." Although the ancient yogis knew of the relationship between the energy centers and the glands, medical science had not yet determined the functions of all the glands. The function of the amygdala, for example, the seat of emotion and memory in the brain, was not verified until 1965, after Alice Bailey's death, so perhaps she was ahead of her time in her understanding of how certain somatic processes worked. But perhaps, like so many, she was simply referring to scientific matters that had become topics of fashionable talk, but that she did not really understand, and was exercising a certain caution in avoiding definiteness while also wishing to seem well-informed. What is certain is that, unfortunately, her explanations are, for most readers, not entirely clear.

Variations in the Chakra System

While the Indic traditions vary among themselves, the schema that Theosophy presents departs from all those traditional Eastern esoteric traditions in some important respects. As we have seen, Yoga and Tantra derived their teachings from the earlier Vedantic concept of two bodies, the sthūla śarīra, which is the visible, material body, and the sūkṣma śarīra, the invisible, nonmaterial subtle body, also known as the linga śarīra, which consists of five kośas (sheaths) or planes of consciousness. In the Theosophical writings, particularly those of C. W. Leadbeater (1854–1934) and Annie Besant (1847–1933), who together established the Adyar School of Theosophy, the emphasis is on a series of seven subtle bodies or vehicles of consciousness, each of which has its own aura and set of chakras.

The translator and scholar Sir John Woodroffe, alias Arthur Avalon, comments on theosophical teachings in his book *The Serpent Power*.

> Though "Theosophical" teaching is largely inspired by Indian ideas, the meaning which it attributes to the Indian terms which it employs is not always that given to these terms by Indians themselves. This is sometimes confusing and misleading, a result which would have been avoided had the writers of this school in all cases adopted their own nomenclature and definitions.[9]

We note that Woodroffe does not dispute the Theosophists' right to devise a system of their own, but clearly regrets their confusing the terminology. He cites a Theosophical work that refers to the subtle body, the linga śarīra, as "the ethereal duplicate." "Elsewhere," he says, "it is called the "astral body," and some statements are made as to the chakras which are not in accordance with the texts with which I am acquainted."[10] (See plates 29 and 30).

Woodroffe comments further that "According to the English author's account,* the cakras are all vortices of 'etheric matter,' apparently of the same kind and subject to the same external influence of the in-rushing

---

*Here, Woodroffe seems to be referring to Annie Besant's book, *Ancient Wisdom*.

seven-fold force of the '*Lógos*' but differing in this, that in each of the *çakras* one or other of their sevenfold forces is predominant."[11] The next part of Woodroffe's argument is not easy to grasp without considerable knowledge of Yoga philosophy, so we shall not comment in this guide for the general reader, but he draws attention to a source of confusion that, given the vagueness and uncertainty of nomenclature apparent throughout the history of the subject, general readers will certainly wish to have pointed out. Many yoga practitioners are puzzled by Woodroffe's statement that the "splenic center" referred to in Theosophical teachings is "not included among the six *chakras* which are dealt with here."[12] His comment also concerns present-day practitioners such as followers of the American healer Barbara Brennan, and practitioners who have studied the work of David Tansley, the British radionics pioneer.

Woodroffe was writing during the early part of the twentieth century. Among today's writers there are different views about whether or not the spleen chakra actually exists and about how it came to be incorporated into chakra theory. The source of the term *spleen chakra* or *splenic chakra* appears to have been C. W. Leadbeater himself, and Woodroffe is at pains to clarify what he sees as a confusion caused by Leadbeater, for he, that is Woodroffe, writes:

> The second *çakra* is sometimes called the Spleen *çakra*. This practice seems to originate in C. W. Leadbeater's book, *The Chakras,* the first book to introduce the *çakras* to the West. However, Leadbeater himself is quite explicit that the Sacral *çakra* (the Indian *svādhiṣṭhāna çakra*) is different from the Spleen *çakra*, which he discusses. He even considers opening the Sacral *çakra* to be disastrous. Leadbeater's description of the Spleen *çakra* bears some relation to the functions attributed to the Spleen in Chinese Medicine (belonging to the Spleen meridian). It is supposed to deal with transporting energy throughout the body. It does not seem to have anything in common with the Western medical understanding of its function in purifying the blood. However, Leadbeater situates the Spleen *çakra* at the spleen, so it has to be concluded that it is incorrect to call the Sacral *çakra* the "*Spleen çakra*."[13]

Yet again, we face uncertainty as to the precise locations and functions of parts of the subtle body. It is an elusive entity, its elusiveness increased by what seem to be careless descriptions by some authors. There may even be further factors. We offer, tentatively, the suggestion that Leadbeater, formerly a cleric in prudish Victorian England, may have regarded the opening of the swādhiṣṭhāna chakra, the chakra concerned with reproduction, as disastrous merely on that account, and even invented a chakra nearby to replace one having a nature so disreputable in his native culture.

An intriguing confirmatory aside to Woodroffe's criticisms of Leadbeater's interpretation and the source of his spleen chakra comes, inadvertently, from Patricia Day Williams, M.D. She states that "many European alchemists used a diagram of a seven-pointed star to map a pathway for human development. In seventeenth-century Bavaria, Gichtel [see plate 30] laid out the seven classical planets within the framework of the human body. . . . He then included a spiral line that, alternating up and down, maps out a pathway to transformation." She then points out that there are various other models of chakras in other traditions where we find a similar pattern, notably in Chinese medicine.[14] Whether the notion of a spleen chakra that has persisted among New Age healers such as Barbara Brennan, whose chakra model is based on Leadbeater's, also arose independently on account of meridians that supply qi (energy) to specific organ systems, including the spleen, or whether the two have a common origin in Leadbeater's views is uncertain.

Leaving the disagreement with Leadbeater behind, we note that Woodroffe finds less to dispute elsewhere, for "many present-day Indian gurus who incorporate *çakras* within their systems of philosophy do not seem to radically disagree with the western view of *çakras,* at least on the key points, and both these eastern and western views have developed from the *Śakta Tantra* school." He then points out that "There are various other models of *çakras* in other traditions, notably in Chinese medicine, and also in Tibetan Buddhism. Even in Jewish *Kabbalah,* the different *Sephiroth* are sometimes associated with parts of the body."[15] We shall examine briefly these variations on the theme.

As we saw in part 1, "Eastern Perspectives," the earliest known mention of chakras is found in the later

Upaniṣads, including specifically the *Brahma Upaniṣad* and the *Yogatattva Upaniṣad*. These Vedic models were adapted in Tibetan Buddhism as Vajrayana theory, and in the Tantric Sakta theory of chakras. It is the Sakta theory of seven main chakras that most people in the West adhere to, either knowingly or unknowingly, and this is largely due to translations of two Indian texts, the *Sat-cakra-Nirupana,* and the *Padaka-Pancaka,* both by that same authority, Sir John Woodroffe.

In the Kabbalah, the different sephiroth are variously translated as spheres, worlds, emanations, or stages of consciousness, and are thus traditionally mapped onto the Tree of Life, which corresponds to the spine. The grouping of the sephiroth into seven levels reveals remarkable correspondences to the seven chakras. The Kabbalah scholar Jay Michaelson emphasizes the importance of all the levels of the tree: "If we imagine the first [upper] three sefirot to be an idea arising in the mind, the second [middle] three to be the stirrings in the heart as it weighs and evaluates it, and the third [lower] three to be the qualities of action that bring it into being, then malchut is its actual being; its manifestation . . . the result."[16] We note the reversal of the upward motion, seen in other systems, from base to crown. Here, emphasis is upon the higher source of being, and the eventual effect of that Great Being upon human embodied life. This seems natural when we recall that the notion of a deity whose very nature is entirely above our own, and who is not to be "likened to wood or stone images," a notion that breaks the ubiquitous hylic pluralism pervading almost all earlier religions, seems to originate in or near the Hebrew world, rather than in the Indic. This difference of perspective, indeed, this great insight, upon our place in the world and the place of Deity above it, will show its importance later in this book.

In chapter 6 we saw that a very similar concept to chakras also exists in Islamic Sufism, as the Laṭā'if-e-Sitta, the Six Subtleties, which are regarded as psychospiritual "organs" or faculties of sensory and suprasensory perception, activation of which makes a person complete.

Attempts have been made to reconcile the systems with each other, and there are some notable successes, even between such divergent traditions as Sakta Tantra, Sufism, and Kabbalism, where chakras, laṭā'if, and sephiroth can seemingly represent the same archetypal spiritual concepts. However, it would be very

difficult to develop a unified coherent chakra science that would integrate all the elements of the various present-day chakrologies,* but, as we understand more about energy and energy fields through scientific investigation, perhaps we shall eventually be able to speak a common language embodying both tradition and experience of the energy centers.[17]

Steiner and the Anthroposophic View

Former secretary of the German chapter of the Theosophical Society, Rudolf Steiner (1861–1925) developed his own spiritual philosophy, and therefore left the Society in 1907. While the Theosophists were oriented toward an Eastern and, specifically, an Indian approach, Steiner's path was based on Christianity and natural science, a path of spiritual development that he felt would enable anyone to have spiritual experiences by practicing rigorous forms of ethical and cognitive self-discipline, concentration, and meditation. One element of the "Eastern" view that he did retain was the teaching that moral development must precede the appearance of the spiritual faculties.

Steiner named his system *Anthroposophy,*† from the Greek *anthrōpos,* "human being," plus *sophia,* "wisdom." This distinguished it from, and perhaps even opposed it to, *Theosophy,* "divine wisdom," also from Greek, *theos,* "god," plus *sophia,* "wisdom." The Anthroposophical Society was inaugurated in 1912. Projects inspired by anthroposophy have included schools, centers for the handicapped, organic farming, and health clinics, of which there are thousands today throughout Europe, America, and Asia, doing practical work based on Steiner's principles. He traveled widely, delivering some

---

Chakrology is a neologism, now included in the Monier Williams Sanskrit-English Dictionary, sometimes applied to the study of chakras by alternative medicine practitioners or esoteric philosophers. The coining of the word followed the need, for there are many different "chakrologies," based on ancient Indian Hindu Tantric esoteric traditions, on New Age interpretations, or on Western occult perceptions, as well as on ancient Greek and Christian references.

†The term was not original, as it had first been used by the German writer, astrologer, and alchemist Heinrich Agrippa von Nettesheim (1486–1535), and later by the German philosopher Immanuel Hermann Fichte (1797–1879).[18]

6,000 lectures throughout Europe, and he wrote thirty books.

Steiner was reputed to be a highly developed seer and his "science of the spirit" was based, he claimed, on direct knowledge and perception of spiritual dimensions. Some of Steiner's spiritual beliefs do not appear to have diverged greatly from those of Theosophy, which, as we have seen, derived its philosophy and practices from older Eastern traditions.[19] For example, Steiner's spiritual disciplines included concentration on an object such as a seed, and control of thoughts, emotions, and will. And, like the "householder yogi," the Steinerian spiritual aspirant was urged not to abandon his personal or social responsibilities. Steiner also emphasized the value of serious cognitive studies as a prerequisite in achieving "knowledge of the higher worlds." Progress on the spiritual path, he believed, depended on the harmonious cultivation of certain qualities, specifically:

Control over one's own thinking
Control over one's will
Composure
Positivity
Impartiality[20]

Steiner's methods of meditation also appear to be substantially the same as traditional Eastern practices. He describes three identifiable stages, but with the essential difference that he considered conventional mysticism to lack the clarity necessary for exact knowledge. Natural science, on the other hand, was, by both definition and declared aim, limited to investigating the natural world. Hence his interest in bringing together science and spirituality through a "super-sensory consciousness" developed through rational thought about spiritual research. He hoped to form a spiritual movement that would free a person from extrinsic spiritual authority by grounding the personality in him- or herself.

Anthroposophy describes the early stages of the evolution of human consciousness as showing an intuitive perception of reality, including clairvoyant perception of spiritual realities. Humanity has progressively evolved an increasing reliance on intellectual faculties and allowed a corresponding loss of intuitive or clairvoyant experiences, which have become atavistic. The increasing intellectualization of consciousness, initially a progressive direction of evolution, has led to excessive reliance on abstraction and loss of contact with both natural and spiritual realities. However, in order to go further, new capacities must be developed that combine the clarity of intellectual thought with the imagination, and beyond this with consciously achieved inspiration and intuitive insight.[21] Steiner's methods for developing these faculties include:

Imagination. Through focusing on symbolic patterns, images, and poetic mantras, the meditator achieves consciously directed "imaginations," which allow sensory phenomena to appear as the expression of underlying beings of a "soul-spiritual" nature.

Inspiration. By overcoming such imaginative pictures, the meditator becomes conscious of the meditative activity itself, which awareness leads to experiences of the expressions of soul-spiritual beings unmediated by sensory phenomena or qualities.

Unification. By intensifying the will forces via exercises such as a chronologically reversed review of the day's events, a further stage of inner independence from sensory experience is achieved, leading to direct contact, even unification, with spiritual beings (intuition), yet without loss of individual awareness.[22]

The Subtle Body in Anthroposophy

In an article in the *Journal of Religion,* Professor Clemen explains:

Both theosophy and anthroposophy contend that man consists not only of three main parts (body, soul, and spirit), but of seven other aspects divided among the three main parts in the following way:

1. The body consists of the "physical," "ethereal," and "astral" bodies, the second and third of which must be described somewhat in detail. The ethereal body is also called the "vital body," for it is the one that gives life and shape to the physical body. As by virtue of the physical body man belongs to the mineral kingdom, so by virtue of the ethereal

body he belongs to the vegetable and animal kingdoms, but while the ethereal body of beasts consists only of powers of growth and propagation the ethereal body of man is mainly the bearer of the habits, dispositions and inclinations of his temperament, character, and memory. The astral body, by contrast, is also called the body of the soul (*Seelenleib*), or body of the sensations (*Empfindungsleib*); but it is also the bearer of the instincts and passions. The ethereal body is common to men, beasts, and plants, the astral only to men and beasts. The ethereal body is not born or freed until the time of the second dentition, the astral appears at the time of puberty.

2. The soul consists of the sensational, intellectual, and conscious soul (*Empfindungs-, Verstandes- u. Bewusstseinseele*). The sensational soul, however, is identical with the body of sensations, and the conscious soul with the first part of the spirit, so in fact the soul consists only of the intellectual soul, from which all thoughts of the outer world arise. It is also called the I-body (*Ichleib*).

3. The spirit consists of the spirit itself (*Geistselbst*), the spirit of life (*Lebensgeist*) and the spirit-man (*Geistmensch*). Dr. Steiner, like Mme. Blavatsky and Mrs. Besant, calls them also by Indian names, which have a different meaning in Sanskrit, namely *manas, buddhi,* and *atma*. With these three parts of the spirit, man partakes of the world of the true, the good, and the beautiful. The spirit, however, like the soul, is found only in man.[23]

Professor Clemen adds: "One might accept all this in spite of its artificiality, if it were to be taken only metaphorically, but according to theosophy and anthroposophy all these parts of man, not the physical body only, can be seen by the clairvoyant, though of course not with the bodily eyes."[24]

In a series of lectures collected under the heading *Founding a Science of the Spirit,* Steiner discusses the transformation of the subtle bodies. He says of the *etheric body:*

Anyone who wants to know the nature of the etheric body by direct vision must be able to maintain his ordinary consciousness intact and "suggest away" the physical body by the strength of his will. He will not, however, be left with an empty space, but will see before him the etheric body glowing with a reddish-blue light like a phantom, whose radiance is a little darker than peach blossom. We never see an etheric body if we "suggest away" a crystal; but in the case of a plant or animal we do, for it is the etheric body that is responsible for nutrition, growth and reproduction.[25]

Is not the etheric body the life force? Steiner describes the *astral body* as the seat of everything we know as desire, passion, and so forth. This, he says, is clear in *straightforward inward self-observation,* requiring no "suggesting away," but he adds that for the initiate the astral body, the third component of a person, can become an outer reality, visible as an egg-shaped cloud that not only surrounds the body, but permeates it. If we "suggest away" the physical body and *also* the etheric body, what we shall see is a delicate cloud of light, inwardly full of movement. Within this cloud or aura the initiate sees every desire, every impulse, as color and form in the astral body. For example, he sees intense passion flashing like rays of lightning out of the astral body. Steiner observes further that the color seen differs from one species to another, but also varies from one individual human to another, and adds "if you train yourself to be sensitive, you will be able to recognize someone's temperament and general disposition by his aura."[26]

Steiner next discusses and expounds the idea that the "I" or ego is unique to each individual, signifying a *personal knowledge* of *ownmost-being* and of *personal* identity with and awareness of it, which each person can assert only of *himself*.* "This attribute makes man

---

*Recall Hume's famous assertion that he could find no "self" but only "impressions" and "ideas." But why would the thinker/seer "see" *itself*? What Steiner and other mystics aver does not contradict Hume, but states that something, or rather some*one,* is found if the person meditates suitably, so entering the necessary state of awareness and *self*-experience. Evidently, Hume never experienced this, though Heidegger, as we saw earlier, seems to acknowledge it. See also Popper and Eccles, pages 102 to 103,[27] and Pitson, commentator on Hume, page 196.[28]

superior to the animals. We must realise the tremendous significance of this word. When Jean Paul* had discovered the 'I' within himself, he knew that he had experienced his immortal being . . ." Steiner describes the ego-body as "a blue, hollow sphere between the eyes, behind the forehead. When a person begins to work on it, rays stream out from this point."[29]

The "I" can exert influence upon the astral body, and, Steiner says, "whatever part of the astral body is thus transformed by the 'I' is called *Manas*. Manas is the fifth part of man's nature," and we come to possess just so much of it as we create by our own efforts.[30] Steiner adds that we can also learn to work upon the etheric body, so attaining buddhi. Our task on this planet, he tells us, is to work "right down to the physical body," the most difficult task of all. In order to do that, we must learn to control the breath and the circulation, to follow consciously the activity of the nerves, and to regulate the processes of thought. He then writes of a person who has carried out the work he has described.

> In theosophical language, a man who has reached this stage is called an Adept; he will then have developed in himself what we call *Atma.*† *Atma* is the seventh member of man's being. . . . In every human being four members are fully formed, the fifth only partly, the sixth and seventh in rudiment only. Physical body, etheric body, astral body, "I" (or ego), Manas, Buddhi, Atma—these are the seven members of man's nature; through them he can participate in three worlds.[31]

Later, he refers to the three worlds‡ as:

_____

*Jean Paul Richter, poet (1763–1825).
†When the word *ātma* occurs in the writings of Eastern traditions and is translated into English it is usually translated as "soul." The cognate German word *seele,* on the other hand, carries a meaning nearer to the English word *mind.*
‡Readers may like to research, in addition to matters directly relevant to the topics of this chapter, other "systems," not necessarily similar to or related to Theosophy or Anthroposophy, which have been referred to by using the phrase "three worlds," but which we have no space to deal with in this book. These include the "system" of philosopher Karl Popper and neuroscientist John Eccles, authors of *The Self and Its Brain,* and ideas dealt with by mathematician and physicist Roger Penrose in the last chapter of his book *Shadows of the Mind.* See the bibliography.

1. The physical world, the scene of human life
2. The astral world or the world of the soul
3. The devachanic world or world of spirit[32]

The Significance of Anthroposophy

Although anthroposophy had its critics, some, like Professor Clemen, who were skeptical of Steiner's claims of clairvoyant abilities, have a grudging respect for his ideas. Clemen himself writes:

> To be sure, some of his ideas are not new and others cannot be put into practice; but at any rate the reduction of all things to a few main principles is worthy of admiration and imitation. . . . So, notwithstanding all the shortcomings and dangers of anthroposophy, perhaps it would not be deplorable if in the near future its influence increased even more than of late. For, as in former times (at the beginning of our era and in the Middle Ages), occultist movements have helped religious progress, so now anthroposophy might pave the way for religious and scientific reforms.[33]

In a more recent review of modern esoteric spirituality, which includes critiques on "The Theosophical Society" and "Rudolf Steiner and Anthroposophy," the reviewer, Arthur Versluis, Fulbright Guest Professor, University of Düsseldorf, notes:

> It is difficult to remain quite as neutral when discussing more modern movements due to the lack of historical distance, but interesting to consider the cultural ramifications of groups whose impact is still being felt on a popular level . . . it may well be that the meeting of spiritual paths— the assimilation not only of one's own spiritual heritage but of that of the human community as a whole—is the distinctive spiritual journey of our time.[34]

FOURTEEN

Energy Healing and the New Age Body

Spirituality is the connecting force or integrating power that unifies all of life. It is what synthesises the total personality and provides energising direction and order.

DAVID C. BAKER, *STUDIES OF THE INNER LIFE:*
THE IMPACT OF SPIRITUALITY ON QUALITY OF LIFE

Since the 1970s, Western esotericism has been regarded as a legitimate academic field of research, scholarship, and education in the universities of Britain, Europe, and America. The many Western traditions, the "esoteric currents," as Antoine Faivre calls them, form a recognizable corpus of work, which encompasses particular worldviews, philosophies, and practices that come under the heading of esotericism, but the categorization and nomenclature themselves are not without difficulties.[1] To begin with, as Wouter Hanegraaff, professor of the history of Hermeticism notes, "the very term 'esotericism' is a particularly loaded one . . . a major cause of confusion (not only among outsiders, but even among specialists) about the nature of the discipline."[2] He points out that there are no less than five meanings in current popular usage. These include the use of the word *esotericism* as:

A synonym of *the occult,* a generic term for those writings that concern the paranormal, the occult sciences, various "exotic" wisdom traditions, contemporary New Age spiritualities, and similar belief systems

Secret and arcane traditions, which make a distinction between initiates and noninitiates

A metaphysical concept that refers to transcendent unity in some exoteric religions

A synonym of *gnosis,* covering various religious phenomena that emphasize experiential rather than rational and dogmatic modes of knowing, and that favor mythical and symbolic over discursive forms of expression

A complex of interrelated currents, including those of Hermeticism, alchemy, Paracelsianism, Rosicrucianism, Kabbalah, Theosophy, and Illuminism, and various related trends during the nineteenth and twentieth centuries.[3]

Hanegraaff does not, in giving his list, tell us in detail what "contemporary New Age spiritualities" consist of, but a number of other writers have identified the subtle body, which, in the West, is usually referred to by the use of the term *energetic model,* as the distinguishing component in what has come to be known as "New Age" spirituality, and they state in particular that "subtle

163

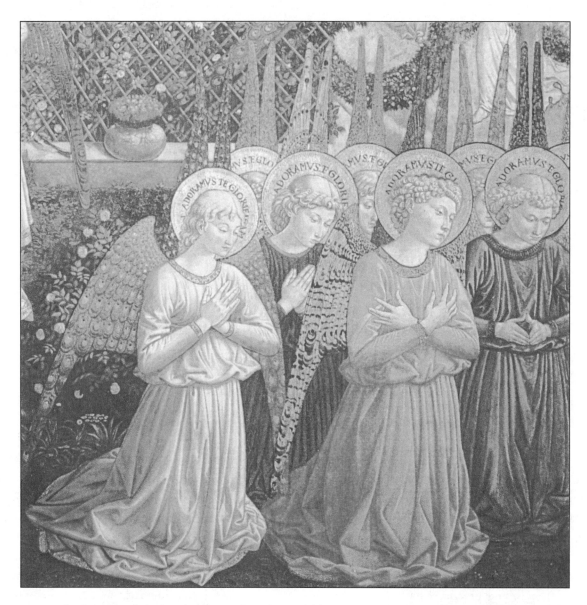

Fig. 14.1. "Halos around the heads of saints have been emblematic conventions in the traditional art of the West . . . For New Agers, however, auras belong not just to saints but to all humans and, indeed, to all physical matter."[4] A particular feature of New Age understanding of the subtle body is that subtle-energy healing can be aided or even administered by healing guides. The descriptions and categorizations show wide cultural variation, of course, for all "gods" are made in the image of the enculturated humans who conceive them, so the Beings to whom these abilities are attributed include a humanoid angelic hierarchy among whom are "ascended masters," deities, and divinities, all invoked in prayer and meditation to provide guidance or intervention in human affairs. Having allowed for human limitation and imagination, we accept, of course, that there may indeed be Superior Beings as well as an *all-encompassing* Great Being, and it is impossible to imagine that such Beings, if they exist, could have *less* "personness" than ourselves. While a scientific outlook has superseded a mythically religious one, science must allow our own personness, so must also allow the probability of superior levels or kinds of personness. Hence, of course, our use of capital initials when referring to them. What is impossible, as always, is to depict such superior personness by terrestrial means. Herein lies the elusiveness of the subtle body by which skeptical recent philosophy has allowed itself to be misled. Detail from Benozzo Gozzoli, *Journey of the Magi*, ca. 1490. (Medici-Riccardi Museum, Florence.)

energy healing" is the dominant mode in the healing repertoire of the "New Age body."

The distinctiveness of the New Age community, says professor Catherine Albanese, is that New Agers are preoccupied with issues about energy and its transmutation into matter. Intellectually dominated by their vision of the new physics, she says, they have seized commonly held notions of Albert Einstein's dicta on matter and energy and used them to formulate a cosmology that articulates their basic religious and philosophical vision. When allowed expression in cultural practice regarding health and healing, this orientation leads its adherents into a world in which religion and therapy mingle freely in ideas and acts that center on energy-phenomena in the human being.[5] In an earlier article, she observed that New Age spirituality refers to "a horizon of meaning" in which she includes the experiential and the sense of connection with ultimates, as with other forms of spirituality, "a horizon patterned to reflect a larger reality" (words that remind us of the anthropic principle and the Hermetic "As above, so below"), which is "ever shifting, transforming itself from moment to moment." To be spiritual in a metaphysical universe, she believes, is to unblock the door and let the waters of life flow through. To put the matter in more contemporary language, it is to be sensitive to subtle energies and to respond to them.[6]

The contemporary view is that the domain of the subtle energies is the aura, the collective term in the West for the emanations from all the layers of the subtle body. The aura was referred to by Plutarch (ca. 50–120 CE) as "revealing the passions and vices in the soul by the variation and movement of its colors," and the purity and spiritual development of a saint was represented in icons in the form of a halo around the head.[7]

Although the language used to describe the aura only became "scientific" about the beginning of the twentieth century, Dr. Walter Kilner's experiments on "the human atmosphere" have resulted in an increasing public awareness. Alongside this development a number of scientists and researchers with far higher scientific credentials, but metaphysical interests as well, have openly acknowledged what, in other quarters, have come to be referred to as "auric sheaths" and "subtle bodies," among them Burr and Northrup,[8] Karagulla,[9] LeShan,[10] Motoyama,[11] Bruyere,[12] Hunt,[13] Tiller,[14] and Schlitz.[15]

Care and Repair of Subtle Bodies

Of particular interest to the healing community is the work of Barbara Brennan, a former NASA scientist, as it "articulates so clearly the texts and contexts that make auric healing worth noticing as contemporary religious therapy of New Age provenance."[16] The map of the human energy field in *Hands of Light* presents Brennan's study of auric sensitivity, a blend of scientific precision and personal experience and experimentation, as a textbook for aspiring practitioners of spiritual, or psychic, healing (see plate 31). Building on scientific concepts derived from quantum physics, interwoven with metaphysical cosmology, Brennan gives practical instructions for the repair of broken and disfigured auras (primarily based on the psychological character types of Wilhelm Reich) and the restoration of well-being.[17]

Brennan's schema of the aura, with its seven energy bodies and associated chakras, adheres to the traditional Eastern model up to a point, but she then adds additional layers, or bodies, of her own, which, she says, go through a process of opening during therapy and have particular roles to play during birth and death: the "haric" level, a key center in Eastern meditation, martial arts, and qigong, which Brennan associates with intentionality and will; and the "core" star level, which she associates with a person's divine essence and the source of creative energy, placed above the solar plexus, in a location that corresponds to that of the Tantric *hṛtpadma* (secret heart).[18]

She also believes that when a person changes his or her belief system this change itself brings about changes in chakra movement and functioning. For Brennan, the aura is the "missing link" between physical medicine and psychotherapy as practiced in the West. Between spirit and matter, she believes, are energy blocks, emotional in nature, which cause physical and spiritual illness. Hence care and repair of the subtle bodies, rather than of the physical body, is the key to well-being. By identifying individual auric patterns the healer can discern the spiritual or emotional causes of physical disease. Some healers also claim to be able to anticipate illnesses from disturbances in the auric patterns that have not yet manifested in physical form, and to be able to avert potential damage.[19]

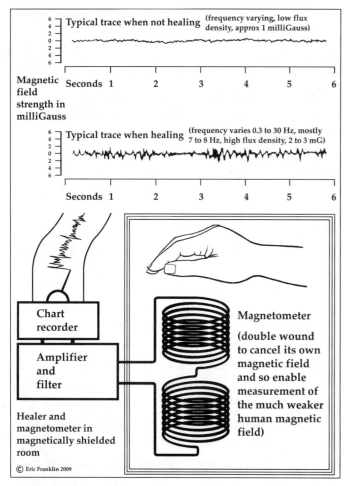

Magnetic field strength in milliGauss

Typical trace when not healing (frequency varying, low flux density, approx 1 milliGauss)

Seconds 1　2　3　4　5　6

Typical trace when healing (frequency varies 0.3 to 30 Hz, mostly 7 to 8 Hz, high flux density, 2 to 3 mG)

Seconds 1　2　3　4　5　6

Chart recorder

Amplifier and filter

Healer and magnetometer in magnetically shielded room

© Eric Franklin 2009

Magnetometer (double wound to cancel its own magnetic field and so enable measurement of the much weaker human magnetic field)

Fig. 14.2. Cellular biologist James Oschman believes that "changes in patients' electromagnetic fields could be due directly to emissions from healers' hands." They produce strong biomagnetic fields that sweep or scan through the same range of frequencies that biomedical researchers find effective for "jump-starting" healing in a variety of hard and soft tissues.[20] The energy coming from the hands can be directed to heal oneself, other humans, animals, or plants. In qigong the hands are considered a moveable zone of energy usable in healing and other purposes.

Reading the Aura

There are now numerous books on the market that give instructions on the reading of auras. The authors present a variety of ideas about what the aura consists of, some of which parallel the Eastern model of the five kośas (sheaths), some the Theosophical model with its additional chakras. Some, such as Barbara Brennan, present schemas of their own.

Joseph Ostram has also presented his own schema. He believes the aura to be a "Double Etheric or Health Aura" formed of three distinct layers: the physical auric body, the etheric auric body, and the vital auric body. He describes the physical auric body as very bright and dense due to physical matter such as mucus and skin particles that are sloughed off the physical body during breathing and movement. The particles are suspended within a field of electromagnetic energy. He believes these particles to be unique to the individual and therefore the means by which animals such as bloodhounds are able to discern and track down specific individuals. This describes something already known to physics and biology. What Ostram and some others add is that in good health this electrochemical band of the aura is bright, clear, and uniform in width as it surrounds the body, and that in ill health it will be seen to bulge near the area affected by disease or injury. Ostram states that this is where ill health can first be seen before any manifestation that can be found by a physician, and that it is often visible before the person shows any other symptom. "In later stages of illness," he says, "the bulging of the physical auric body will appear to disrupt the etheric auric body (causing a hole) and the vital auric body (reducing radiance)."[21]

Ostram ascribes certain characteristics to the next layer of the aura, the etheric auric body, that remind us of the Eastern concept of the sūkṣma śarīra or linga śarīra. He says that it is the matrix upon which the physical body exists; without this matrix the physical body begins to decay and eventually disintegrate. At the moment of death, the etheric double and its auric emanations (the etheric auric body) carry off the soul energy to other levels of existence in the nonphysical world. Very often those who have been declared physically dead, but are subsequently revived, report floating above their physical body, claiming they saw their body below, surrounded by frantic medical personnel trying to resuscitate it. But they felt that "out of body" as they were, they still had a *complete* body [my emphasis]. In fact they usually report having very little concern for the physical vehicle below them.[22] "In diagnosing the severity with which an illness has affected an area," Ostram states that "the vital auric body is very helpful. Areas of disruption due to disease or illness are drained of vital energy. This causes the normally straight radiant lines of energy to droop, eventually falling to the innermost portion of this auric body in an often chaotic and matted fashion . . ." which not only inhibits the flow of vital force but also causes the tissues to decay or atrophy.

Ostram then discusses the relationship between the vital auric body, the emotional bodies, and the chakras.[23]

The vital auric body, he claims, touches the astral or emotional auric body and expands into it at times of high vitality. This is an important relationship because the vital auric body also acts to absorb emotional disruptions, pulling them into the inner layers of the aura and sending them for processing to the appropriate chakra or energy vortex. Each chakra deals with a specific kind of energy. For example, another person's resentment aimed at us can become lodged in our astral auric body where, if it is not dealt with, it will be drawn in by the vital auric body, and will reduce vitality.

Ostram then explains how the damaging change can be passed to the second (sacral), third (solar plexus), and fourth (heart) chakras, affecting the physical organs of those regions, and can eventually manifest on the physical plane as intestinal, stomach, or heart problems. He observes that when emotional disruptions are ignored or "stuffed," they have to manifest on the physical plane to get our attention. He believes we would all be better off if we dealt with our anger and resentments and other emotional issues before they manifested as sickness or death.[24] This understanding reminds us of Wilhelm Reich's psychology, which also seeks to link the psychological with the somatic.

Psychological Themes of the Chakras

One of the problems in understanding the subtle body is, as we have just seen, that in the West, just as in the East, different terms are used by different healers. It is not always easy to grasp their particular perception of the subtle body, how it functions, and how they experience it. Part of this problem arises from the fact that not all healers have come to their knowledge of the subtle body through yoga and meditation practice but have "arrived" from different directions, from having a natural ability to heal, for instance, or via a creative life. Some healers have no intellectual framework at all, and work through their subtle sense perception, in much the same way as yoga practitioners do. We saw this in chapter 5. Such healers just "know" or "feel" when healing has begun and when it ends. Others follow an understanding adapted to their particular discipline. Hence we find that the layers or "levels" of the subtle body, its

kośas (sheaths), chakras (energy centers or vortices), and nadis (energy currents or streams), are described using different terms and explanations depending on the type of therapy employed.

An alternative therapist may see the process differently from a spiritual healer or a transpersonal psychologist, and their intentions, though ultimately directed to the same goal, the healing of the client, may even invoke a different kind of process. Some healers and practitioners become a locus of concentrated psychospiritual energy or, as Feuerstein, whom we quoted in chapter 3, puts it, they are converted from "low-energy systems" to "high-energy systems" through the energy at work in the subtle body itself. Furthermore, despite the differences in the terms that healers and therapists use to describe what they do, and the differences of level or layer from which the healing is believed to come, there is a common consensus that certain recognizable changes occur that alter their own consciousness and enable them to influence the consciousness of others.

One psychotherapist comments that emphasis in these therapies is usually on bringing about an integration of mental, emotional, physical, and spiritual levels through hands-on work, which creates in the client a heightened experience of his or her subtle body. This is distinct from psychotherapy, which works explicitly with the *relationship* between the client and the therapist. Only a few schools of psychotherapy work explicitly with the subtle body as an energetic phenomenon and then usually through a particular experience such as countertransference.[25]

Jung stated his belief that the term *subtle body* should refer to that part of the unconscious that becomes more and more nearly identical with the functioning of the human body, growing darker and darker and ending in the utter darkness of matter.[26] What this means, from the analyst's viewpoint, is that our unconscious thoughts and feelings exist in the subtle body and the less access we have to them at the higher levels the greater the likelihood that they will be crystallized as physical structure and physical symptoms. In becoming denser, Jung says, the patterns are pressing up against the limits of our conscious mind. This somatizing process is a step toward embodiment, and away from the more continuous dissection into layers of the subtle body, and thus a move toward wholeness.[27]

According to the psychotherapist Phoebe Payne and psychiatrist Laurence Bendit, who are also parapsychologists, the chakra is a vortical energy form created by two streams of energy weaving together.[28] The *motor stream* flows in the spinal cord, is thrown out from the center, and flows toward the periphery in a widening spiral. The *sensory* or receptive stream, impinging on the surface of the etheric body, spirals inward, narrowing as it goes. These two spirals flow parallel to one another, but in opposite directions. They may be compared to interlocking screw threads, in that one may be said to run in the grooves of the other and give an impression of spinning. It is important that these two streams are coordinated with one another. If the motor, or outgoing, field is weak, the person is vulnerable to psychic invasion or shock. An individual with a depleted or unstable energy field is easily overwhelmed by another person's psychic energy.

It is a common belief among energy healers that the chakras have specific psychological themes. As chakras are understood to be the organizing centers for the reception, assimilation, and transmission of life energies, and to have physical, psychological, and spiritual issues associated with them, they are widely regarded as the ideal schema through which imbalances and disturbances in energy can be adjusted to restore well-being.[29] This model of the chakras, some therapists have found, helps them to understand how they take in information about their clients (and vice versa), and process it as sensations, feelings, fantasies, images, and, ultimately, as interpretation and intervention. The energy that is processed through a chakra is then distributed through the body or discharged from it. Perhaps information that we block out—because it threatens to overwhelm us in some way—can hang around in our subtle bodies, potentially accumulating to the point where we become exhausted or ill.[30]

Reiki Healing

One of the most popular and widespread forms of New Age healing is the Japanese system of Reiki, a title that is usually explained as meaning "universal energy," because it is derived from a Chinese term meaning "spiritual power." Etymologically, *ki* means "life energy," and *rei* has several meanings including "feeling of mystery,"

"ethereal atmosphere," and "sense of the Divine," but does not mean "universal," as claimed by many Reiki practitioners. The word *rei* as used in relation to Reiki is popularly believed to mean divine knowledge or spiritual consciousness. This suggests that an aspect of the Reiki energy partakes of sentient divine consciousness and, it is claimed, understands each person completely, knows the cause of the illness, and knows what to do to facilitate the person's healing.

Reiki is a form of hands-on healing developed in 1922 by Dr. Mikao Usui, who claimed to have received the ability to heal "without energy depletion" after three weeks of fasting and meditation on Mount Kurama. The main characteristic of Reiki is that the hands of the practitioner are placed on the client's body over the areas that correspond to the chakras. It differs from "spiritual healing" and its Indian cousin "prānic healing," in that Reiki practitioners are "initiated" into a quasi-esoteric system of three stages or "degrees," which involves being given certain symbols or symbolic images to visualize during treatment to enhance the flow of healing energy.

It is hard to say whether use of these enhancement symbols in Reiki treatments produces different results from other forms of hands-on healing because it is dif-

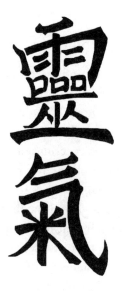

Fig. 14.3. Here, the Japanese name Reiki is written in Chinese characters, providing an instance of a common practice known as *kanji*. The word *kanji* combines *kan*, "Chinese," and *ji*, "character." The *kanji* ideograms for Reiki convey many levels of meaning, ranging from the mundane to the highly esoteric.

ficult to find independent studies of Reiki to compare with the large corpus of experimental work already done with spiritual healing.[31] Exaggerated claims have been made by some Reiki practitioners, many of whom have no other therapeutic or medical training. Statements have been made to the effect that "Reiki is a special kind of life force that is only channeled by someone who has been attuned to it" and "healers who have not received the Reiki attunement from a Reiki Master are not using Reiki but some other kind of energy." Such claims do no service to Reiki, especially since its effectiveness has not been established, either in the long term or in cases of serious illness. Further, if, as it seems, Reiki practitioners acknowledge that other healers use a different energy, the question of which procedure is the more effective should be answered by careful analysis of results. However, despite the lack of proper assessment, it appears to be widely recognized in the therapeutic community that Reiki can work alongside other forms of therapy.

Reiki bases its healing modality on the traditional Indian model of the seven main corporeal chakras, but numerous variations of this model have emerged from the various Reiki schools. The variant models include, in some cases, additional energy centers that extend "up" to the universe and "down" to the earth, a version that continues the correspondence with the Indian systems, since they also have such additional chakras. There are also untested depictions of interconnections between human and cosmic energy fields, and some practitioners believe they can tap into "intergalactic" or "interplanetary" energies, whatever those terms may mean. As in all forms of therapy and spirituality, there is a spectrum of beliefs that ranges from the sublime to the mundane and the totally imaginary. However, there is a common consensus that most people gain benefit from Reiki treatment. Reported benefits include a deep sense of relaxation and increased well-being, relief of aches and pains from minor chronic ailments, and an enhanced ability to cope with stressful life changes and traumatic experience. At the very least, it seems to do no harm and has no known side-effects.

How Does Reiki Work?

The theory is that the Reiki practitioner guides the healing energy through the subtle pathways of the energy

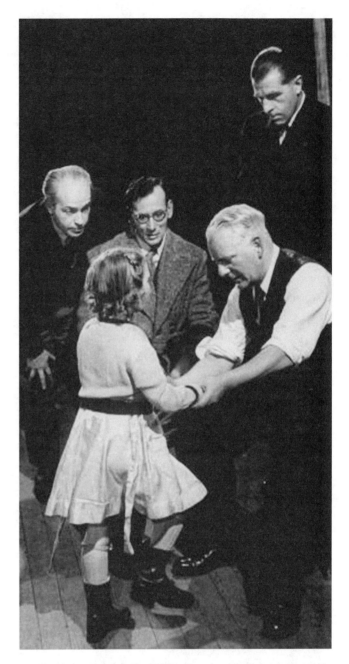

Fig. 14.4. The famous English healer Harry Edwards at work. The placement of hands in both spiritual healing and Reiki follows the chakra system from the top downward. Two or more healers may be present in both systems to intensify the healing process. (Time Life, Inc. www.gettyimages.com.)

body—a description reminiscent of the Indian nadis and the Chinese system of meridians—removing blocks and restoring the flow of the vital energy current so that the organs and tissues can resume their normal functioning. Since life-force energy is influenced by thoughts and feelings and, as we have seen in previous chapters, can be negatively influenced, at both conscious and unconscious levels, by traumatic experiences and negative thoughts about oneself and the world, charging the affected parts of the energy field with "positive" energy is believed to raise the "vibratory level of the energy field" in and around the physical body, clearing and healing the energy pathways and allowing the life force to flow in a healthy and natural way (see plate 32). In practice, the Reiki healer claims to become a channel for the healing energy, the process apparently similar to that described by Olga and Ambrose Worrall, who will be mentioned in chapter 16.

An interesting outcome of the Reiki experience is that some clients report that they have become more sensitive and intuitive, more receptive to "higher" levels of consciousness, and even that they are beginning to develop healing abilities themselves. Some practitioners report experiences similar to those experienced by mystics and yogis, of being surrounded by light and of being in the "divine presence," or of being supported by guides, guardians, or angels during the healing process. What seems clear, therefore, is that some "New Age" healers are able to enter altered states of being that have been accessed by others over the centuries, and, whatever their beliefs about how they get there, are rediscovering the path to the One.

It was Jung who developed the idea that the subtle body is the medium through which projections are transmitted. University of Texas assistant professor of history Bret E. Carroll explains that the psychotherapist is "always embroiled in the client's dynamic," and needs to be involved in this way in order to get an "insight."[32] Somatic countertransference can be viewed as conscious use of a capacity for or tendency toward resonance with the client. "By taking the position of therapist you are implicitly agreeing to subject yourself to the distorting effect of the client's particular energy field in order to understand it (this does not preclude the client's attempts to do the same for the therapist, nor the fact that therapists have plenty of "distortions" of their own)." Professor Carroll also says that information can be transported between persons via any of the subtle body layers and at "different levels of force and velocity," and these differences account for the varieties of experience and of the resulting definitions of countertransference.[33] In his paper "On the Subtle Body Concept in Clinical Practice," Zurich-trained psychoanalyst Nathan

Schwartz-Salant remarks that "the subtle body may be projected and imaginally perceived as operating between people. Furthermore the intermediate subtle body realm can be a conjoined body, made up of the individual subtle bodies of two people."[34] This seems a particularly important point with regard to the character of our relationship with the "subtle world," the "above," as a whole.

Healing Guides

A feature of spiritual healing in the New Age is the relationship with spirit guides. Some healers claim that they receive their knowledge about clients' illnesses through guides or guardians who are present during the healing, or through whom they "channel" information. Some of these guides are said to be "guardian angels," who provide lifetime support and protection, while other guides come and go at different periods and life crises. This is one of the areas where traditional Christianity and spiritualism, a religious system whose adherents believe the spirits of the dead communicate with the living through a medium, appear to meet, although there are major differences between the two religions. "Orthodox" religion generally plays down the role of angels, for example, regarding a person's direct relationship with God as far more important than any relationship with an intermediary, whereas for spiritualists their dealings with their guides are very significant.[35]

Different views are held in different traditions, both Eastern and Western, as to whether guides are discarnate humans who have transcended the human state and have "survived" after their deaths, or are beings who have never incarnated as humans, such as angels are usually conceived to be. Some spiritualists believe that discarnate entities are involved in the process of providing both the diagnosis and the healing energy to help the patient. Present-day practices have their antecedents in the spiritualist movement of the mid-nineteenth century, when spiritualist mediums held séances in which they entered trance states and, claiming to be aided by "spirit guides," diagnosed and prescribed remedies, many of them from the conventional pharmacological and technological repertoire of the day.[36] The parapsychologist Donald Watson points out that this is by no means a solely modern phenomenon. The Neo-Platonists of

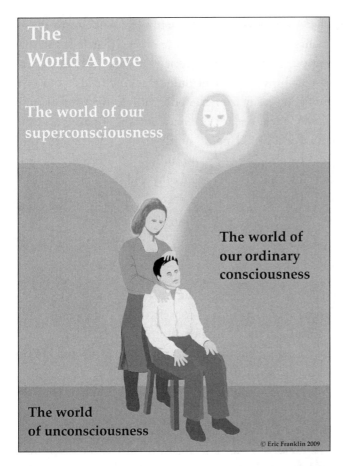

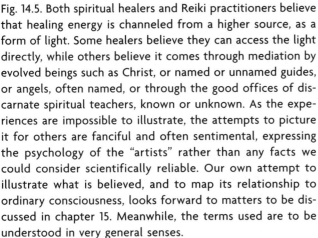

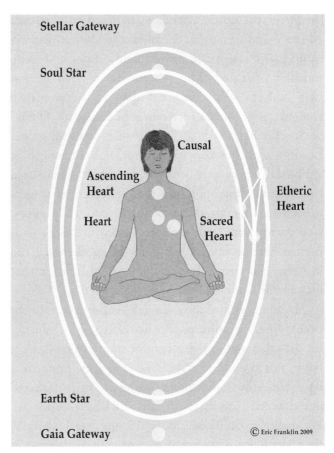

Fig. 14.5. Both spiritual healers and Reiki practitioners believe that healing energy is channeled from a higher source, as a form of light. Some healers believe they can access the light directly, while others believe it comes through mediation by evolved beings such as Christ, or named or unnamed guides, or angels, often named, or through the good offices of discarnate spiritual teachers, known or unknown. As the experiences are impossible to illustrate, the attempts to picture it for others are fanciful and often sentimental, expressing the psychology of the "artists" rather than any facts we could consider scientifically reliable. Our own attempt to illustrate what is believed, and to map its relationship to ordinary consciousness, looks forward to matters to be discussed in chapter 15. Meanwhile, the terms used are to be understood in very general senses.

Fig. 14.6. The "New Age Body" presents a schema of the subtle body extended into realms beyond the standard healing model of seven chakras. These are referred to by some Reiki schools as "transpersonal" and include the "soul star" (above the head) and the "Gaia gateway" (below the feet), both of which appeared in the Indian system centuries ago. Some of the additional Reiki chakras may be rediscoveries of ancient knowledge. The claim that "Reiki permeates the universe and the entire reality" may be an allusion to samādhi or nirvāna, concepts that are held in common by healers and meditators, as studies have shown; or it may even be the experience of the quantum interconnectedness of the physical universe, a matter that needs further research and will be discussed in chapter 15.

the second century CE practiced something similar to the spiritualist séance, though entities whom modern spiritualists consider to be discarnate *human* entities, formerly living humans, were perceived by the Neo-Platonists to be gods and daemons.[37]

Brennan, too, acknowledges that guidance plays a part in her work. She describes how, as her life unfolded, the "unseen hand" that led her became more and more perceptible. At first, she sensed it only vaguely. Then

she began to see spiritual beings, as if in a vision. Later she began to hear them talking to her and to feel them touch her. She now accepts that she has a guide. "I can see, feel and hear him."[38]

Barbara Brennan and some others have, as well as a paranormal awareness of other beings, the advantage of understanding spiritual healing through the so-called "New Physics." In the nineteenth century, models of energetic healing conformed with the then-accepted theory of the ether, a medium believed to permeate all space and to be that in which the ubiquitous electromagnetic transverse waves (such as light and radio waves) propagated. The concept of an ether *of that kind* had to be abandoned following the empirical demonstration of the correctness of Einstein's Theory of Special Relativity of 1905, which showed, astonishingly, that the velocity of light, not the length of a physical object, is a constant, the object's measured length depending upon how the instrument that measures it is moving relative to that object. This theory, well corroborated and accepted, need not occupy us further here, as our interest is in the subtle body, and in particular in the further understanding of it that may accrue from study of healing.

During much of the twentieth century and into the twenty-first, quantum physics has offered a "substitute" for the ether, not as a medium for transmission of light waves, nor as a means of sending "messages" faster than light, but rather as a kind of "static" or "instantaneous" interconnectedness that is, in itself, still largely mysterious. We shall give details in chapter 15, and briefly describe the scientific evidence before discussing the consequences for the concept of a subtle body, indeed, a whole "level" of subtle being. Here, we can return to Albanese's opinion, not of science per se, but her view that observation does seem to provide a measure of confirmation of metaphysical experience. What is especially important about the aura, she says, in the context of what she calls "metaphysical practical narration," is that it can be manipulated, and so healed.[39] We believe this is true, but find Albanese's acknowledgement of it a little too grudging.

Albanese sees that although Brennan was an aeronautics and space administration physicist, a profession deeply grounded in modern science and technology, her spiritual healing work is grounded in a nineteenth century Theosophical model of subtle bodies. Adding

that "metaphysicians are manifestly sensitive to movement and change," Albanese claims that it is for that reason, that Brennan, Hunt (Dr. Valerie Hunt, scientist and investigator of human energy fields), and others "glide easily from the physical into the psychological mode where science becomes an ally," finding order in the world by "bringing subtle-energy science into spirit and by nudging body into mind," so "neutralizing wild terrain, changing its geography and making the spirit a safe country in which to travel."[40] This language seems a little more vague than anyone based in science would approve, and present efforts to bring physics and psychology together are worthy of higher praise than Albanese gives. It is a little surprising to find her, a professor of religion, more skeptical with regard to support from science for matters such as consciousness and intentionality in healing, and therefore of subtle levels of being, than an increasing number of respected scientists and philosophers of science.

Here, we cite just two: Wolfgang Pauli, one of the founders of quantum physics, who said, "We should now proceed to find a neutral, or unitarian, language *in which every concept we use is applicable as well to the unconscious as to matter* [my emphasis], in order to overcome this wrong view that the unconscious psyche and matter are two things,"[41] an endeavor of which both Herbert Dingle and Carl Jung approve; and Karl Popper, who, despite the disparagement of the notion by its own originator, Gilbert Ryle, openly acknowledged that "I believe in the Ghost in the Machine."[42] A revolution in science that brought the loss of the ether, a purely physical postulate, never observed and so never proved existent, made way for the greatest imaginable gain, support from physics itself for the existence of the subtle body, an entity having, no matter how Ryle might have reacted against the claim, at least some affinity with that Ghost. Our next chapter will explain.

FIFTEEN

Science, Philosophy, and the Subtle Body

Sooner or later nuclear physics and the psychology of the unconscious will draw closely together as both of them independently of one another and from opposite directions, push forward into transcendental territory. . . . Psyche cannot be totally different from matter for how otherwise could it move matter? And matter cannot be alien to psyche, for how else could matter produce psyche? Psyche and matter exist in the same world, and each partakes of the other, otherwise any reciprocal action would be impossible. If research could only advance far enough, therefore, we should arrive at an ultimate agreement between physical and psychological concepts. Our present attempts may be bold, but I believe they are on the right lines.

C. G. JUNG, "PSYCHOLOGICAL TYPES" IN VOL. 6, *COLLECTED WORKS*

This passage from Jung raises many questions* that cannot be asked, let alone answered, until a very broad and safe groundwork has been laid. Then they must be approached with both daring and caution if anything of worth is to be achieved. The unification Jung seeks seems a worthy objective, for true knowledge must surely constitute a single and harmonious whole, embracing all subjects. Physicists, along with the less conservative among religious thinkers, have been to the fore in the search for such a synthesis, but the task can never be completed until certain linguistic difficulties produced by humankind's division of knowledge into subjects, each with its own specific language, have been resolved. We make no apology, therefore, for dealing first with these. It is the alternative course of ignoring such problems and plunging directly into complex matters without regard for their semantic foundations that would require apology to the reader.

Linguistic barriers to mutual understanding are among the most obstinate of all difficulties, yet, curiously, words are, in themselves, utterly irrelevant. The problem is simply this: experts from different fields use

---

*Here is a clue to questions that could be asked of Jung: the philosopher Alfred Ayer argued that "It is no more surprising that there should be causal connections between mental and physical phenomena than that there should be such connections between purely physical phenomena."[1] We must inquire *in what sense* mind might have a physical basis, and might consider Ayer's statement alongside Voltaire's assertion that being born twice is no more surprising than being born once.

words in different ways, and therefore fail to communicate with each other. Since we are concerned with realities, not with the words by which we refer to them, it is clear that refusal to translate from one expert's language into another's before drawing conclusions about the realities themselves leaves the linguistic barrier in place and so vitiates the whole project. The problem has another aspect, for a spurious synthesis can always be, and often is, claimed by commentators whose use of words is so imprecise that it conceals crucial differences of intended meaning between those whose words they quote in support of their own contentions. In effect, they are then *mis*quoting and misusing their sources. Allowing the meanings of words to slip and slide by refusing to agree upon consistent usages at the earliest opportunity allows delusive parallels to be claimed upon merely verbal evidence, and utterly foundationless unifications between systems of ideas to be asserted on those delusive verbal grounds. Writers guilty of this negligence have nothing to offer us but the perpetuation of old uncertainties and old misunderstandings. We hope to remain innocent of such sins by taking a totally different path. New knowledge has always entered a preexisting broader culture that it modified, bringing its own consequences and raising new questions. These questions led back to the antecedent understanding, which was reexamined in that new and broader context, and by a kind of spiral progress the body of human knowledge, and the modes and metaphors by which it was understood and interpreted, perpetually changed and grew.

When understanding is unclear language becomes unclear and, once language has become unclear, the inaccurate linguistic usages themselves prevent accurate understanding by hearer or reader. Often a vicious downward spiral into total incomprehensibility is created. That ancient writers have, in just this way, left us a legacy of unclear references has been shown many times in this book. Here, we add that, despite the claims of some who should know better, understanding *always* precedes language, *never* the reverse. If it were not so we could never question the correctness of a linguistic statement for it would be interpreted in the best available way and so be automatically (if mistakenly) accepted as correct, if also as clumsy. It is only our preexisting understanding or an understanding instantly perceived in the moment of hearing or reading that enables us to recognize that the

form of words that has been presented to us cannot carry the intended meaning. If understanding did not precede and supervene over verbal forms at all stages we could never, having once learned a language, be in doubt as to the meaning of a verbal utterance, nor, again, would we ever struggle to find the right words, nor, finally, would we be able to say anything effectively, least of all express fine nuances of meaning. We are always aware of the discrepancy between meanings and the words we assemble to express them—or, if not, we are beings of remarkably crude sensibility. If meaning did not supervene in consciousness over the words used to convey that meaning we could also never *know* that our utterances were inaccurate, for if that were so no one would be comparing knowledge with description and finding the description wanting. But we are frequently conscious of this process occurring, which confirms the primacy of meaning. The notion that language precedes understanding we believe to be nonsense of the worst order, and that language precedes consciousness frankly stupid, though we do not deny that language is a means to the *enhancement* of an existing consciousness, nor deny that consciousness, once present, immediately perceives meanings and so immediately seeks to conceptualize those meanings using a preverbal language *sense*. How can those who hold the view that language precedes consciousness and meaning explain the frequent difficulty of expressing ourselves with the sharpness with which we hold the thought we wish to express? If thought *were itself words* we could never *have* such difficulty, let alone *know that* we were having the difficulty. There are times when the most articulate cast about helplessly for *le môt juste* or struggle to be understood by others, while those less accurately conscious of what they want to say are content to make and hear vague utterance. The self, in all instances of verbal difficulty, is conscious both of what it wants to express and of its difficulty in expressing it in words. If words preceded consciousness, this experience would be impossible, for words, not realities, would then themselves become realities *constitutive of* the perceived world of which we are conscious, whereas we are all well aware of the mismatch between the world's realities and verbal realities. The whole relationship of words to things would then radically change; unless, of course, the promulgators of the ideas we reject are simply not thinking very carefully, or are not expressing themselves very well. We repeat our promise to remain innocent of such sins.

This long chapter, given the rigor required, the breadth and complexity of its totally interwoven subject matters, and the linguistic problems, is far too brief. Nevertheless, we shall hurry very slowly, presenting ideas as they arise, exploring their contexts and following the natural, self-referring growth of our knowledge, an organic progress rather than an organized tabulation of statements. We shall, nonetheless, make many statements, some very forthright indeed, as we explain the nature of science, describe some of its methods, sound alerts for nonscientists who have to deal with it, and explain some scientific ideas relating to the subtle body that are often misunderstood and misrepresented to the reading public. We give evidence for the reality of a subtle body, and quote briefly a few authorities. Along the way we shall make detours as necessary into philosophy per se, and then resume our discussion. No more could be done in the space we have, but the bibliography suggests further reading.

We have begun, then, with Jung, and, of necessity, used existing ill-defined words, but do so fully aware that we must redefine usage in the light of discovery. Perhaps all that is clear at this point is that this chapter attempts the almost impossible multiple task of finding mutual understanding between various experts, each accustomed to his or her own "word game" and then—only then—attempts to find a veridical synthesis from their understandings, not of words, which are merely the necessary tools of communication, but of the entities to which they point by means of their words.

The Meeting of Physics and Psychology

Jung is surely right to set as an ultimate objective the correlation of psychology with physics and, of course, of physics with psychology. At least one eminent physicist contemporary with Jung agreed. In 1937 Herbert Dingle published *Through Science to Philosophy,* in which he writes the following intriguing passage.

Originally, the experiences which are the ultimate subject-matter of biology and psychology are [mostly]* indistinguishable from the experi-

---

*Dingle has a footnote making this reservation.

ences dealt with by physics. They are excluded from physics because science chooses, as a practical device, so to treat them in order to maintain the very satisfactory correlations it can then establish. If a critic were to object that this is an unfair act, that it is illegitimate to claim victory over the phenomena of motion* when, by a sort of Pride's Purge, every movement that does not obey the so-called laws is eliminated—I think he is unanswerable by one who maintains that science is discovering objective laws. For the position is not merely that the laws of motion are not applicable to the excluded phenomena; they are applicable, and when applied are found to be violated. They tell me that the movements of a given mass in given surroundings can be calculated. I put the given mass in the given surroundings, and find that if it is a dead fly the calculations are verified, and if it is a living fly they are not. It is not that in the latter case I cannot determine the mass or the other necessary circumstances; I can, and I find that the requirements of the laws are violated. Only when we recognize that the procedure of science throughout is an active endeavor to create something, and not a passive endeavor to discern something, can we make it intelligible. As a statement of some characteristic of objective nature, the laws of motion are false; as a record of success in the task of making our experience rational, they are true.[2]

Dingle reminds us again and again throughout the book that science is "the application of reason to experience," and a more succinct definition of science would be difficult to find. It is salutary, then, to find that his statements turn lay understandings of science on their heads, but in so doing they show that science is, by extending itself as Dingle suggests, free to investigate what it is that enables a living fly to disobey the "laws" that control a dead one. Science is not what the layperson thinks it is, nor even what many thinkers, experts in their own fields,

---

*Dingle here means *all* motions, including, of course, those of living organisms, and is pointing out that only the motions of nonliving physical systems obey the laws of motion as formulated by Newton (for classical physics), and later reformulated relativistically by Einstein.

believe it to be. It is not the discovery of "laws of physics," which are inherently "out there," totally independent of us and inflexibly controlling everything that happens in the world as they silently wait to be recognized, dusted off, and worshiped in words (or even in mathematical equations). Science is the human process of producing hypotheses that will, like crutches, enable us to make a halting progress toward a holistic, correlated understanding of those phenomena, and only those phenomena, of our experiential *world-about** *which our senses can observe* and, within the limits of our possibly erroneous beliefs as to what constitutes logic, to make usable correlations. The "laws" it produces are of only partial application, and the further search for a unification of science with other disciplines remains incomplete now, just as it was when Jung and Dingle first called for it seventy years ago.

We note at once that humankind must have been "doing science" as so defined for a very long time indeed, that even newborn babies do it, and that it has undergone a number of revolutions. Science as practiced every day by babies is not a matter of verbal or mathematical theorizing, but of prelinguistic *understanding, interpreting, and intending.* Accordingly, adult discovery of reality may be more a matter of *interpretative picturing* than of words. Einstein tells us that he found it so, which reminds us yet again to give our concept-percepts of reality precedence over our subsequent attempts to describe them verbally, or even by mathematics. Not all have understood the difference between the picturing of reality by rational contemplation and imagination on the one hand and, on the other, the verbal analysis of preexisting descriptive texts or the imposition of mathematics that does not fit the facts observed. Before passing on we shall allow a little space to an example.

Gilbert Ryle's book *The Concept of Mind,* first published in 1949, has been very influential, which is why we have chosen it for adverse comment. Despite claiming to analyze our very nature as living beings Ryle gives us a discussion of the subject that is not merely nonempirical and nonscientific but is grounded almost entirely in our use of language. He writes disparagingly of the dualist view

of our nature, to which he variously refers as "the Official Doctrine" and "the official theory," saying "I shall often speak of it, with deliberate abusiveness, as 'the dogma of the Ghost in the Machine.'"[3] Curiously, he does not even define the meaning of his own phrase, but the reader discerns that he is referring to the belief that each of us is a mechanical body containing a nonmaterial real self, the *res cogitans* or "thinking thing" postulated by Descartes. It is this nonmaterial and nonmechanical entity that Ryle denies, and disparagingly calls the "Ghost."

However, by the end of the paragraph concerned Ryle has made a great mistake and so derailed the whole book. Accusing Descartes of making what he calls a "category-mistake," he makes a far worse category error himself. Ryle makes the dubious claim that Descartes had grounded his view that we are dual beings in a belief that mental events will be subject to laws that differ from, but nonetheless run parallel to, the *mechanical* laws believed by Descartes and his contemporaries to hold sway over the world of physics. So Descartes (according to Ryle) misgrounded his dualistic view of mind and body in a kind of "paramechanical *non*mechanicalism." However, whether Descartes gave sufficient attention to the question whether the soul or mind or spirit *could* be (let alone actually was) under the kind of *rigid* law then believed to rule the physical world need not detain us, for it is an oxymoron to say that an *autonomous* being could be under rigid law. More importantly, as we now know, and as Ryle in 1949 ought to have known, the physical world *itself* does not display the kind of mechanical law in which Descartes believed, three and a half centuries ago, and he certainly believed himself to be an autonomous Being with freedom of choice, just as Dingle's living fly evidently did, for he thought of himself as a *res cogitans,* a *thinking thing.* A *thinking* thing clearly lays claim to the autonomy of thinking for itself. The question of paramechanical *non*mechanicalism is therefore doubly irrelevant to our quest. We are looking, rather, for that thinking thing. However, its relevance *here* is that Ryle then admits, just as Descartes also saw, that mental events *do* differ from what Ryle calls "mechanical" events. Immediately, then, Ryle ought to admit that we do have two categories of event. What he fails to realize is that this immediately restores Descartes' claim to be a thinking thing, which might indeed be a nonphysical (because nonmechanical) Ghost in the (mechanical) Machine. Thus, even if Descartes had misgrounded his

---

*The phrase "world-about" translates one often used by Martin Heidegger, the phenomenologist philosopher, to whose understandings we shall frequently refer.

dualistic view of the mind in a kind of "paramechanical *non*mechanicalism," his *conclusion* might nonetheless be correct, the true ground of any dualistic view simply being other than that which (according to Ryle) Descartes had asserted. Having missed this, Ryle goes on to perpetuate his own error by veering off into discussion of verbal usages that, as we have said, are utterly irrelevant to any inquiry as to *what we are* as Beings since that can only be a matter for empirical science. Questions regarding the soul or subtle body are questions of fact, not of the categories of our thinking processes. Thus misled by his own antireligious prejudices, Ryle makes an error of the very kind he warns his readers against, and so misses the truth of "the Ghost in the Machine." Popper and Eccles, authors of *The Self and Its Brain,* thought "the Ghost in the Machine" a *good* description of our being.

In the section headed "Afterthoughts" to chapter 7 of *The Concept of Mind,* which Ryle entitles "Sensation and Observation," he rightly finds a difference between perceptions of the body itself (including its own sense organs) *as the object of perception,* and perceptions of the world-about as *perceptions made using the body's sense organs,* yet he cannot even discern that this duality *is* the difference he has found. The thoughtful reader discerns it for himself, unspokenly present among Ryle's words. Perhaps his failure is unsurprising, for nothing is better compatible with a dualistic interpretation of our being than precisely *this* sensible distinction between precisely *these* different experiences, namely experience of our being *from "inside" it,* and our experience of the world "outside" the body (for which we have already used and shall often use the Heideggerian phrase *der Umwelt,* translated as "the world-about"), which is gained *via the physical body's external sense organs.* For the dualist, believing that a being inhabits a body that thus becomes a lived body is compatible with there being a perceptible difference between the experience of the body *itself* and the experience of *the world* obtained *via* the body. Ryle admits the difference of experience, by implication, but his antireligious and antispiritual agenda is all too discernible in his failure to make this simple analysis. Instead, he embarks, as is his habit throughout *The Concept of Mind,* on an inconclusive analysis of our uses of language.

Like a number of more recent philosophers he continually asserts that there are no grounds for what he calls the Official Doctrine of dualism, while never proving his assertion and always circumlocuting evidence of our duality whenever it confronts him. He even admits he cannot account satisfactorily for his failure to speak with precision on these aspects of his case. The final sentence of his chapter 7 shows how he can allow himself such gross and obvious error. He does it by refusing ever to enter the arena of reality, instead confining himself to words and our uses of them, for he writes: "I do not know what more is to be said about the logical grammar of such words, save that there is much more to be said." No, there is not, at least not by Ryle. How *common* usage and abusage of words, a patently *pre*scientific, *counter*scientific use of them, could tell us anything about reality is beyond imagination. Words are *fundamentally and irredeemably irrelevant* to the matters of reality we have in hand in this book. Of course, we see perfectly clearly that many people's concepts are impaired by verbal misusage, and have already expressed this belief, but maintain that Ryle himself is among them.

Ryle deserves no more attention than this, especially as we have little space, and we feel no duty to him or to other authors who maintain similar views beyond including his book in the bibliography. A bibliographical entry is not always a recommendation. His prejudices were his tragedy, for the wrong stance that mars *The Concept of Mind* obscures his insight that idealism and materialism are also dogmas arising from categorial misconceptions.[4] What Ryle fails to see is that such unifications of seeming opposites are themselves dualisms, the duality aligned differently from expectation. As we shall see, much later in this chapter, Shah Wali Allah is not alone in successfully unifying dualism with monistic views, and even "matter" and "spirit" find unity when the correct viewpoint is chosen. What remains is the question of what livingness is, but the route to our answer will, perforce, occupy many pages.

Words, Reality, and Logic*

In *Projection and Recollection in Jungian Psychology,* Marie-Louise von Franz says, "In Western cultural history

---

*Readers familiar with philosophy of the past century will see that this heading paraphrases (though not intentionally on our part) the title of Alfred Ayer's book *Language, Truth, and Logic,* and does so with sound reason. Ayer later saw and acknowledged a few errors in his book, but the greater part of it is sound, over seventy years after its first publication.

the transpsychic has been described sometimes as spirit, sometimes as matter. Theologians and philosophers are more concerned with the former, physicists with the latter."[5] But what precisely is meant by these words? What are these entities, "the transpsychic," "spirit," and "matter," *in themselves*? Scientists and philosophers prefer the simplest available explanation of any observation, in accordance with the principle known as "Occam's Razor." The scientist's view would be that our topic, the subtle body, *if there be such,* will prove to be the entity we find it necessary to postulate in order to explain all the observed facts, and perhaps a few more. Whether we shall find the words *spirit* or *matter* serviceable remains to be decided when all the observations made have been explained by a theory having explanatory power equal to that task.

So here, illustrated by von Franz's words, is one of the main categorial, semantic, and premethodological questions regarding the subtle body. We have drawn attention to the general philosophical question, and should now attend to it in its own specific detail. If the subtle body has "real" existence, of what does it consist? Is it a single, simple, entity, or has it parts? If it proves necessary to postulate that it has parts, of what do the parts consist? Given these uncertainties, what tests will disclose to us what we want to know, and with what *provisional* expectations should we frame the question of what *reality* a subtle body might be? *Qu'est-ce que c'est?* What *is* it that it is? Only when we have the answer, perhaps as a conception not yet verbalizable, can we ask what *terms* we should apply to it. If we do not yet know *that* a subtle body exists, nor *of what* it consists if it does exist, we are clearly not yet entitled to describe it, so the words *spirit* and *matter* are at best presumptive and tendentious, at worst meaningless and misleading, for they signify only this: that we might believe, on purely *logical* grounds, that *if* there is an entity that could *properly* be called a subtle body *it could not consist of what the physical body consists of.* But this trite piece of logic, necessarily, but trivially, valid, merely states a verbal truism, an analytical truth *about words,* that is merely contingent upon reality, *if even that.* It tells us *nothing at all* about the subtle body. It means only that *if* "subtle" is differentiable from "physical" then physical and subtle are, by virtue of that difference, not the same.

What philosophers warn us against is that such trivial, automatically true *verbal* structures, empty of all

truth, are, despite their emptiness, capable of producing powerful delusions, persuading us of the reality of entities for which we have invented *names,* but the *existence* and *true nature* of which (if they are real at all) could only be verified by pragmatic, empirical tests quite outside the realms of verbal analysis, linguistic theory, or, for that matter, poetry or ordinary speech. The question of the nature of the "real world" itself we must leave until later, despite the fact that it is, at bottom, this question that von Franz raises, but only implicitly and tacitly, when she writes of *spirit* and *matter.*

However, our intention is not to criticize von Franz for using words that may indeed be unsuitably defined in the word game of popular discourse and quite differently defined in the word games of different specialists, but to remind ourselves of the need to avoid certain mindsets produced by the unavoidable use of long-familiar words, and to maintain instead an openness that shall not be bewitched by words. Wittgenstein, who conceived the notion of the "word game," puts the point aphoristically at the end of paragraph 339 of his *Philosophical Investigations:* "An unsuitable type of expression is a sure means of remaining in a state of confusion." Von Franz's statement starts with an unguarded assumption that the terms *spirit* and *matter* are already correctly defined and consensually understood, but this may not be the case. Questions about realities cannot begin to be answered until consensus regarding verbal meanings has been achieved, yet (this is our next important point) these meanings cannot themselves be settled until the facts about the realities are known. This seeming circularity, as we have seen, is inherent in the ongoing process of science, whether or not it expands as Dingle and Jung suggest. Newly established facts shift the meanings of preexisting words by a kind of nonvicious "progressive circularity" or "recursive forward-rolling spiral," which we have mentioned already in another connection, and which will prove an impasse only if we are unaware of it and are careless in verbal usage. All usages are provisional, and must be revised whenever we reach a conclusion concerning a relevant reality.

The War of the Word Games

The verbal precision now seen to be necessary is far from our everyday mode of discourse, but we have to get our investigation started, so let us accept von Franz's *pre-*

sumption that there is, in her word game, a "transpsychic" that in other word games is conceived of as "spirit" or as "matter," any traditional distinctions between these terms notwithstanding. Theologians and philosophers *may,* as von Franz claims, be more disposed to speak of "spirit," physicists keener to analyze "matter," and these words *may* denote the same entity, as the first of her two sentences seems to suggest, but her second sentence seems opposed to the first, appearing to *presume* that spirit and matter are *not* the same. One wonders, therefore, whether von Franz's thinking itself is naïvely grounded in the traditional opposition, and, in view of her seeming unawareness of the conflict between her first sentence and her second, whether her thinking is precise enough to serve the purpose of finding common understanding between the parties. One also suspects that, like so many others, she does not quite grasp what Dingle is trying to tell us about what science is, and what it is not.

It is a small part of the present movement toward Dingle's aim of an integral science (though he did not use that term himself) that, a few decades after von Franz, some physicists ask whether knowledge from realms that were earlier excluded from physics is, after all, relevant to its world and, therefore, to the twenty-first century expanded edition of its word game. Wolfgang Pauli was one of the earliest of these, famously saying, "We should now proceed to find a neutral, or unitarian, language in which every concept we use is applicable as well to the unconscious as to matter, in order to overcome this wrong view that the unconscious psyche and matter are two things."[6] Von Franz was referring to the same topic in saying that "what was once regarded as the *opposition* between spirit and matter turns up again in contemporary physics as a discussion of the *relation between* consciousness (or Mind) and matter."[7]

Undogmatically correct use of words such as *spirit* and *matter* is necessary, indeed *so* necessary that, far from rushing to define them, as we might be expected to do, we shall do precisely the reverse, leaving them open until they define themselves in the light of an inquiry ranging over several areas of human discovery, which will tell us what the words *ought to* mean. *That* is a question for empirical science, expanded as Dingle, Jung, and Pauli envisage, but probably for an expanded empirical science *alone.* It is certainly not a question for

philosophers of language. They warn of the linguistic dangers, and we recognize the truth of what they say, but that is the end of their task, as many of them would agree. We are seeking realities, and hoping to conceive them as they truly are. Our next set of questions, then, is to ask what science is, how it works, what its problems are, and how those problems (including the conceptual and verbal ones pointed out by philosophers) are to be overcome.

What Is Science in Practice?

Science proceeds by asking questions and testing for answers, which are then considered. The questions must often be reframed in the light of the answers received. Competent and honest scientists are aware of this inherent tentativeness and uncertainty, for it is the raison d'être of their craft. We are trying to find out what we do not know. But, as Heidegger convincingly maintains, our very perceptions of the world are inevitably colored by our mode of being in it and by the understanding of the world-about that a Being* here in the world has. This limits even what we can imagine, and therefore limits our formulation of hypotheses. We do not so much see objects "preexisting" in the world but rather see in the world-about only those things *that have referential relations to us (and so also to each other).* The world as we see it is what our *way of* seeing permits or causes us to see. If things existing out there in the world had no relation to us at all, and were of no interest to us, if they could not be seen by us *as* this, or *as* that, we would not see them as "things" at all. "Thingness" comes into being in, and as a part of, our consciousness of the world-about. This way of being constitutes an intentional stance, a *being-toward* the world, which "finds" *things-which-relate-to-us* and so constructs its world. Of course, we cannot, here, study Heidegger in detail, but his view is highly relevant to questions about the nature of our being in the physical world, and we shall often refer to it.

Popper's name is rarely heard in conjunction with Heidegger's, yet he expresses an entirely similar understanding in *The Self and Its Brain,* where he tells us that every observation and experiment we perform is

---

*Translators use initial capitals for Heidegger's "Dasein," "Being-in-the-world," and related phrases. He writes of "the being of Beings," confirming the necessity for these capitals in English.

impregnated with theory and interpreted in accordance with some theory, for we observe only what catches our attention on account of its relevance to our problems, or biological situation, our expectations, or our plans for action. It is not only our observational instruments that are based on theories we hold (we shall say more about this), for our very sense organs, without which we can observe nothing at all, provide us with hypotheses.

Popper goes so far as to say, emphasizing his point by using italics, that all our sense organs have anticipatory theory genetically incorporated. He explains what he means by reference to the frog's eye-brain system, which does not even notice a fly within its field of view unless the fly moves. When a movement occurs, the frog's musculature instantly extends its tongue to catch the prey, even in flight. Popper says that our sense organs have been produced by adaptation, in effect incorporating theories. For the frog, a main theory of life is: "If it moves across my field of view it is a tasty fly." Theories, Popper says, are prior to observation, and therefore cannot be *merely* the result of repeated observation. In life and in science we *first* have a hypothesis, an expectation, a tentative view, and *then* we presume its truth and act accordingly, or, if we are sufficiently thoughtful and concerned (which traits almost define the scientist), we do not take the hypothesis for true until we have *tested* it by repeated observation and analysis of the results.[8]

Heidegger agrees, describing a similar *unified* process, which has the identifiable features of, first, a *sensing,* then an *understanding* of a world *in which Being is already present, having been "thrown" there* (a conception to which we shall return), and finally an act of *interpretation,* and, he says, these are already operating in the most inattentive and naïve interaction with the world. The interpretation, both philosophers agree, may be very seriously erroneous, but it *is* nonetheless a proto-scientific hypothesis, for it is out of the same kind of interpretative thinking, however much matured, that our formal science springs. Thus, even a baby, learning by experience what its world-about contains, has to start with a hypothesis of some kind, albeit unformed, intuitive, unverbalized, even subconscious. No sense can be made of the world without this *already actively hypothesizing* kind of awareness. The baby does *not* need words to react in this way to the world-about, but we, being adult language-users, might attempt to verbalize one

example of a baby's hypothesizing as: "If I make a grab in the direction of that fuzzy orange patch I shall find I am pulling Teddy into my mouth," and we experienced adults never ask, indeed *cannot meaningfully* ask, any question without some conception of how the object of our inquiry works, or what it is to be seen *as,* or what we could *use* it for.

To ask any question that has no such referential relations would be to utter obvious nonsense. Indeed, our world, of which our Being-in-the-world is already an inseparable "part," *consists of* these referential, sensible, meaningful relations, and if our everyday maxim were *not* something resembling "When *in* the world one must *live as* a being in the world," our behavior would be seen by those around as rather odd. This being the context, the reality of our world-about, we feel it would be ridiculous to ask, "Would it hurt these chairs if we were to repaint them?" While such events might form the basis of fantasies such as Ravel's opera *L'Enfant et les Sortilèges,* and, while we knowingly manufacture automatons to amuse or disturb the mind, to ask the question in seriousness would be to bring into doubt the deeply embedded axiom that there is a distinction between *Beings* and *nonbeings.* We are Beings, and the chairs are not. The chairs *have* a mode of being, of course, but our point is that a chair's mode of being is very seriously different from *our* way of being. It is precisely this grounding presumption, this axiom-for-living, indeed this axiom-for-*the*-living (not for chairs), that can, when it stirs our consciousness, provide amusement or derision according to context. However, it is important to realize that it *is* an assumption, and our main task is to bring it out of its everyday obscurity and examine it, for it contains an obvious secret usually overlooked, and willfully obscured by many present-day philosophers.

We also tend to take our own intentionality as a given, and do not see chairs or any of that class of entity we call "things" as Beings that have *their own* intentionality, let alone as having intentions like ours. The presence of intentionality seems a valid item of evidence in justifying the distinction we make between Beings and things. This is very obvious, but worthy of being called to our attention, for we persistently let it fall into the obscurity of *presumption.* We are scarcely aware that we, being Beings, *use* our intentionality, and we envisage chairs as things—not as Beings—for sitting in, and we make them for this purpose. This is obvious, yet not quite as trite as it seems, for it leads us to inquire into that obvious secret. Why are we so *sure* that the idea of a chair feeling pain if we paint it is ridiculous? The answer is surely that we *see* (and thereafter presume) the differentiation, the duality, between Beings and things, a difference that is less stressed by most philosophers than one might expect it to be.

Why is this question not seen, even by philosophers such as Heidegger, as needing to be explored, and needing such alertness, not least for the very reason that the answer *is* almost always presumed, and then forgotten, along with its consequences. We do not *maintain* awareness of it, and so are duped by philosophy that denies the difference between beinghood and thinghood. But does not the apparent *truth* of that presumption that Beings and things are different in their very essence prompt the question of the reality of the subtle body and the further question of *what* the subtle body *is*? But we take it for granted that the body is matter, the same matter as the chair, so why, or how, are Beings different from things? We shall return to this question, but by a spiraling route, for our discussion must first lead us elsewhere.

The Problem of Bias

As soon as we examine our practical approach to discovery, we realize that no observer is unbiased, for all experiment is necessarily grounded in *pre*conception, in a bias toward one view rather than another. Here, then, is the first problem of science, and it is built into the very nature of our being. We prejudge, and we are sometimes wrong. The very act of framing a testable hypothesis produces a situation of tentative or incipient prejudice that limits the frame of reference of the experiment even as it also calls into question the very preconception on which the experiment is based. We may have to redesign the experiment.

But this is not all. We should also ponder the less obvious fact that to be biased is to live in the past, something that comes to us all too naturally, for it is our very way of being. Our consciousness of "self" is largely consciousness of the past of the self, though alongside this is a looking-forward into the future.* Working under the

influence of the unavoidable bias of past ideas is difficult, necessitating the progressive circularity, described earlier, of hypothesis, experiment, refutation, reexperiment, and new hypothesis. If bias is unacknowledged it may go beyond the innocent and unavoidable level and become willful, as in the case of entrenched opposition to newly published work, of which Copernicus's heliocentric theory and Einstein's two theories of relativity provide famous examples. Such bias exerts a malign influence over related experimental design, and can be dishonestly used to exclude automatically what the proponent of an alternative hypothesis is claiming. Results supporting the opponent's view can be precluded by the dishonest foresight of ensuring that the experiment excludes any measurement or analysis of results that would confirm the unwelcome interpretation.*

The results of such biased experimental design, selective observation, and skewed interpretation are often paraded as scientific disproof of an opposing view when they are nothing of the kind, but only an unscientific expression of the prejudices of scientists and, sometimes, of philosophers. What starts as unsuspected bias, whether due to our fundamental way of being or to ill-considered opinion, can harden into prejudice and breed deliberate and knowing dishonesty. So the unwary scientist faces an insidious danger within himself: "Seek, and you shall find" *whatever you are looking for,* but unless you are careful it will be at the cost of blindness to all else, *which may include the truth.* Science history is full of such delusions.

The Scientist's Own Mind as a Problem for Science

We must, and can, guard against being misled by bias, but other problems are less tractable. This is particularly true of the scientific study of ourselves, and therefore of the study of the postulated entity "the subtle body," for that subtle body, if in any sense a real entity, must be part of what we each experience or think of as "myself," no matter what the reality of that "self" may ultimately

---

*Heidegger has much to say on these matters in *Being and Time*. Division Two of the book, beginning with numbered section 45, is particularly relevant, and his treatment is so full that no short reference can be given here.

*Rupert Sheldrake gives an example of tendentious bias in *Dogs That Know When Their Owners Are Coming Home* (London: Arrow, 2000). For context it will be best to read the whole of his second chapter, beginning on page 16. On page 46 he gives details of a series of observations and adds a note (note 22) on page 274.

prove to be. The problem for the science of "subjective," that is *personal,* experience, our experience *as Experiencers,* is inherent, the problem of an irremovable, not merely an attitudinal, bias, and must be handled with even greater care than the forms of bias with which we have already dealt. We are not researching ourselves as an "extraterrestrial" being would do, nor, indeed, as a cat would. The questions we shall ask ourselves in this chapter are determined by what we are, and a person studying her or his *own* being cannot avoid influencing both the data and the interpretation of it. We are trying to interpret *ourselves,* so the data is as changeable as we are, and we who observe are altered by the data even as we gather it, and as we gather it we cause it to change yet further.

Furthermore, we cannot find ourselves in the data, but only the data in ourselves, nor can we find ourselves in the brain being studied, even if it is our own brain. Observing and recording data from our own brain does not produce or duplicate "us." If we look at our brain we cannot thereby shake hands with our double. We are conspicuous by our absolute absence from both the brain before us and the data recorded from it. A sense of *personal being* simply does not fit those *merely physical* entities. A certain kind of dualism is therefore unavoidable, even if "selfness" has somehow emerged from neural complexity (which in any case many, including ourselves, deny). There seem, here, to be at least two stages or levels at which selfhood is lost to view, put at a distance from the observer (even the observer of him- or herself), and also at least two stages where we might make mistakes of observation and interpretation, perhaps even a circular and infinite vicious regress, error-prone at every step, not the single step of conscious observing-cum-interpreting apparent in our observations of the world-about. Here, we have to examine not just the brain (or mind) but the brain (or mind) as its own user of brain (or mind). We allow ourselves to write such a sentence because it is important that we grasp how fundamental this complexity of self-involvement is. We want to discover, reliably, the relationship between what we term *mind* and *brain,* and between *mind* and *body.* Should they be distinguished? While we would all affirm that we (whatever "we" are) do *sense* our own personhood, whether we use that word or the word *self* or any other word to denote that which we sense, it is difficult to see

how what we would feel to be *evidence of* our own *personhood* (which is not mere existence) could arise solely out of the brain, a physical entity, even if the brain were all there is, with no subtle entity associated with it. Should we not see the evidence we have as evidence of our *not* being *merely* what observations and records find? What, then, is the value of this feeling, this *personal* feeling, that we are *persons,* not brain-systems? Neuroscience does not show us persons, but only electrical impulses in, and the structure of, a soft, moist, mass of jellylike animal tissue. The *person* who interprets the data about the brain feels himself "outside" the brain being studied, even when the electroencephalograph is attached to his own head. We can't ask encephalograms questions about the *person* whose mappings they are, and even an infinitely large pile of encephalograms does not amount to a person, and fails even to hear our questions, let alone speak any replies. Personhood is *experience* of something as "myself," *my* personness, *my* distinct unity, *my* autonomy, indeed, *my* privacy. Nothing resulting from observation of brains has ever been that. Our very sense of "I-ness" is therefore evidence of a subtle, nonmaterial mode of being, but tells us nothing yet of its nature or origin.

There have been attempts by physicalist philosophers to solve the problem by resort to ad hoc postulates that raise more questions than they answer. We shall deal with some of them shortly. There can be no salvation for neurophysiological explanations of consciousness, let alone of the sense of personhood, in focusing narrowly upon the brain, for brains are undeniably physical, both as objects and as functioning systems, while personhood is a category of being, which, no matter what it will prove to *be,* is an entity lying entirely outside the physical. It is a category error to confuse them. Look for electrical impulses in the brain and electrical impulses is what you will find; indeed, it is all you will find, but where is the conscious person? You did not look for a person, and that is why you did not find a person, nor even some deficient, if also conscious, automaton. If dogma decrees that you must find him or her in, and only in, the brain, the problem will be how to ask the brain to disclose him or her. What you are seeking, a personal self, does not experience itself as a brain, or as being *in* a brain, and cannot be asked to step out from the brain and show itself. All it could do (*via* the brain and the connected motor nerves and muscles) is make the body jump up and down and shout "I'm *here, in here!*" Alternatively, of course, you might deny that there is any self to be found, that it is a chimera, unreal, a puff of self-deluding imagination, but this is not what we feel, and feeling, as we shall see, is a more important witness than the physicalist sciences can either discover or admit. And it is also not-of-the-physical-world, a fact of some importance.

At the *level* of selfness, within the *category* of selfness, it is the *experiences* of selfness that must be accepted as veridical. Posing physiological questions via physiological experiments is undoubtedly useful for other purposes, but it prejudges or precludes what it is our task *not* to prejudge or preclude, but to *discover*. Physiological descriptions of the brain are merely *correlative to* selfhood, personness, the experience of "I," and yield, at best, partial descriptions, for the question is wrongly put, excluding a priori the most important fact of all, that personhood is something *felt,* something *experienced,* and is *itself* an entity we have emotions about. The self has feelings about itself. As Heidegger puts it, we are Beings for whom our being is an issue.[9] It matters to us.

The residual question seems to be whether the sense of self derives from the brain per se, or is present with but essentially independent of it. We venture to suggest that neuroscience, by its very structure, is incapable of devising any experiment that could answer this question, for it has excluded any *personal* answer a priori, both by its methods and because the very quest shows the category error just pointed out. Selfness is a totally different kind, or level, of "thing" from brain, *even if it arises naturally and totally from brain.* Neuroscience tells us a great deal about the brain, but nothing about the Being. In Heideggerian terms, we are *not* the ground of our own Being, but our Being *is* the being of this ground. We are one with a way of being that is bigger than ourselves. In the yogic traditions this is expressed as "Tat twam asi." In Pauline terms, "our citizenship is in heaven" (Philippians 3.20), not here on earth. We trust this chapter will, before it ends, provide an understanding of our being that unifies the insights of our prescientific past and those of a science that is itself expanding as the future unfolds.

The problem might be described as one of a puzzling convolvement of entities of different categories, or levels, of reality. Earlier, we mentioned a possible source of light upon the problem. The sense we each have of being a "self" or "person" or "mind" seems to include an element of will or intention, of ability to "cause things." Even Dingle's fly seems to *show* intention, rather than subservience to prescriptive "laws of motion," even if it has not sufficient consciousness to *experience* its intentionality as such. It seems to be able to cause itself to go toward food, for instance. As Dingle says, the dead fly is another matter, its movements predictable by physics, so we can surely say at least this: that the empirically observed livingness and deadness of bodies demonstrate in some quite serious way different states of being and might be expected to correlate closely with any subtle body that exists. In what does the difference consist? Biology has given us no incisive answer, for while personhood seems immediately absent, the physical body *itself* does not immediately and suddenly show a difference after an organism is observed to have died. It does so only gradually. Surgeons even impose "standstill," surely in some real aspects and in physicalist terms a temporary death, upon patients while operating on their brains, and resuscitation succeeds when the operation is over. So what change is it that occurs in the empirical observable we call "dying"? The physical does not give an answer, so the true answer may have nothing to do with physical biology, but the answer would surely give real meaning to the phrase "subtle body" and even begin to enable us to say what it is that the subtle body *is,* whether "imaginary" or "real," material or not, emergent from physical complexity or independently substantive.

It is important to recognize that if, in researching the brain and consciousness, we allow the word *mind* to slip in to replace the word *brain* (or vice versa), as we did some pages back (though we drew attention to the fact by an unusual sentence construction), we make an unwarranted assumption, and may obscure the very truth we seek, by unwittingly making *either* the *presumption* that there is a distinguishable subtle body *or* the *presumption* that there is not. The terms *mind* and *brain* may not be interchangeable in even the smallest degree, and we allow avoidable bias if we let ourselves think that they are. Our intuitive sense, our experience of ourselves, which caused us to invent the two words, was that neither of them is sufficient to define our way of being on its own. We intuitively believe that brain and mind are not one thing, yet ignorance of their true distinction forces us to use the words interchangeably. The problem is to find a way to test and analyze this belief.

Taking Stock and Looking Around
The Problems, the Tools for Solving Them, and a New Departure

Recent consciousness has become intrigued by a concept, hinted at a page or two back, that has been dubbed the *strange loop,* a topological oddity, as it seems to our Western-logical consciousness, which is, nonetheless, claimed to be ubiquitous in our world. The oddity lies in this, that, crudely speaking, when a strange loop is present things apparently *cause each other.* Perhaps we should state this differently: *when* things *cause each other* we name the structure of the resulting causal system a "strange loop" because, for our Western linear-logical way of thinking, such an entity is unexpected. Many, confronted with this notion, ask whether causation can ever be mutual, quoting the ancient dogma *post hoc ergo propter hoc* (since it happens after something else it must be caused by that thing). Differently again, the view might be stated as "There are causes in the world that seem themselves to be caused by the entities they cause."

The important questions in testing the hypothesis of the strange loop are indeed whether the alleged entities are in any sense real, and, if so, whether they are in any sense causal-in-the-real-world, and, if that too, what they signify. What is their true role in the elucidation of our being? Facts in the world cause ideas in the minds that are in the world, and these minds then cause many of the facts in the world, which then cause ideas in the minds . . . and so on. Perhaps, if "mere ideas" are causative entities, it is our accepted logic that is not beyond criticism, for more substantial than the inadequacies of language is the realization among quantum physicists that causation in the world seems, now, to work in a mutual way or even to be a fiction. That is very odd indeed for the scientific consciousness that produced classical physics, for linear causation was for several centuries the central dogma of Western science and all its undeniable successes were triumphs of linear logic applied to observations. Now linear causation is being questioned. Does this situation ratify the notion of the strange loop via

a kind of *convolved* or mutual causation? This notion, alien to the classical physics of Western awareness, might not seem so to holistic thinkers from further East, and from further back in history, just as it might seem justified within the new quantum physics disclosed to the Western mind from the last years of the nineteenth century onward. The rest of this book provides a survey of the Eastern and earlier Western sources as they have contributed to human apprehension of the notion of a subtle body. In the present chapter we are attempting to place those beliefs into the same word game as Western science, and vice versa, by modifying, legitimately, of course, whatever we need in order to achieve a unification. This unification, if we can make it, is what we shall regard as true. We have Dingle's authority, Pauli's request, and Jung's consent to do this. Is the strange loop a legitimate part of this new science, or a delusion as great as its nonlogicality suggests?

A point to note here is that something long sensed by humans can, on coming before a more focused mode of awareness, be *seen-as* in a new way, and so be interpreted in a new way, with unexpected consequences. The strange loop might be such an entity, its oddity not in the strange loop itself but in our having failed, in the West, to perceive and understand "convolved causation" long ago. Let us try to understand it now. If A cannot happen unless B, which depends upon C, which only occurs when D, nothing seems strange and we think we have reason to ascribe a clear line of causation from D to A. If, by contrast, A depends upon B, which only happens if C, which depends upon D, which cannot happen unless B, we have a strange loop and may need to reassess the very grounds of physics, or logic, or even mathematics. The "system" has referred back to itself in a manner that causality cannot explain, circularizing at least a part of the purported causal process. This produces disquiet in the rational mind.

The perceived problem is especially severe if A, B, C, and D are not at the same level of reality, or, to put the matter in other words, do not have the same *type* of thingness, for strange loops are claimed to intercross between entities conceived to exist at different levels, imagined or real, such as *mental* events and *physical* events. While twentieth-century science largely, if not entirely, rejected the belief, we all act as if we believe that mental events have a *downward* causative effect upon material events, the belief epitomized in the popular concept of "the power of mind over matter." This causality, as we customarily see it, runs in the opposite direction to the *upward* causation acknowledged by classical physics. Strange loops, if they are real entities, result from such complexities of causal process. Let us hold this understanding in mind while we approach the whole matter from another direction.

In chapter 1 of *The Concept of Mind* Ryle admits that there are both what he calls mechanical causes of corporeal movements and mental causes of such movements, yet claims "it makes no sense to conjoin or disjoin the two." However, reality conjoins them. Our concept of mind should be grounded in our observation of the world, not in our grammatical habits, which are themselves contingent upon and in large measure the result of those observations—and may, indeed, be mapped *inaccurately* from observation. Why tolerate two stages of potential inaccuracy when one can be avoided? If the concepts of mental causation and mechanical causation are themselves valid, as Ryle himself acknowledges by the very fact that he uses them, their conjunction is simply their presence alongside each other here in the world of our being and experience, and that conjunction in reality is a fact to which we are entitled to tailor our language, whereas the converse is not the case. Heidegger and Popper, of at least equal standing with Ryle, agree that meaning precedes language, and, clearly, maps the reality with which language deals. So, since our language should follow reality, not the other way round, why should we not also conjoin these concepts in our thinking and speaking? Why should we not accept a schema *describing* reality, which *does* conjoin what reality itself does not hesitate to conjoin, then, if this presents us with *strange* (for example, top-down) causations, *accept* them and seek a schema *explaining* the multilevel reality in which those causations seem no longer strange but part of the wholeness of truth?

Do we have a world in which we cannot even "make sense" of conjunctions of mental and mechanical causations, as Ryle claims, or one that contains, as an essential and efficacious feature, precisely such *complex* "causations"? It is not difficult to prove Ryle wrong and to demonstrate our point, for if I swing my knee while the doctor taps it with his hammer, two kinds of movement occur simultaneously: the swinging willed by me, my

mind, and the sudden jerk brought about by the doctor via nerves within my body that I cannot mindfully control. We have no problem in considering both movements perfectly well explained, the one a result of mental (downward) causation mediated via the nervous system, the other merely "mechanical" (to use Ryle's word). We can even think of both lines of causation at once, indeed at both causal levels at once, and legitimately explain the events using one level, the other, or both, as the facts show to be appropriate. Further, the doctor could, with nothing more than my acquiescence, set my leg swinging himself, and I can tap my own knee, while swinging my leg or not, and in either case obtain the reflex action. So what reality conjoins let not Ryle put asunder.

A further illustration might be given by the simple question: Did my car descend the hill because the handbrake failed while I was not there to react to its failure, or because I choicefully drove down the hill? In both examples, causation can start with the mind or within the ordinary processes of unimpeded physics. The cosmic importance of this simple statement will appear later in this chapter.

Can Ryle defend himself? His sentence reads, "But I am saying that the phrase 'there occur mental processes' does not mean the same sort of thing as 'there occur physical processes' and, *therefore* [my italics], that it makes no sense to conjoin or disjoin the two."[10] But Ryle's *conclusion* is wrong, as we have just shown. Reality clearly contains both events caused without the intervention of our minds and events initiated by our minds, and this is true whatever mind *itself* actually *is*. The only fact that seems to support Ryle is the mere tautology, circularity, and truism, an example of the *empty necessity of verbal logic* that we condemned some pages back, that mental processes, being different from mechanical processes, are not the same as each other. Is this marvelous truth what philosophy in 1949 was for? So much for the first part of his sentence. The second part, that it "makes no sense to conjoin or disjoin the two" is, frankly, nonsense, as our examples and innumerable others show. Reality conjoins within itself what Ryle claims it is nonsense to conjoin in our thinking and speaking. Our intellectual duty in this dispute is to give judgment for reality, not for Ryle, and to ensure that linguistic usage follows reality, not the other way round.

What Ryle predicates upon the conceived dissimilarity

of two entities does *not* prevent either or both those entities from causing events in the physical world. In fact, what Ryle himself admits to be true is clear prima facie evidence for a certain kind of dualism, a duality of levels of cause, living and choiceful causation descending from what, for that very reason, we conceive to be the "higher" place, and physical and predictable causation compelled by the "lower" realm of physical laws, as acknowledged by Dingle and all physicists. This duality, ever-present in our experience, is highly relevant to our search for the subtle body, but it is precisely what Ryle's book, taken as a whole, seeks to deny. However, he cannot support his view since all the evidence points the other way, while he *looks* the other way, *choosing* an opposite perspective to avoid that evidence. He admits the difference, even claims the difference is one of conceptual category (though others would consider it a difference of *causal level*), yet he circumnavigates the obvious explanation that there are indeed two *real* categories, two *kinds,* or, at the very least, two *levels* or two *degrees of complexity* of causation in the situation. He sees a real duality staring him in the face, and denies its facticity by resort to a criticism of *verbal style.* This must seem astonishing, so we need to prove our point, and ask the reader to forgive the time it will take.

One of Ryle's examples of what he would call a category error, thereby ostensively defining that term, describes a person "coming home in a sedan chair, in a flood of tears," which contains neither a solecism nor a conflation of causal categories. The reader is invited to consult Ryle's book and see for him- or herself that my repetition of the word *in* has removed even the purported category error and shown it to arise from a mere misjudgment of verbal style by the person responsible for the laughable "She came home in a flood of tears and a sedan chair," which Ryle cites as his major example of such error.[11] Yet even this *stylistically* clumsy wording is defensible as a proper usage. It uses just one occurrence of the word *in* distributed over two distinct instances of "in-ness," one instance material or physical (in the sedan chair), the other metaphorical, conceptual, mental (in tears). This is how we would all understand the sentence, merely smiling at its linguistic oddity. In logical terms, this sentence construction is simply analogous to a Boolean operator, a device of logic, which we shall shortly define ostensively by giving a real-world illus-

tration. Unsurprisingly, the examples by which Ryle attempts to persuade us of his view are all merely *solecistic verbal misusages,* which are quite irrelevant. When did the structure and use of language *precede or supervene* the expression of meaning, and when did language have the power to cancel facts? Ryle's argument fails because it is merely verbal, and he shows himself either deliberately dishonest or jaw-droppingly ignorant of a rather simple level of science. He makes a dogmatic assertion on grounds of mere linguistic usage of his prejudice regarding a scientific question he is totally unqualified to consider. His failure to distinguish between reality and verbal description is also atavistic, primitive in the pejorative sense, a throwback to an old and narrow consciousness quite unworthy of human beings of the twenty-first century. We *all* know that language maps very inadequately onto reality, and that the unskillful misuse it (and are misled by it), so how can anyone hope to prove *empirical facts about realities* when the only support for his argument is the solecistic, indeed the merely *stylistic,* inadequacies of certain *verbal usages*?

It is remarkable that Ryle, in the middle of the twentieth century, seems to have been so unaware of the mathematics and the logic of a century earlier, already in his day long since in use, and even applied in the material world, in the simple electronics of the 1940s. Some two-gang electric switches are material-world Boolean operators. While two ordinary electric switches may be mounted in one fixture, and still be worked independently because each has its own toggle, there is a very common kind of double switch, the single toggle of which works two switches that are electrically separate but are simply mounted side by side so that the two quite distinct circuits are switched on or off simultaneously. Many rotary switches are of this type. Any single switch operating two or more circuits in parallel is a Boolean operator. Another example is the combined electric switch and water tap, mounted on one shaft so that they are always both on or both off. If the water flows, it is heated; when the flow is stopped the heating also stops. Computers contain vast numbers of Boolean operators, but these, of course, are invisible to us, known only to expert technicians. In the stylistically poor, but not ungrammatical, sentence cited earlier, the word *in* is applied in just this way to two different facts at once and, in logical terms, is therefore a Boolean operator.

The lady returns home in a sedan chair and in tears. So what point is Ryle making? If we give the whole passage more scrutiny than it rewards we discover two things: that Ryle has assumed what he claims he will prove, namely that it is an error to envisage a Ghost in the Machine; and that everything he has to say about the matter is in fact irrelevant to what can only be a scientific, not a linguistic or even a philosophical, question. The question of how we should use the word *in* with reference to sedan chairs and emotional states concerns science and philosophy only insofar as both endeavors should seek clarity of expression.

The important conclusion is that incommensurables can and do have causal relations in the real world, acting both upward and downward. This is inexplicable for physicalists, who, to escape the difficulty, have resorted (with what success we shall soon discover) to the invention of the concept of the strange loop. So we shall set Ryle aside, but examine this new purported entity closely. Despite the crassness and dishonesty of Ryle's thinking, he has been influential, and his legacy is inhibition in thinking for physicists who have been conditioned to pay certain philosophers the respect their bombast demands rather than the respect they are worth. More recent books than Ryle's show the same philosophical arrogance and tendency to dogmatize without *relevant* evidence. Both the strange loop, if "real," and Boolean logic, which acknowledges that a single cause can bring about changes in two objects that themselves have no connection, both discredit Ryle, but this Rylean diversion has nonetheless had purpose in showing that causation *can* come by different routes and from different levels of cause, and *multiple* causation of one and the same action is not merely possible but frequent. We ask only that the reader note that we have *not* claimed that the obvious multiplicity of possible causes for movements of the knee proves the presence of any strange loop among those causes.

Should we, then, discarding Ryle, rush to the opposing camp, willing to embrace any argument that proves him irrelevant, such as the possibility that the strange loop, with its inherent complexities of causation, is a real-world entity? Probably not, for if we were, uncritically, to acknowledge strange loops everywhere we look, we should be left with no rational understanding of anything. Should we not, instead, continue to use the logic of our experience, tracing lines of apparent causation, namely the correlations described by Dingle as the achievements of science, and accepting *them* as valid explanations, while accepting unexpected causal convolutions—strange loops—if, and only if, we find we have no "straight-line" explanation that is adequate? This is surely wise. However, setting up the strange loop in opposition to Ryle has had another purpose, for it has brought face to face two attempts to discredit dualism, which are *incompatible with each other* and therefore cannot both be true.

Maturer thinking than that of the physicalists suggests that we should hold a dynamic balance between linear causation and convolved or mutual causation, acknowledging that each expresses simply a *viewpoint* on reality. This is a new notion, and important, for many of the causative realities of our Being-in-the-world are indeed ideas, mental constructs, each giving rise to a *point of view,* a perspective, and thence *an intentional stance, a motivation.* These multilevel causations may, but will not necessarily, contain strange loops. From mere differences of perspective, differences of viewpoint, have arisen the feud between dualism and monism, wars of religion, and rival scientific hypotheses, to name but three manifestations. Our beliefs themselves are, seen in this context, causal. They are *realities* and they bring about real effects, which lead some to accept the notion of strange loops, yet simple linear causes (the *only* interest of science in earlier centuries) also abound in the world of what Heidegger calls our "view-about" (*Umsicht*). As we progress through this chapter this difficult balancing of alternative perspectives will become easier, as the supraperspectival view of Jean Gebser, and indeed of all of today's integralist thinkers, slowly supervenes within our minds.

A Closer Look at Strange Loops

So now we are ready to go further, leaving Rylean philosophy far behind, first by questioning the very notion of causation itself, and later by raising the related question of whether many systems currently seen as strange loops might not be rendered linear-logical by a shift not in their facts but in our view of their interrelationships and causes.

We noted that Ryle seemed unable to cite realities to support his argument, and it is a little surprising to find that the exponents of strange loops are also not well able either to define them or to give examples. We believe that while they may have cause for concern over the concept itself, they should not trouble over any verbal difficulties. There are questions that are best solved by contemplation of images, or contemplation of consciousness itself, rather than by Wittgensteinian word games or Rylean riddles, which are doomed to fail for they are *unavoidably clumsy,* mere mappings *abstracted from* the realities that the scientist researches and the meditator knows directly, both without depending on words. Why pore over the map if you can *see* the territory? However, attempts have been made to define the *strange loop* in words, not least by Douglas Hofstadter, author of the famous book *Gödel, Escher, Bach.* One of his attempts, in his later book *I Am a Strange Loop,* runs as follows:

> And yet when I say "strange loop," I have something else in mind, a less concrete, more elusive notion. What I mean by "strange loop" is—here goes a first stab, anyway—not a physical circuit but an abstract loop in which, in the series of stages that constitute the cycling-around, there is a shift from one level of abstraction (or structure) to another, which feels like an upward movement in a hierarchy, and yet somehow the successive "upward" shifts turn out to give rise to a closed cycle. That is, despite one's sense of departing ever further from one's origin, one winds up, to one's shock, exactly where one had started out. In short, a "strange loop" is a paradoxical level-crossing feedback loop.[12]

Strangely, or perhaps not so strangely, one looks in vain for convincing examples of strange loops in Hofstadter's works. Is the very notion of the strange loop in difficulties? Another attempted definition, on the Wikipedia website, says "a 'strange loop' arises when, by moving up or down through a hierarchical system, one finds oneself back where one started. 'Strange loops' may involve self-reference and paradox." Our own attempt might be to say that a strange loop is understandable as a circularity that tangles a hierarchy. A *tangled* hierarchy is one in which the levels are confused because the *dependencies* are ordered in a nonrectilinear way. The hierarchy is tangled into a strange loop, higher entities (such

as the perspectives of humans) depending on lower (such as empirical facts and physical processes), but also bringing about effects of their own at those lower levels, all the causes and effects occurring simultaneously. So our own phrase to describe such a structure, replacing the paradoxically causal notion of the strange loop, would be that its parts show *interdependency of being* since *everything involved is happening at the same time.* But is there anything strange about this structure of intercausality? We think not, for it is simply a description of how Heidegger's Being-in-the-world works. Even its hint of uncaused timelessness does not seem alien to our way of being, especially when we also contemplate the sense that what we see as empirical facts might depend on our consciousness since the very concept of "empirical fact" *must* depend in some way upon our human way of seeing the world-about, which is a function *of which we are conscious.* But, again, we see no *strangeness* here. It is our everyday experience. Only those who deny the reality of consciousness itself, or think it a mere epiphenomenon of physical existence, would consider either complex causation or a seemingly timeless world-contemplating consciousness to be *strange.*

On looking again at figure 2.6 (on page 19) the reader will see that Yggdrasil, to be conceived as a picture of human consciousness, shows a door leading directly from the *under*world to the *summit* of the Norse equivalent of "Mount Meru," and the outer branches of the Tree of Life reach to the same height as those of the central trunk, totally surrounding the everyday world, passing through and round it because that everyday world-about is *less real to the observing mind* than the multileveled tree of the whole and self-aware self *itself.* The very phrase "self-aware self itself" is chosen to suggest the recursive, self-observing and self-referring nature we find ourselves to have, and the self-understanding that created Yggdrasil in the Nordic mind certainly evinces the multiple causations we have noted before. It also certainly shows "bottom-up" causation, with the resulting enlightenment "at the top," but, being the most fully conscious part, that elevated enlightenment then shows itself causative in a downward direction, making choices, and changing the physical world in which it stands. The *self* is the center of the world of the living. But is this whole structure a *strange* loop? Again it does not seem so. It seems only to illustrate, as Freud might have pointed out, the reality within ourselves of mental content of which "we" are unconscious but which might rise within us and so influence our very ordinary and unstrange downward-and-outward conscious mental functioning.

Where, then, are the boundaries of the entity I call "myself"? "I" seem to *include* functionings of which "I" am not conscious, but "I" also seem to *be* an "I," which is indeed conscious of its own "I-ness" *and* of its world-about, and which sees "I myself-ness" and "world-about" as distinct from each other, even if as distinct-within-a-Whole. If "I-ness" is a *part* of "my" Whole, that whole might indeed be causally convolved or internally self-interdependent for its being-as-a-Whole. The question then becomes how we define *livingness* and whether, since my conscious self-ness is not coextensive with what is undoubtedly *my own* unconscious functioning, my whole-ness as a living being might not be dual or even multiplex.

In attempting to illuminate a belief common among

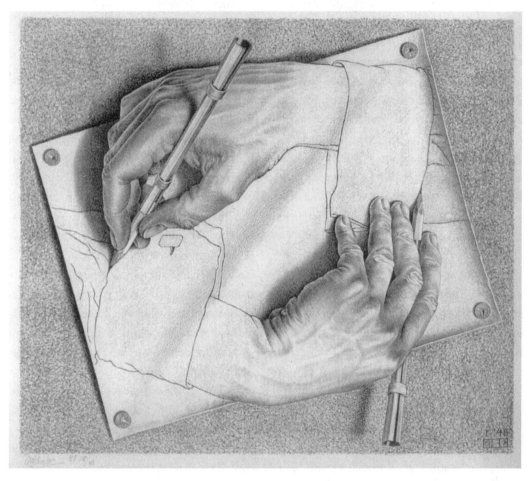

Fig. 15.1. Escher's famous hands, even before they are fully "there," need each other in order to be there. He imagines them as bringing each other into being, as causing each other. Some would claim that his illustration pictures a strange loop, but this is not the case. The hands are not at different levels of reality, except in the rather strained sense that *each* must *precede* the other in order for *either* to *come into* being. This might, however, be said to illustrate *our* notion of mutual dependency, or interdependency, of being. Escher's drawing does not illustrate a strange loop, let alone provide an instance of one, for the only shift of levels in it is the normal one between the creator of the drawing (clearly the upper level) and the drawing itself. This is willed and conscious downward causation again, the bête noir of the physicalist. Escher does not show *himself wielding the hand* that draws another hand, but *only* two such hands. Mary Cassatt painted Monet painting, and Escher, intriguing though the image is, has similarly simply drawn his own hand drawing his own hand. This is not strange, and it is nearer to a Platonic notion than to the convolved—or confused—emergentism of the physicalist's strange loop. We should ask whether genuine strange loops really exist, for if we do not detect and reject nongenuine strange loops we impair our ability to understand and explain anything at all.

physicists and mathematicians (though abhorred by language-bound philosophers) we cannot avoid using causal and temporal language since that is all we have at present. We have to say that a "mutual causation" such as Escher illustrates, which might seem impossible to our *time-ly* consciousness of our world, might "occur" in another "place" where "things" "already" exist in a higher reality, a Platonic *eternal* world, time*less*ly containing all potentials for being. This schema has been unfashionable for centuries, but whence, if not from such a "world," arise the a priori rock-solid self-consistencies of mathematics? And whence our Being, able to grasp those truths? It is this question that we keep open, and seek to answer. Our physical world-about, by contrast, is a world of *time-ly processes,* such as the ticking of a clock or the jumping of excited electrons from level to level within the atom, or yesterday's stroll in the park that provides pleasant memories for our consciousness today.

Recall that Dingle says that science is a creation, not a discovery, a creation of the human mind. Now creativity, mathematics, physics, and psychology merge in a union that might show mutual dependencies between entities and between levels, just as Yggdrasil confuses levels and is a Whole produced by observation, imagination, and conflation, as we saw in chapter 2. But this does not seem to justify the notion of the strange loop. Science is likewise observation, imagination, and the explicative conflation that Dingle calls correlation. Like all other world trees, Yggdrasil is located at the center of the contemplative's universe, the center of solipsistic consciousness, that meeting place of "I am" and of "As above, so below," of simultaneous looking "up" and looking "down," and its trunk, like the meditator's own spine, is a vertical axis around which the nine worlds of Norse myth lie. It is also the Vedic Axis. Now it shows that its nature is the same as that of science itself.

All these constructs are inventions of the human mind, which, we believe, is finding itself to be coexistent not only with the everyday, obvious, physical world-about but also with an unseen but directly experienced level, which Heidegger describes as its "ownmost" essential self. But it is not a strange loop, for its causations can be rationally understood without invoking convolutions alien to our ordinary everyday being or even to our sense of linear logic. The purported strange loop, then, is as elusive as its name suggests. Our own rather different

notion of interdependency of being may be more useful, and there is an evident interdependence between twentieth century mathematical logic and a very old idea only recently revived after centuries of neglect that is more relevant still. We shall return to this question near the end of the chapter.

Is Causation Causal, and Do Processes Process?

Whatever the eventual resolution of the problem of strange loops and interdependencies of being we should not shrink from the possibility that a baffling oddity, whether false or true, heralds a great leap in understanding. After all, such surprises have happened before, as in the gestation of Einstein's special theory of relativity in the unpromising womb of a vexing anomaly in earlier theory and the failure of experiment to resolve it. Like some other blessings, the nontemporal, noncausal notion of interdependency of being has come to us in disguise, incomprehensible until we espouse two other concepts of modern physics, quantum interconnectedness and the quantum vacuum, of which we shall say more. But what could it be that claims to thrust causal logic aside, replacing it with what may seem, in lame words, a mere "seeing" that *things are as they are* and that that is the *reason why* they are as they are? Is *this* facile nontemporal antiexplanation going to be the *ultimate* truth? Such a way of thinking seems, at first, entirely unacceptable. It is circular, perverse in its exclusion of all logical process or argument. Children object when their parents impose "reasons" of this kind. Its interest is in the fact that it is existential, not causal. We cannot quite preclude the possibility that while it scarcely *explains* it, it may accurately *describe* the way things "be." *Explanation* could then lie a step further on, or, rather, a step higher.

Great forward leaps arise, often, out of looking back, as the French *Reculer pour mieux sauter* reminds us. We must accept a turmoil of ideas, excluding none, if we are to sort out science and its relationships in any useful way. If we look back at that earlier Eastern consciousness, which maintained its equanimity in the face of a hazily discerned complexity at the root of humanity's being, pronouncing "Thou art That," we do so, now, with a more focused consciousness. Is future science, then, dependent upon a new perspective? That seemingly reasonable question is somewhat misconceived because it assumes that the present mode of human consciousness is equal to the present task of science, and that it will continue to operate when psychology and physics draw closer. Jean Gebser, author of *The Ever-Present Origin,* would deny both these presumptions. Interdependency of being will become clearer to us if, as Gebser claims, a change from a "perspectival" to an "aperspectival" consciousness is in progress. Linear logic will become merely a special (very simple, and not dishonored) limiting case within an aperspectival view of the cosmos.

Perhaps, to convey his meaning to those who have not read Gebser, we might use the words *supraperspectival,* or *holistic,* or *global,* or *integral* to characterize the enhanced consciousness he foresees. No strangeness would remain in any loop, whether causal or existential, which we could see *from all perspectives at once,* that is, aperspectivally, or, putting it better, *without* a perspective, as if from "above" perspective itself, from a "perspective" *without* position, without even metaphorical "position," that is without "pastness" or "bias"—*without* all the difficulties we have been considering—a "perspective" of "I see" and of "just is" so all-encompassing that it is in fact no perspective at all, but engulfs perspectivity itself in an Indra's Net of all-seeing. The confusion in which our thinking finds itself when faced with the strange loop, or the lesser confusion that "interdependency of being" might engender, is itself one of the problems of science. Indeed, it is a barrier to science, alongside the aforementioned biases of various kinds and causes, but the notion of the aperspectival, too, must await its place, and time, much later in this chapter, for our survey of the problems of "doing science" are not yet exhausted.

Indeed, the problem seems to deepen, for science, as it begins to acknowledge the possibility of "downward causation," sees ipso facto that psychological factors *might influence what is observed even as an experiment proceeds.* Is this a troublesome complication, or does it fit with aperspectivity and mutual causation? If, as has been habitual for some centuries, we demand to trace single lines of causation, such as mere "pushes and pulls," we have to ask what kind of causation it is that can apparently interfere with experiments without physical contact with the apparatus? How does *that* work? Newton would have emphatically denied the very possibility. Can we provide examples? We scarcely have space for examples, but many readers will be aware of Jung's "synchronicity," of "the Pauli effect" and similar odd events, and

we have all read something of poltergeists and miracles of healing. Perhaps in an expanded science harmonizing physics and psychology such phenomena will not seem odd at all. The apparent possibility of an influence upon experiment by "mind" alone (the term is used provisionally) is, of course, far deeper than the self-trickery, mentioned earlier, of tendentious experimental *prior design* or biased *interpretation* of results.

What concerns us here is far more important to the question of the subtle body, namely the fact that the mind, whatever the mind proves to be, *appears sometimes to take an active, even an executive, part in physical events that are "objectively" observed, and might therefore influence experimental results themselves.* The study of such a process of *active influence,* if the facts asserted are confirmed, will be of great use in combining physics and psychology into one correlated science, though the conceptual and experimental difficulties are immense, for reasons we have given. If substantiated, active influence by mind *without* visible "pushing and pulling" will necessarily be *actions by a subtle level of our being,* evidence of a *reality* that today's limited physics (which explains the movements of Dingle's fly only when it is dead), would have to categorize as *nonphysical,* and therefore accept as evidence of a *subtle* body.

We shall later give two illuminating case histories, but until we have looked into the fundamental nature of the physical world, inquiring whether it can include or accommodate a level we would wish to call *subtle,* or wish to describe using von Franz's word *spirit,* we can claim no *certainty* about this question. Let us turn, then, to an uncertainty of a very different kind, the *technically defined* uncertainty inherent in quantum physics, which many believe grounds the possibility of minds, and of their being-here-in-*this*-(physical)-world at all.

Uncertainty in Science and in Everyday Experience
"Willing" Certainty Out of Uncertainty

Although the topic here is quantum physics itself we shall preserve consistency with the rest of the book by appraising uncertainty in quantum physics always in relation to our quest for the subtle body, but without violence to proper understanding of the physics *qua* physics. It has been suggested that if the mind intervenes causally in the physical world it is via a "flexibility," which has been described in mathematical terms and is known as "Heisenberg's uncertainty principle." However, there are three distinguishable levels of uncertainty in experimental work so we must first understand those levels, at least in simple terms that will illuminate points to be made later regarding the subtle body.

The First Level of Uncertainty

The first level of uncertainty is easily dealt with and we need not give it much space. It is simply the inherent inaccuracy of all measurement. If you place a ruler alongside a piece of wood you can "read off" its length by visual inspection. Use a magnifying glass and you will find the original measurement not quite accurate after all. Magnify still more and you will find the marks on the ruler no longer narrow enough to measure to, and the ends of the piece of wood will have become "woolly," positionally vague. The ruler simply *is not* the object being measured. That object is *itself* and its "size" (if it has a size) is *its own* size, not that of the ruler. If you feel this statement odd or banal perhaps you should ponder it a little longer. So much more would have to be said if this were a book about mathematics, but we must move on. An *exact* mapping from object to ruler is simply impossible, and the belief that it is possible is a misconception, based on the common belief that "numbers are accurate: words are not." An experimenter therefore makes many measurements, and uses the mean value of many results when making a final assessment.

The story is told of the mathematics graduate who turned to experimental physics and was given an assignment by his professor. He set up the necessary equipment and made some measurements. After an hour he presented himself in the professor's office with his results. The professor, surprised to see him, asked, "How many sets of measurements did you make?" "Three," said the mathematician. "Come back when you've done a thousand," the professor replied. This points to an important difference, often overlooked, between mathematics and science. Mathematics is a system of *necessary* truths of a *logical* kind, arguably a priori, and having reference to or ground in *eternal truths*. Some mathematicians believe their world is the Platonic world of Ideas that we described in an historical context in chapter 11. While mathematics provides theories of probability (we shall

shortly meet one such theory that has *two* mathematical statements or descriptions), it is not in itself the messy and inherently inaccurate *technology* of material-world measurement of physical entities and their interactions. Even when dealing with probability, mathematics *itself* is *precise*.

Here we must deal with a frequently met misunderstanding. While mathematical treatment of probability is precise, and while *any* arithmetical expression is *in itself* precise, the *correspondence between* reality and its attempted mathematical description may not, even in theory, be capable of precision. As perceived by us, a mathematical statement of quantity automatically *looks* accurate, but the impression may be false, for in many situations in our world there is no guarantee of the *validity*, the real-world-valid *meaningfulness*, let alone of the further requirement of accuracy of quantification, of the resulting *statement* of *quantity*. The *statement*, the attempted mathematization itself, may be inappropriate. Many entities are not measurable *at all*, and even for measurables the very concept of *absolute accuracy of measurement* is a fiction, a delusion.

The Second Level of Uncertainty and Its Historical Context

We must give far more space to the other two levels of uncertainty since one of them is crucial to belief in a subtle body, while the other is a shallow impostor, which must be understood so that it can be removed from our line of sight. The second level of uncertainty in science relates, like the first, to practical difficulties in measurement, but only with regard to measurement of what are referred to as "mass points," in other words single *particles* or small ensembles of *particles*. Theoretical physicist and mathematician Werner Heisenberg formulated the mathematics, known as "matrix mechanics," which *describes*, and in many senses solves, the *practical* problem but leaves without satisfactory answer a very deep *conceptual* problem with very deep empirical and theoretical implications.

Heisenberg wrestled for several years with the philosophical problems, and came to believe there must be a *third*, much deeper, indeterminacy, subsisting not in measurement as such or in inadequate measurement techniques, but in *physical reality itself*. Note that his matrix mechanics was now established, and that it dealt with particles. Heisenberg had no further mathematical description to offer to describe any other kind of physical process than the *movements of particles,* and he therefore lacked a mathematical description of his postulated deeper, *real unpredictability in the physical world.* We must be careful to grasp the distinction if we are to understand the full implications to be disclosed later in this chapter. It was as if Heisenberg were stranded, unable to conceptualize or define what he suspected. But help was at hand, for the deep, real unpredictability suspected by Heisenberg had been mathematically formulated by wave mechanics, a treatment of the propagation of *waves,* not particles, worked out by Erwin Schrödinger and presented in a range of equations generically known to the nonspecialist as "the Schrödinger equation." *These* equations, these *wave* equations, had *built into their very nature* the *real* unpredictability-of-future, which Heisenberg had discerned lying beyond the measurability problems (which we acknowledge we have yet to describe, for here we are narrating the historical situation in theoretical science of the mid 1920s).

The two mathematical descriptions, Schrödinger's and Heisenberg's, are quite distinct, but are also entirely compatible. We shall therefore avoid any gap in our own exposition of uncertainty by dealing with Schrödinger's wave equations and their consequences for the concept of the subtle body after describing the "shallow" Heisenberg uncertainty but before bringing in the third, "deep" Heisenberg uncertainty, of which, once Schrödinger has been understood, little more will need to be said. This sequence will develop the relevant ideas in the most comprehensible way, and we shall draw out those ideas by describing the practical experiments that were based upon the mathematics, and that confirmed the correctness of both wave and particle descriptions.

Heisenberg's early formulations of the idea of uncertainty grew out of his mathematical treatment of what were essentially practical problems in measuring such parameters as the velocity or position of single particles by means of other single particles as they interacted with them. If we wish to measure the position, at a particular instant, of a single electron we might shoot a photon at it and measure the time it takes for the photon to reflect back to the measuring apparatus. After measuring this time-lag we can calculate the electron's position relative to the measuring apparatus at the moment of the collision. The photon will be able to "count" the electron's distance from the measuring apparatus, using its own wavelength as the unit of distance, and do so, crudely speaking, to the nearest multiple of that wavelength, but no more finely than that, so the shorter the wavelength of the photon, the more accurately the electron's position can be established.

Readers who, at this point, want to protest that we are speaking of a photon as a particle, yet imputing to it a wavelength, something particles seem most unlikely to have, are asked their indulgence for this impropriety, for here we have not merely the *shallow* problem of inadequate language to contend with but also a *deep* inadequacy of concept. How are we to think of electrons and photons, as particles or as waves? Clearly, from the divergent evidence of experiment, they might be neither, but of some other nature unimaginable to us; but we must have conceptual tools for thinking about them, however blunt. So we shall *think* of them as neither, but *speak* of them as either, *according to the experimental situation.* This seems disingenuous, but experiment itself has shown it to be valid procedure, and the deep reason for it will eventually appear. For the present it does compound the anomaly of which readers might wish to complain, so we assure them that the final understanding will deal with the linguistic, the practical, and the conceptual difficulties and even provide clear evidence for the real existence of a subtle body of a kind more grand by far than the medieval conception of an individual immortal soul, but we require *many* more pages before we can reach that haven with solid ground beneath our feet at every step. This chapter is constructing itself by assembling first the component ideas of a new kind of Whole, then clearing away excrescences of misunderstanding from those ideas, and finally assembling the newly cleaned components into what we trust will be a Wholeness more nearly true than any that human thought has devised in earlier eras. Meanwhile, we must continue the discussion of the practical physics of measurement, for that is the only possible next step if the final construct is to stand, but we offer two routes to do so. Readers wishing to contemplate the theoretical questions in some depth may like to read the text boxes and study the diagrams. Others may prefer to proceed with the main text.

We resume our main narrative, then, by acknowledging the difficulty inherent in any attempt to establish the electron's position. By colliding with the electron and bouncing off it, that is, by the very act of measuring the electron's position, the photon has thrust the electron off its course or, in more technical terms, has altered its momentum.* The shorter the wavelength of the photon the more accurately it will determine the electron's position, but the shorter the wavelength the higher the photon's energy. The higher its energy the more it disturbs the electron's momentum as it bounces off it. So if the photon has a short wavelength it confines our knowledge of the position of the electron within closer limits than a long-wave photon could, but because a short-wave photon has higher energy it disturbs the electron's momentum more than a long-wave photon would because it transfers more energy to the electron in the collision. Thus, if we measure the position accurately using a short-wave high-energy photon we have to accept that the momentum, if measured at the same instant (or the "next instant"), will be less accurately measured because the electron is being (or has already been) more severely disturbed; and vice versa. The accuracies of the two measurements are inversely related; if one is accurate the other is automatically and unavoidably disturbed, and therefore less accurate, and this situation is inescapable, imposed by the very nature of the measuring processes and the measured items involved.

These are *natural* processes. We simply *use* them, arranging them, observing them, and interpreting them, for our own purposes. The same reciprocal relation regarding accuracy applies to *all* measurements of single particles and often to measurements of much larger entities. In principle, it applies to classical† physics just as

much as to quantum physics, though in classical physics it could rarely be important because most classical measurements are of much "heavier" entities and measuring them applies a relatively extremely soft touch, which scarcely disturbs them at all. If you measure the position of a building using a modern laser rangefinder, the light that performs the act of measuring does not move the building very much. A small spot of light bounces back from the enormous mass of the building, having exerted a pressure upon it so small that no human hand placed in the beam could even feel it (though it *would* damage the eye). However, in quantum physics, crudely speaking the physics of the very small, it is usually single particles, or assemblages of relatively few particles, that are measured, and the measuring particle (or wave) is of the same order of size as the particle it measures. Their interaction is like a collision of planets and extremely disturbing to the entity being "measured."* With a variety of small but unavoidable verbal and rational imprecisions, this is the "shallow" second uncertainty, a simple and gross fact of the technology of the measurement of single particles.

The question now is *why* things are this way. What sort of reality is it that works like this? This is the question Heisenberg, who knew of Schrödinger's wave-mechanical equations and their prediction of multiple possible outcomes from particle-scale actions, asked himself, and if we are to understand it we, too, should look at the matter at a deeper level than the layperson usually troubles to do.

Approaching the Third Level of Uncertainty
The Relevance of the Philosophy of Our Being

The shallow second level of uncertainty is a very real fact of science, with serious consequences for our access to accurate knowledge of the quantum world of the very small, and Heisenberg and others were, of course, well aware of the impossibility of simultaneous accurate measurement of all the *potentially* measurable quantities relating to single particles, such as the pair usually cited, position and momentum. It was precisely this

---

*Speed in a specified direction is termed *velocity,* and *momentum* is a measure of the energy of a particle that takes into account both its velocity and its mass.
†*Classical* physics is the physics of deterministic "laws" abstracted from everyday experience; it was superseded by the discovery of the quantization of all physical action and the realization that the true "laws" of physics (if there are any such) are not predictors of fixed effects but only laws of *probability*-of-effect. It is in the resulting "slack" of undeterminedness that, many believe, mind finds scope for free will. This is its crucial relevance to the quest for the subtle body. But quantization itself lies outside the scope of this book. Interested readers may like to research the work of Max Planck and others concerning "black body radiation" in the last years of the nineteenth century and the earliest years of the twentieth.

*You can get a vague and unquantified impression of this by firing a flashgun toward a sheet of cellophane held about an inch in front of it. Most people are very surprised to see that the light "rattles" the cellophane. Sunlight presses against your sunroom window, and bends it, before it succeeds in pushing through.

The "Shallow" Heisenberg Uncertainty

The "shallow" Heisenberg uncertainty is merely a matter of measurements even though they are considered to be measurements of *real* interactions between *real* wavicles. The position of an electron relative to the measuring apparatus itself (all such measurement is from some such reference body) can be determined by projecting an electromagnetic wave at it and timing the arrival of the wave at a sensing device after it has been reflected back. This is shown, very schematically, in diagram 1 of figure 15.2. On the (always false but not always important) assumption that the electron is not accelerated or decelerated by its collision with the photon, this allows a measurement of the electron's position that is accurate to the nearest whole wavelength of the radiation used. An accurate measurement, illustrated in diagram 2, thus requires a short-wave photon, but, ipso facto, such a photon has high energy and therefore disturbs the electron's velocity (and its momentum) more than an inaccurate measurement using a low-energy long-wave photon, as in diagram 3, would have done. Simultaneous or even near-simultaneous measurements of position and momentum, or of any *mutually influencing* variables, known as *conjugate* variables, therefore cannot all be highly accurate. A measurement of velocity and a measurement of position are mutually related in this way, since both involve change of position in space. In any pair of measurements of conjugate variables, one measurement or the other is seriously falsified because the electron has been disturbed *in the relevant way* (e.g. its position in space) by whichever measurement takes place earlier, no matter how minute the time lapse between the measurements.

This explanation might be characterized as being in the "early quantum" style, that is, according to early understandings of quantum physics, roughly prior to the 1920s. The question is whether the "early quantum" schema is all there is to the matter. This book cannot give space to an exhaustive answer, but must restrict itself to those aspects of the physics that most concern the quest for the subtle body.

However, explanations, like descriptions, are of different "depths" and different *accuracy of mapping onto reality*. We could have given, as a macro-scale, crudely *classical*, understanding, an explanation stating that once the first parameter has been measured the disturbance brought about by the necessary collision has altered *the whole of the electron's*

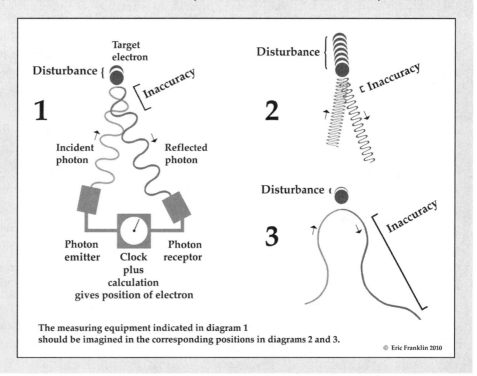

Fig. 15.2. Using a photon to measure the position of an electron: the "shallow" Heisenberg uncertainty.

future trajectory, so rendering invalid, or at least suspect, *all* measurements later than the first of any group of parameters originally intended to be measured *whether at the same instant or in succession*. This classical-style explanation of the uncertainty involved when two or more parameters are measured is at least cogent and intelligible. However, the *intelligibility-for-humans* of an explanation does not guarantee that the explanation presents a *truthful correspondence with reality*. Once the quantization of all physical action had been discovered such explanations could no longer satisfy the criterion of correspondence between word or meaning on the one hand and natural fact or reality on the other. No one who does not start with this realization has the smallest hope of understanding physics, quantum or classical.

In any measuring system such as the one depicted here, the reflected photon that bounces away after its collision with the electron has (in all but very special experimental situations far outside the scope of this book) a lower energy and, ipso facto, a longer wavelength, than the incident photon. This is because the photon's disturbance of the electron *is* the transfer of a quantum of the photon's energy to the electron. After any collision the reflected photon is less energetic than it was before the collision, and its wavelength is therefore longer. This is acknowledged in the diagram by showing each reflected photon-wave with a longer wavelength than the incident photon-wave.

Whatever the explanatory schema, whether classical or quantum, deep or shallow, verbalizable or only picturable, the margins of uncertainty of any two measurements of conjugate variables are in a kind of inverse relation to each other, inaccuracy in all post-disturbance measurements being unavoidable, but, beyond this fundamental fact, thoughtful readers may also have realized that, as explanations, not only our "classical style" account, but even our very carefully worded "early quantum" account, and our equally considered diagram, are inherently, and unavoidably, flawed. The diagram is highly schematic and uses conventional signs to represent electrons and photon waves. While their

use is unavoidable, these signs can be as seriously misleading as imprecise verbal language. Perhaps the most serious inadequacy of the representation is the inconsistency of showing the photons as transverse Maxwellian propagating waves, but the electrons as classical solids. This perpetuates the totally false distinction we, as sensing biological organisms, make between "matter" and "radiation," based on the different sensitivities of our bodies, at least in everyday situations, to impacts of electromagnetic waves such as light or heat as contrasted with impacts of matter, such as "solid objects" like stones. All these confessed anomalies of description are clues to the nature of the "deep" Heisenberg uncertainty, which requires of us a radically different conception of reality itself, not merely an awareness of the technology of measurement or of the even more banal problems of devising explanations and illustrations of scientific ideas. To remove the flaws of "shallow" explanations is, in effect, to retrace the thinking that gave rise to Heisenberg's uncertainty principle.

Heisenberg was well aware of the problem of mismatch between our concepts and reality, and his contemplations over many years suggested to him that *all* explanations resembling those given here are too "shallow." He believed that, even if the measurements *could* be made simultaneously, some kind of reciprocal uncertainty relationship would *still* be present between them. He suspected that the reason was a far "deeper" indeterminacy, subsisting not in measurement or measurement techniques, but in physical reality itself, which required "deeper" explanation than any merely technological, albeit insuperable, problem of simultaneous measurement with zero disturbance. These merely technological problems were, inconveniently, masking from view a future evolution of reality, which was *fundamentally* uncertain, undetermined. However, it was Schrödinger's *wave* mechanics that confirmed this, for Heisenberg's treatment for *particles* could never do so. This is why we have to deal with Schrödinger's work alongside our treatment of Heisenberg's. So the third, deep, level of *Heisenberg's* uncertainty principle relates to phenomena that *Schrödinger* described in a range of equations that are generically known to the nonspecialist as "the Schrödinger equation." With almost a century's hindsight, we can see why this is necessarily the case. Waves are probabilistic, *unde-termined*, evolving possibilities; that is their nature and, indeed, their purpose, as will become clear. Particles are *post-determination* entities. Heisenberg

knew the "deep" nature of the uncertainty he was looking for, but it could not be found among enti-ties that were themselves the result of *the process of determination*, but only in their *as-yet-undetermined* precursors, which were, of course, waves. Repeated readings of our text will, we trust, place a clear *pic-ture* of this in the mind of every reader.

second uncertainty that Heisenberg's matrix mechan-ics described, but he felt, perhaps in part on account of Schrödinger's work, that something more fundamental than the mere technology of measurement was present, an *inherent unpredictability* within the *very nature* of our physical world, an unpredictability so deep that it meant, roughly speaking, that the very concept of the measurability of particles was merely a presumptive fic-tion carried over from our everyday-world experience of measuring rather gross "things" such as cues and bil-liard balls or magnets and iron filings as they pushed or pulled each other around the macro-world of classical physics. The change of viewpoint from that of classi-cal physics, that is *mechanism,* needed to grasp the *deep* Heisenberg uncertainty is so great that we must follow an epicycle into philosophy and an examination of our ways of thinking before we return to physics itself. Readers as yet unfamiliar with the thinking underlying quantum physics will not attain the new view without considering this section with care *before* attempting to proceed further. So far, we have traveled on rails, but quantum physics is nothing like classical physics. Now we must fly.

The deep, third uncertainty, by contrast with the shallow second, results from a *nonexistence.* Position, momentum, and all other quantum particle measurables *do not exist* and therefore cannot be measured until they are measured; and perhaps even *the particle itself* (if there are such things as particles) does not exist. The reader must excuse this arresting syntax for something funda-mental, if also shocking and almost unsayable, is being said, and will be more fully explained in the follow-ing pages. Many, even today, would stoutly insist that the very conception we attempt to convey is irrational, and claim that our statement of it violates the laws of syntax and *therefore* cannot be true, but they would be

wrong, victims of that *word*-bound *fact*-denying reason-ing, which schoolchildren (and the philosopher Ryle and his successors) have so often evinced, a certitude born of *verbal conditioning and grammar,* which has forgotten that there is *a-reality-beyond-the-words*. The ancients fell victim to this same semiconsciousness, this same eleva-tion of *Logos,* the Word, the *mesmerizing* word, above reality, a reality kept remote and unknowable by the very words that named it, and present-day philosophers who concentrate on language and meaning are continu-ing this hallowed and hollow tradition. Heisenberg did not fall into this error, and, like so many of the greatest scientists, was his own philosopher.

Today, we should regard falling prey to bewitchment by words a careless naïveté, and, even worse, as atavistic. It is a mode of the ancient mythic consciousness, aided and abetted by mental consciousness, that should have no place in today's analyses of reality. Linguists ana-lyze "meaning" but only gnostics have the experience of *knowing.* What is required of us is what Einstein always brought to his own contemplative theorizing, a pictur-ing imagination. We can often picture what we cannot say. Those who claim, as many have done, that if we are unable to express a thought in words we do not have that thought at all are simply wrong, their own think-ing, not ours, limited by words and their claim in fact advertising their failure to understand anything at any level higher than the verbal, and hence the mythic, or possibly the rudimentarily mental. Words are *not* reality, nor do they even represent it satisfactorily, and if all a person knew were words that person would know noth-ing. It is a *reality-beyond-the-words* that we are seeking to understand and describe. All that should be claimed for language is that *if* a thought can be expressed in words it can be expressed *clearly* by *well-chosen and well-ordered* words, which is not at all the same claim. Further, the verbal *usage* of claiming that a particle is not there to be measured until it is measured *seems* irrational *only* because we have wrong ideas both about the physical world and about *causation,* and hence have misleading linguistic habits, all three being leftovers from mentalist science, that of the mechanistic classical "solidity" of huge aggregates of particles as "things" in the everyday world, which push and pull each other around before our view. Quantum physics is nothing like this.

Our next logical step, then, is to combine in *imagination* Schrödinger's vision of how waves evolve over time with Heisenberg's vision of a deep undecidedness hidden within the "solid reality" of particles. Note first how the compatibility between two radically different mathematical descriptions, Heisenberg's quantum-mechanical treatment and Schrödinger's classically deterministic wave mechanics, suggests that both theories have value. They corroborate each other, and it is this corroborated *uncertainty-of-future* in quantum-level physical interactions that supports the notion of the subtle body. Of course, experiment was required, to test the predictions and provide further corroboration. Schrödinger's *wave* equations are *descriptions,* given *before* the event, *predictions* of the *possibilities* of the future evolution of a present state out-from (Greek εκ) which *one* new reality will "stand forth" as a solid thing, so being made *phenomenally* (Greek φαινομενον) real in *our* world-about. Heisenberg's mathematics of *mass-point* measurement pertains to that reality, defining the leeway available at any moment in each "measurable" of that reality-making process, according to the "state of fixedness" of the *other* potential measurables. The two descriptions are entirely compatible. It is as if Heisenberg, contemplating the "reciprocal inaccuracy" of particle measurements revealed by his matrix mechanics, intuited the deep uncertainty-of-*future* that Schrödinger saw staring out at him from his very differently grounded wave mechanics, which predicts the *possibility* of many outcomes, each with a different degree of probability, but none fixed *until fixed.* The question is how this "fixing" of reality is done, and Pauli has already given us a hint.

Among the influences on Heisenberg's thought was a famous, and, in its time, rather puzzling, experiment known as the "double slit experiment." (See several diagrams illustrating this experiment in figure 15.3 within the boxed text starting on page 199.) It had first been performed as long ago as 1801, by Thomas Young, in a simple macro-world form using everyday apparatus, which would not have revealed anything of interest to us in our search for the subtle body but had enough importance for physics to have been repeated a number of times, with refinements and developments, until as recently as 1989. We shall describe a relevant version, though only in the briefest outline, for that is all we have space for, and all we need, though a more detailed description is provided in the text box.

A beam of light is projected toward a screen with two parallel slits in it. The slits have to be microscopically fine and close together to produce the characteristic effect. The beam passes through the slits, travels on, and finally impinges on a second screen beyond. On the second screen we see a distinct pattern of alternate light and dark bands, parallel with the slits. This pattern is caused by what is known as constructive and destructive "interference" between light waves passing through the two slits, as illustrated and discussed in some detail in figure 15.3. What was shocking was that a modern version of Young's experiment showed that if *just one* photon at a time, just *one* quantum of light at a time, was projected toward the first screen, with its two slits, and passed through and fell upon the second screen, the same clear interference pattern built up, light particle by light particle, over time. Each single photon, *each* particle of light energy, seemed to be acting like a wave, the front of which could rationally be considered to pass through *both* slits simultaneously, whereas a single *particle* could surely not do so. (We remind the reader that we are bound to speak of waves and particles according to the experimental conditions, and, of course, according to our limited powers of conceptualization.) The interference pattern on the second screen had to be taken as evidence of the presence of a wavefront, not of a particle. The wavefront, split by the slits, spread out as two related fronts beyond the slits, and so produced the pattern as its peaks and troughs intersected at the second screen. Since (in our human conception) only a wave could do this, there was no particle after all. Alternatively, since this process also occurred *over time,* that is, *one* particle at a time, one might surmise that each particle passed only through one slit but, to our very great surprise, each particle acted in such a way that, *over a time period,* the aggregate of all their individual histories gave the *same* pattern as waves would give.

The Double Slit Experiment

What is the double slit experiment, and what does it tell us about ourselves as living Beings and the world in which we find ourselves? Why is a bit of simple technology on the physicist's bench considered relevant to the question of our very nature as Beings, or if not that then at least to our nature as Beings-*in-this-world*? Is the belief that the experiment gives us such insight justified? Before we can even address these questions we are immediately faced with the human being's unknowingness, of which Dingle reminded us. Consideration of the problem shows how little science as it really is resembles the person-in-the-street's conception of it. Not only that, but we must first understand something of the philosophical hinterland of the experiment, and that hinterland is ourselves, for it is *our* experiment, performed by *our* hands and eyes. *Our Being* affects it. What is our place, relative to the experiment, its apparatus, its originating hypothesis, its practicalities? Here, in what might seem the simplest of physical actions, the passage of light (or electrons, or atoms, or even molecules) through a hole, the integrity of our explanatory conceptualization is compromised at the first step, and at every succeeding step, by our need to vacillate between description as if of "waves" (like those large-scale everyday undulations we see as water flows round obstacles) and the quite different line-like trajectories that lumps like baseballs seem to trace as we watch them flying through the air.

Our own nature first restricts the explanations we can find, and then decides whether, having invented them, we can believe them. Explanation, to fulfill the meaning of that word itself, has to make sense *to us,* it has to tell *us* a convincing story within *our* possible ways of thinking. Deepening even this huge uncertainty, we also have to recognize what Heidegger asserts, that our very nature is *Dasein,** translatable as "Being *there*," an unusual term, already in use in German philosophy before Heidegger's adoption of it, which asserts the *existence* of our Being. It is (emphatically) there, it is undeniably a *real* being. This concept is not unlike Descartes' "thinking thing"

*See figure 15.6.

that cannot doubt its own existence, but the "seeing" of Dasein is restricted, by *its own* concepts and percepts, to *its own world-about*-as-it-*appears-to-it*-to-be, which includes, of course, the very phenomena we now wish to fix conceptually, and which so effectively resist conceptualization. Thus we live not merely in uncertainty as to which concept to apply, particle or wave, but within a *real* circularity, a *circular* reality, an *inter*dependency of being, with us on the one hand, the world on the other, that is to say we live *within the confined state of a selfness, which is inextricably amid its world* (which is entirely *un*like what Descartes believed about us and the world). We are not observers of a world from outside that world. We are inside our world, trying to explain it, our sense organs are inside our world, sensing it, and in a rather important if nonsubstantive sense, the world is inside us. This might seem to help our search for explication of what happens in that world in which we *are,* but it does the opposite, for, as well as its sense organs being incapable, unaided, of the *microscopic* view we now need (for example to see what happens to tiny postulated entities we call electrons), our conceptualizing *itself* is dual, and neither of our available modes of seeing (seeing waves and seeing particles) provides us with a convincing certainty, for when we perform experiments *both* show themselves true and both show themselves *incomplete.*

Furthermore, the *we* who feel the pressing need and wish to understand are not the mechanism of observation but the Observer, and *ourselves* mercurially elusive. Despite their convolvement, Dasein and the world *are* distinguishable, not one and the same. There *is* a chasm, but it is not to be conceived as lying between self and world, where Descartes placed it, but, by a far smaller shift than many believe, simply *within* a subjective *whole-"me"-as-a-Being-within-this-world,* which world, just as Descartes believed, includes the physical body. As we explained, *the world* has simply come within the "us" (as well as the "us" being in the world), a relationship that makes no difference whatever to the reality of an indwelling livingness (of whatever name and character). The chasm therefore demarcates what Ryle recognized as "mechanical" from what he recognized as "mental," but, by being precisely this, proves the exact converse of what he claimed, that there *is* a ghost (livingness) in the machine (world).

So the problems of explaining to us, in our complexity and our quasi-schizophrenia of fallible self-analysis, what happens in the double slit experiment (and many others) are exceedingly complex. Richard Feynman averred that, given deep thought, the double slit experiment would reveal to the thinker the whole of quantum physics. As we said, we cannot explain the evidence arriving before our senses from the world-about in simple terms but only by a vacillation between segments of explanation, which seem incompatible with each other. Perhaps, then, the wavicles we postulate are real, perhaps *they, themselves* vacillate, *really* performing, not just seeming to perform, the alternative behaviors we have to postulate as wave-like and particle-like, but we cannot know this, the world we want to describe being hidden from us even though we are so deeply convolved with it. We have absolutely no *direct* experience of the world, notwithstanding that the world is in us and we in it, having only experience of selfness and its mental contents. We *imagine* what occurs at the scale of tiny entities passing through tiny slits in screens as analogous to what we see in the large-scale world, such as water passing through gaps, or around obstacles in its path, but we also need to invoke an image resembling that of single grains of blown sand following unique tra-

jectories through space. Yet further, we need the notion of expansion in every direction from a point origin surrounding an ever-increasing globular volume of space, as if of a spherical balloon being blown up, which is, crudely speaking, the basic metaphor used in the concept of fields. The resulting explanation seems a mish-mash of disingenuous fables, and unless reality itself does have the wave-particle duality we think we see, our explanation is indeed a fable, but we offer it, with all its accompanying caveats, with absolute honesty. Consciousness will grow, but now, still near the beginning of the twenty-first century, the kind of picture we give here remains the best that laypeople who are neither professional scientists nor mathematicians can yet behold. So we illustrate three schemata, wave, particle, and field, as an aid to imagination, but remind readers that all verbal and graphic explanations are gross approximations, clumsy mappings, mere analogies, for what *really* happens is hidden from us even though it envelops us. But note what follows: we, in our innermost Beingness, cannot, therefore, be of the same nature as the world we observe. This new realization will become the focus of attention later. Here, we ground our eventual conclusions by dealing as properly as we can with the physics, and with the philosophy underlying it.

In diagram 1 of figure 15.3 we show a source of waves and the wavefront expanding from it in all directions into the surrounding space. What we show is a section, of course, of this three-dimensional

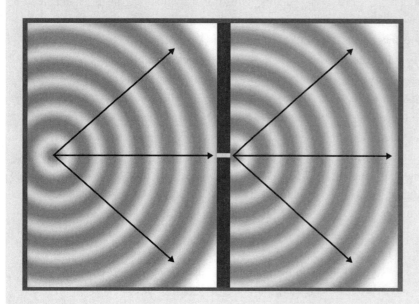

Fig. 15.3. The double slit experiment: Diagram 1

ever-growing sphere. The wavefront reaches a barrier with a very small hole in it. Most of the wave energy reflects back from or is absorbed by the barrier (neither of these processes is shown) but a very narrow "beam" passes through the hole, the matter around the hole dragging at the waves as they attempt to pass and absorbing some of the energy, but once free of this incipient interaction with matter the energy that remains free begins a similar spherical expansion as a new wavefront. We could not have given ourselves such an explanation until the notion of rectilinear propagation and the notion of an expanding field had been invented. Note the word authorized by Dingle. Science is a creation, an invention designed to explain, not the discovery of laws that have no exceptions. The explanation works, in some ways, but not all. An alternative involves the belief that the energy is emitted by the source as single, discrete particles. This we do not illustrate because the observable results are similar, but this version of the experiment forces us to accept the paradox that the energy behaves both as a wave and as a stream of particles. More is said in our main text.

Diagram 2 of figure 15.3 shows, again schematically and with only a tentative relationship with what really happens, the situation when there are two slits (microscopically close together) in the screen blocking the path of the expanding wavefront or, in the other parable, blocking the stream of energy particles projected one at a time from the source. Here, two new wavefronts emerge, one from each slit, and their pulsing highs and lows of energy superimpose as the two fronts move forward instant by instant. As the *paths* of the two wavefronts are not quite in coincidence, their *peaks and troughs* also fail to coincide at every instant, doing so only periodically, so a pattern results. If, in the diagram, we interpret each bright ring as the energy-peak of the pulsing wave we see that when peak superimposes onto peak (as at B) their energies add together and a bright band appears on the screen. This is indicated in our diagram by the panel to the right. When peak superimposes onto trough (as at A) we have a zero sum situation, the net energy reducing to zero, and the screen in these areas, receiving no energy, remains dark. This effect of destructive interference whenever trough coincides with peak and constructive interference when peaks coincide is also shown schematically in diagram 3 on page 202.

Diagram 2a, on page 202, is offered as an alternative, which may be easier to interpret than diagram 2. Here, we use a different graphical convention, but to represent exactly the same process. We show the emerging energy waves not as an expanding sphere but as if each consisted of individual "rays" (each would be a radius of that sphere) having the same wavelength, and it will be seen that the upper superimposition of rays is in phase as it impinges upon the screen, while the lower is out of phase at the screen. The in-phase situation is that of constructive interference, and gives the bright band shown in the right-hand panel (representing the screen), while the lower, out-of-phase situation, destructive interference, cancels the energy so that nothing can show

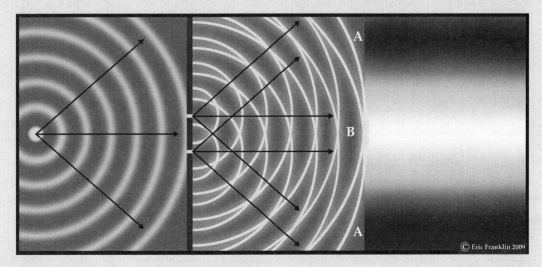

Fig. 15.3. The double slit experiment: Diagram 2

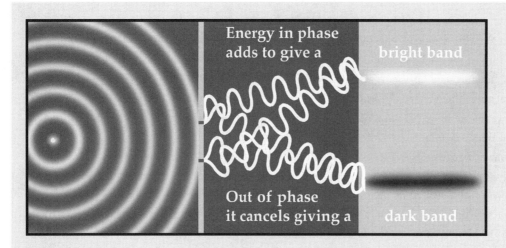

Fig. 15.3. The double slit
experiment: Diagram 2a

Energy in phase adds to give a bright band

Out of phase it cancels giving a dark band

Fig. 15.3. The double slit experiment: Diagram 3. Waves that are in phase with each other sum their energy. This is illustrated at 1, where the black wavy line indicates the resulting intensified wave. Waves that are out of phase nullify each other, as illustrated at 2, where the straight horizontal black line suggests the null energy level. This wave process pervades the whole physical cosmos yet is invisible to us in everyday life. The apparent cancellation of out-of-phase energy raises an important question about invisible levels of physical reality, and Tonomura's experiment investigated this, confirming the reality of a huge reservoir of energy at an invisible level of the world. Nullified energy is conserved but falls into this invisible level of reality. This further matter is dealt with later in this chapter.

1 CONSTRUCTIVE INTERFERENCE
(mutual addition of in-phase energies)

In-phase waves fuse to give high-amplitude wave in our sensible physical world

2 DESTRUCTIVE INTERFERENCE
(mutual subtraction of out-of-phase energies)

Mutually nullifying waves show zero sensible-world energy. Energy drops into potential field

on that area of the screen, which therefore remains dark.

An intriguing question, to be dealt with later, is what happens to cancelled energy, for the very notion seems to deny the truth of an accepted prin-

ciple, that energy is always conserved. Where does the cancelled energy go? The answer is highly pertinent to the question of our nature as Beings-in-the-world and, indeed, the nature of the physical world itself.

What *linked* the particles if *this* explanation were correct? The implications were deeply shocking.

Just as shocking was the discovery that when instead of light energy an experimenter used electrons, which were also considered to be particles, but particles of matter, not of energy, similar interference patterns could be seen, and, again, there were interference patterns when the electrons were projected toward and through the slits only one at a time. Not only did each single photon of light energy show itself to be a wave, but the electron,

a particle of matter, did the same, proving itself a wave, not a particle. Matter and energy suddenly seemed much more like each other than classical physicists (and the present-day layperson) had thought, each seeming to present its own polar duality between waveness and particleness, a kind of diversity-in-unity. And, oddly, it was their interaction *as waves* that seemed to *produce* their "real" presence as particles.

Faced with these conflations of opposites within a single reality one might wonder what would become of the concepts "spirit" and "matter" as used by scientists and theologians, referred to by von Franz in the short quotation given many pages ago. The reader will understand why we declined to define them before gaining at least some clarity on *how* to define them. The Copenhagen Convention of 1926 had published an interpretation of quantum physics, to which we are referring here, albeit sketchily, that is sufficiently accurate for our purposes. It was already familiar to physicists before von Franz began to write. Theologians were perhaps a little slower to acquaint themselves with the shocking new ideas. Language, of course, lagged far behind, and still does, each word hauling with it aggregations of old meaning it would have to shed if nonspecialists were not henceforth to be misled. In addition to the linguistic problems, bewildering dualities and complementarities in physical reality (at least as it is observed and measured by us) surely have consequences for the validity of any concept of dualism or monism, wheresoever applied, and therefore also for the verbal distinction between "subtle" and "material" by which we refer to postulated entities such as the kośas, soul as distinguished from body, mind, aura, and many others. Perhaps the ancient arguments about the nature of humanity's Being fought between the champions of monism and those of dualism were misconceived. Might not both monism and dualism be correct, each in its own sphere, each at its own level, each true, *but according to viewpoint*? Shah Wali Allah, as we saw in chapter 6, evolved a synthesis of the dualistic and monistic Sufi views of his day, and the myriad Hindu schools included beliefs at every point on the continuum between strong monism and strong dualism. Does not the answer to this question depend simply upon our choice of the level at which to investigate, and so arrive at a verdict, which is in reality arbitrary, for if we had chosen another viewpoint we would have made a different analysis? So Sankara and Madhva might be reconciled at last.

We hinted earlier that our interpretation of that other duality, between linear, often temporal, causation on the one hand, interdependency of being on the other, might also change according to viewpoint. Today, the physicists' quest for a "theory of everything" openly and avowedly seeks to explain the duality produced by what is termed a *broken symmetry* by devising a higher-order theory under which phenomena at the level of duality,

each having its own law, find unification under a single higher law, which is valid only when that higher part of the possible range of physical conditions obtains. In the rest of the range the duality appears, and with it the two laws. Thus, in the present example, *applicable to the world-about in which we live and move,* we have one law for particles of matter, one for waves of energy. The big bang hypothesis describes an emergence out from singularity into duality, which then divides further, producing further dualities. The emergence of biological species follows the same pattern, a pattern that Taoism discerned several millennia ago. This is also the way human creativity works, divergently, from where we are now to a future containing more realized possibilities than the present, for example from a musical germ idea, which is not likely to be new, to its full flowering in a development that *is* new, telling a symphonic story, which, however much it somewhat resembles other works, is indeed unique. Perhaps it works this way because this is how our universe itself evolved, we being one with the cosmos. We are at home in a universe in which we are a natural product and which, for that reason, permits us to live and to be what we are. This is the anthropic principle. The universe we *see* is the universe we *be*, but it works the other way round as well, for the universe we be is the only universe we can see, for our way of being dictates our way of seeing. There is an interdependency of being between us and our home universe. We reflect the universe and it reflects us back to ourselves when we observe it. This is Heidegger's Being-in-the-world, in which there are other Beings like us.* We wonder, if the anthropic principle is a valid interpretation, whether we had some part in the creation of the universe, in the big bang that brought us, long afterward, to our *biological* birth, possible only on a planet having the moderate temperature range of ours. We hint, here, at further ideas to be brought forward later. Meanwhile, being human, we look back at the origin of the universe and see it in the only way we can, using our senses and our minds, as progressive breaches of symmetry, phenomenalizing to our view first the two, then the thousand things, then the ten thousand things,

---

*We note, in passing, though the point is important, deserving its own book, that this is the objective ground of ethics, of the belief that I must *not* hurt you, and *must* help you when you are in need.

though these seemingly diverse interpretations remain merely facets of one reality. The only universe we can see is the universe we, being what we are within it, are able to see. However, as our consciousness develops we may see it in a fuller way, an idea already mooted with regard to Gebser's views. Does our thinking, ever-present in some *timeless* realm in which *interdependency*-of-being would have the power that causation seems to have here in our everyday world, *actively make* the big bang (retrospectively, of course, as viewed from the present epoch), or did it *happen,* eventually producing *us,* with our divergent way of thinking, as a product of its own divergings? Which is cause, and which is caused? The question is mind-numbing in its awesomeness and in its difficulty, yet not without point. The traditional concept of temporal causation, cause preceding effect, has begun to fail, as we predicted some pages back. Perhaps Aristotle's "final cause," the future objective that brings about its own bringing-about by reaching back into what, once that objective has been achieved, will have become the past, is valid, after all. And time *is not,* yet, in its not-being, is all one. This riddle we cannot pursue in this book.

Modifying Our View of Causation, and the Consequences for Language

So causation has come to be in doubt. A concept of interdependency of being for which time is somehow an irrelevancy has replaced even Aristotle's teleological final cause. So we do not claim that "singularity X plus condition Y *causes* duality Z," but discounting causation does not reduce such a sentence to meaninglessness. It can be salvaged. Language, the communication of the human way of thinking, offers an alternative of a grammatically valid kind familiar to all of us from schooldays, not the subject-verb-object sentence, which *is* causal, describing a *transitive action,* but its contemplative alternative, the nontransitive explicative *complementary* or *existential* sentence, which asserts that "An A is a B." We *can* say that, in all our observations, whenever X and Y are observed, Z is also observable, for such a sentence is neither an unprovable assertion of causation nor an empty truism. Humans create language to express the way humans think. This mainly verbal aside is important for our capacity to comprehend *the part of the observer* in *all* our interactions with the world, including scientific experiment, and

with this firmer grasp we must return to the double slit experiment, this time to discover why it is relevant to our quest for the subtle body.

The Double Slit Experiment and the Nature of Matter

Particles cannot interfere to make the patterns seen in the double slit experiment. Interference can be produced only between intersecting wavefronts. Ergo, we conclude that, just as with light particles and waves, each electron, too, was in fact a wave when it self-interfered beyond the slits and so fell in patterned distribution on the second screen. Now came the next shock. If the experimenter "measured" the electron passing through the system, the interference pattern instantly disappeared. An electron that had been intercepted by something other than itself, in even the lightest way, was no longer a wave after the interception, for it no longer did what waves do. Physicists could not detect the electron wave *in any way at all* without it instantly ceasing to be a wave. The electron *qua* particle comes into being when we detect it. *The world-about comes into being when we detect it.*

Now a bold conjecture could be made. The electron wave had become a particle, and the only available explanation of that extreme and sudden change was its interaction, no matter how slight, with something else. Waves spread without limit, filling the universe, overlapping, reinforcing, cancelling, but always still waves, nonsolid, not "clogging up" the universe, unless an interaction turns them into particles, which are components of "solid" reality. Have we not, some of us, met something like this before? Though not quite the same, it nonetheless reminds us of a question raised by Descartes, the scientist-philosopher of the seventeenth century who was among the first to move away from scholastic views of the universe toward the science of today. His views on our nature are now almost universally derided rather than being sifted to "test all things, and hold fast to that which is good," as the apostle Paul advised, and as every philosopher and every scientist is bound by his professional claims to do. However, the seeming unreality of the wave-world, contrasted with the "solidity" of the apparent, phenomenal, matter-world of everyday experience reminds us of the Cartesian doubt about the reality of the external world. True, Descartes' reasons for doubting have little relevance to modern questions concerning the deep structure of the world, or to our quest for the subtle body, but the superficial similarity between the notions is intriguing.

What, in his *sense of being,* persuaded Descartes to doubt the "reality" of what his *sense organs* told him lay "out there"? The Heideggerian view, which we see no reason to reject, is that our Being *includes* the world in which we exist. We are each in a polar duality-in-oneness, a part-to-whole duality, with the world in which we have our being. It is not a world-over-there, separate from "myself" and from all other "selves," and quite possibly even non-existent, as Descartes suggested, rationally enough, if also wrongly, but a world with which my I-ness and each other person's I-ness is already one. Our being *is* what Heidegger calls Being-in-the-world.

For both philosophers, whether the world around us (which must include our bodies) is material or non-material is a further question, which we can set aside, especially as the very meaning or definition of the word *material* or *matter* (as opposed to *spirit*) is precisely what is questioned by the physics of the double slit experiment, and, we recall, by Pauli, who asserted that the unconscious psyche and matter are not two things. But we do have to beware the temptation to reject a right idea simply because it shallowly resembles a wrong one. Perhaps Descartes' discredited idea is not wholly wrong but simply needs adjustment, a bringing up to date. Did not the whole of physics, as it stood just before 1900, need adjustment, including even the ideas of the great Newton? And, after they had almost all been adjusted, were they not reinstated, but now as limiting cases of the new relativistic and quantum physics?

The bold conjecture, which we now rephrase a little, is this: In the sense that is valid in the realm of our Being-in-the-world, matter comes into being only as it is observed. This strongly suggests that the observer, if a being with even the smallest degree of freedom of will (which would make it a Being), will also prove to have a commensurate executive power. We shall say more on this in the appropriate place. Meanwhile, we acknowledge the apparent recklessness of reasserting a supposedly discredited view in an educated world dominated by twentieth-century philosophy, but cite the evident indifference, for the quantum entities themselves, between what the human consciousness describes as observing or measuring, on the one hand, and, on the other, being

intercepted by other particles or waves. What happens to the quantum entities themselves is the same, as scientists and philosophers will agree, vehemently resisting any claim that particles are aware of what happens to them, and resisting still more the notion that, being aware, particles react according to whether there is, in some instances, a mind manipulating them or they are merely being jostled by mindless, random movements of other particles.

But did we not find that, while an automatic movement will occur if any object strikes the human knee in a particular way, what we think of as human will can also lie hidden behind that effect? It proves nothing against belief in a multileveled cosmos influenced by Will that examination of the knee's jerk by the physicist, acting within his or her circumscribed world, would yield a merely material explanation that excludes both the doctor's will and the patient's permission. That circumscription of science's frame of reference, noted by Dingle in the hope that it would one day cease, has had pernicious effect, for even more to be rejected, many physicists and philosophers would say, is the notion that some Great Mind fills the universe and that, therefore, no collision of particles is entirely devoid of Mind's awareness or even control. This notion, however, is entirely acceptable to many other scientists. True or not, such conceptions presuppose a physical world that is not causally closed, but *can be interfered with from outside itself as normally defined.* This is a notion of huge importance, and we draw attention to it in preparation for a fuller development later in this chapter. So, at their own level, particles and waves seem unaware of us as possible causers of their motions, and, indeed, we seem to cause relatively little change in the world, but while we do seem aware of the physical world before us, and sometimes act upon it, it shows no evidence that it sees us as we "cause" events to occur in it. Perhaps we are missing something, a kind of mindliness unlike ours and indiscernible by us, at work in the physical world, but what we *cannot* miss is that there is a *difference* in the way of being of the material world and the way of being we, including cats and dogs and every entity we recognize as living, experience.

However, the uncontrolled, uninfluenced actions of particles are not without nonrandom effects of their own, for understanding wave and particle interactions shows us how what we see as solid objects come into being and hold together. Their particles perpetually react with each other, as if measuring each other, *creating* each other's positions and speeds, and, as energy particles are continually exchanged, the *group* energy, the *potential object's* speed and position, a macro-world phenomenon, becomes equalized and coordinated throughout the *aggregating mass* of particles, so that the solid thing *thus coming into being* does not fly apart but begins to move as one chunk. Crystallization is an easily imagined instance of this. Each particle's neighbor particles are "looking at it" and so drawing the entity together *as* what we, on observing it, shall *see as* an entity. This aggregation takes place in precisely the same way, and the whole physical world coheres, by such "forces," whether *we* observe it or not. With regard to the question of the fundamental existence of the physical world, the world that is to us our world-about, we are superfluous, our we-ness *as* observers being outside the world of physics per se. Coherence between particles by physical forces is also the guarantee of the persistence of physical entities, whether *we* are looking at them or not. *Their particles are "looking at each other" and do not need our conscious (or unconscious) regard to hold them together.* This suggests that most philosophical questions concerning the existence of the external world and of the necessity or otherwise of an observer of it have been ill-founded, and the solution to the alleged conundrum might well be provided not by the philosophy, which has hitherto failed to solve them, but by science, and, indeed, turn out to be strongly dualistic. This chapter will show that the recent failure of dualism to satisfy some minds is not the result of its having been tried and having been shown to fail but that the versions tried have been too weak, too much like the hylic pluralism of much earlier cultures than ours. It is the strongest possible dualism that succeeds, providing the deep explanatory power (to use Popper's phrase) that the problem needs. We look at the physical universe *via* our sensory bodies, but that *observation process alone* does not normally affect the physical world itself because the observer is not itself part of the physical world.

Alternatively, the view would have to be that while our observing minds are indeed in-the-world, in both the everyday sense and Heidegger's sense, that very fact would imply that within that physical world which is "external" to ourselves there is a greater mind sustaining it in its physicality. We could not protest that there can be no such mind because we do not see or otherwise sense it, for our own minds are also undetectable by our senses. Perhaps it is in the nature of minds to be invisible, unamenable to the five bodily senses, and this, too, is rational, for as we conceive it, it is the mind that *uses* the senses. Mind is not itself a sense organ, or even one of the senses; it is, however, in some real sense, the Senser of the sensible. Thus, as we have said, dualistic and antidualistic interpretations coexist as *perspectives upon* a Whole Being that seems multilayered.

We shall raise later the question of whether our *intentional mode of being* can affect the physical world. More relevant here is the belief that the whole physical universe seems to be connected and made whole *by its own internal self-regard.* This is what we have called an interdependency of being, and the physicists' conception is not entirely new, for in the Indian traditions this self-observing unity was Indra's Net, imagined a very long time ago. We could say that the physical universe *is* because it *sees itself.* As we conceive this, suddenly the oddity of the strange loop falls neatly into place, though, we believe, by showing the notion flawed. The whole long-problematical idea of causality (grounded in our wrong conception of time) dissolves, becoming that same *mutuality between being and being caused to be* which we have advocated in its place. It would, of course, be better to say "being and being seen to be being," for that expression, though still imperfect, does at least remove the offending idea of linear, temporal, causation that our awareness of the timeless has now called into question. The implications of such a view are vast, and this complex chapter, as it rolls forward, seeks progressively to open up such a view, giving reasons, so eliminating any strange loops that are merely products of miscomprehension while preserving those few, if any, which by their reality maintain their necessity.

In pleading for the reader's patience we point out that it is humanity's physical-world inability to grasp conceptions *straight-away-as-a-top-down-AND-bottom-up-whole,* and the linearity of verbal language itself, which require this fugue-like, reiterative, cyclical development of the ideas. We cannot say everything at once, and, language and imagination being the imperfect tools they are, what we do say, at each stage, is incomplete, or only approximately true. Heidegger wrote *Being and*

Time in this way, unable to expound the whole of a new view in just one process. He continually returned later to matters that, perforce, had been only partially elucidated earlier. The whole history of human culture has developed in a similar "rotatory" way, competing interpretations of our cosmos gaining approval and losing it as further understanding accepted new views of ideas earlier discarded. Our contention is that opposing views will often both prove true, their consistency with each other obscured meanwhile by their incompleteness and lingering inaccuracy, so, at every stage, modifications are required. What matters, then, is the timeless, perspectiveless, and integral understanding toward which this chapter is heading, and which, we trust, will justify its slowly evolving form, and the reader's patience.

The evidence is that the physical world as understood by Newton is largely predictable, but not causally closed, the world of the broader physics now being built by both theoretical and experimental physicists still less so. The distinction to be made between one quantum interaction and another is not in the physical world per se, for we detect no difference *there,* but rather in their primary causation, for some interactions are, we believe, chosen by or even grounded in our conscious intentionality, which is itself accompanied by our sense of the genuineness of our freedom of choice. That polarity, alone, without recourse to any other notion, is more than sufficient to suggest the presence of a part-to-whole duality. The Heideggerian Being-in-the-world we have often mentioned is describable as dipolar and as showing a difference of consciousness between Beings at its one pole and its evidently less-aware components, such as *things-for* (German *zeug*), which exist at its other pole, which is the world-about. This very conception bespeaks both our intentionality and what some would immediately term our matter-spirit dual constitution. We, as the reader will recall, decline to use those terms in that prescriptive way until doing so has become unavoidable.

The question remaining open is whether this duality is to be regarded as emerging as a strange loop from the physical world alone, for it is believed by some to be a product of complexity, consciousness being merely a by-product of that complexity, or whether the duality results from an infiltration into the physical world of something higher, which, being already a consciousness, shows a supervisory and downwardly executive capacity in that world? Will the physical world itself afford us any clue as to which view is correct? En route to the offering of an answer we must now circle back and resume the laying of sound scientific foundations.

Schrödinger's Wave-World

Accordingly, as our next step forward we return to Erwin Schrödinger. As all the great scientists have been well aware of the philosophical questions and implications arising from their work, and have given answers, returning to Schrödinger is a more reliable next step than any offered by philosophers who are not also scientists, and who therefore rely too heavily upon language and linguistic linear logic, so losing touch with the realities they claim to analyze. We have already noted that Schrödinger's equations describe a wave-world entirely compatible with Heisenberg's particle-world, which fact provides a degree of mutual corroboration of each theory by the other. The results of double slit experiments not only support the correctness of both theoretical descriptions, but even show under what circumstances each will be instanced in any experiment. Yet further, the double slit results are compatible with the notion that wave and particle are not merely mutable the one into the other but that the physical world is carrying out such mutations perpetually.

However, that last verbal construct is not as accurate as we would like. We would rather say that the physical world *is in its very being* a seething mass of mutations of that kind. It is *itself* a wave-particle dual entity. Some waves become particles, and waves of light, which we consider to be energy, and particles of matter, themselves crystallized out from energy, interact to make the physical world. Particles also revert to their wave state continually, as their circumstances allow. (Even these careful statements are inadequate, but for the moment we shall be content with them.)

This being the nature of the physical universe we wish to know the consequences for our search for a subtle body of the commutability of waves and particles. Earlier, we characterized Schrödinger's mathematics as describing the future evolution of waves, and hinted at a relationship with Heisenberg's notions of an *inherent* uncertainty in the physical world. The uncertainty of outcome is indicated in Schrödinger's equations by the fact that they each have no *single* result. They predict only the probabilities of a wide range of *possible* outcomes.

They predict them precisely and deterministically (which is *not* inconsistent with the probabilistic nature of the equations); but solving a Schrödinger equation gives no single numerical quantity, and so predicts no single, determinate real-world outcome. The solution stops short of specifying, let alone causing, any one reality. It gives a "superposition" of many *possible* outcomes, each of which has a different, specific and calculable, *probability* of becoming actual, and, as the wave evolution proceeds in the real world, the "pile" of resultant waves, being waves, even interfere with each other to provide whole ranges of other potential outcomes. The situation is vaguely like the sounding of the diminished triad in tonal music, which produces an emotional hesitation, a pregnant pause, a taking stock before proceeding, which can be resolved by going *almost anywhere*. Not only do Schrödinger's equations each allow or offer a very wide range of final realities, but they refuse to *choose* any of them, as the double slit experiment shows, for the wave evolution requires an interception from *outside* its own "waveness" to *actualize* any of the possibilities in the material world.

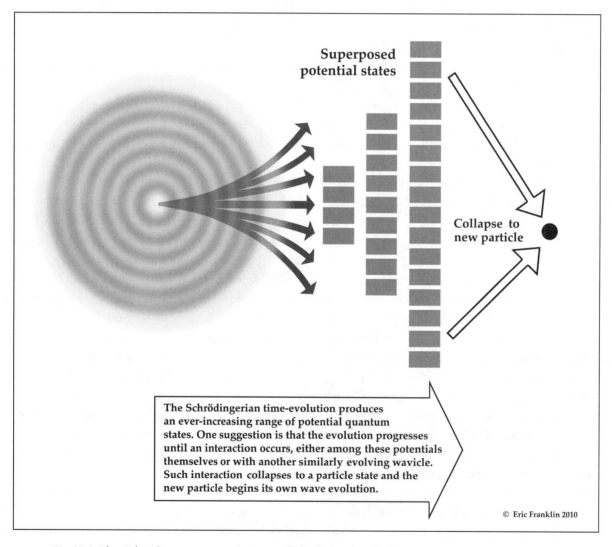

Superposed potential states

Collapse to new particle

The Schrödingerian time-evolution produces an ever-increasing range of potential quantum states. One suggestion is that the evolution progresses until an interaction occurs, either among these potentials themselves or with another similarly evolving wavicle. Such interaction collapses to a particle state and the new particle begins its own wave evolution.

© Eric Franklin 2010

Fig. 15.4. The Schrödinger wave evolution is difficult to elucidate graphically. This is our attempt to illustrate the development over time of that multiplicity of possibilities which awaits the interaction in the physical world that will render one of them "real" as a particle. Of course, by far the most probable outcome in most instances is the *persistence* of the particle out from which the original wave evolved. In such cases, when no interaction with another developing wavefront is offered or accepted the original wavefront interacts within itself and collapses back to the original particle. A new wavefront then emerges and the cycle can, in cases such as the unreactive atom of gold or platinum, continue almost indefinitely without change in the source particle. This illustration should be considered in conjunction with figure 15.5.

The Deep Heisenberg Uncertainty

Heisenberg's matrix mechanics shows how measurements of the positions, speeds, and so on of the postulated entities we call particles are influenced, even falsified, by other measurements. Schrödinger's wave mechanics relates to the alternative postulate of waves by describing their evolution over time. The two descriptions are compatible, and seem to be equivalent, and they also *seem to be* equally valid as mappings onto *reality*, but Heisenberg, Schrödinger, and many others questioned what reality it might be that lay behind their mathematical formulations. They considered the question of whether their mathematical or visual or even merely verbal attempts to parallel observation by devising such descriptions was producing descriptions of *real events* or was merely furnishing parallels, which might make correct predictions while in fact showing no valid correspondence with reality. Such hypotheses could be considered successful only in a merely *instrumental* sense. They would work as predictors, as a clockwork mechanism with a circular dial and two pointers works as a teller of the position of the sun on cloudy days, when you could not just look and see, or at night. The scheme of the Ptolemaic universe with its complex planetary motions

was merely instrumental in this sense. While it was a perfectly good instrument of *prediction* its *explanatory* power was *zero*. It would tell you where and when any particular planet might be seen in the sky, but it had no power to explain how or why this would be the case. There was another problem in devising descriptions of reality. Reality has always been bigger than theory. We could make statements about reality, but no bundle of statements ever amounted to the reality itself. In fact, the chasm between description and reality even related to the ancient problem of hylic pluralism, the question of *what it is* that the matter of the world actually *is,* and of whether there was, in addition, something quite different, which we would call spirit. We cannot delay here to remind the reader of all the hypothesized levels of reality and unreality the human mind had conjectured over the millennia. Some sense of this will be gleaned from the rest of this book. But looking out upon the world and realizing that it yielded less knowledge of itself than was, hypothetically, there to be known suggests a hiatus of being between our world and ourselves as Seers. That curious fact relates to our quest for the subtle body, but we must return to Heisenberg.

Fig. 15.5. Interactions between waves in the Schrödinger probability-wave evolution produce particles. Measurements made "within" or "amid" these processes are uncertain, this uncertainty being Heisenberg's concern in devising his matrix mechanics to define mathematically the impossibility of accurate simultaneous measurement of all the related parameters. A main concern was whether the uncertainty resulted from a feature of the evolving *reality,* or was *nothing more than* a problem of *measurement.*

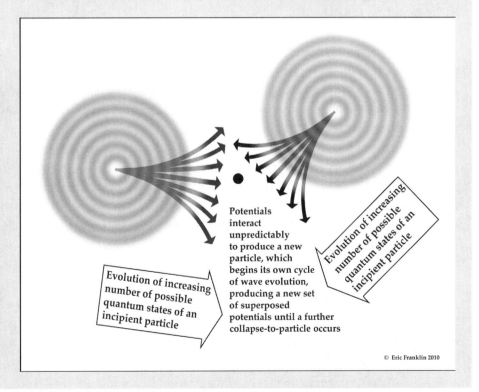

Evolution of increasing number of possible quantum states of an incipient particle

Potentials interact unpredictably to produce a new particle, which begins its own cycle of wave evolution, producing a new set of superposed potentials until a further collapse-to-particle occurs

Evolution of increasing number of possible quantum states of an incipient particle

© Eric Franklin 2010

He faced the whole range of questions as to what should be considered *real*. He could not be content with producing a piece of mathematics that was only instrumental. The *postulates* were particles and waves, and we had observations, though some of them were surprising, and now we had mathematical descriptions that seemed to fit. But had we got the *postulates* right in the first place? Was it legitimate to work backward from a mathematics that fits observations to regarding as real that entity of which the mathematics would be true? Reality, *at least as we perceive it*, seems to hover between the two states of matter and wave, and to be an ever-changing mixture of them. However, there is a circularity, for our ways of *perception* of reality influence our *conceptualizations*, and our *conceptualizations* influence our *perceptions*, and so modify our scientific postulates and hypotheses. Then there is another circularity, for we are trapped within the small circle of our powers of observation, our imagination, and our intellect, and even though we are here-in-the-world-of-our-own-Being we cannot even fully observe the world in which we are. This is surprising, if our *whole* nature is physically material. Would we not have expected to be able to observe *everything,* or if not to observe everything then to be *unaware* that there might be anything that we could not observe? We are undoubtedly limited, but we are not *so* limited. We do have senses, and imagination, and intellect. The facts, then, seem rather the other way: we *do* realize that we are, in some sense, capable of "seeing" far more than our living here-in-this-physical-world allows us to see. The very occultness of the physical, which is so apparent regarding our present topic, suggests strongly that we as observers are permitted by our physical senses only a very limited view even of *our own* world-about. This, too, seems to support a dualistic view of our total Being, for we are clearly distinct from the world, and, again, we must return to the physics.

What we conceptualize as matter is what we experience as solid, even if so finely divided as to be sensed as gas, the atmosphere being an ever-present example, while the postulated *non*material cause of the movement of matter is named energy.

However, these macro-world crude, everyday distinctions fail utterly when we extend our bodily senses using instruments capable of far finer perception of, or interaction with, the world than our bodily senses give us. When we use such equipment we find that energy can appear as waves or as particles, and matter likewise appears as waves or as particles. Special relativity theory predicted not just this *similarity* between the dual phenomena of waveness and particleness but an even deeper *equivalence* of matter and energy, and experiments (such as the uranium bomb) confirmed this equivalence. So what we had formerly conceived to be distinct entities, energy and matter, are, in fact, not merely of similar, seemingly dual, kind, but are even commutable the one into the other. However, our *understanding* has never yet succeeded in replacing the matter concept and the energy concept with any other *single* concept, and therefore our understanding *itself*, with its various verbal, numerical, and visual re-presentations of what is being understood, oscillates among paradoxical, conflicting conceptions and puzzling notions. Why is this? Is the duality only in our limitation in perceptive powers, or in that which we perceive, the real world-about? The concept of wave-particle duality and the concept of matter-energy duality are *inventions of the Being out of whose consciousness those concepts have arisen*. Further, we note that our mathematics, in Heideggerian terms the *zeug* or "thing-for" of all measured physics, its ground and chief tool, supports *both* the notion of particles and the notion of waves. The hypotheses of Schrödinger and Heisenberg *each* describe *only one* conception, but *both* conceptions make testable, reliable predictions in the world, the one for waves (whether of matter or of energy), the other for particles (whether of matter or of energy). The wave-particle duality thus shows itself more fundamental than, indeed to be the ground of, the matter-energy duality, which, as we have pointed out, is in part a delusion suffered by humans on account of the differing modes of operation of their bodily sense organs. We shall therefore concern ourselves here only with wave-particle duality since it applies to both matter and energy.

Support from two branches of mathematics

(the matrix mechanics of Heisenberg and the wave mechanics of Schrödinger) suggests the reality of the entities postulated by *both* the wave conception *and* the particle conception, and, indeed, the truth of both those conceptions. *Both* are to be recognized as products of our *Being-in-the-world,* yet they also seem to be what we usually describe as "objectively real." What we "see" as an external reality is, to some degree and in some ways, decided by our Being, but the duality in the world-about seems real, not merely a mispercept of our imagination. It is probably not by mere chance that Heidegger's *Being and Time,* a book that explores the phenomenon of our Being-here, was written at precisely the point in European history when Schrödinger's wave mechanics and Heisenberg's uncertainty principle came into being, namely the middle 1920s. Ideas, sometimes approachable from widely diverse starting points and expressible in either or both mathematical and nonmathematical media, are "in the air" at the same period, and, in due course, show themselves to be facets of one truth. So we have, yet again, a unity in duality and a duality in unity, namely the physical world of waves and particles, and a part-to-whole duality, our Being-here-in-that-world. The mixing and oscillating interchange of these two apparently real states, particle and wave, *in that same physical world in which we have our Being-in-the-world* suggest a *real,* and deep, indeterminacy within ourselves as *Beings-in-the-world-who-observe-the-world.* This, then, is the deep Heisenberg uncertainty *as it shows itself to us in the world of our Being.* It is present in the physical world, but it is also present in us *as physical beings,* in either the very same way or in an analogous way. The physical world itself is dual, in this way, while the "we" who observe the physical world do not observe it either completely or directly, and therefore may be of yet another nature, producing yet *another* duality, between that observing "we" and the world. We, who observe, may not be *necessary* to the instant-by-instant evolution of the physical world, but we *are* certainly *involved in* the evolution of the physical world, not least as agents of change in it. This, too, is a dualistic picture, and, we believe, just as unavoidable as the wave-particle duality and the part-to-whole duality of *Being-in-the-*

world. We, whatever we may prove to be, are in a part-to-whole duality with the *world-about.* We must return from our *conceptions of* physics, and of ourselves in the physical world, to physics *itself* as *mathematics* reveals it.

The Schrödingerian wave evolution is conceived as the development "over time" of an ever-expanding three-dimensional sphere of the energy that is the equivalent of, and the prerequisite for the formation of, a particle of matter. Our illustration, by contrast with the four-dimensional evolving reality, has to be both two-dimensional and static. This is not the only problem of representation. It needs to be understood that a process that is extremely difficult for physicists themselves to describe or conceive, whether in verbal or mathematical or visual terms, is even more difficult to describe and illustrate graphically for the general reader. We trust that those who ponder our figures 15.4 and 15.5 will forgive their unavoidable inadequacies. The mathematician and theoretical physicist Roger Penrose, who, writing for those who already have a knowledge of the science, succeeds magnificently in his *verbal* endeavor, discusses, in section 6.8 of *Shadows of the Mind,* the possibility that an interaction between two sufficiently different superposed states-of-*potential,* that is, states of the ongoing ever-expanding sphere of Schrödingerian *probability*-waves (see fig. 15.4), produces a clash (our word) sufficiently severe to bring the expansion to a halt (our phrase) so that its energy, which cannot be destroyed, collapses inward (again, our phrase) into a real particle at a particular point in space. We attempt here to render such a process of "reality-making" visualizable, and with no apology for the unavoidably poor analogy between our diagram and what really happens when, as we have put it, the universe observes itself and so brings itself into physically real being. In conceptions such as this matter shows itself to be as much a process as a thing. As the *process* must be regarded as real if matter *itself* is regarded as real, the moment-by-moment succession of *states* of the *ongoing process* before the collapse to a particle takes place is necessarily also real, but despite being real it is *inherently uncertain,* as already explained at some length. In other words, the process is real but it is a real *process-going-forward-into-the-unknown,* with no *static "lumps"* of realness. The classical concept of solids and pushes is inadequate. The process, *as it is in its processing,* is not merely unmeasurable and unpredictable (for measuring *the process* brings it, just for an instant, to a sudden stop as *a quasi-classical particle*), but uncertain and undetermined in the deeply real sense we have tried to describe. The universe, then, is conceived by most physicists as at least partly, perhaps wholly, undetermined, and as being continuously brought to a determinate state of "reality" instant by instant, by what we have termed reality-making interactions within itself.

We should be careful to note that this succession of instants *is* the process *itself,* the process of *becoming* the universe in its *next, and momentary* future state. This succession of instants is not a process *running alongside* an independently running, wholly separate physical time. *There is no such thing as time.* Time is simply our invention, a vague notion unsurely based in our observations and memories of changes, which take place in our *world-about.* The most primordial of these is, of course, the daily motion of the sun from east to west across the sky above the visible earth. The time of physics *is* the *process itself* of any *ongoing changingness.* There *may* be another time running *behind* the physical world, of which we may be unable to discover anything at all, but there is no time-as-such *within* it. The so-called time *of,* or time *within,* the physical world *is* the *physical world's own processes of change.* The process of making particles out-from an immediately past instantaneous state of the process of changingness and potential seems to take place globally, throughout the universe, and to do so without the intervention of our consciousness, but, being undetermined at least to some degree, the evolution of the universe might be influenceable by consciousness, and with some palpable effect even if the effect be attenuated by distance. However, evidence given elsewhere in this book suggests that such influence is not only real but can even operate *without* diminution over distance. This, if the case, would be an action more firmly inherent in *fundamental* reality than most of the matters with which

twentieth-century physics ever concerned itself. An underlying potential field of standing waves was postulated by the pioneers of electromagnetic theory in the later nineteenth century, but was rarely investigated. Ervin Laszlo calls it the A-field (for Akashic Field), referring to the ancient Indic notion of the ākāśa. Others describe it as a field of potential waves, as the "zero-point field" or as the "quantum potential field." Tonomura's experiment, as we shall see, has confirmed its reality. The ramifications of the discovery are surprisingly wide. If consciousness can wield influence over physical reality—and our experience already suggests that we do wield at least some freedom of will in this way—humans are immediately faced by the challenge of ethics, and without the possibility of denying that the individual's ethical responsibility is global, for we are, *ipso facto,* all globally connected. Heidegger considers that one of the *essential, inherent* modes of our Being-in-the-world is what he terms "being-with with others in the world." These are new ideas, to be examined later in the chapter.

Let us return to physics *per se* and explore the Schrödingerian wave-evolution and its consequences a little further. Unless its progress is interrupted, the evolution is an ever-ongoing expansion. It spreads over time and eventually fills *all of space,* an intriguing fact we should retain until its significance can be drawn out, later in this chapter. If a particle's evolution of future probabilities is stopped very early, either by a clash among those probabilities themselves (see fig. 15.4) or by an interaction with another particle (fig. 15.5) the original particle is, roughly speaking, maintained in being, not dissolving into a newly evolving wave having many future possibilities of its own, though the *quantum state,* the energy-state, of the maintained particle will be changed by at least one quantum in every interaction it experiences. (A quantum change is what such an interaction *is.*) The particle may be "held in place" in this way by that type of physical interaction that we call a chemical bond. This happens, for example, inside a salt crystal, which, as a very large entity undergoing myriad interactions among its own particles, remains, when considered *as a whole,* much as it was in its earlier history. In living matter, despite a great deal of its structure also being crystalline, certain kinds of changes, such as the metabolic processes themselves, take place more freely, opening up the question of whether the complexity of the organism *per se* allows the operation of will, which in turn raises the question of whether that will comes into being and operation only as a part of the physical complexity or has some independence of existence and operation. It is here that the physics finds its next point of relevance to the subtle body. However, if one insists, as some do, that complexity alone suffices for consciousness to appear in any conglomeration of matter we have to ask the further question *how* complexity alone would generate first consciousness itself, and then a free will of a kind the operation of which persuades the system *itself* within which the free movements are occurring that it is *itself* a self that is conscious *of itself as a self*. We could even ask: Whence the *concept* "self"? The bare claim, often made, that this kind of self-reference within a sufficiently complex system is, first, an adequate explanation of the *fact* of consciousness and then an adequate description of what consciousness actually *is* fails utterly to demonstrate *how* this could come to be so. It is mere assertion, and experience suggests it is false. Our computers are full of *self-referring* processes, the type of complexity said to generate consciousness, yet they do not seem to be conscious even to the minutest degree. Hence our claim, against Feuerstein, Jung, and many others, that consciousness is *not* an emergent phenomenon of physical complexity and that a form of vitalism that takes account of modern science is required if our conscious-beingness is to be understood at all.

Prediction of the superposed *probabilities* is, as we must stress, precise and deterministic, but it stops short by offering a range of *open potentials-to-become-a-particle*.

So now the question has become "Which reality, and why?" And other questions follow. Are *we* involved, as part of our Being-in-the-world, in choosing which reality appears? Do conversions of a myriad piled-up probabilities, each "pile" becoming one particle, perpetually bring forth, quantum instant by quantum instant, the world of our experience? It seems so, for just such *singleness* of reality is precisely what *our* reality *is,* for it is a *single* situation that we experience as our everyday world. "Singleness," as we apply the word here, seems an inherent characteristic of *our* experienced reality. We do not see the moon simultaneously in two or more places in the sky, nor see two cars on the drive with the same registration number, though, interestingly, we can *imagine* both those situations, showing that our directable awareness is *not* fixed as the physical world is fixed. It is as if our Being lives in the Schrödinger equation, *before* the choice of particle-reality is made, rather than in the reality-of-particles that does finally result from the interference from outside. Readers will forgive our explaining that this is a somewhat *poetic* notion, not to be taken as a truth of physics (which Dingle showed to be a narrow system of explanations) but merely as that way of "seeing" Ourselves-in-the-world which might be correct in portraying us as a kind of Being who is, at least to a degree, "above" or "outside" the world in which it lives, and therefore able to influence its future. Which reality and why may in many instances be decided by us. How would this come about?

The mathematical descriptions devised by Heisenberg and Schrödinger seem to describe the same real process, though each describes only one phase of it. Schrödinger's wave mechanics describes the probabilistic evolution of the waves out from which particles emerge and back into which they eventually evaporate. Heisenberg's matrix mechanics describes the measurability of the states of the particles. Despite the overwhelming probability that they describe aspects of one complex process, we humans find ourselves able to picture the reality only as having two facets, each difficult to unify with the other, one being the concept of propagating wave fields, described by Schrödinger, the other the concept of particles in a range of possible quantized states, described by Heisenberg. However, the difficulty is much reduced by the understanding given by Penrose in *Shadows of the Mind,* in which he suggests a process by which the wave evolution expands freely over time until halted by an interference that causes a collapse back to the particle state, the future potentials of which immediately begin to redevelop and superpose as the process continuously evolves yet further. This is mentioned in more detail in the text box on pages 209-13.

If we are to attempt a valid answer to the question of how manipulation of matter by will might come about we must avoid naïve assumptions about both ourselves as Beings-in-the-world and the world-about itself that we see around us. Note how we have put this. Humans had invented, or discovered, the mathematical patterns that had then been found by experiment to fit the observations of what was taken to be an underlying physical reality. Postulated description and interpreted reality seemed to confirm each other's validity, and belief in the famous wave-particle duality of quantum physics became if not obligatory then certainly highly rational. But there is something in the process that we must take care to note. The whole concept is a human (mathematical) view of a human (observational) view of a postulated "reality," which is in fact an invisible unknown. The whole structure of fact and interpretation is, in a very real sense, *internal to and convolved with the human mind that creates it.* The mathematics parallels a *human* view out upon the world, which sees only those entities that can be *seen-as* in some way that relates meaningfully to us as Beings-in-the-world. The *duality in the mathematics* even parallels dualities in our *view of* the world, for the reality of the world-about is one that we humans have found ourselves able to picture *only* as having two facets, each difficult to unify with the other. There are many such dichotomies in the human Umsicht, the human view out-upon-the-world, not least those between matter and spirit, and between self and world. These we deal with elsewhere in this chapter, but note how fundamental to our *way of being* Beings-in-the-world our own nature is. We see ourselves, *our own* dualities, "out there" in the world, but we also see ourselves, our own dualities, *as if* those dualities were deep dualities *of the world itself.* Is all bipolarity, all duality, *inside* us? Here, our concern is a bipolarity within physics, within human application of reason to experience, as Dingle put it, between the concept of propagating wave fields and the concept of particles in a range of possible quantized states of excitation. Penrose's suggestion, as we saw, deals convincingly with this duality as far as its physical-only aspect is concerned. The reader will recall that he suggests a process by which (in our own words) a free wave evolution over "time" spreads and is halted by a "recompaction" into the particle state, the potential futures of which then begin again to reexpand and superpose.

We remind the reader that this duality of *conception* relates to the nature of our *perception,* of our bodily senses, for had their relative sensitivities been different we might never have made a distinction between "matter" and "energy," and so might have been capable of a different conception of what we see as waves and particles. This often-neglected fact has deep significance with regard to our way of being as intelligent animals in the physical world. The wave-particle duality and the matter-energy duality are unavoidable for us as we are constituted. No matter how a Higher Being might unify the two ways in which we are able to see, *for us* the dualism is "true."

The "shallow" second level of the Heisenberg uncertainty indicated that we cannot measure both the momentum and the position of a quantum-scale entity with high precision because measurement of the one disturbs measurement of the other. With Schrödinger's description of wave evolution in mind, we see that there is a far more fundamental unfixedness. The world is waves until an event of observation/interaction/measurement produces particles. As we have seen, these are, physically, all the same kind of event, though we stand as observer to some of them. Until such an event, until a "reality-making," there are no quantities to be measured. There is no precise position because there is no particle. Waves extend throughout all space, so cannot have definable position. They are "fields." Only a particle, a "mass point," has position. Its position varies with time, so the particle is also said to have *momentum,* imparted to it by any *energy,* any photon, it has absorbed. Photons, alias electromagnetic energy waves, have (we could say they inherently *are*) energy-of-movement, moving at the *constant* speed of light until impeded by or absorbed into matter. Matter, by contrast, might be described as "energy frozen into thingness." So the momentum of any particle is produced by the electromagnetic wave that has been absorbed by it, so causing it to move, the energy that, as it was absorbed, overcame the *inertia* of the *stationary* particle.

Being-in-the-world

Heidegger's *Being and Time* is a long and difficult work, originally in a German that is often idiomatic and, beyond that, even strains the conventions of grammar, revives old usages, and creates neologisms in its attempt to convey insights of great subtlety, which current language cannot encompass. It subtly adjusts, rather than destroys, intuitive vernacular perceptions of our existence and nature in such a way as to show that our Being—in the original the word is *Dasein*—is a unitary, yet complex, consciousness that includes, rather than merely observes, the world that surrounds us and into which we find ourselves thrown. This consciousness suffers angst on account of its sense of vulnerability, as if knowing that here in this world it is far from home. In the world we each have an "ownmost" mode of being, which is uniquely true-to-self, and a social mode which Heidegger styles the "they-self." (Please see also fig. 15.14.) Accordingly, one of our modes of being is, he says, "being-with with others in the world." Our world *itself* is not so much a totally separate physical substrate for the life of an embodied soul (though we believe this ancient intuition to be nonetheless fundamentally correct) but is *itself constituted by* our perceptions of and relations with it. Thus, according to Heidegger, each Dasein, each *essential Being,* is, in the *practical* realities in which it finds itself, Being-*in-this-world.*

As a first step toward grasping Heidegger's conception we could say that each of us is constituted as a being by being "there" in the *existential* sense in which we say, even of an idea, "It's *there*—you can't deny it!" *not* in the *topological* sense in which something is *there* in *that* place rather than *here* alongside us. This notion of a Being that first *exists* (it is *there*) but then does its living in a world *without which neither Dasein itself nor that world would have the characters that we see them to have,* distinguishes Heidegger's view strongly from that of Descartes. Descartes believed our Being to be a totally isolated, conscious thinkingness, a thinking thing, chasmically separated from a matter-world with which it shared nothing at all. Heidegger analyzes and describes our way of *being-there-in-the-world,* but believes that the prenatal past and our future after death are alike shrouded in the deepest obscurity, and therefore beyond comment. On this question, we assert that

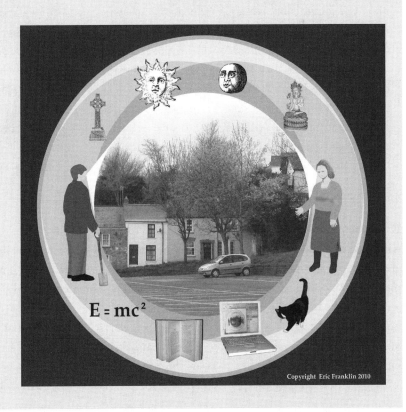

Fig. 15.6. An attempt to illustrate Being-in-the-world

some part of each of us is independently alive before birth and after death and *is* the essential *livingness* evinced throughout the life of each Dasein, which is "thrown" here to sojourn for the "wholeness" of its lifetime in this world. This chapter is assembling some of the evidence for our view.

One does not have to adopt the extreme emergentist position in order to dissociate oneself from the extreme dualism of Descartes. It is the comprehensive middle view, differently, but just as strongly, dualistic as that of Descartes, a view that recognizes dualities within unities and unities within dualities, that finally shows itself to be correct. The view we advocate is that our being is a unitary experiencing entity, but we are *alive* here on account of being Beings whose *natural* "place" is elsewhere, whose *very nature* is *to be,* and therefore subsists in an "elsewhere" from which we are estranged and that, as part of that estrangement, is hidden from us during our angst-ridden sojourn on this planet. This differs somewhat from Descartes' interpretation, but it is *radically* different from any view that believes that life arises from physical organic complexity. Organic complexity is simply necessary if life is to be lived *here in the phenomenal world* (of which organic complexity is an essential feature) and if the living being is to reveal itself to other Dasein who are also living here in the phenomenal world in those organic bodies that are the *only* apparatus the physical world offers for Dasein to be *here* at all.

This account scarcely does justice to Heidegger, and neither Heidegger's concept nor Descartes' lends itself to illustration. Our attempt centers a little too heavily upon Heidegger's contention that our Being-in-the-world consists of our referential relations with what we see (or otherwise sense) as our world-about. He, like Schopenhauer before him, points out that, unless we find that entities have a *relatedness-to-ourselves* as we look out upon the world, they cannot even become objects of perception for us. We simply do not see what is not meaningful for us. We show (in what became, as we worked on the illustration, almost a mandala, capable of being used as an object of contemplation) a representative sample of the myriad things-for in the world, including our fellow animals, religious, scientific, and mathematical concepts, mundane work tools, and, of course, other people, other Dasein, *here with us* in this same world. Thus it is *sense, understood and interpreted by us,* which constitutes our *world-as-we-see-and-experience-it.* While the outer world in its substantiality is asserted, the world of our being is in an equally real sense within us.

This looks forward to the thinking of Gebser, who suggests that our capabilities as perceivers will themselves increase, enabling us to have, for the first time, a greater, more-encompassing, overview, beyond our present discrete perspectives, which new way of seeing will allow the phenomenalization, the appearance, or revelation, out-from the numinous of "new" objects of perception in our world-about. The world itself (understood in Heidegger's sense) will enlarge *as the human mind enlarges.* We believe the new conception will, its current unfamiliarity notwithstanding, be essentially a re-turning, a re-volution, of the ongoing spiral process-of-becoming of the cosmos, a *new* and enhanced Neo-Platonic purview, a new phase of the perennial philosophy.

At this depth, then, the matter-energy duality can legitimately be considered "true," though in any reasonably advanced physics textbook this explanation would be made more precise. Our point is that electromagnetic energy, light, becomes the energy component of the momentum of particles when it becomes *trapped in matter.* This picture has an almost eerie familiarity. The *human* thinking that has given us the Schrödinger equation and the Heisenberg uncertainty principle also gave us, earlier in our history, the concept of an opposition, or at least a distinction, between light and "gross matter." The ideas are fundamentally the same, not necessarily because the universe cannot contain any different structure (for perhaps it contains an infinity of different structures, im*percept*ible to our senses and therefore un*know*able to us), but rather because *we* can think in no other way. In what sense, then, can any such ideas be true? They are true *for us,* constituted as we are as Beings-of-our-kind-in-this-kind-of-world, the only world we can see because it is inherently part of that dipole of self-in-the-world, which we each, and *severally*, experience. This is mere truism, of course, because we can assert no causation in it, but it is an illuminating truism, for, as so often, it provides further information about its subject. It is another complementary sentence, telling us that an A is a B (there can be no logical objection to that), and it invites what is, for many, a new view of ourselves.

When quantum physics was new, in the 1920s, physicists spoke with some embarrassment about the unresolved problem of "wave-particle dualism," as if some single understanding, which at the time eluded us, would, if only we could imagine it, produce a unified theory and supersede the apparent duality. Physicists still wanted a classical kind of simplicity, and were not happy with the vacillating duality of waves and particles that Schrödinger, Heisenberg, and the modernized double slit experiment presented for their belief. In due course the words *wave* and *particle* were conflated as the neologism *wavicle,* as if in readiness for the new theory, yet, nearly ninety years on, there has been much progress but this particular theory has not arrived. Instead, even the seemingly solid components of the physical world have dissolved still further into an unimaginableness far beyond mere intangibility. So we wonder whether a new theory is as necessary as many physicists believe, for wave-particle duality presents no problem to a rational, if unfashionable, understanding of our being, which seems to have greater explanatory power than any other attempt of which we are aware.

Scientists wishing to discover how, in the universe itself, the matter-energy duality may have arisen, postulate an epoch very shortly after the big bang when the ongoing changing of the conditions brought about a "decoupling" of particles (crudely speaking slow-moving matter) from waves (energy, always moving at the velocity of light). With reference to such hypotheses, we have pointed out that all dualisms find unity at higher levels in an analogous way, so our way of being parallels our hypotheses about the nature and structure of the universe in which we have our being. Consider, then, what follows: The duality in our present perceptions may be unavoidable, irresolvable, not merely because it is inevitable *as the fruit of our human thinking* but *because there is a real duality in the universe as it is now,* and we, as Beings-in-*the-world-as-it-is-now,* are the product of that current state of the universe and therefore *think in ways that derive from the real duality within which we live.* This expands notions hinted at earlier as this chapter follows its natural forward spiral.

Our situation of Being-here-in-this-world is, then, a further example of an interdependency of being. The universe seemed, to the ancients, who were totally self-centered, to be human-shaped because they saw it in the way that was natural to their way of being. Today, we reverse this, and, perhaps unwisely, we invoke causation. The doctrine has its nuanced varieties, of course, but most would agree, in broad terms, that the universe, being of a certain design, has bred us as beings (or as Beings) who see it as *it* requires (for mechanistic "reasons"), and this is why we see the dualities we are pointing out. However, the perceptive reader will note how the acknowledgement of dualities is *necessary a priori,* and is not dependent on our particular monist or dualist perspectives upon our nature. Of course, as an "argument," what we are saying is circular, but that is the very point we are making. The *argument* is that the situation being understood is one that *makes circular argument both unavoidable and true.* The nature of that entity, which includes us and which we call the universe, is that of an interdependency of being. The "argument" is, nonetheless, *also* causal(!), for we are children of the universe, and *therefore* we think and "see" in the universe's own way. It contains what we can only interpret as dualities, and we are by nature categorizers, analysts, finders of distinctions, which are, of course, dualities, and of temporal sequences that are, of course, conceived by time-ly Beings such as us to be causal. Post hoc ergo propter hoc is, for us, a *natural* way to think.

We live at a "low" level where there are many dualities, but can imagine the state in which every duality resolves into a more comprehensive unity. The physicist's "symmetry break" is the mathematical description of just such a descending transition from one to two that occurred in the very early universe and seems to have left traces in us. It is therefore no surprise that we find dualities everywhere we look, and, for the same reason, there is no ultimate validity in any argument between dualism and monism. This situation results from antecedents that produced *both* matter and energy as *both* waves and particles, and also produced us (in some sense of the word "produced") as Beings of matter *and* mind who are able to perceive *these* truths, but (at least as yet) no others. We are convolved with our universe, which is convolved with us. This being the truth for us, we may already have ready-to-hand an explanation of our *lack* of a *unified* explanation of waves and particles, and a deeper, Heideggerian, conception of Jung and Dingle's quest for greater correlation between human *self*-understanding and our understanding of the *world-about*. These are indeed aspects of one science, and this must become increasingly apparent, eventually even axiomatic, for any new holistic science.

We suggest that Being-in-the-world is one of a number of new, twentieth-century dualisms-in-unity, a part-to-whole polar duality having very little in common with Descartes' concept of a *total* separateness between being and world, which was a duality so chasmic that even the reality of the external world itself could be doubted. We do not doubt that the world-about exists, but the question of whether it has an *essential nature* we would want to call "real" rather than "ideal," while undeniably open, is unimportant and misleading. Neither matter nor energy is "real" in the everyday sense that the door we bump into is real for us. We must not confuse, in our thinking, the *conceptually* different *levels* of a multiplicity of "realities" that are *all* perfectly real *in their own terms*. This, no doubt, is what Ryle ought to have said, or even really wished to say, but being no scientist, failed to say. What we contend is that, regardless of whether Descartes or Heidegger is right, dualistic views at our level of life cannot be denied. They are simply bottom-up views, to be contrasted with top-down views, which are monistic.

Quantum Indeterminacy and the Possibility of Real Freedom of Will

If the physical world is not undetermined we cannot change it. If we *knew* we could not act choicefully we would not argue for any kind of *subtle* being related to, but substantively distinguishable from, physical being. All events, including our purported free decisions and voluntary actions, would then simply be physical events *not* caused by us in any autonomous sense of the word *us* and the sense of our own autonomy and personhood would itself be a delusion, or, at most, a powerless epiphe-

nomenon of physical being that did not constitute evidence for any such autonomous "us." We must therefore acknowledge the *logical* possibility of our presuming the existence of what we seek, a self-directing consciousness, when we merely *conceive the notion* of an autonomous self without justification from any empirical observation we could make *within the physical world*. Many assert that this is indeed our situation, but is it a *real* possibility that we have no power of decision, as opposed to a merely *logical* possibility? How, if, on their own testimony, they lack the ability to make such an assertion *by choice*, do they make the assertion? They must be caused to make it by the physical world. If so, what is their assertion worth? And if so, our own opposed assertion must be worth just as much, or just as little, and it would be puzzling to find that a merely physical, merely machinelike world would not act consistently with itself but contradict itself in this way.

And there is more to be said. We believe our capacity for decision making is real, for our being able to *conceive* of an "unphysical" freedom, which, according to the assertion that the ability is *not* real, could not exist anywhere within what (again according to the assertion) is a *merely* physical world, would be a most astonishing self-transcendence by that world. If our being and actions really were *wholly* constituted by and *wholly* determined by the physical world we would (ex hypothesi) be *wholly* physical beings who lacked both the imagined autonomy and the autonomous imagination. We doubt whether such beings could have the imagination to imagine autonomy, and believe they would be unable to feel the deprivation imposed by its lack. Could such beings even be conscious, let alone beings who seem to themselves to be makers of decisions? We believe not. They would be helplessly drawn along through a history or causal cascade of mere physical processes of which, too, they would be unaware. Note, therefore, how our sense of possessing a real ability to make executive decisions *is itself evidence of the truth of the claim* that we are *not* wholly physical beings but have some autonomous freedom and power over physics. How could automatons *conceive of* an ability *so alien to* their very *constitution as* automatons, as mere *stuff* complying with the so-called "laws of physics"? Of course, the emergentists argue against this, but our argument is far more powerful than at first it seems, for we should recall that the so-called laws of physics *are themselves the product of our thought*. If we were automatons, the very laws of physics, which (it is claimed) deny us autonomy, could not be relied upon as true, for the laws would then have been made or discovered by automatons, whose evidence we could not trust. Perhaps the responsible automatons *had* autonomy *until* they made or discovered the law that they were unfree? This would be a novel interpretation of the myth of the fall of man.

The conclusion of the purported argument against our autonomy denies its own implied premise that we were capable of free consideration of the evidence. A verdict that we are automatons could therefore not be relied upon. If logical (and probably also real) problems are to be avoided it is intuitively and logically necessary to postulate that we have real choice. Those who want to claim that our purported freedom of will is not real have to claim that laws of physics that we extracted from the world prove us to be *automatons who could not have made such abstractions.* But in fact, as Herbert Dingle knew and every living fly knows, the laws of physics made by inquisitive humankind are *not even* the sum total of the processes inherent in the realm of physical action, and *all* the entities we consider to be "living" are precisely those that give us empirical evidence that they *refuse to obey the so-called laws.* Only some very *flexible* form of emergentism still seems capable of standing against our claim to full autonomy-of-action-within-the-limits-of-the-physical-world and even greater autonomy of imagination.

Now follows a further step. We have established that we are *at least* the *acknowledgers of the possibility* of free decision-making, and we have questioned whether we could even *know of* such a possibility, even *imagine* it, unless, *whether recognizing it for what it was or not,* we *actually experienced the ability itself?* Note what we have now done. We have distanced our own *self*-awareness from the argument, appealing not to *knowledge followed by action* but only to *experience,* to *happenings that happen to people* according to laws of physics (or not) of which they are not the instigators but *merely aware;* and still the argument holds. The very act of mere acknowledgment is itself the *making of a choice to believe that of which one is aware,* and it seems a *free* choice, not least since some *refuse* to choose to believe it.

Here, as so often in this spirally evolving chapter,

we adumbrate a hypothesis we shall develop, adding "threads" as we go, within a later turn of that spiral. In order to explain to our own satisfaction our sense of self we may find it necessary to postulate a reality beyond even an extended world of physics, a reality that is currently all-but-invisible to us on account of the physical world itself standing in our line of sight. The first tree in an avenue might obscure all those beyond, and, indeed, hide from us the living person standing beyond the further end of the avenue, or even between the trees. This is a powerful and attractive image to those who believe vitalism and dualism are not errors, but notions in need of reinvestigation and, no doubt, a little modification.

Even if our consciousness were, despite our experiencing it, helpless or passive, it would be *at least* an emergent property of the physical world, and entitled to *at least* a minimal recognition as a higher-order entity in its own right. The other possibility, an executive self-directing consciousness, riding in, but also above, a physical world of which it is *not* a part, would be better described as transcendent than as emergent. Recent science has already embraced related ideas, as mentioned earlier, for a complex of levels within physics is perceptible in the unification theories that describe how a multiplicity of physical "laws" under certain conditions is continuous, reaching out through the necessary "breaches of symmetry," with a singularity of law under other conditions. This structure is in line with the Taoist conception of the "ten thousand things" as emanations at our level out from the one true Tao.*

Reality and Sign
A Wide-Ranging Exploration

This new topic may seem distant from what we have just discussed, but the connection is closer than might be thought, only an adjustment of view being required for the next stage of our complex argument. Consciousness has long been a maker of signs, and the smallness of our mental capacity, faced with the immensity of reality, has long been the ground of the need to make them. But

---

*In its first chapter the *Tao Te Ching* says of the Tao: "Nameless, it is the origin of Heaven and Earth; named, it is the Mother of the ten thousand Beings." Readers are referred to *The Daoist Body* by Kristofer Schipper, translated into English by Karen Duval, of which details are given in the bibliography.

many of humanity's accumulated signs are inaccurate. We are perpetually trying to separate reality from false representation and false interpretation, so an understanding is undeniably important if progress toward the aims and objectives of this chapter is to be maintained. When a project takes one into new and unfamiliar realms, as our subject may well do, it is necessary to re-equip for strange terrain ahead. Misleading signs from the past must not be allowed to misdirect our present thinking.

Since science is a human construct, both its limits and its scope defined by our Being, what succeeds when applied to current physical theory may continue to succeed even if physics can combine with psychology and biology in the manner advocated by Dingle. It will still be *our* science, the science of *humans* as we find ourselves to be. Many physicists already acknowledge the importance of consciousness within their world, and its importance is not invalidated, but rather confirmed, by the experiential recognition that such thinking arises within our very being. It is thinking of precisely the same *type* as that of the Neo-Platonists, for physicists, too, seek an immanent-*and*-transcendent unity, even if it is now conceived as a "grand unified theory" of the physical world, able to subsume under one entity the plurality of our world as experienced by us, including, of course, the laws of physics, which we have extracted from certain *experiences* of that world that we control, namely *experiments*. Note how this is put, for while physicists hope to describe that world *as it is*, it is recognized that our science is always limited to *making a limited range of statements* about the world, and no range of statements, *even if not inherently limited,* could ever *be* the reality referred to or described.

There are two points here, the existential one and the linguistic/semantic one. We need to be clear about both, for there are philosophers who concern themselves solely with such problems as the meanings of sentences who deny that science is limited to what our senses do, or in principle could, tell us, and their own utterances suggest that they believe that the presentation of a full-enough verbal description could bring about the described experience itself. The artist, the composer, the seer, fall *speechless* (how ironic and how right!) at such willful blindness and such apparently shameless demonstration of these philosophers' lack of the rel-

evant *experience*. How can one prefer a program note, a description—if it amounts even to that—to the performance of the music itself, the living, moving real *experience,* the *real* language, the *real* communication, the only reason the music came into being at all? Music can only be experienced *as music*. Like the joke that has to be explained, music is destroyed by description. Music is music, not descriptions of harmonic progressions and contrapuntal interweavings, not a verbal narrative of its story, or meaning, nor yet is it the score. Again, what some would regard as trite truisms constitute a powerful rebuttal of philosophical error, a rebuke to the very people who most insist that such statements are trite. They are not.

Even though our Being-in-the-world *includes* the world within which it *is*, the mind, that is the awareness we each have of our experience of self, is smaller, having only a limited view upon the physical world, *as if viewing it from outside*. Further, the mind, the consciousness, objectifies its own "subjective" experience, *fabricating* a "Self to experience its experience," which, installing that Self within itself, it then sets up in opposition to the "world." This constructed objectification effectively displaces what Heidegger calls "a genuine pre-phenomenological experience" of the "I," a process that does not remove the physical reality of the world (as Descartes might have claimed) for it is merely a viewpoint upon the world made by the mind's, indeed, by the "bare consciousness's," perception of itself.[13] Meditators will be aware of Heidegger's notion, but might well describe it differently.

This deserves introspection, for one of our main points here is that words cannot, without being pondered, convey what is being meant. Words are *about* some reality, or, of course, are meaningless. Expanding the same point, the mind's higher-level separation of "self" from world-about can never *encompass* the physical *world-as-such*, which it seeks to understand and define. The very process of this objectivizing way of thinking would prevent this even if it were not *inherently impossible* to bridge the category gap between *any* reality and *any* verbal construction. None of us could claim that our scientific *description* of a tree, for example, is even complete, let alone that it *constitutes* the tree, especially when we consider Sophy Burnham's account of her experience of knowing a tree *as if she had been the tree herself* (see chapter 18). Most descriptions would stop short at a record of the color and texture of the outside of the trunk, ignoring even easily knowable characteristics of it that are usually hidden from immediate view, such as the tree's interior structure and chemical composition.

We might name the tree, as if the mere short-form that is its name could stand in for exhaustive personal *experience* of it in its *being,* which, of course, it can never do, though it is failing to grasp precisely *this* truth that has produced most of humankind's still-lingering magical and mythical confusion between word and reality. This conflation is a relic, usually undiscerned by its perpetrators, of an early mode of humankind's consciousness, still alive and arrogantly thriving both in the consciousness of box-ticking administrators and in the unsuspecting minds of many present-day philosophers. In reality it is the same as the historically documented confusion of levels or categories between mere name or representation and actual essence. This severe limitation of mental process is also related to idolatry, to sympathetic magic, and to ritualistic religion, of course. Integral consciousness must rise above such limitations.

As recently as the era of photography people from certain cultures complained, upon discovering that a photograph had been taken, that their souls had been stolen and carried off in the camera. If this were so should not their souls have *felt* themselves being sucked *into* the camera and trapped there? How, after the click of the shutter, and aware of what had happened, did the person remain outside the camera, and able to voice the complaint? Alternatively, how could the person be so unaware of her own soul as to have to *believe,* rather than to *experience,* its capture and abduction by the camera? And how would the photographic print of the *outward appearance* of the person as recorded via the lens *be* the *soul?* Would multiple prints prove that the stolen soul was, since its abduction, now procreating replicas of itself? Would not a painted portrait or other likeness also be a stolen soul? Such level-conflating consciousness is ally to the belief that figurines stuck with pins by malicious minds have not just a psychological power, but a direct physical effectiveness like that of a hammer upon a nail. One might wonder what, in the ancient world of gods made in the image of men, were the real roots of the prohibition within more than one religious tradition against making any molten or graven image to fall down in worship of it.

Confusion of levels has always reigned supreme in the human mind, and to this day lawyers knowingly make unethical use of the proclivity in every court, while poets use it a little more honorably. One of our chief duties now is to sort the levels out, refusing to perpetuate their conflation, or the parallel conflation of sign with reality. The question (at which we hinted earlier but must still postpone answering) is this: Are strange loops (which confuse levels) a *mis*explanation or an *incomplete* explanation? Putting the same question differently, do we have an explanatory schema in which what appear to some as strange loops disentangle themselves, so proving the very notion invalid?

We were saying, earlier, that no description is complete, and still less is it the reality that it describes. In fact, descriptions, we now see, are signs, and, like all other signs, inherently inadequate. Description cannot *encompass* or *contain* or *be* (in *any* sense of those words) the item described, and it is also inaccurate, a mere *mapping,* for the description is words or other symbols, not the *thing itself.* Terrain is not printed paper, music is not the score. The need to avoid improper conflation of incommensurables, which so concerned Ryle, is not merely a matter of language-use, as he saw it, but, far more importantly, a matter of perceiving clearly the categorial division between merely linguistic "entities" and *real* entities. Only when this division is clearly seen could any strange loop suggesting the reality of downward causation by human will come into view at all. Language, as a structure "in the mind"—whatever it is that mind is—may have the power to produce physical effects, but, we suspect, only when consciousness, acting as a causal agent, makes choices based on linguistic utterances, and, in consequence, actively intervenes. This is a looped causation, no doubt, but it is not a *strange* loop. We do not wish to anticipate later developments, but let us tentatively take this view and discover where it leads, whether to a hideous coil of strange loops so intertwined as to defeat all understanding, or to a schema having great explanatory power because it examines all the evidence, holds fast to what is recognized as the success of physical science, and straightens out as many apparent strange loops as it can.

Let us turn back a little way and ask: How did confusions between reality and mere sign ever arise? Briefly, the answer must be that human consciousness in due course created language, but, having made that remarkable achievement, was nonetheless itself so little developed that the *sound* of the linguistic label thereafter evoked an experience *as if* of the reality itself. A verbal sign could never *be* that reality, but for a long time humans living in a state we might now liken to perpetual dreaming confused sign with reality, and we still struggle with the relics of that archaic consciousness. The rightly despised "box-ticking" of today's social administration systems, mentioned earlier, is just such a relic. The confusion between commodities and their fiscal values is another. For eons humans have struggled with their inability to separate *thing-itself* from linguistic *tag*. We still see it in the inability of many people to ask themselves, or even to understand, the question "What *is* it that it is?" The problem is exacerbated and perpetuated, as always, by human laziness, letting words, mere signs, stand in for the *understanding, contemplating, and beholding* of what is before us in the world-about.

Let us here put forth a riddle, to be explained later (though observant readers will also see that we have hinted at it before): the physical world, being self-sufficiently itself, observing itself and *therefore* being, understands *itself* perfectly, yet *we* do *not* understand it perfectly. So might not our failure to understand the physical world perfectly arise because our observing Being is not in and of the physical world that it observes? This seems at least possible, the current intense opposition to dualistic views of our nature notwithstanding. We shall have more to say, for the realization that observation and description, and therefore science, are all severely limited has vast consequences. Here, we shall content ourselves with repeating that science is *not* a complete description of the world, nor ever makes that claim, but only *a record of those statements that we believe we can truthfully make about the world.*

Further, we only know what we know, and there may be more things in heaven and earth than are known in our philosophy. There may be aspects even of *physical* reality with which we could never even become acquainted, let alone gain deep knowledge, though this statement might require a slight redefinition of the word *physical*, to extend it beyond what we sense and know to what we do not sense and therefore do not know, but which may be of a *similar* (i.e. a physical) *kind*. What we mean is that there may be parameters, even entities, similar to those we know and categorize as "physical," but for which we have *no sense organ and therefore no sense and therefore no experience and therefore no concept and therefore no word.* We cannot even conceive what such parameters or entities would be, nor what instruments would measure them. We have to be content to acknowledge that such matters would not be physical *for us*, for (of course!) in regard to any such entity we would not even know *what it is* that we did not know, and we could form no prior hypothesis regarding it that we could then test to prove that it was (or was not) what we had thought. If the physical world has parameters beyond what our bodily senses sense we can never even know *of* them, let alone *conceive* what they might *be*, still less describe them or construct means of measuring them. Hence Dingle's cautionary statements that, for example, "light" and "photons," "electrons," and "waves" are all *postulated* entities, necessarily invoked by our logic if we are to be able to frame descriptions and make correlations between experiences.*

Signs without Corresponding Realities
Perhaps the Most Delusive of All, yet Revealing the Nature of Science

As a thought experiment, we might *try* to invent a "parameter" that has no relation whatever to the sensations acquired via our bodily senses. Is this even possible? We believe not. However, for the sake of the thought experiment, if I were to attempt to imagine something to measure, which is not *in principle amenable to a natural sensing ability of the human body (all of which we already know by millennia of experience)*, I would find it impossible to invest the idea with any meaning not already known; the name I would have to invent for it would be not merely otiose, but fantasy, and probably self-advertisingly ridiculous. It would not even have the reality of a unicorn, for we can at least imagine that species, similar as it is to the horse, the precise number of its horns within the imagination even of a very small child, especially one who has seen a picture of a rhinoc-

---

*See Dingle, *Through Science to Philosophy*, page 292. Readers are alerted to the fact that in the relevant paragraph and almost the whole book Dingle uses the word *molecule* in the special sense he explains on page 50, a sense in which the advocates of atomistic logic also use it. No doubt he hoped to be understood by them.

eros. But if my imagination attempts to enter empty, unobserved regions of the world and I, being no specialist in such matters, purport to invent a concept, and so ask "What is the 'squalification coefficient' of the monoclinic sulfur crystal?" any physical chemist will immediately know me to be at best naïve and misinformed, at worst a fool. There is, within our experienceable physical world, our phenomenal world, no such entity or process as "squalification." It can therefore have neither meaning nor any associated mathematization expressible as its "coefficient." To ask whether there is a third crystalline form of sulfur, additional to the rhombic and monoclinic forms, would *not* be meaningless in the same way, for an answer is imaginable, and might have an observable correlate in the world. But I cannot tell you what "squalification" *is,* or even could be, and my failure is not due to your great knowledge of the crystallization of sulfur (though you may have that knowledge) or to my ignorance of the physical chemistry of sulfur, but to my total inability to *imagine* what *any* phenomenon outside the grasp of my *senses* could be. *So I cannot invest the invented word with any meaningful correlation with reality, and therefore cannot describe it using other words.* "Squalification" does not exist. Nonetheless, "squalification" *looks* very much like a word, but in reality it is not *even* a word. It is an embarrassing, irritating impostor, *pretending to be* a word. "Unicorn" has content, but no correlative in the world-about in the sense in which "horse" has a correlative, but "squalification" has *no content at all* and *no possible correlative knowable by us* (which is why the invented "word" is so irritating to us). Even babies rarely use sounds meaninglessly. As Heidegger claims, meaning precedes words, the contrary claims of some notwithstanding.

So while Wittgenstein is undoubtedly right to point out that language bewitches our thought unless we are careful to avoid such delusion, the far more fundamental point is Heidegger's claim that understanding and interpretation of the world-about arise prior to all language, and in fact bring language into being and use. If there is nothing "out there" (or "in here") for us to understand there can be no understanding, nor, therefore, any words expressing any understanding. We understand the world-about via our senses, and *we* interpret it to ascertain its referential relations with *ourselves.* The world-about is the other pole of our Being.

There are four further important truths to be grasped about the thought experiment regarding the "squalification coefficient." First, I certainly cannot *measure or observe* "squalification." *I do not even know what I would be attempting to measure or observe.* Second, *I could therefore not design equipment to observe or measure the (nonexistent, pretended) "squalification."** For the purposes of science, these privations constitute strong a priori *dis*qualification of the pseudoword. Nevertheless (our third point) the absence of a phenomenon-within-our-world does not preclude the possibility that there could be a process resembling the physical processes that *are* known to us, but *outside* the limited realm of our *experiencing sensitivities,* and *therefore* also outside the realm of our imagination. Then, fourthly, and following from our third point, there could be a subtle "something"— for *subtle* is a word we could then justifiably use—*outside* our physics and therefore outside our knowledge, *yet able to influence our world.* It is *this* mind-opening realization, rather than any other point, which raises the thought experiment about "squalification" above the realm of the silly, and makes it worthwhile. It teaches us a great deal about the nature of science and our practice of it. Moreover, we shall see that there *is* a situation of this type in real physics. We have mentioned it already, for it *may* be what the ancients termed the ākāśa. The evidence is currently largely indirect, though some individuals may have a more nearly direct sense of it, and Tonomura has now demonstrated a related reality by an experiment within the realm of physics of such subtlety that the occultness of the entity has been overcome and physical-world processes that had been obscuring it have been drawn aside. We shall describe the experiment in detail later.

That there could be a subtle entity *outside* our physics and therefore outside our knowledge, *yet able to*

*Readers aware of diagnostic practices such as radionics, and suspecting our opposition, will be much relieved to read what we shall say later. We trust it will suffice here to remark that the apostle Paul says "spiritual things are spiritually discerned," and add that some such discernments are facilitated by *diversion of conscious awareness* away from the true objective of the inquiry toward objects that merely occupy or absorb a meditative kind of attention and so set the unconscious mind free to discern the answer independently, not via the intellect, but intuitively, while the intellect is distracted elsewhere.

influence our world argues for dualism, in our usage of the term, for it places the observing mind outside the physical world, whether transcendently or immanently. It is worth noting, wryly, that Gilbert Ryle effectively admits that mind is nonmaterial, not seeming to realize that this strongly suggests the dualism he sets out to disprove. However, he can do no other, for by removing "mind" from the category of physical entities into a different realm (which different realm he fails to define) he makes it a pole of a duality with that physical world from which he removes it. He would have to admit that the duality, which he acknowledges between mind and physical world, exists whether mind is real or imaginary, immanent or transcendent, part of physical reality or part of a strange (or unstrange) loop transcending physical reality. He consumes over five pages of *The Concept of Mind* giving banal, obfuscatory, and elementary examples of merely verbal unrelated category errors, yet ends the chapter without clarifying the argument he set out to state. Of course, no one can clarify error.

What Is an "I"?

Our being is Being-in-the-physical-world-about, and we are limited by it, but, we suggest, with one important and very instructive freedom. We have an internal "sense of being there *as a Being*," which is difficult to describe because, isolated from other manifestations of consciousness, it is a blank experience. We are "there" *regardless of any other thing or thought*. The sensation of this can even be a listless experience of *being bored with our own conscious being-there* unless we have some focus for our interest, which, of course, will normally use the bodily senses, while the conscious self itself has no external sense organ *of its own,* nor even an internal sense organ unless, possibly, a kind of telepathic sense that might use some part or parts of the brain. No doubt a person who does not wish to use any external sense organ yet wishes to avoid boredom will find him- or herself meditating! We are sure of our sense of sight, for we experience it and can even prove which organs are organs of sight by covering and uncovering our eyes, the simplest of empirical tests, but how could we become sure of an interior, invisible, intangible sense, which no other person can "see" and which we cannot prove "objectively real" by shutting and re-opening its sense organ? We would be trying to look at consciousness *itself,* with its sense of "I-ness,"

which we could not do by "shutting and re-opening consciousness," for how would we observe our consciousness while in the "shut-down" state of *un*consciousness? And no other person can observe our consciousness for us.

Of course, memory convinces each of us of our reality as a self, and of the continuity and development of that self, but Hume found this a problem, claiming, famously, that he could not find any unitary, stable self when he looked for it introspectively, but (in our own words) *found only what his consciousness was conscious of, not any sort of conscious self per se.*[14] But Heidegger's point is that we *are* each of us aware of being a Being in his existential sense *whether we have a current focus of interest or not,* but when we do focus our attention on something other than ourselves awareness of ourselves becomes "transparent" just as awareness of a tool in the hand fades into "transparency" so long as it is functioning correctly. We become "lost" in our own doings and makings. So why would Hume expect to discover anything other than *impressions he was receiving from the external world*? He would discover *himself* only if he were *not* receiving such impressions. He was the Seer of what he saw, but would he *rationally* expect to see Himself-the-Seer seeing what he was seeing (and presumably see Himself within that scene seeing Himself seeing Himself—and so on)? Do our physical eyes see *themselves*? Does the tongue taste *itself*? No more need a self see itself when it sees something or receives any other impression from the world-about. When, by contrast, the self is meditating or merely listlessly awake it experiences itself *in* and *as* its *Being-there,* something of which it *is* aware without focus on anything else. And, of course, no one can deny the additional facts, their apparent opposition being merely a matter of verbal usages, that the self (whatever it is) is *not* always "the same" because it changes and develops, yet *is* always "the same" because for each one of us it is *my* "pure consciousness," not yours. Unlike Hume we see no problem in this, and, for any who still believe Hume raises a worthwhile question, Heidegger explains it.

We are each conscious of being conscious, and therefore cannot rationally doubt the reality of consciousness. The unanswered questions are what consciousness *is,* and what, if anything, constitutes an "I." Earlier, we considered Heidegger's view that no separate "self," independent of the world-about in Descartes' extreme sense, seemed to be required. Here, having moved our own argument forward, we offer the firmer view that whatever its constitution, the "I" may, after all, be more distinguishable and more worthy of categorization as "real" than Heidegger allows. We are searching for the subtle body *itself,* but Heidegger's project in writing *Being and Time* was not to search for the *nature* of our being-as-Beings but only for *the sense or meaning of* our being. His book gives a kind of fundamentally deep psychology of humans as they are, here in the world. Popper and Eccles go further, for they certainly held the view that the self is an *entity* present in the biological system, supervising much of what that biological system does. Both Popper and Heidegger are notable philosophers, so their view of the questions we are posing may be important, and we must investigate, not least because our quest for the subtle body, while it poses empirical questions, does so in a philosophical context.

Heidegger's View of Our Being

While accepting many of Heidegger's insights and schematic explanations as a fundamental, ontological *psychology* of our *being-as-living-Beings-in-the-world,* or, since *psychology* seems not quite the right term, as an introspective survey of our modes of awareness, we nonetheless continually ask ourselves how far, in pursuing the *science of the subtle body,* it is possible to travel with Heidegger, and whether at some point it will be necessary to part company from him. After doubt-casting adumbrations earlier in *Being and Time,* such as numbered section 47, the answer finally reveals itself in chapter 5, numbered section 72, where Heidegger concerns himself with the "historicality" of Dasein (the human being, the Being that is *there*), a broad concept, which, for him, includes Dasein's spreading-over-time, the continuity, unchanged and uninterrupted, of its *identity and essence,* and its *self-recognition and recollection* despite the changes that undeniably occur along the way both in Dasein itself and in its world. Hence, of course, the topic of the "historicity" of Dasein though the word is not a happy translation, as we shall see. Heidegger asserts "Dasein does not exist as the sum of the momentary actualities of Experiences which come along successively and disappear."[15] This seems to suggest that, some of his other utterances notwithstanding, Heidegger accepts the notion that Dasein, the Being that is *there,* is in the nor-

mal sense of the words an *entity* and, moreover, an entity having *continuous* existence, *not* merely a succession of discrete momentary *events* with no *person* participating. The *continuous entity* that he attests *is,* therefore, what *we, in our normal everyday usage, term a "person."* If this is indeed his belief, we agree, though we may differ from him in our understanding of the *reason why* this is the case.

The constancy-and-continuity-of-identity-through-change, along with the question which is fundamental to it of how consciousness appears (as in the Greek word εκ) *out-from-within* our Being-*there* (Dasein), is to this day acknowledged by most philosophers to be one of their greatest problems, "the great mystery" as one of their number once admitted to me in personal discussion. Heidegger agrees with those philosophers who believe we need an explanation of our continuity-of-identity, for he says, "The question of Dasein's 'connectedness' is the ontological problem of Dasein's historizing."[16] A translator and exponent of Heidegger with whom I am personally acquainted rejects the translation "historizing" as obfuscatory, substituting "happening," or the phrase "coming to pass." Philosophers, then, acknowledge that they do not understand how Daseins happen, or come to pass, or how, having happened, they continue throughout their lives to be *recognizably themselves.* What is it that makes *you* continuously *your*self, and *me* continuously *my*self? One wonders why the majority of philosophers find this question so puzzling. We have given a partial answer already, and shall add more, not least because it is surely an empirical question, of which that same expert Heideggerian remarked, "There is very little that is empirical in philosophy." Perhaps, then, philosophers themselves should agree it is not a problem for them to answer, yet philosophers do presume to make pronouncements on the matter, so we need to investigate a little further.

Many contemporary philosophers of mind believe, with Heidegger, that if *they* are to find an acceptable explanation of our continuity as Beings-in-the-world it will depend largely on our concept of time, so we, in this chapter of this book, are compelled to make the briefest detour into that question that will serve our purpose. As it happens, the result is crucial, and unequivocal in its support for our view over that of the majority of recent philosophers, but in expounding this view we must, of course, begin at the beginning. Aristotle conceived time to be a succession of *nows,* which continually arrive from the unrealized future and disappear in an instant into an oblivion, which we call the past. This is a somewhat schematic, abstract, mathematical conception of time, with no psychological component, no influence from any recognition of self. Heidegger agrees, though in chapter 6 of *Being and Time* he reinterprets the Aristotelian view in an attempt to accommodate it to his own ideas. In chapter 5 and the early sections of chapter 6 he risks a conflation, and, we venture to suggest, is unwise to do so, between the *mathematical* Aristotelian understanding and a pervasive *psychological* aspect, which he examines with great insight and at length in sections 79 and 80. The two species of time would be better handled completely separately until they could be brought together in a final synthesis. However, choosing a different course, he first adds to the longstanding confusion in the human mind between personal time-*sense* and objective time-*measure* and then attempts to separate the mixture out again. In chapter 5, section 72, where his concern is our historicality, he tells us that when that long Aristotelian succession of nows leaves a remainder behind in the world the relic passes not into the oblivion, which, according to Aristotle, swallows every now as soon as it arrives, but into history, so *remaining* in the world, but, whatever its earlier status had been, now only in a diminished relationship with us, which he styles its "presence-at-hand." It is, he would say, no longer "*ready*-to-hand," as if for us to *use,* even if it had once been ready-to-hand in this sense. However, there are expert expositors of Heidegger who dispute the validity of his distinction between "present-at-hand" and "ready-to-hand." As if aware of his vulnerability to this criticism Heidegger does make, as we do, a *stronger* distinction between the presence-at-hand and readiness-to-hand of things-in-the-world on the one side, and Dasein itself, the Being that is *there-in-its-world,* on the other side, so acknowledging, though less emphatically than we do, the difference, indeed the polar *duality,* between being merely a present and possibly useful *thing-in-the-world* and being a living *Being-in-the-world.*

Returning to notions expressed in section 9, Heidegger begins section 79 with the perhaps unusually clear statement that "Dasein exists *as an entity* [my italics] for which, in its Being, that Being is itself an *issue.*"[17]

Back in numbered section 72 he had even spoken of "the question of the constancy of the Self, which we defined as the "who" of Dasein," yet if you were to ask most contemporary professors of philosophy, including Heideggerians, what kind of entity the "who" of Dasein *is* you would be scathingly told that the question is empirical, and therefore of no concern, and that in any case it makes no sense because it presupposes a substantive "I," which everyone knows does not exist. One is told that this posited "self" or "I" is like the "it" of the statement "It is raining," and, like the *reification* of the it that rains, the *reification* of the I that is the Being-that-is-*there* is a gross error of the philosophically unsophisticated mind, which has allowed itself to be bewitched by language. In repudiating and refuting this we first acknowledge, as do Freud and all his followers, that nonfundamental artificial, shallow, and *changeable* ego selves are concocted by each of us as a means of survival as members of a pain-inflicting society and as an internalization of parental influence, but patiently point out that these merely psychological *constructs* are too *shallow* to be the *fundamental* entity either we or Heidegger have in view. We are concerned in this book with our nature and constitution, not with the changeable day-to-day modes of our psychological lives. Regarding the *fundamental* question of our *fundamental* essence, our very *being-as-Beings,* we could not more strongly disagree with the willful and extreme claim that there is no self in our Being-here-in-the-world. Heidegger, himself one of the philosophers, affirms its *existence,* as we have seen. Only its *nature* remains to be discovered and elucidated. So we point out first that the use of "It is raining" as an analogical argument against the reality of the self fails on all counts, firstly because there is none of the alleged bewitchment by language in it, but merely a convention of speech, which every reasonably intelligent person already understands. The it of "it is raining" is simply an everyday short form of verbal communication, equivalent to the mathematician's "Let us henceforth denote this complex expression by A," for a meteorological process, which the scientist will fully explain to us, not merely intelligibly but also convincingly, at any level from that of the schoolchild to that of the professor of physics. He will say that the it that rains is the atmosphere, and describe in quantified detail, which can be tested by experiment, those atmospheric conditions that are conducive to raining. He might then explain at a deeper level how an aerosol forms, and how a drop in temperature causes coagulation of its droplets into drops of water too heavy for their now proportionately smaller surface area to continue to hold them in suspension in the air. They fall as rain. The it of "It is raining" is thus a very real it, not at all a linguistic construct that deludes, even though the person in the street could not explain what it is. Philosophers who use such illustrations as "It is raining" as if they supported their dogmatic rejection of dualistic interpretations of our fundamental nature are either dishonest or naïvely mistaken. Nor only that, for they should see without our help how contrary to their own purpose the analogy with raining is, for if it had any bearing at all the reality of the pronominal it that rains would support the notion of the substantive I because a black cloud can properly be the very real and substantive subject of that pronoun, and will obligingly prove its reality by dropping rain on any philosopher who has taken no notice of the sky and has left his umbrella back home. The self is just as real as the black cloud.

So, as Heidegger clearly states that Dasein exists *as an entity* and refers to the "who" of Dasein, our next inquiry must discover what it is that Heidegger substitutes for the continuous substantive self that most recent philosophers have rejected as an illusion. In *Being and Time* Heidegger contends for a view of each Dasein as a *Whole,* which is eventually completed by its ultimate and "unsurpassable" possibility, its *cessation,* its dying. Since, according to Heidegger (and we agree), time "is not," is not a thing-in-itself, the future, the present, and the past of each Dasein must, as Dasein lives, somehow exist "contemporaneously." The reader will understand that we are constrained by language to use a temporal term of a matter that should be described in *un*-timely or time-*less* terms, which language lacks. In this way, being a Whole either replaces or displaces being a soul, but we ask why Heidegger would wish to put forward his postulate of Wholes instead of the postulate of the substantive self, or soul. Are they not equivalent, behind their different names? We suggest that he wants to hold on to some aspects of the traditional belief while withholding his assent from certain Neo-Platonic conceptions of eternity-of-being, which he wishes to circumnavigate in silence. It is a curious fact that Neo-Platonists and their beliefs are never mentioned in *Being and Time,* while the philosophy of Aristotle and Augustine and the much more recent writings of Kant, Hegel, Schopenhauer, Nietzsche, and others are often referred to.

Heidegger has prepared his readers for his interpretation of our being as Wholes, earlier in the book, but, as our conclusion will show, we are under no obligation to review this material. Now, in beginning section 72, he first makes a number of assertions, some very obscure, but explains none of them either by empirical fact or by logical argument from any accepted fact. Then, since he wants to maintain his doctrine of Wholes, which show the continuity and identity over time that is so mysterious to philosophers, Heidegger seeks a *metaphor* (not an entity) that will specifically *oppose* the atomistic conception of time as a sequence of *nows,* which is described by Aristotle, a *verbal metaphor* that will characterize the *continuity-of-being-from-birth-to-death* that is his postulated Wholeness of Dasein, and therefore also the Wholeness of Being-in-the-world, but he stops short of addressing the empirical question of *what* any such Dasein would, in the real world, *have to* be. Putting it another way, which Ryle would doubtless think sufficient, while we do not, Heidegger seeks, and finds, a metaphor that functions, linguistically, *only adjectivally,* silently leaving unaddressed the empirical question, the question of the *noun* to which the adjective applies and *without which the adjective would itself have to be reified if it were to make any grammatical sense.* Thus Heidegger lights upon the notion of "stretching-over," in the belief that its application will *explain,* rather than merely describe, the continuousness of our Being-a-Whole by contrasting the simple concept of an unbroken elasticity, a "stretched-over-ness," with the granularity of the Aristotelian time sequence of discrete nows, which granularity, as we saw earlier, he *denies* is the nature of Dasein. So now we are forced to ask what, qua thing-in-itself, a "stretched-over-*ness,*" apparently a mere quality, could *be?* Are we to accept the silly claim that Dasein *is* a "stretched-over," pretending that the adjective is a noun? It is questions of this grammatically improper sort, not empirical questions, that are meaningless. The obvious and necessary question is "What is it that is thus stretched over the lifetime of Dasein, the Being-that-is-*there*?"

Why do we insist, against the purported vast authority of most philosophers, that this is the proper question? The answer is obvious. In the *real* world (rather than in the immaterial world of philosophers' thoughts) the postulated Heideggerian Whole *has to be* of a different substance from that world itself for his own adjectival stretched-over-ness to apply to it at all. The adjective "stretched-over" is, by Heidegger's own stipulative definition, not applicable to the physical world of the *physical, granular* Aristotelian time-of-the-*physical*-world. If the world of granular time is any kind of reality, no matter how gross, no matter how ethereal, and if time has, by that same definition, the character of *not* stretching over its particles, it must at least be different from any reality that *does* have a stretched-over nature.

Because most philosophers are so insistent in their rejection of dualistic views we must press our argument with an alternative statement of it. However un*thing*ly a thing it was, the stretched-over thing *would have to be whatever it is that the "who" of Dasein is,* which *makes* Dasein, or at least its "who," a thing, albeit a *nonphysical* thing, for *continuous, unbroken stretchedness* is asserted to be the *distinguishing* feature of Dasein among the nows of discrete time. Acknowledging this difference would allow Heidegger to extricate Dasein from the realm of Aristotelian, physical, *discontinuous* time *without modifying the Aristotelian view itself.* However, Heidegger chooses not to take this openly dualistic course, preferring the contrary procedure of *reinterpreting Aristotle* in the light of *the continuity of Dasein,* which he does in chapter 6. The question therefore becomes whether the Aristotelian view that time is a discontinuity of successive nows is correct or incorrect, for this will decide whether or not Heidegger can legitimately reinterpret him in order to bring Aristotle over into his world-of-Beings-who-are-continuously-stretched-over-Wholes. However, it is in fact immaterial in which camp Aristotle eventually stands, for physics has given us an unequivocal answer, independently of Aristotelian thoughts from the protoscientific world of millennia ago. The physical world does indeed proceed by a sequence of halting, discrete nows. We call them quantum states, with *unexistent* quantum leaps between them. So the Aristotelian conception of time *is* a correct description of physical time, and therefore need not be reinterpreted.

However, this view invites the ire of philosophers, for physics is empirical, giving answers that philosophers regard as irrelevant, or even meaningless, at least within their own proper realm. So instead of accepting the rational consequences of his own understanding and accommodating it instead to the discoveries about the world that physicists were already making in the 1920s when he was writing *Being and Time,* Heidegger hurries past to other matters, leaving us to realize for ourselves that the continuity he himself imputes to Dasein is precisely that feature that, if he is right, shows Dasein (or at least some part of Dasein) to be of *different* essence from the physical world of granular time. This is necessarily a dualistic interpretation, but it is necessary to accept it regardless of any interpretation or reinterpretation of Aristotle's sequence of nows. Aristotle is irrelevant.

Putting the matter another way, the dividedness into discrete parts that Aristotle believes is shown by time is precisely what Heidegger *denies* to be a feature of Dasein, so if Dasein is "stretched-over and continuous," *not* showing the discontinuities that characterize the physical world in which clock time, not psychological time, predominates, Dasein, or at least some crucial component of it, *must* be *non*physical. Whether it is a large part of us or only a small part, which is thus stretched over the wholeness of a life, its presence somewhere in our Being is inferable from observation of the phenomenal world. You do remain yourself for life, through all its changes, and I do remain myself. Thus we have the simple truism that a life is as long as the observed livingness of the Dasein in question. Furthermore, in a manner suggestive of the presence of the Heideggerian stretched-over-ness, which can only be nonphysical, Dasein does indeed *remember* physical events that have passed off the scene into history, and does indeed *foresee* future events and states *that have never yet occurred or existed,* yet it is the *impossibility* of any such *nonphysical* entity that most philosophers are at pains to assert. We assert its *necessity,* and, having shown sound reason from the writing of a great philosopher, are justified in seeking it. This whole book centers upon this search.

So we ask whether Heidegger admits as true at least some of the claims of dualists, including the claim that there is a part of our Being-in-the-world that exists *continuously,* not as a succession of indivisible, discrete events, and therefore might even precede and perpetuate its life *outside* its *physically visible* limits at birth and death? If so, he has been misrepresented by his own advocates. Alternatively, is he making a paradoxical, indeed, self-inconsistent special plea for a view that, by accommodating Aristotelian discontinuous time to Dasein's continuous way of being, rather than the reverse, endangers his own avowed intention of proving Dasein's *distinct, nonparticulate, stretched-over wholeness* spanning the world-about of discrete nows? Which way does he want it? He certainly comes close in section 72 to admitting that Dasein is a self-like Being in some intelligible sense when he tells us that "With the analysis of the specific movement and persistence which belong to Dasein's historizing (better translated as "happening," or "coming-to-pass") we come back . . . to . . . the question of the constancy of the Self, which we defined as the 'who' of Dasein." He chooses to refrain from specifying *what* the being of Dasein actually *is*, except that it is some kind of "who," and to reinterpret Aristotle in an attempt to avoid the otherwise unavoidable dualism of admitting that Dasein, or some part of it, is a soul, spanning Aristotle's discrete time by its foresight and memory and its assertion of selfhood. But accommodating Aristotle to his notion of a stretched-over-Wholeness-of-Dasein does not get rid of physics or change the physical world, and the alternative of accepting *without* reinterpretation Aristotle's correct description of (physical) time as a succession of nows also fails to alter either physics or the physical world. Therefore, if the Self, the "who" of Dasein, is (or has) a constancy or persistence that neither physical time nor physical matter shows, how can we believe that Dasein is a *physical* entity?* After so much has been said, this Heideggerian Whole, this (undefined and innominate) "stretched-over," still looks very much like the traditional immaterial soul, if in merely adjectival rather than the appropriate nominal verbal garb. We apologize to readers for whom our argument need not have been repeated.

What conclusions can we draw? Perhaps Heidegger is a dualist who needs to be saved from mistaken expositors. Perhaps he is afraid of antidualistic criticism by fellow philosophers and, as a result, guilty of equivocation, or even of self-contradiction. If that seems unlikely, perhaps he is simply wrong on some points. Perhaps, like Wittgenstein, he is often unclear. Perhaps he is simply very confused, especially in section 72 and related passages where he mixes conceptions of physical and psycho-

logical time, the time of the quantum-jumping, ticking and self-measuring, material world and the time-sense of the consciousness. Curiously, it was concerning this very same chapter 5 of *Being and Time* that an expositor and translator of Heidegger remarked to a group among whom I sat that "The philosophy here is superficial, but it is a brave man who criticizes Heidegger publicly, and I am not a brave man." We, by contrast, do not hesitate to point out Heidegger's errors. It is unsurprising that they concern questions of fact, matters of empirical science, for science was no more Heidegger's specialism than it was Ryle's, and no wonder also that it is precisely here that philosophers themselves disdain to tread, for it is the battlefield on which they have, throughout history, been defeated time and time again by the advance of science.

Leaving Heidegger Behind

We shall continue to quote Heidegger, but with reservations and without adulation, for even his most expert apologists acknowledge that he is not always right. Of course, what we say here does not do justice to Heidegger's *Being and Time* as a whole, but shows only that he is unreliable in those parts of it that concern our search for rational description of and, so far as may be possible, proven truth about our being *itself*. Before proceeding, we add one final reproof to the many philosophers who will disagree with us. It is this. Without empirical fact, a very minor concern for present-day philosophers, there could never have been any philosophy at all. No one could arrive at the truth of our fundamental being without first doing the relevant science, and it is extreme arrogance to claim to reveal truth without first amassing and assessing the scientific, the empirical, evidence for one's philosophical claims.

In resuming our own efforts toward that end we remark that perhaps even our essential "I-ness" has more than one level. Perhaps it is even a strange loop, as many now believe, strongly combining physical matter (the body in the world) with the intangible yet undeniable exercise of autonomous will in that world. What can we say of this? Our being is, perhaps, the "Experiencer of the experiencing of being a Being." Such a form of words has at least the merit of *defining* it without risk of error in identifying its *constitution*, and the further merit of being a testable hypothesis. If

---

*Figure 16.2 is an illustration of the contrast between the two species of time.

we take a further step to discover more we might wonder whether our experience of a private sense of what it is to *be,* and of *what it is that we are,* could be the elusive "spirituality" of which von Franz and many others speak, but about the reality of which many are unsure. Perhaps spirituality is simply what we experience as I-ness when we are conscious, especially when our awareness is turned within ourselves and, for a while, withdrawn from the worldly concerns of the external world-about? Even the body becomes external to the Being in this context of meditative consciousness. So perhaps I-ness is indeed an entity-of-conscious-ideas, *which exerts its will downward upon the physical.*

But *how* has such a Being, if our suggestion is correct, come to be conscious? Let us discuss the notion further, for not all of us are meditators, and the ideas involved here are not familiar to every reader. Might not an *unconscious* machine work in just the same way as a Being if filled with the same data? We looked at the Schrödinger equation and Heisenberg's uncertainty principle, and concluded they might be relevant to just such an entity as a self-aware "I." So perhaps spirituality is what we find when we are alertly conscious, but are focusing on our being-conscious itself, rather than on some external matter or concern; what we find when we *maintain* consciousness, but withdraw from *sensory* experience via the bodily sense organs into a direct experience of "ourselves" alone. The reader will recall that we mentioned this earlier. Note that this self-experience would have the structure of a loop of self-*reference,* self-*observation,* self-*experience,* and so would be analogous to the measurement, observation, and interference that we noted earlier, occurring in the physical world. We also noted that this seems to be the nature of our Being *itself,* but here we see it with that other loop, the physical body, temporarily switched out of range. This is "As above, so below" and the notion is more relevant than we might expect, both to us—whatever it is that "we" shall prove to be—and to mathematics.

The self-examination required to investigate consciousness and spirituality is intractable only because we have not made this analysis sufficiently clearly, and because consciousness is itself the only tool we can use in its own investigation. No wonder our consciousness and our "spiritual" nature have always been inscru-

table, but that difficulty constitutes not the slightest reason to deny the existence of the very being that, unless it existed *in some such functional sense as we have described,* could not even make the denial. Being in a position to make the denial proves the denial false. We saw earlier that the physical world is more a process than a thing, so it may be literally true that each of us *is* the-(process-of)-thinking-that-one-*is*-and-that-one-is-*thinking,* a notion not far removed from Descartes' "Cogito, ergo sum," but one that does not entail his absolute separation of self from world. As always, we acknowledge the verbal difficulties in conveying ideas that are subtly different from long-familiar notions, and, in this instance, cut short the probably fruitless chasing after verbal precision so that we can try instead to *discover by introspection, a nonverbal process, what it is that our Being is,* and from what its existence arises. That such Being *exists* is in doubt only for the deluded or the adamantly prejudiced.

We need to take stock before proceeding. At this point we acknowledge three things: the possibility of what we cannot in principle observe; the proviso that if the entity we have called our Being is not physical as we experience, define, and verbally describe the physical, we shall not find *direct* evidence of it in the physical realm as so defined; and that this very fact, should we find *indirect* evidence of it in the physical world, would be evidence that such an entity does indeed exist, but *not,* indeed, *necessarily* not, in the physical world as we know it. Here, we suggest, is a very important point. The *indirectness* of all evidence for the "spiritual" (except, of course, spiritual experience itself, for the experiencer him- or herself) and the elusiveness of consciousness per se (the very characteristics that lead some to deny their reality) is itself evidence that they *are real,* but *are not* physical. They seem to be above the physical, even to exercise some measure of control over it, and there may also be entities *below* the physical, a notion of which we shall say more.

Returning to our present thread, we ask why we should expect or try to find "Being" or "spirituality" within the world of the narrow study we call physics? Either physics must expand in unexpected directions, though, as we saw earlier, it is impossible to predict how this might be possible, or (we think this far more likely) we must look within a different realm and in a different way.* The ways of the physical world simply will not do. This fact itself supports a dualistic interpretation, the other part of *this* duality being *non*physical, not a polarity *within* the physical, and so able to "think outside the box" of the physical world. Imagination is important, and, as suggested earlier in a slightly different context, perhaps being conscious of "bare consciousness," so contemplating *consciousness itself,* will serve? Is not this what we call "meditation," a different, open, and imaginative mode of being conscious? Gebser would certainly think so. Might not the meditative state be the realm or locus of spiritual discernment, the everyday-physical being allowed to drop out of consciousness, so opening the way of the spirit, whether from a higher reach of *this* realm or from a *higher* realm? Are our present-day categorizations still valid, or do we need to set them aside so that a more comprehensive view can appear?

The Disclosure of Consciousness within the World of Emanation and Immanence

Perhaps we can now attempt a cautious, provisional fitting together of ourselves as Beings who sense ourselves *as* "ourselves" with what our looking out upon the world (our science) has taught us. When a conscious human sets up apparatus and switches it on, so causing an interaction between wavicles that would not otherwise have occurred, the intervention alters the whole future of the universe by an exercise of human will. Humans, animals, even Dingle's living fly, fix the single "real-world" outcome of the Schrödinger evolution, enforcing the "collapse to a particle" of the multiplex of probabilities that his mathematics describes. Our willed intervention "demands" a particle to replace his "pile" of alternative waves. By choice we bring particles out of a cloud of

mere probability into what, in our perceptional world, our sense organs persuade us has sufficient sensibleness to be what we, by reason of that sufficiency of sensation, call "reality." Recall that our *physical* reality is our *sensible* reality, what our sense organs tell us, directly or via instruments, no more, no less. All else is metaphysical, perhaps just as real, but its essence, its "what it *is* that it is," unknowable to us.

However (resuming our argument), to do to one particle what a stone's constituent particles are mutually and continuously doing to each other, holding the stone together, and presumably doing so *without* knowing it, seems a derisibly minute magic power for a human being to boast. What we must note, however, is that this "magic" is inherent in our very nature, for we do this myriad times *in every action we take.* Whether our acts seem small or great they all require us to use a more or less conscious will, which is to some degree separate from, though still *in some sense* within, the physical world. A few paragraphs back we noted our habit of evolving social "selves," each an evanescent artifice of the mind, if also effectual. Here, we see something different, more fundamental, more *real* in all normal usage of that word.

Now we may view matters from the position of the psychologist, the student of the *psychic* world. Doing so, we find a parallel with that "necessity of existence" within the *physical* world, which, at least so far as we can *see* within that world, results less from linear causation following an inexplicable first cause than from *mutual interdependencies of being,* from *apparently* strange loops that question the very notions of time and causality. There are alternative perspectives upon the two poles of our Being-in-the-world. There is our view of the physical world "as it is" (which we call science) and the view of ourselves "as we find ourselves to be" (which perhaps we might call the view of a spiritual science that is not yet in full flower). However, following our present lines of thought we are led to perceive that even the physical world is not *caused,* except in that special sense that the word *cause* was devised specifically to *deny,* namely its own *just-being-there,* and to think that we, similarly, are not caused but, rather, are ourselves causes, agents of free will, of intentionality, here in the physical world, albeit restrained by limits, which, for the most part, that world sets. Left to itself, the physical world acts in its habitual

---

*This might seem to deny Dingle's claim that physics must come into correlation with psychology, but this is not so. What Dingle asks for is more complete correlation of ideas and language *within* science. He is not speaking of metaphysical matters, that is, of any matter that is *inherently beyond* any scientific knowledge that humans, on account of their limitations in sense perception and logic, are capable of discovering. Science can *always* learn *more* facts, but it cannot learn *any* facts of a *kind* that is beyond the scope of its thinking and its senses, extended where necessary with instruments devised to parallel those natural senses. Insofar as the body itself is sensitive to electromagnetic radiations, a fact belatedly acknowledged by mainstream scientists, this is even true of instruments for measuring such radiations.

way, as if obeying laws, but *we,* throughout our lives, act as Living Beings, interfering in the world, not by forcing it to exceed its own possibilities (which are, of course, vast) but to make it choose among those possibilities and so act in ways probability alone would not have brought about. This is top-down causation, abhorred by some philosophers. Very occasionally, we even make the world act in ways that surprise us, for it seems, very occasionally, to act in an almost capricious way. But the caprice is ours if, when this happens, it results from our "obeying" voluntary *non*laws of our own devising. Being here-in-the-world, we are, of course, *usually* passive observers of the world's *usually uninfluenced,* indeed, within-itself-deterministic, Schrödingerian evolution, and our powers of intention are limited, though not extinguished, by the physical world-about. Another facet of the same truth is that here in this world we are *compromised,* our intentions often thwarted by the near-unity probabilities that physics stubbornly imposes. If we are to understand our place in the world we must hold these two scenarios in balance in our minds.

Nothing remotely like these considerations entered the thoughts of classical physicists, and this is precisely why Descartes' view of our being and Newton's view of the physical world are inadequate. They are divorced from each other. So, just as with relativity, just as with wave-particle indeterminacy and complementarity, it has always been earlier paradigms, the preexisting physics, not the obdurate newly observed facts, that had to change, and, about a century ago, we began to espouse the quantum world. It is not quantum physics that is impossible to understand, as some say, but classical physics, for classical physics contains no place for *us.* It must, therefore, be wrong (no matter what our essential nature) and we can no more truly *understand* what is not correct than, as we remarked earlier in another connection, we can clarify error.

Let us try to put all the apparent facts together, and imagine the totality. If the physical world is held in being by its own self-regard through interactions of waves and exchanges of particles, the mind or consciousness (our terms still undefined) now seems just as "real" as the physical world, for that physical world has been shown to be more than a little "dreamlike." But mind or consciousness, whatever it is that it is, has a *kind* of reality that is sufficiently different from *physical* realness to

show not a single one of the normal physical attributes of mass, weight (which are not the same), inertia, and electromagnetic intercommunication. While this fact does not constitute proof of any claim that goes beyond the fact itself, we have already discussed the matter with some thoroughness, and it is therefore rational to conclude immediately that consciousness is *nonphysical*. However, we shall look further into the whole matter, and before moving on we should also remind ourselves that consciousness is nonphysical in two distinct senses. It is nonphysical for the empirical reasons we have been describing, and shall soon augment, but it was, at least until recently, also *nonphysical by physicists' own definition*. As Dingle says, we excluded ourselves and living flies when we imposed restrictions on physics so that we could fabricate a system of mechanistic laws. Only by the correlation between the sciences that Dingle wished for is it at last becoming a matter for a reexpanded and open-minded physics that might accept mind as a real and active agency. Curiously, some physicists, along with a minority of twentieth-century electrobiologists, despised in their own time, have themselves led the way into investigation of consciousness, for the earlier limited physics had itself begun to point them in that direction. While an open-minded physics is now coming into being, we cannot immediately expect an open-minded science, for most biologists still follow that *old* physics and resist what they see as a return to vitalism in the recent wider investigations. However, that resistance is based only on dogma, not on observation. Recall the movements of Dingle's fly and our claim, based on our own observed experience, to be capable of choiceful action. These point to a separable livingness in live Beings rather than to physical mechanism, and, we say again, it was physical mechanism itself that led some to think a broader physics necessary.

The question therefore becomes: What is the *structure* of the living being, and what are its *differences* from the not-living being? We acknowledge that physical complexity is a component of that structure, but claim that it *cannot* be the whole. The reasoning is very simple, but perhaps a little subtle. Certainly I have *never* heard it advanced, though I doubt that my own thinking can be entirely original. A probable reason for the unfamiliarity of the argument is not difficult to find, for the assumption in discussions of the origin of life is *always* the physicalist presumption that it came about when complex molecules were first synthesized. This closedness of mind precludes from the start even faintly vitalistic or dualistic explanations. But the argument is no less impressive for being rarely, if ever, heard. It is simply this: if it is clear that chairs, and even the most complex computers, are not living, while we are, then, by observation and, following observation, by the framing of a definition of living and nonliving that describes *circumscriptively* the observed differences, it will be in *comparing two states of ourselves* that we shall find the understanding we seek, *not* in comparing ourselves with chairs, or even with the most advanced computers, *for they show only one state.* What two states of ourselves should we compare? The answer is obvious: the living state and the not-living state, for we claim to have a very clear impression of the difference. Even philosophers, for whom *nothing* should be obvious, have claimed in my hearing that *this* difference *is* obvious! We shall develop this intriguing view further at the end of the chapter.

Know Thine Enemy
The Science and the Culture We Are Leaving Behind

Before proceeding it will be useful, if also rather sobering, to look back at the physics, and, indeed, the whole cultural milieu of human knowledge that we are finally leaving behind, and to see again, clearly, the reasons why we are turning our backs on it. By an all-too-real category error, some physicists, even today, and most philosophers and biologists, still attempt to explain our consciousness *using the terms of a physics that, as a constituting fact of its own formulation, deliberately excluded from its concern the very phenomenon that is now to be examined and explained.* This is an astonishingly naïve error. By its own self-imposed limitation, science could then give an explanation only of the *physical* components of consciousness (if any) or, more irrelevant still, a *mapping* in *physical* terms of *non*physical terrain. We cannot rationally make this *stipulative* kind of definition of any matter not yet known, and taking the product of any such procedure as a full, exhaustively defining description of any entity restrictively predefines what is to be investigated and discovered. Such a procedure is as silly, as totally off the point, as an explanation of music to the congenitally deaf by means of training them in score

reading. It is no wonder, then, that Heidegger stresses, perhaps overstresses, the anti-Cartesian view that our very being is Being-*in-the-world,* not Being-"*in*"-but-in-*isolation-from* the world.

A Circular, or Spiral, Tour of Human Consciousness

Any answer to the question of what consciousness *is* that the outdated *physics-without-consciousness* could ever have given would necessarily be a *totally* misleading, fundamentally *irrelevant* description of the *physical correlates of* consciousness, *not* of consciousness *itself.* We might produce such a map, a kind of picture, but it would certainly fail to represent the territory. How could we expect to produce a viable explanation of consciousness by means of a science that had deliberately ignored consciousness and whose very "laws" had been discovered only by its exclusion? Nevertheless, and partly by a self-imposed isolation of physicists from other, "softer" scientists, the belief was, for a very long time, that consciousness, if it is to become a subject for physical science at all, must be explained by yesterday's unexpanded physics, and by such physics *alone,* and, of course, by the fashionable reductionist biology, the practitioners of which chose a mechanistic course aping that of the old narrow physics and eschewing any hint of "religion" or "the spiritual." But this presumed what the attempt was meant to test, namely the assertion that consciousness, notwithstanding that it was specifically excluded from physics *because it defied reductionist understanding and because if it had not been excluded there could have been no physics at all,* is, nonetheless, physical *in this same restricted sense.* Please pause to see the huge inherent inconsistency that is lurking here. If consciousness was physical *in the same sense in which the world-about was physical* why had there ever been a need to exclude it? The *pre*sumption, the dogma that consciousness has a wholly physical, or even a wholly physiological, explanation is the grossest of all *logical* blunders, as well as a scientific blunder, yet the vast majority of recent and current authors have continued to make it. If narrowly defined physics could have explained consciousness, music would *be* a pattern of black marks on paper (but with no one conscious to read them, let alone to hear in the imagination the sound itself).

The opposition to the notion of independent

conscious entities mounted by most biologists on the supposedly safe ground of a classical physics that had, by its own choice, no authority on the question is, nonetheless, understandable. The error is explained by Western history, by the huge harm done during the past half millennium by an ignorant ecclesiastical authoritarianism that had itself discarded much of Neo-Platonism and against which a Faustian scientific pride and prejudice increasingly arrayed themselves. This battle, almost surreal because ultimately irrelevant to truth, between two self-appointed Grand Inquisitors, indeed, two bigoted Grand Ignorances, blighted and delayed the scientific investigation of consciousness. Further, the claim that consciousness would be explained by physics assumed, indeed, *pre*sumed, the truth of a view it claimed not yet to hold but to be trying to discover. This further astonishing blunder would preclude a priori both the expansion of physics per se and the very lines of investigation and interpretation that are relevant here, which *further* preclusion would merely perpetuate the vast ignorance on both sides of the battle between ecclesiastical authority and early science. Note that these presumptions are *circular in logical structure,* as preclusions imposed by the closed mind always are. They are *false* strange loops, *wrongly* imputed interdependencies of being. The closed mind *is* one that assumes it is already right and investigates, or pretends to investigate, only in this discoloring light. It is no wonder, then, that today we see too eager an acceptance of strange loops that, seen differently and so exposed as fraudulent, might untangle themselves to reveal the dreaded dualism. We have more to say, later. Here, it is sufficient to remind the reader that strange loops should be accepted only when there is no other explanation, for too ready an acceptance of them itself encourages their proliferation of mysteries that in fact will usually prove chimerical. We saw earlier that if the whole world were strange loops we could have no proper understanding of anything. The very fact that we find them strange should suggest that there is something in the situation that we are failing to understand, so the establishment of a new strange loop always risks closing off a line of inquiry into something not yet understood. This, as we see when we ponder the matter, is precisely the error that ancient inward-turned anthropomorphic science always made. Today's

science is equally anthropomorphic, but over the millennia the human mind has itself expanded, allowing us greater real explanatory power in understanding the phenomena of our world-about. We must learn the lessons of the past, and never close off scientific inquiry itself, nor close our minds to the discoveries it makes.

Such closings-off are, sadly, not uncommon even now. We mentioned earlier the prejudiced ill-design of some experiments. One present-day school of scientists and philosophers does perceive, at least dimly, the blunders we have just described, for its members advocate escape from the otherwise unavoidable dualist and vitalist consequences by denying the very *existence* of consciousness. This is surely dishonest, and demands an even more extreme reductionist materialism than the damaging reductionism of most scientific theory since Descartes. At most, the advocates of such views claim, consciousness is mere epiphenomenon, arising by chance out of the complexity of brains. Some even believe we fool ourselves by thinking of ourselves as conscious. We wonder how any person who understands the proper use of language and has a grasp of verbal logic can hold such a view. It violates both language itself and language use, for those who deny the reality of consciousness do so *by an exercise of consciousness* (how else?). *Whatever it is* that consciousness *is,* and whatever its source or sources, it *exists*. It is *an experience had by humans, and ipso facto an empirical fact*. As soon as you are aware of the *problem of* consciousness you have already proved the *reality* of consciousness within yourself, *for that awareness-of-being-aware is what consciousness is*. This realization is the ground of Descartes' "Cogito, ergo sum," and with a few small provisos it remains valid, despite its many critics. What would not be proved is "Cogito, ergo ego sum," in which the emphatic "ego" modifies the meaning to "I think, therefore I am a Self." This, of course, raises the question of what a "Self" would consist in, and how it would be distinguished from any other selves who might be alongside one in the world. But the reality of consciousness per se is empirically established by nothing more than the experience of experiencing, whether there is an ego self, or any other self-constructed sense of egoistic being, or not.

Accordingly, the next question is: What *is* it that consciousness *is*? Consciousness is as real as Being-in-the-world, which is *also* experience, and seems no more dreamlike, no more unreal, than physics itself, insofar as we can know it, for, as we have already seen, from the time of Newton physics has become increasingly occult and its postulated entities less and less real-in-our-everyday-experiential-way. It is therefore physics that must take note of Dingle and Pauli, and expand its frontiers, as far as it can (but no further). It will then, of course, immediately meet its ghosts, among them the antiecclesiastical and unscientific Ryle's "Ghost in the Machine," in which, like the scientists and philosophers he and others have misled, *he* did not believe (though Popper and Eccles did). It is the ghost, the conscious whatever-it-is-that-is-aware-of-itself, that is writing this book, and your own similar, and very real, ghost of consciousness, which, the writers hope, is enjoying reading it.

This brings us circling back to a question that passed before us earlier, of whether even our conscious will is, in deep reality, dictated to us by the physical world, making us mere automatons *without our even realizing it.* In countenancing the *logical* possibility of our being mere automatons, however unlikely to be true in reality, we must test this extreme form of the view that consciousness is merely an emergent phenomenon arising out of the complexity of physical organisms. As they become more complex, the argument goes, parts of brains are able to act in recursive ways, referring to other parts in a cyclical way, which thus forms a loop, possibly a strange loop, of self-reference. It is asserted that the self-reference is, or somehow becomes, consciousness, though the manner in which this is believed to happen and the reason why it should happen are never explained. This, we suggest, is already a strong clue to the delusiveness of the view, and Popper would agree. A bare assertion such as this has no explanatory power. It needs the reliable witness of stubborn facts. Whatever their disagreements over detail, this is the type of view espoused by Paul Davies, Daniel Dennett, and Douglas Hofstadter, though in our view their attempted explanations all fail, and even within their own camp there have been dissenters.

In *I Am a Strange Loop* Hofstadter writes as follows, and we can use his words as an example for comment.

What drove all this—my core inner passion— was a burning desire to see unveiled the secrets of human mentation, to come to understand how

it could be that trillions of silent, synchronized scintillations taking place every second inside a human skull enable a person to think, to perceive, to remember, to create and to feel.[18]

Apart from the reader's uncertainty as to what the phrase "enable a person" should be taken to mean, this is entirely acceptable, admirable, but for one huge and fundamental error. Hofstadter *presumes* that "the brain enables the person," that all the human functions and experiences he mentions are the products of the human brain. *Was not this the question to be investigated?*

When we turn to the question of what he means by "scintillations . . . enable a person to think . . ." we cannot miss the fact that, having *assumed* that these scintillations in the brain will explain everything he is investigating he has nonetheless also implicitly assumed the real existence of "persons." In other words he has already *assumed the answer to* something that in fact he *must* or *ought to be investigating,* the fundamental question of *what* a person *is,* not merely the question of *whether* a person is. He tacitly assumes the reality of a kind of Being that *we* assert *does* indeed exist, yet on the basis of his own premises he ought to be questioning its reality, for he is *assuming* that the whole of the conscious experience of the purported "persons" consists absolutely of processes in the brain (which we deny). No wonder the link between brain and person puzzles him, for he has overlooked his own presumptions regarding it. Why does he expect to prove a *physicalist* explanation of consciousness (as resulting from scintillations in the brain), which depends on the *same* assumption that persons are real as is made by vitalist or dualist opponents who deny that brain is sufficient? What vitalists and dualists assert to be a hiatus between brain and Being that *they* can easily acknowledge remains, for Hofstadter, the same inexplicable hiatus, demanding, in *his* view, an explanation he and all others of his persuasion recognize still eludes them. Hence, of course, his question. Our own opinion is that his books do not answer it. Roger Penrose, a very considerable mind in mathematics and science whom we shall quote, has at least an equal depth of understanding, and leaves the same question open.

When chairs are physical, but fairly obviously not conscious, we have no ground to assume a priori that the consciousness we show, even though we are physical beings, is itself *solely and entirely* physical. The tentative presumption, the testable hypothesis, should be the converse, that our consciousness is not at all likely to be merely physical. When we examine the work of writers who hold that consciousness emerges out of complexity we find no evidence of the truth of their claim. This is unsurprising, for there is no *independent,* noncircular and nonstrangely looping reason to believe that complexity could, itself, be sufficient. The fact that the presumed article of faith is not being proved is hidden by those of the emergentist persuasion by repeating the *assertion* as often as possible, author and reader alike not noticing the failure to describe any *process* by which a complex machine might, by complexity alone, gain consciousness. The belief is an unfounded dogma, as its endless repetition without proof suggests, its only honorable possibility of salvation being to regard it as an unprovable axiom. But the unprovable assertion that complexity makes consciousness could never be accepted as an axiom for if it were true it would be *itself a consequence of what is to be investigated* and therefore *cannot* be allowed as a part of the evidence. To make it such would be to take the notion of strange loops a very long way too far.

The assertion that consciousness emerges from complexity is unproved. Accordingly, could not the intellectual opposition, including many shades of dualists, claim the opposite with no less ground, that the complexity of a system cannot produce an entity that transcends that system in the specifically personal way that consciousness seems to transcend the physical world? The relation of conscious personhood and brain seems of a different order from those senses in which a fully assembled machine is greater than the sum of its parts. The person seems above the brain, using it, while the assembled machine, useless until complete, is *still* useless without an operator and a power supply. The brain, the physicalists themselves are forced to admit, is itself *only the machine.* While conclusive *logical* proof seems difficult at this point, *empirical* evidence to be given later will certainly help us decide.

However, logic is certainly relevant, and some readers will know that here we are close to the realm of mathematical logic. We glimpse it as we glimpse a stretch of road ahead and above us as it spirals up from the valley toward a mountain pass. After giving the empirical evidence, our chapter will discuss the perhaps surprising

relevance of mathematical logic to the subtle body, and so draw toward its conclusion.

Meanwhile, we need to pause again, and take stock. It seems unlikely that we are automatons, for, as we have said already, we have a strong sense of our own autonomy, a sense of being-a-*self-determining*-self. Tables and chairs, even complex computers, do *not* seem to share that sense, the evidence being that they do *not* act as we do even though they are here alongside us in the world. They do obey the "laws" of physics, as observation of them confirms. This verges on truism, of course, for the establishment of those so-called laws of physics was made on the ground of precisely such observations of the actions of *inanimate* things, which, today, we take for granted. We also take for granted our own very different behavior, the difference being so *reliable,* and so clear. Although, as we have seen, this, too, is almost mere truism, grounded in the *exclusion* of living organisms from the earlier restricted physics, it is no less for that a valid induction from the facts, confirmed and consistently reconfirmed, if never proved, by huge numbers of careful observations. We, while living, may dance in the street, but tables and chairs do not.

If a chair in Ravel's opera *L'Enfant et les Sortilèges,* or a plastic Father Christmas in the superstore, were to sing we would not attribute our outward observation of the singing to inward consciousness of any kind in the chair or plastic figure. Moreover, Father Christmas's voice, imitating ours, emanates from the plastic figure by means of far simpler circuitry installed within it than the circuitry of our brains and tongues. So even *very* simple machines *can* imitate, *outwardly,* human *outward* behavior, and do so more or less accurately, but we still do not impute consciousness to them. We know that they only act as they do because we humans have installed programming to operate mechanisms that were also understood, designed, and made *by us.* Were record players conscious? We think not. Yet they sang to us. Today's computers, far more complex, even use processes of quantum physics without seeming to gain consciousness. Only certain very poor software programs "think" *they* know better than I do what *I* want to write. But those poor programs (and the much better ones) were devised by *human* minds. Nonetheless, the inspired and creative human author still reigns supreme for the machines are not conscious. At what point, then, does outward behavior become reliable evidence even of inner consciousness, let alone of an inner Being? Is it ever reliable? The evidence available is, as always in such matters, indirect, but what we find suggests a number of further ideas. Let us examine, in at least a preliminary way, a few of these.

First we note that the *appearance of* consciousness can be installed into a machine by a Being of what we would certainly have to consider a "higher" type. This is "as above, so below" in yet another of its manifestations. It is top-down causation, dogmatically repudiated by mechanistic science. It is also both interference from outside the lower-level system and an installing-into-and-indwelling of that lower-level system by a higher-order entity. This is true whether the indwelling entity is an organization of, a patterning of, the substance of the lower entity or a distinct kind of substance. Turning toward empirical evidence we see that human consciousness is not extinguished when it withdraws very deeply into the coma state, from which it often reemerges intact as the physical body repairs itself. On emerging from coma some sufferers tell us they have been normally, fully conscious, but unable to work the machine of the body, including its limb muscles and speech organs. Sufferers of certain diseases of the brain are also well aware of what they wish to say, but merely unable to express the conventionally correct, comprehensible sound of it because cells on the brain's left side are damaged. Evidence from within the person is, therefore, ambiguous. Why, then, should we accept without full explanatory corroboration the dogma that our own consciousness *is* or even *is the result of* nothing more than the complexity of interconnection of our brain cells? The phenomena of coma and dementia suggest otherwise.

If we look more closely at this evidence we find it sufficient to generate an explanatory hypothesis. Note that we have evidence that the consciousness *itself* is not diminished by the failure of the physical body. The only relevant fact we have is that the person's ability to communicate in the physical world is impaired. Might not the barrier that prevents dementia sufferers and persons in the coma state communicating in ways that would prove their consciousness to others in the world pass progressively deeper within the progressively failing physical system until the consciousness *itself*, unimpaired but unable to remain functional within the body, were finally "squeezed out" from it, to exist independently? There is no reason to believe that conscious existence could not continue, for the physical world has now become irrelevant for the consciousness concerned. Arguing that unembodied consciousness is impossible assumes what it seeks to prove, namely that the physical is essential. It is circular argument, and therefore no argument at all. We have no evidence whatever that consciousness does not persist after dementia or death occurs. Dementia and coma themselves provide a measure of evidence that the opposite is the case, that consciousness is in reality quite independent of body. This manner of disembodied survival could even be true of something as seemingly insubstantial as a mere pattern or map of *the person as formerly known-in-the-world*. Please ponder our chosen phraseology. Any pattern that withdraws would be unable to communicate further with the physical world *because it no longer had control of the physical machine of the body,* but the world into which any such pattern withdraws from our physical world might be a world in which *such patterns are the true realities.* Perhaps we might postulate that it is a "world of thought." This schema has the virtue of rationality and simplicity. It even has explanatory power, while the assertion that consciousness is the result of physical complexity alone has no such power. A suggestion we shall leave without comment at this stage is that the pattern from one life might become the morphogenetic field for a subsequent life.

Once the person's consciousness is unable to communicate further with the physical world there can be *no direct physical evidence* either that such a thought-being had ever been present or that it had now departed. But no one could *prove* that it had *not* been present in the body while the body was still seen as alive. The erstwhile evidence of "aliveness" itself tends rather to prove that it *had* been present. What, then, *is* the end of life, and of what is the end of life the evidence? That the brain is essential for functioning *in the physical world* is beyond all rational doubt, but those who hold opposing views cannot prove invalid the view we have described. A pure consciousness, unable any longer to communicate its presence via a damaged brain, might simply leave to dwell elsewhere. We could not know, for we, our normal observational powers limited to *this* world, could not *observe* the occurrence. As we said, for the present we shall treat our own view as unproved, but the problem of explaining how complexity per se could produce consciousness also remains insoluble for those who advocate it.

What is beyond argument is that we and Dingle's fly, despite living down here in the physical world, do not obey the "laws" of classical physics, but seem, rather, to use the freedoms, the *un*lawfulness(!), of quantum physics. *This autonomy,* whether physical or supraphysical, whether relative or absolute, is the *defining difference,* then, between what we categorize as "things" and what we call "living beings." Along with our being Beings, not things, comes the sense of the reality of our power of autonomous action, limited though it is. We noted earlier the bipolar structure linking Being-in-the-world and world itself. There are many Beings in the world, your "I" and my "I" among them, but very simple empirical investigation shows that tables and chairs are not Beings, though cats and dogs are. Even flies are Beings, as Dingle's distinction between their behavior when alive and when dead attests. The question might, as we saw above, become that of whether consciousness is an emergent property of our bodies or a separate kind of "thing." We have suggested it is separate, but, of course, we shall bear in mind the possibility that it will prove to be both, *according to the level of our viewpoint,* such categorization itself, as well as the realities, being then in question. There may be levels of consciousness, some nearer the physical than others. But what would a "consciousness-thing" *be*? We deliberately use the very general word *thing,* for we do not want to prejudge what the nature of consciousness itself may be, nor its relationship with the physical body or with the being of Beings. However, what we have said holds open the possibility that it may prove itself very definitely not physical, and very definitely autonomous.

Understanding the Nature of Bodily Actions
Their Limits and Their Possible Extensions

The *willed* operation of the physical body normally *takes place where the body is, literally within its reach.* Where else could it, *normally,* take place? This simply *is* our normal bodily experience, *functionally and ostensively so defined by that experience itself.* The vast majority of the actions of which we are aware are first willed, then body-mediated, and ultimately body-limited, for just as we can imagine, sense, and measure *only* what the body

could, at least in principle, *sense* using its external sense organs, so we can *operate upon* the *physical* world *only* in analogous ways, either using the available movements of the body directly or by harnessing the physical world itself in the form of tools to perform actions that are, of necessity and in *absolutely every case,* entirely similar *in principle* to the body's own willed actions even if beyond the strength or reach or delicacy of the unaided body's movements. Nothing else can *ever* be done; nothing else can *ever* be imagined. This limitation of our Being is inherent and irremovable, yet it is one that, because we are, perforce, so accustomed to it, we rarely realize is present and operating. Thus, what we are adding here extends the sphere of the truths that arose from the thought experiment about "squalification" and shows that they have even wider application. In every case, what tools do for us has the same nature as the bodily actions of which we are capable, and we can neither imagine other purposes nor conceive or make tools that would be required for any purpose outside that range. Just as our range of conceptualization is limited by the range of information that arrives from the bodily senses, so also our actions, whether physical or imaginary, whether unaided or requiring equipment, are limited to what *in principle* the body itself can do.

The parallel between what the body can do and what tools can do holds even in the case of exotic machines such as spacecraft. The telephone and all its more modern extensions, such as the internet, work in this parallel way, using our ears or, via our computers, our eyes, without exception limited to operations paralleling the body's own capacities. Printing machines print words, but we could, and once did, write all our books. A woodsaw is only an extension of the hand, but far more efficient for its purpose than our fingernails, and even a perfume or spice from far around the world reaches our sense of smell or taste either via the body's own capacity to move or via some extension thereof that is entirely the same in principle. Transport systems from spice-road camels to aircraft and even telecommunication satellites simply mimic or enhance what the body itself could do. Even the equipment devised by scientists fits this pattern, slightly extended, for it similarly improves our observational abilities but observes nothing at all that, in principle, the body's senses could not observe or (here is the slight extension) the human mind interpret in a "body-centered" kind of way. Hence even our *concepts* of wave and particle are incompatible, or at best complementary, *because they originated in the differing sensitivities of our bodily sense organs* and the categorization of them *as different* that we created to explain them, and then continued to use in the era of modern physics. All tools, even tools of thought, are conceptions of our hypothesizing minds, which, having observed *ourselves,* extend our natural, bodily capacities. This is true even when we use our minds to outwit less capable minds-in-the-world, for we could fish with our bare hands but have found it more effective to ply a rod and line with guileful skill, persuading a fish to feed on the bait instead of trying to apprehend its slippery body when, on account of that very action, *its own will* would be to escape, not to feed.

Yet inputs to and outputs from the body seem each to show one exception to their normal co-extensiveness with the body. Telepathy, clairvoyance, and a number of related phenomena are inputs not mediated via any *external* bodily sense organ, and intentionality, normally *expressed* via the body's movements, would, if used alone, *bypass all body parts* and become instead an interior intention to carry out not the usual local action, whether using the body or technological extensions of it, but an equivalent effect spatially displaced from the body and, so far as our senses could confirm, *unbridged by anything physical.* The intention would be to realize an output beyond the body's reach, to "teleport" the physical effect to a distant place. Attempts to act in this way seem on occasion to succeed, and some human Beings seem better at it than others. Such efforts of will usually have a different purpose from our habitual actions, for we do not usually intend remote instances of the customary pushes and pulls of classical physics but to bring about effects that would not be everyday events even if bodily touch were involved, such as the healing of another's body, or mind, or even one's own.

Such a force-for-human-action-at-a-distance, whether within classical physics or requiring quantum effects, or even entirely extraphysical, has long been believed real, if also rarely seen and even more rarely proved, as the history of humankind's magic shows. If just one instance seemed irrefutable under the scrutiny of today's science the claim to use intentionality as a force-in-itself, *without the body's aid,* would have to be taken very seriously

indeed, not explained away by the subtle verbiage of skeptical philosophy. Of course, the question whether such phenomena take place by "spiritual" (as yet unidentified) means or "physical" (known) means, such as electromagnetism, would be a matter for an investigation not merely of effects-recordable-within-the-physical-world (i.e. measurements made using technical means) but also (as we have already seen) of *the correct application of those words,* because what, *seen as and in itself,* needs to be categorized as parts of *physics* might include "higher" and "lower" levels *within* physics than we have yet confirmed. We would reserve the word *spiritual* only for events *not* explicable within physics. The two ordinarily unobservable exceptions, telepathy and psychokinesis, have only recently received the close scrutiny they deserve, at least by Western scientists. The questions, then, are: Do we have evidence of the reality of a power of intentionality acting without the body? and: Do we have any hint as to the nature and mode of operation of any such power?

The question of telepathy is now settled in favor of its reality in all but the most prejudiced minds. The wider question of the whole range of "willed outputs beyond the body" has already attracted a great deal of research, far more than is generally acknowledged, and evidence is accumulating. As the question is important and topical we shall make brief mention of particular sources of information. James Oschman, in his book *Energy Medicine: The Scientific Basis,* gives his reasons for believing that present-day physics is probably about to discover *within itself* a "mechanism" for willed-action-at-a-distance.[19] If he is right, many skeptics will fall silent. We shall mention Oschman and others again. As Popper reminded us, many pages ago, bodily senses and actions have been with us for millennia, in his view breeding the baby's increasing familiarity with its own powers, then vernacular science, later, considered and rational hypotheses, eventually today's focused, planned, and organized research with stringent testing and measurement, and, during that history, huge numbers of the material-world extensions of bodily sense that we call "apparatus." Popper believes that evolution has produced in all species inherent patterns amounting to a kind of a priori scientific theory offering a range of perceptions and actions with respect to the world-about of the organism concerned. We mentioned earlier his view of the fly-catching capacity of the frog, programmed to catch live flies even though it ignores motionless ones. In similar ways, he said, all our sense organs have anticipatory theory genetically incorporated. This, however, is the point at which we disagree with him. Our dualism is a stronger form of dualism than his. We think it is no more possible to explain a genetic information bank of the kind he posits than to explain how consciousness could arise automatically from complexity. The body itself, including the brain, is, we believe, probably scarcely changed from many millennia ago. Our view is that when a baby is born into this world of becoming, the nonphysical pattern, or morphogenetic field (or perhaps we should even use the word *spirit*), of the baby has already in it, regardless of biological constitution in any of its aspects, knowledge it will need of its new world-about. Thus, we believe, spiritual evolution leads biological evolution, not the other way round. The human baby, scientific from birth, develops almost automatically its inborn familiarity with the powers of its own Being-in-the-world. So we circle back to our two questions: Is there evidence of a power of human intentionality acting without the body and, if so, what are its nature and mode of operation? Curiously, what we see the body do sheds light on this question of what the body cannot do, but sometimes happens nonetheless.

Consciousness and Experiment

Since these questions are our present concern, this is the place to describe a famous series of experiments, its results crucial to the question of what "we" might consist of, whether merely "gross matter" living under the "laws of physics," or, at least in part, something a little more "subtle" and a little less restricted. But we must approach with caution. The experiments and their consequences have often been misunderstood. Some commentators with a journalist's level of understanding of science are tempted to claim that Alain Aspect's Paris experiments of 1981 to 1982 proved the existence of a spirit world of which we are a living, active, executant part. In some cases, the claim may even result from a rash, presumptive misunderstanding to the effect that it was *consciousness* that *produced* Aspect's experimental results *by interfering psychically in what happened,* rather than that consciousness *merely arranged*

the experimental apparatus, which then performed as normal.

Such confusion may have arisen from a related confusion regarding the distinct question, valid in itself, that we have ourselves just raised, the question of whether consciousness, intentionality, *might* alter the future of the world and thereby the outcome of any experiment performed in the world. The question certainly *relates to* Aspect's result (though no more than it relates to all other events in the universe) and it is the reason we want to look at his experiments, but we shall pursue it only after we have dealt with the experiments *as simple physics.*

No disrespect is intended by our use of the word *simple,* for the equipment needed if the experiments were to give reliable results beyond the range of inherent inaccuracy and error was sophisticated indeed. For example, the photon detectors available to Aspect in 1981 were barely capable of what was required. Nevertheless, the experiment gave an unequivocal result, and what it does provide is a *crucial* but *preliminary* step *entirely within the physical world* but *allowing us to anticipate* that there *could be* a "spirit" world *of which we are a living and active part* and that *because the double slit experiment and Schrödinger's and Heisenberg's mathematics had shown that the physical world is not fully predetermined* "we" (whatever "we" are) might even be able to change its future development by willed acts *or even by acts of will.* But scientific corroboration of these further objectives, even if possible at all, would require many steps beyond Aspect's and the double slit experiments themselves. We shall therefore avoid confused journalistic overenthusiasm and deal with Aspect's Paris experiment first as pure physics.

Through the middle years of the twentieth century dispute continued between the proponents of the classical, *causal* physics (which, to the surprise of most laypersons, includes Einstein's relativity) and the advocates of the new *indeterministic* quantum physics, supported by Heisenberg's principle of uncertainty, Bohr's formulation of the same matter, and Schrödinger's *differently grounded and classical* (though probabilistic) wave-mechanical theory, which we explored earlier. Resolving the dispute would require elegant experiments to decide between Einstein's famous assertion that "God does not play dice"—effectively the claim that the physical world is not only *entirely* deterministic but also *causally closed* (that is beyond the possibility of capricious or unlawful interference from *outside itself*)—and the belief that quantum indeterminacy is an *inherent* and *utterly ordinary* part of the physical world. Such indeterminacy is a central postulate of the interpretation of quantum physics published after the Copenhagen Convention of 1926.

The experiments required were far beyond the technical limits of the equipment available when the dispute between classical and quantum physics first arose, but by 1966 theoretical physicist John Bell had made and published the calculations and predictions that enabled the necessary testable hypothesis to be framed and the technical requirements of the future experiment to be specified. In simplistic terms, Einstein's theory and quantum theory made different predictions of the behavior of pairs of particles that had been generated in one particle-level interaction. What experimental measurements showed would decide between Einstein's determinism and the indeterminism of quantum theory. Finally, as the 1980s arrived, equipment that would make the required measurements reliably and accurately began to become available. We shall describe the essentials of a version of the experiment using matters familiar to us from the double slit experiment. There is, however, an important difference. In the double slit experiment just *one* quantum, propagating as a wavefront, interferes with itself to produce a pattern until an interaction with the wave "collapses" it to form a particle. In Aspect's experiment *two* wavicles are generated, but from one event, and it is their relationship *with each other* as they move *apart* at the velocity of light after that simultaneous generation that is investigated. But before we can proceed we must present a few ideas.

What Are "Quantum Entanglement" and "Action at a Distance"?

Generally, if two particles are produced by an intra-atomic or interatomic event they will form a "spin pair." *In simple terms,* this means that as the particles are generated and "released" they rebound from each other, repelling each other as described by one of Newton's laws of motion: "Action and reaction are equal and opposite." This is true of both the linear movement as the particles travel away from each other, and of their rotational

movement or "spin." The spins of "spin pairs" are generated in "opposite sense," one particle rebounding away from the other and spinning "clockwise" as it goes, the other rebounding and spinning "counterclockwise." This linear and rotational "balance" conserves the total energy present through the whole sequence of events. Particles thus generated by a single event are said to be "entangled" with each other. Aspect sought to establish what *physical reality* the newly postulated "entanglement" *actually was,* so far as it could be known by what it *did* and how it seemed to work, and *so* to discover the answer to his *central* question, whether communication faster than the velocity of light could be proved between entangled particles, for *only* an unassailable demonstration of a *faster-than-light connection or communication* would prove that the postulated "quantum interconnectedness" was operating across the space between the entangled particles. As always, here we acknowledge the conceptual difficulty presented by the wave-particle duality; the particles will at first be waves. Only interference from outside will convert them into particles. This interference is, in fact, the central event in Aspect's experiment, as we shall now see.

The essence of the experiment is that the two jointly generated (entangled) traveling waves are emitted from a source, and their wavefronts are allowed to propagate away for some distance. An interaction is then imposed upon *one* of the mutually receding waves, collapsing it to a particle. *At this instant* the other wave, which has not been forced to collapse, remains a wave. The question is: What now happens to the second entangled wave, with which nothing from "outside" has interfered? Does it, too, collapse to a particle, in harmony with the first wave's collapse, and if so, *when* does the collapse happen? There should not be a "reduction" or "collapse" from wave to particle *earlier than* the arrival of an "instruction to become a particle," which "message," if it occurs at all, would (according to classical physics and Einstein) arrive *at, or even below, the velocity of light* from the wave that had collapsed to the particle state. The reason given by Einstein that such a message could travel *no faster* from point to point than the speed of light was that the mathematics of relativity *require* that nothing in the physical world other than *massless energy* (that is, electromagnetic radiation, light itself) is able to travel at, let alone faster than, this velocity.

All matter particles have (or, in relativity theory, *are*) *inertial mass,* and therefore resist acceleration; this resistance, this mass, increases exponentially the faster the particle of matter moves. Hence, the velocity of *massless* light is a *limiting maximum* velocity imposed on any "*mass* particle" in the prequantum classical-relativistic physical world. Faster-than-light communication is therefore axiomatically *impossible* if relativity and classical, determinate, causal physics are both correct. Already, by 1926, relativity was firmly established as correct for the physical world as then known. So, in any entangled generation of two "wavicles" no "instruction" from the wave that had already been forced to condense to a particle and show its spin could be received by the second wave earlier than a pulse of electromagnetic energy, light, could arrive. If, however, Aspect's measurements showed that the second particle *had* appeared and *had* taken up the opposite spin to the first, at a moment *earlier than a message-at-the-velocity-of-light could have arrived from the first particle,* he would have proved the reality of a connection between the particles of some *other* kind than light, that is other than electromagnetic radiation. This link would either be a *communication* that traveled faster than light or a *connectedness* that did not need to travel at all, an ever-present influence always *there* and always in touch with *elsewhere,* no matter how distant. As always, words are inadequate and potentially very misleading, but perhaps one might think of the connectedness as an all-pervading static force, or even as an "executive ether."

In the text box accompanying figure 15.7 we describe a version of Aspect's experiment that follows naturally from our description, given earlier, of the behavior of light waves and electron waves in the double slit experiment, but other versions of the experiment are possible, measuring a variety of parameters, and some of these have been carried out. In the best-known version Aspect used the characteristic forward movement of transverse waves, which resembles the wriggling motion of a snake. So long as it is not impeded, the wavefront of light expands in *all* directions, but when it encounters a barrier, which offers a kind of molecular-level slit-like way through, the light polarizes itself at the correct angle, passes through, and thereafter moves onward in that same plane. This polarization angle can, of course, be measured. In this way Aspect tested the entanglement

of two photons (light waves) by enforcing the *polarization* of the first, with simultaneous observation of the entangled second photon to see whether it instantly showed any particular polarization. The second photon did indeed *instantly* assume the same polarization as the first, despite the fact that no "message at the speed of light" could have reached it, a result impossible to explain using the classical physics of Einstein.

This was evidence of an *interconnectedness* operating faster than light, or even instantaneously. In attempting to describe a reality that stretches our imaginative powers and lies far beyond the power of language, we have to use a form of words that seems an oxymoron. If it were instantaneous it would be a kind of *just is,* a *state* of the universe's very being, not a process at all, albeit an *active* state that is impossible to visualize, a kind of *timelessly changeless activity* unlike the *temporal processes* of classical physics. Further, Aspect's result would either require an extension of physics, to understand what in all earlier physics had seemed impossible, or the immense conjecture that there is, *beyond all physics as sensed by us,* an all-encompassing Indra's Net holding *instantaneous* discourse with itself over huge *physical* distances, yet allowing those *physical* changes to influence its timelessly quasi-unchanging self. Verbal thinkers will have extreme difficulty in *picturing* this idea, but *picturable* it is. It even amounts to a testable hypothesis, as Tonomura recently, and others living a century before him, knew. We shall deal with Tonomura's closely related experiment later.

Which interpretation of Aspect's results should be adopted might rest in some of its aspects upon nothing more than linguistics, but the redefinition of the scope of physics would be more important, not least because that *real* level might involve phenomena already known, such as distant viewing and clairvoyance, that, although once thought impossible by scientists and certainly inexplicable by classical physics, have nonetheless been attested by witnesses throughout history. It is here, and only contingently (for other areas of physics that are more directly relevant would have to concur), that Aspect's experiment might, beyond its own intentions and purview, support belief in entities invisible to us yet convolved with our physical world, whether *in and of* it or *outside* it despite being in the same "place" and, if outside, nonetheless *capable of influencing it* from outside. Such influences

Aspect's Paris Experiment

Aspect's experiment can be performed in a variety of ways, of which one is illustrated here, in a considerably simplified and somewhat schematic form. This explanation is also very brief, but states the main facts and reveals the line of reasoning.

Pairs of entangled photons are generated in and emitted from the source S, and allowed to fly along fiber optic cables laid out in opposite directions. These cables are not shown in our diagram, the photons that travel along them being indicated by the usual symbol for wavefronts and (after the polarizers) the symbol for transverse propagating waves. The use of fiber optic guides ensures that the photon wavefronts cannot expand as they would in vacuo, overlap, and so interfere directly with each other, and that they reach a considerable distance from each other (about 13 meters, as Aspect measured it, equal to about 14 yards) before any interaction (measurement) is imposed upon them. The photons, as emitted by the source, are unpolarized, that is, they are indeterminate in respect of the plane in space of their transverse vibration, and the angles of the polarizers are set by the experimenters prior to each run of the experiment.

While the photons are actually in flight (relatively slowly, through glass, not vacuum) the two electromagnetic switches, controlled by a nuclear random number generator, are reset. This ensures that (assuming normal temporal causation) the setting of the switches has not affected the emission or travel of the photons—they are already on their way before their paths are chosen by the switches. The switching of the electromagnetic fields in the switches (one controlling each photon) changes each photon's path, and, given sufficient length of optical cable, does so fast enough to choose the route before the photon

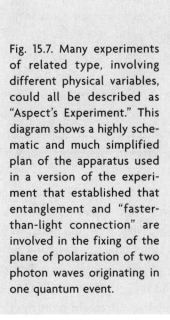

Fig. 15.7. Many experiments of related type, involving different physical variables, could all be described as "Aspect's Experiment." This diagram shows a highly schematic and much simplified plan of the apparatus used in a version of the experiment that established that entanglement and "faster-than-light connection" are involved in the fixing of the plane of polarization of two photon waves originating in one quantum event.

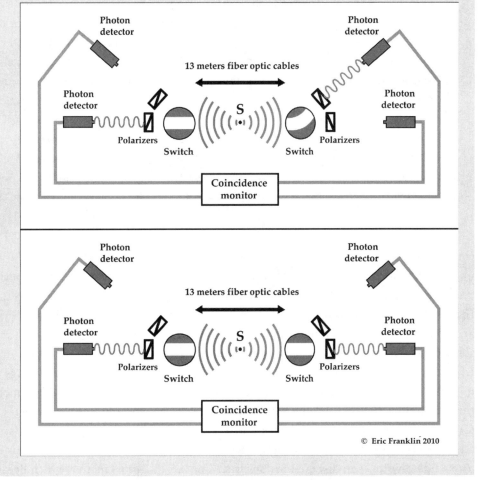

© Eric Franklin 2010

arrives. The two polarizers in one arm of the apparatus have been preset at different angles, and the angles of the polarizers in the other arm have been set to match. On each of the two fiber optic paths the choice of polarizer takes place in time to determine which of the two polarizers ahead of each flying photon the photon will pass through, and, therefore, which of the two photon detectors beyond the polarizers will receive each photon. As each wavefront (photon) approaches its polarizer it has no well-defined polarization, but the polarizer interacts with it, in effect "measuring" it *with respect to its polarization,* forcing the photon-wave to vibrate in the plane at which the polarizer has been preset by the experimenters. The coincidence monitor registers every photon, effectively recording whether each photon was received, which photon detector received each photon, and when, and the angles of the polarizers.

There are four possible pairings of the paths that the paired photons can follow. These pairings are determined by the random number generator that controls the switches. We show one path-pairing in each of our two diagrams. On the basis of what is shown, the other possible pairings can easily be imagined. The tabulated list of results provided by the coincidence monitor correlates all the information about every photon, pair by pair, including the preset angles of polarization of each photon in each pair. The crucial question is to discover, by analysis of the listed data provided by the coincidence monitor, whether the polarization angle actually shown by each photon correlates with the polarization shown by its entangled partner. If *both* photons of an entangled pair are found to have arrived, and to have done so via polarizers set to the same angle, the crucial correlation will have been established because the two originally unpolarized photons will, by some means, have taken on the same polarization angle.

Aspect and his colleagues found a correlation fully equal to 1 between the polarization angles of the members of each pair of photons. In every single instance, an exceedingly rare result in scientific experiment, when a photon interacted with its polarizer and took up the set polarization angle, the other photon of the same entangled pair must have been already making the same "adjustment" as it arrived at its own polarizer. Whenever the preset angle of the two polarizers was the same, both photons passed through unimpeded and were registered by the coincidence monitor, and whenever the preset angles were not the same one wavefront was blocked by its polarizer because a polarization had already been imposed upon it by the other photon of the pair. Many runs of the experiment were made, with the polarizers set at different angles. Since no "instruction" to take up any particular polarization could have been passed, even at the speed at which electromagnetic radiation might, hypothetically, have travelled from the one photon to the other, the conclusion was that a "quantum interconnectedness" acting faster than light—perhaps even instantly, timelessly—was present. The result does not, of course, prove the existence of a subtle body, but it certainly has consequences for any full understanding of our "Being-here" in the physical world.

could hardly be denied a place within physics, so our universe would have to be acknowledged to be causally unclosed *or* to be larger than heretofore. The pervading Indra's Net–like field would then be seen as "higher" and top-down causation might seem more credible to some thinkers than it has recently been. According to what the *nature* of the connectedness proved to be, one might decide this question by reexamining the definition of physics (though nothing would alter the newly established facts). What seemed to us sufficiently different from preexisting physics might then be *defined as* outside physics, perhaps even as "spiritual," or, *if it* *proved investigable in a similar manner to earlier physics,* we might prefer to consider it as *within* a *redefined and extended* physics. This is, of course, the ancient question of hylic pluralism, raising its head once more, but with a modern face.

So we, ourselves, in our deep essence, might come to be considered Beings who were *outside* a new physics that could not accommodate what we found ourselves to be, or we might be Beings functioning in a *higher level of a broader physics* than any physics we had known before. As we remarked, this is the ancient problem of fine and gross matter, which became in more recent centuries the question of spirit and matter. In either case, we would have the duty of understanding ourselves by creating a *science of Being* or a *science of spirituality,* to complement the *science of physics.* So we see that the ancient concept of the *meta*physical might not yet be obsolete, and we also have a *logical* possibility, *but no more,* of a conscious, self-directing subtle body.

Had Aspect's experiments, despite the realities described by Schrödinger's probability-wave equations and Heisenberg's uncertainty principle, given results in accord with classical determinacy none of these speculations would have been possible (though a result so inconsistent with those other well-established parts of physics would have been extremely odd). Such results would have suggested the *im*possibility of *any* way of being above that of tables and chairs, and would have shown that freedom of choice in human action was utter delusion. If that had been the result we would, to answer a question raised earlier, be automatons, *even if we did not know it.* Belief that we had at our voluntary disposal any form of free will that could be considered real would have become impossible to justify, and the conclusion that we are mere automatons, mere pawns of mere physics, despite our being conscious, would have been unavoidable. But this very *line of thought* would then be bizarre, incredible, for we would have to explain how organisms *without* ever having experienced freedom could not merely *imagine* freedom, but could also *question* whether that freedom itself was *real* or *delusory.* The ability to pose *this* question is the ability to *imagine two worlds,* the *real* world-about, and a world in which *imagination itself and also its products* were the *realities.* That ability, which we clearly have, would, in a world of automatons, have been distinctly odd. Whence would have come our ability to imagine what we could *never,* even hypothetically, experience?

But none of that had happened. Aspect had demonstrated quantum interconnection, and it harmonized perfectly with quantum indeterminacy. Human will might, therefore, now survive to find tenancy in the interconnectedness of the cosmos, a "higher," more "subtle" (or more "fundamental") level of physics than Newton ever imagined; or even to fly to realms of Being outside and far above physics itself. While in no way directly concerned with it, Aspect's experiment had also, of course, opened wider the door to the acceptance as

rational of scientific investigation of consciousness and its powers, and had thereby advanced both Dingle's aim of better correlations *within* physics and his further aim of correlation between psychology, biology, and physics. Belief that there is a subtle body was now at least respectable, defensible if as yet unproved, but questions of what a conscious subtle body might *be,* whether it existed within physics or outside it, and how it might react with the physical world, *including the world of the physical body itself,* remained, of course, to be investigated.

Before leaving the Paris experiment we shall let Aspect speak for himself in a short quotation from the end of his talk in memory of John Bell, in Vienna in December 2000, which he humbly entitled "Bell's Theorem: The Naïve View of an Experimentalist."[20] We need not edit Aspect's slightly quaint English, and need not understand the whole of his conclusion. Its relevance to the possibility of a subtle body will be clear without an advanced grasp of the physics.

> We have nowadays an impressive amount of sensitive experiments where Bell's inequalities have been clearly violated. Moreover, the results are in excellent agreement with the quantum mechanical predictions including all the known features of the real experiment. Each of the remaining loopholes has been separately closed, [Aspect gives references] and although yet more ideal experiments are still desirable, it is legitimate to discuss the consequences of the rejection of supplementary parameter theories obeying Einstein's causality. It may be concluded that quantum mechanics has some non-locality in it, and that this non-local character is vindicated by experiments.[21]

Active connection over large distances between quantum particles such as photons generated as "entangled pairs" that have then moved far apart, an interconnection that many had long thought possible, was now effectively proved. "Entanglement" is a real, observable phenomenon, and requires explanation in accordance with quantum physics, Newton's deterministic physics being inadequate. Indeed, Aspect goes a little further, saying that—and we note his choice of words—"a pair of entangled photons must be considered a single global object . . ." They are a single global object *despite huge distance between them.* Therefore, causality in a sense not too distant from our everyday understanding of that term should operate between them. Aspect's statement therefore implies the *possibility* (subject to demonstration) that claims of the effectiveness of human intentionality, for example in healing, and of "spiritual" healing *at a distance* may be true, though we have no reason to believe that Aspect and his team had any intention themselves to become involved in such speculation or any investigation of it.

We allow ourselves a final verbatim quotation, for which Aspect's own report used italics, so we shall do so here. Clearly, he wished to emphasize his point, and we wish to add one of our own. He says *"We must be grateful to John Bell for having shown us that philosophical questions about the nature of reality could be translated into a problem for physicists, where naïve experimentalists can contribute."*[22]

Our point is that this is a view that even some Wittgensteinian philosophers, among the less likely, one might think, to espouse such a view, now begin to accept. Among them is Harri Wettstein, an article by whom is listed in the bibliography. Wettstein suggests that philosophers should be more prepared than they are to "soil their hands" with empirical investigation. It is a welcome suggestion, centuries overdue, and the more so because a Wittgensteinian makes it. However, we doubt whether Gilbert Ryle would have approved scientific (empirical) investigations that would surely overturn his verbally based dogmas, sweeping them aside as irrelevant.

Where Do We Stand Now? The Consequences for Life of Aspect's Result
A Discursive Survey before Proceeding

Aspect's experiment and, before it, the double slit experiment have given rise to the suggestion, and the hope, that mind (we acknowledge an as-yet undefined term) is an instrument of free control of the natural world. The double slit experiment and the related theoretical descriptions by Schrödinger and Heisenberg have been discussed. We ask now what Aspect has added. He has demonstrated the reality of quantum connection over distances that, within the laboratory, are large, and later experiments have shown the same connectedness over distances measured in kilometers, with no evidence of

diminution over those distances. Of the classical four forces, two, electromagnetism and gravity, decay exponentially over distance according to an inverse square law, while the intranuclear forces decay even more steeply and are effectively zero outside each atomic nucleus in which they operate. The connection now established by Aspect is quite unlike these forces, their effects so familiar to us in our everyday world-about, for his interconnection is utterly insensible for us. Nothing happening within his apparatus could be observed by the unaided human senses. The connectedness is nonetheless certainly real, though the evidence for it is doubly indirect, and Aspect needed sophisticated equipment to find it. It is no wonder that earlier science did not find, or even look for, it. While mystics had asserted its reality no one else had sensed it, and we may rationally wonder whether the quantum interconnectedness may be *in some sense* completely outside our world, *non*spatial, or whether it may occupy a "space" completely distinct from, yet somehow contiguous with, our space, or, again, be "spatial" in a very different way totally unfamiliar to us here in our spatial and temporal physical world, in which our natural tendency is to think of space as that which contains things, rather than of an emptiness, a void. We note that the notion of the quintessential ākāśa, however we may rename it, has entered here.

Further, quantum *interconnection,* indeed *interconnection over physical-world distance,* now proved by Aspect, goes hand in hand with quantum *indeterminacy,* already demonstrated by other experiments and supported by both Heisenberg's uncertainty principle and Schrödinger's wave equations. This affords us a broader view, one containing greater possibilities, of our place as Beings-in-the-physical-world. That greater breadth of view has consequences. Our world-about *itself* is no longer what it was because *our view of it* has changed, and our Being-in-it is also, ipso facto, changed. If our Being is an executive force, as we have suggested earlier, the change in our conception of the world-about will itself bring *changes in our actions and expectations in that world.* Even the so-called laws of physics may change. These speculations run far ahead of the solid ground as yet beneath our feet, but we can glimpse the enlarged vista even from a distance. Stepping carefully, then, let us survey this broader vista, beginning, as rational investigation always does, with what seems currently beyond our rational doubt. Those certainties now include Aspect's result.

As human knowledge grows it becomes clearer that any discussion must widen naturally until it encompasses everything. Acknowledging this, we must, however reluctantly, pass by fascinating possibilities, pursuing only what relates directly to the search for the subtle body. We make a new start, then, with the *physical* body.

What, or Who, Works the Physical Body?

It is a truism worth stating that we humans have, from the dawn of self-awareness and even in its vaguest and most dreamlike modes, exercised control over *physical* processes using *physical* means, just as Dingle's fly has done, the fly presumably doing so without self-knowledge enough to conceive the truism. What is different, today, is our understanding of such matters, the recognition that *something real* might underlie that truism, and that the controller may be of a nature quite distinct from that of the controlled. As science develops, the minds of those of us who ponder the consequences open to new perceptions and concepts, and their capabilities within the world increase, even though human bodies remain as they have long been.* This does not constitute proof of the ideas that arise, of course, but it is entirely compatible with notions of mind-body or spirit-body duality. What is new is that we now know better what we are doing, and can do it with greater self-awareness, and, as James Oschman, Larry Dossey, and many others, some dualists or vitalists, others not, assure us, we can investigate intentionality and what may be nonphysical control of the world, in modern scientific ways. We should look, then, at how we live in our bodies, in preparation for a more comprehensive grasp of what and who we are.

We have always operated the physical body in the same way, of course, often purposefully, but largely as unreflectively as the fly, and the extension of the process by, for example, holding something in the hand, which we manipulate, makes no difference in principle to the nature of the action. To see a stone *as* a tool to crack a marrow bone, as prehistoric man doubtless often did, is, in Heidegger's words, to see the stone as a "thing-for" (German *zeug*). Use of what we call a prosthesis is entirely the same in principle. We choose the word to show that any artifact enabling humanly willed action (such as an artificial limb) is entirely akin to the humble stone, or (perhaps a more startling realization) to the limb it has replaced, or even to the whole natural body. A microscope is only a tool for extending the range of the eyes. When it becomes possible, a digital camera installed in place of a natural eye that has failed will be just the same in principle. A piano provides, via the arms and fingers, a means of intentionally externalizing the expressive feelings of the musical mind, the product entering, via the ears, the mind that then experiences the music, whether that of composer, performer, or audience. Manipulating material to make some object, such as clay for a pot, is entirely the same, physically speaking, when using the hand itself as it is when using a separate tool, such as a spatula, to shape the clay. We must never allow ourselves to be misled—bewitched, as Wittgenstein describes it—by the contrast in usage between the words for natural limbs and words such as *prosthesis*. The body itself is undeniably a set of tools, those of a human differing from those of a cat, or a horse, bestowing different abilities and imposing different limitations, so if any tool attached to the body is a prosthesis, the body itself is, in essence, a prosthesis of the mind. Door handles are designed for operation by our hands, and the cat, intellectually fully able to intend the same action of opening the door, finds the handles not well-designed for its paws, or, of course, its paws not well-designed for the handles, yet succeeds in opening the door when we affix a device suitably designed for it to use. The question of whether the mind is an emergent property of the physical or a supraphysical operator of physical machines (such as bodies and spatulas) is still open, as we saw earlier, and is difficult to resolve, but this is not essentially a matter for dispute between monist and dualist views for, as we showed, the traditional strong distinction between monist and dualist interpretations of the

---

*We put the matter this way because the unreflective person, using, for example, today's technology with no thought of how it came into his hands, no awareness of the difference between his world and that of primitive humans, does not share the expansion of mind that the thoughtful can enjoy. Many people despise their modern birthright by ignoring what might expand the mind, others abuse it, having taken it for granted. Primitive humans, who were, we think, as intelligent as ourselves, had simply not discovered enough to think our thoughts, yet may not have lacked spirituality in the way in which, despite our easier access to understanding, many seem content to do today.

living world is itself naïve and unnecessary and mainly a matter of viewpoint, of perspective, of categorization, of the setting of conceptual boundaries between things we see, perhaps erroneously, as separate. What, we might ask, *is* a "thing?" In the present context the only true duality seems to be that between living Being and unliving *thing,* as we have remarked before, and the stubborn question is the one just raised yet again, whether Being emerges out of matter or has its subsistence elsewhere, merely *living in* matter.

The Powers of the Age to Come

What, then, can we expect in the future, enlightened and encouraged by science's discoveries? Equipped with an understanding of quantum physics we should be able to demonstrate at least some degree of control of quantum processes, in both passively perceptive and autonomously active modes, taking the opportunity, by free choice alone, to *direct* Schrödinger's indeterminate wave-world, and do so over large distances using Aspect's spaceless and lossless quantum interconnection. *Conscious,* at last, of the facts of the quantum-physical world, we should now feel empowered to *extend* this operation of *conscious* will *as a choice-making and directive power,* just as we have, for many millennia, used the body itself and so manipulated by physical means gross and graspable physical things that are within reach of the body. Both anecdotal records and laboratory tests give evidence of the reality, if also of the rarity of its use, of an ability to influence events at a distance without obvious technical means, and to sense physical objects at a distance without the use of such means.

Seeing at a distance is not seeing with "eyes on stalks," a gross error resulting from a total confusion of the various *levels* of the physical or greater-than-physical world in the minds of many philosophers, but seeing *without* eyes and *without* hindrance by intervening physical-world things or distance. Why would the Seer need eyes? Its very *nature* is to see. It does so *without* tools, *without* prostheses, *without* reference to physical space, since its very nature is either nonphysical or subtly physical. Aspect has now proved not subtle seeing itself (of course) but the invisible level of the physical world at which subtle seeing *might* (subject to confirmation from further research) occur. From the well-known work of J. B. Rhine, one of the first scientific investigators of

what we now call parapsychology, in the 1930s to the present, innumerable experiments and personal accounts have provided evidence. There is a further category of evidence from out-of-body experience and near-death experience that has increased in volume and reliability following recent advances in resuscitation techniques. Such evidence is also too well known to require us to give references or to comment here. This evidence is more strongly suggestive of a *real duality* somewhere within our *being-alive*ness, for the claim is that Being has a *fuller* consciousness when that conscious Seer is *outside* the body than we normally have during our familiar body-life. The body enables only as a prosthesis enables. Its *nature* is not to enable but to restrict, and seeing without eyes is in at least some ways a more capable process than seeing with eyes. We even have reason to suggest a reversed version of the part-to-whole duality noted earlier, for it seems that consciousness is, when, on rare occasions, it is allowed its full natural scope, larger than the body, for in some not inconceivable manner it simultaneously contains the body and is limited by the body. The being-lived body is *smaller* than the Heideggerian Dasein, the living Being who is *there,* not the reverse.

The postulate of an extended physics versus the postulate of a *meta*physical living Being, if we may verbalize it thus, is the running battle of our era, just as it has been throughout the history of hylic pluralism. But the word *versus* may be wrong: perhaps we have here yet another situation of "both and," rather than one of "either or." Perhaps our being as embodied humans walking the earth contains modes of being at both these levels. The concepts of ka, ba, and akh, etheric body, astral body, ānanda-maya-kośa, jīvan-mukta, and many others, are very far from new. Perhaps they will now become acceptable, at least in translation, even to Western science.

The Apparent Strange Loop of a More Highly Conscious Consciousness

Here, as so often, we join Dingle and Jung's quest for a unified science, but, immediately, we are plunged into philosophical speculation regarding the aim and vision of science. Since the question of the nature of the reality of the *cosmos* is inextricably connected with the same question about the *subtle body,* we are bound to find space for an extension of each question into the realm of the other. We shall do this via the long-standing philosophical "problem," mentioned earlier, of whether the world exists only when being observed by a conscious observer. Some might consider this a silly preoccupation, long ago dismissed from the minds of serious philosophers, but the question of the world and the observer has ramifications, today, which keep the ancient pseudoproblem alive, perhaps as more than an entertaining diversion.

Heidegger's view, mentioned earlier, is that our very nature is of Being-in-the-world, a *unitary* phenomenon, though nonetheless complex *within* its unity. In keeping with this perceptual-conceptual view, we have mentioned already the growing evidence that human powers extend beyond what we have for long taken to be their everyday limits. Where does such evidence take us? Certainly into modified questions grounded in modified hypotheses. For example: Have "powers" capable of wider use been quietly at work, perhaps via a *subtle* body mediating *between* will and the physical world? We have acknowledged this idea already, for it merely rephrases the earlier question of whether there is a ghost operating the body-machine. What is new here is the further question: Do we have any evidence that such powers have been, habitually, perhaps even necessarily, at work in matters taken hitherto to be "merely normal" and "merely physical"?

Let us reexamine our most recent example (though the double slit experiment would have served us just as well). Aspect's experiment *was* carried out by *the conscious beings* professeur Aspect and his assistants, albeit with the most honorable of *detached* intentions. We did hint at this before, but coming upon the matter again, along our present line of approach, shows us that this seemingly fatuous truism is in fact rather startling. It suddenly faces us with something we have long ignored, the fact that we conscious beings of the twenty-first century can *never* perform an experiment *without* consciously intending to do so. The experimenters went about their work deliberately and consciously, and if they had *not* consciously *intended* to do so the experiment would not have been performed at all. Further, Aspect and his colleagues made their measurements in a manner as detached from human wishes as any interaction between a human and the world can be, intending neither physical nor psychic interference with the procedures. Indeed, there was a further distancing between experimenter and

apparatus, for we saw that in so sophisticated an experiment *none* of the observations could have been made by the human body unaided. All needed instruments, prostheses. If human will *had* affected the measurements by any other means than the familiar everyday causations we all use and expect to work predictably, human will had affected *all* measurements in such ways since the dawn of science, and would always do so. This they did not prove, nor disprove, for, of course, they had not set out to test it.

However, this problem *is* important *for us*. Whether or not human consciousness *itself, and acting alone,* can intervene to change the direction of normal physical events would be relevant to any concept of the subtle body because a positive answer would suggest that even the *physical* body either included or was associated with a kind of executive presence that not only works the physical body, but also sometimes extends or travels far beyond its visible boundary, the skin. Such an extension, whether within physics or outside it, would certainly justify the use of the word *subtle*.

We are "there," looking out upon the world, and conceiving and acting out our intentions regarding it. No experiment we perform escapes our *presence,* our *scrutiny,* and our *will*. The relationship between world and consciousness, taken for granted and ignored every day of the thousands of years during which our consciousness has developed, may now be very different from what we have habitually assumed. It may be causative, yet also optional, for example. And it may change. So we can, and must, meaningfully ask whether Aspect's *intention* did affect his *results*. It is banal in the extreme, yet necessary, to remind ourselves that he and his team did not perform the experiments unconsciously. Only stones can do that, for even flies show intention and some degree of awareness. When stones and flies, alive or dead, show effects that humans can then see, they *simply become part of the unconscious apparatus of experiments performed by human consciousness*. However unconsciously passive the material side of it, the consciousness-to-physical-world dipole is, at its pole of Being-there, deliberative and active, as the human-in-the-world goes about its customary "doings and makings." Human intentionality is, now, in the dawning of Gebser's integral consciousness, an ever-present "principle," even a kind of "force." Aspect's experiments could not and would not have taken place at all had he not intended them. The double slit experiment was also done by intention. So was your opening of this book. Intentionality, in the world of conscious beings, is universal, going hand in hand with understanding, with interpretation of the world, with manipulation of it. Indeed, the presence of those observable, inferable, actions is taken as proof of the presence and reality of the intentionality itself. In this context yet another word requires redefinition. That word is *experiment,* for all conscious, reflective, action is, in a universal and global sense, experiment, producing new insights and changed futures containing actions previously unplanned. Evolving consciousness, it seems, is at the very center of it all, at least for our species, for it is its own driver.*

When, long ago, in the state of Gebser's "magical consciousness," the inventor of the wheel watched as a rounded stone came free and rolled down a hill, he or she unwittingly carried out an experiment (of which the stone, too, was doubtless unaware) and "saw" its result and further possibilities without having even sought them. This was not the fully conscious Popperian ideal of present-day scientific method, for his analysis of the process lay in the then far future of the human world, but it worked in a similar way. The ancient observer of stones and slopes took it for granted that nothing would move without some kind of visible or inferable interference by a *living* being, perhaps even a god. The god *itself* was a postulate to explain *unfamiliar* movements, which could not otherwise be explained. The scarcely conscious prior hypothesis was, approximately, that if no animal or human was seen to cause movement no movement would happen, unless the invisible (and unpredictable and often bad-tempered) god of rolling boulders intervened. To this day we are startled by sudden movements and remain apprehensive if no visible cause comes into view. To invent the rolling *wheel* was a further step, awaiting humankind's awakening.

The everyday observation being that stones on the hillside would *not* move, ancient man did not conceive a rational hypothesis based on earlier experience concerning the possible causes of their unexpected movements, as we would try to do today, but in a moment of vision

he nonetheless saw what he would have seen if he *had* first thought of the downward-moving stone, but when he then *interpreted* what he had seen and repeated the experiment by dislodging another stone at the top of a hill to "see what it (or the god in it) would do" he *did* have the hypothesis that it might do what the first stone had done, and he *did* test that hypothesis, in his rough-and-ready way, and found it true. "Stones have a strong wish to go downhill" (or something like it) became one of the scientific theories of his age.

The wheel was *still* not yet in view. That required the further step, alien to many philosophers, but not to Einstein or Beethoven, of *imagination*. Perhaps, much later, this protoscientist's descendents began to sort out the realization that he had discovered a whole suite of facts, not just one, that rounded stones roll whereas pieces of slate only slide, that slates don't even slide unless the hill is very steep, and they are so lazy that they often grind to a halt, while round stones are so happy to have been set free, at last, that they often dance and skip as they descend. It may even have been realized, dimly, that it might not be the stone-god's personality alone that caused the downward, accelerating, happy saltarello, but that there might be something or someone, some "spirit of happy downness" pulling everything, including the observer's body, in the direction his own bodily senses already knew as "down." Whether he had any *word* for "down" is irrelevant, for the immediate sensation of "downness" in the body sufficed, and was already familiar.

However, "down" was sometimes painful or worse for humans, especially if the journey was long but you got there quickly, so perhaps the theory was soon modified, "down" being not always happy, but simply the *proper* place for stones, while humans aspired toward the place to which smoke went, the abode, therefore, of the gods, hidden in the dazzling haze of the heavenly Above. This might have seemed to explain the pain, for humans, of falling in the opposite direction to that of *aspiration*. Science, in those days, was a very "spiritual" matter. Falling down was not a movement toward the gods (who lived on Mount Olympus, or above the summit of Mount Meru) and was punishable by them. It hurt. This kind of notion was, of course, still a part of science as late as Aristotle. He needs, today, to be regarded with suspicion, for his views on causation are

---

*One is reminded of the apostle Paul's words in Romans 8.19–23.

beginning, at last, to seem very little better than the prehistoric theories we have just invented.

Toward a More Complete Completeness, a More Comprehending Comprehension

In this discursive and wide-ranging chapter we have already glimpsed the notion of the self-regarding timeless (and therefore acausal) "just-isness" of the world, noting that the whole physical universe seems to be connected and made whole *by its own internal self-regard.* This inward-turned-ness is a kind of *completeness,* and a kind of *consistency* (of which states we shall say more), and notable for its non-self-destructive tendency. That universal multiplex of loops of interdependent being, Indra's Net, does indeed catch all, and shows each item to all the other items and itself. It is a kind of "set of all sets, including itself, the whole, and even the empty set," a kind of mathematical all-in-one, *no matter how anomalous it may, in some respects, appear to be.* Such seemingly paradoxical notions relate to thoughts that will bring this evolving chapter to its climax.

Today, we are too aware for archaic, magical, mythical, anthropomorphic hypothesizing to occur, unless, perhaps, a gifted, aware, but unsophisticated, very young child might have similar experience, but some of us may be more aware still, on the verge of noticing phenomena hitherto missed by the majority. Schopenhauer and Heidegger assure us that beings in the world could not even be objects of our perception unless, as they disclose themselves to us out-from the world-about, they do so because, indeed, *only* because, they have some interest for or relevance or meaningfulness to us. Our relatedness to them reveals them to us *as themselves,* but as *themselves as they seem to us,* for it is this phenomenal nature and only this that we perceive. We have only a severely limited range of senses to observe them, so *in* themselves they might be rather different. Attention to these beings, or entities, out there in the world-about is, in an initially bewildering sense, a two-way transaction between self and world, questioning our present-day conception of causation. Hence Heidegger's notion of Being-in-the-world, which we have characterized as a part-to-whole dipole, a new dualism conceived to exist within the obviously *non*dual context of the Whole.

Adding to the Heideggerian account of our apperception of the world-about, we have Gebser's assurance, mentioned earlier, that humankind, over millennia, developed first what he terms *archaic* consciousness, then *magical* consciousness, next *mythic* consciousness, then the currently prevalent *mental* consciousness. Within this latest mode of consciousness he sees an unperspectival worldview followed, from about 1500 CE in the West, by a perspectival view. He goes on to claim that we are now developing what he calls aperspectival consciousness, an *all-round* view *transcending* the current perspectival, partial, viewpointed kinds of observation, and that this most recent and still-emerging development heralds what he calls *integral* consciousness, which will be available to us alongside the preexisting modes. In chapter 18 we shall develop such concepts further, for the advocates of "Spiral Dynamics" have made a similar understanding central to their own explanatory schemes. So we should note again that Gebser sees these mutations of consciousness not as a historical succession and supercession, but as an *accumulation* of different ways of being conscious. Consciousness is not one mode of awareness, but a whole suite of tools, each with its typical ways of experiencing and its own objects of "view." Therefore, as we become aware that we have these modes, and as new modes are added, we should begin to use them, each for its own range of purposes. Musical composition, for instance (to the surprise of those who do not understand it), needs a primarily mythic, storytelling consciousness. Integral consciousness, moreover, may offer something attributed formerly only to God, an awareness that does not cross space or take time doing so in order to see what is far away, or even what is future or past. Quantum interconnectedness or other phenomena of modern physics may make this possible; as we become aware of them, and so include them in our intending, they may even make the operation of integral consciousness voluntary.*

Gebser sees the new integral consciousness as

---

*Again, the reader is asked to excuse the limitations imposed by existing language, and to excuse our resisting the temptation to turn aside into discussion of the philosophical problems produced by the inability of spatiotemporal terminology from the past to express new concepts that transcend space and time. Such verbal philosophy is a useless, self-impeding diversion, practiced, since they perceive nothing else, by those who have no reimaginative vision for what is being communicated. We are concerned with the ideas and the realities, not with the outdated and clumsy language we are all constrained to use.

working aperspectivally, having no single limiting perspective because it comprehends all perspectives in one all-seeing global grasp-of-mind. Jung and Dingle's quest for a union between their disciplines fits neatly with this quest. Perhaps only such a consciousness could build the expanded and integrated psycho-bio-physics that Jung and Dingle envisaged. Perhaps that very quest will, of itself, not merely necessitate, but even provide us with, the already-expanded consciousness required to discover both the expanded physics *and that expanded consciousness itself,* for consciousness *is* awareness of itself *as* awareness of things other than itself. If this abdication of causation seems irrational it will serve to illustrate the very effect we are now seeking to transcend, the blighting of insightful vision when linear, causal logic is applied to realms now being glimpsed in which such logic cannot be usefully applied at all. The physical universe is already seen as seeing itself and so as "bringing itself about." Language fails, of course, for "bringing something about" sounds like the description of a process rather than of a state or manner of being, but earlier we described this "seeing itself and so being" and are familiar with the notion. Further, we may come into possession not just of enhanced understanding or knowledge, but even of the enhanced powers we have spoken of already, for what we notice, in the self-seeing and self-connected quantum universe, and find to be "new" as we "do science" today and think about what we observe, we may develop into an ability to perform freely within, and control by will, the greater world revealed to us by that very same expanded understanding. Our Being-in-the-world grows with us, and our world-about grows as our consciousness grows. Awareness of an encompassing world without the trappings of physical causation may produce in our minds a conflation of "cause" with "effect," possibly *outdating altogether the current related usages of both terms* even within our physical world, for this everyday level of understanding was probably always wrong, if only we could have seen it. Post hoc ergo propter hoc (*after* this, therefore *because of* this) was probably never true, but merely seemed so in a world enslaved to a temporal perspective. Linear logic is a natural development in such a world. Here, Aristotle may seem more right than elsewhere, for he at least perceived the *teleological* concept of the "*final*

cause," the end toward which "causation" tended, conceiving it as a kind of causal pull by the future back upon the present. It was a first step, useful, quasi-correct but nevertheless quite wrong in its deep essence, and he should have seen it, for the concept of final cause compromised the very notions it relied upon, those of time and causality itself. The future must already exist, in some sense, for it "causes" progress from the present toward itself. Progress toward a final state is conceived as taking place "because of" that final state's *already-existingness.* So the so-called causal reality is better conceived as we have suggested, as an interdependency of being, which concept, appropriately aperspectival with respect to time, is entirely *present-tense.* We need, now, a far more mature view than Aristotle's, in line with the new Gebserian aperspectivalism.

The World without Us and with Us

So we remove, as expected, the pseudoproblem of the world's continued existence when "no one is observing it," for this is never the case. It is its own observer, the bringer into the *being-a-Whole* that its own being *is,* and we come with it, but, because we are "time-ly" beings, limited to "now," to "foresight," and to "memory" (the things that led Aristotle halfway to the truth, but left him stranded there), the question of the extent of the powers of consciousness and intention now comes to the fore, and is undeniably relevant to the concept of the subtle body. Let us look more closely, then, at intentionality, and at the "space" and "time" in which it has to work.

All our senses are neither more nor less than those that have defined physics. Physics is *our* product, fashioned according to *our* capacities and limitations. It is therefore impossible to make direct observation by physical methods of any *nonphysical* entity, yet, knowing ourselves limited but sensing also that we are not ourselves entirely physical, we cannot deny that there may be myriad realities that are not physical, either by the present definition or by any possible expansion of it. We cannot make physical observations of our "spiritual" parts, even if (or even *though*) such exist, because all our observational techniques are, by reason of our nature, precisely those that define physics, namely our bodily senses, extended in range, but not in nature, by instruments; de facto this automatically excludes all else. We invented the very word *spiritual because* we sensed inwardly that physics did *not* comprehend everything of which we are *aware*. This is why attempts to detect ghosts in haunted buildings by *physical* means always fall short of discovering *non*physical beings. The spiritual is therefore *discriminated* (rather than defined in the true sense of the word) precisely and automatically by its being "the normally unobservable," which makes it "*meta*physics." It is *essentially* unobservable, unless the inner sense, which has no sense organ (what we might term "our sense of selfness itself"), has precisely the kind of power we seek, a power of direct, organless receptivity and intentionality, a capacity not mediated by the physical body. By now, all this is familiar. The question is where we should go next, and the answer is clear.

Is There Such a Thing as Action Entirely *without the Body?*

The only possibility of a testable empirical question regarding an essentially unobservable entity would be whether "mind" or "spirit" (something real but unobservable by physical means and therefore neither apperceived nor defined) can exist or act *only* when the healthy body exists, or whether we can find strong evidence of its acting *outside* the body, *independently of* the body. As we have stressed before, only such actions by a *non*physical entity having effects *within* the physical world, instances of a kind of psychokinesis, could be so investigated, for *we can examine it only from within our physical world even if its real existence is outside that world.* This would be, of necessity, indirect evidence, but such evidence is no more indirect than the evidence I have that in whatever sense I exist you also exist. Such evidence would support a *necessary hypothesis* of the real presence and real action of *something* that seems to be truly *meta*physical, just as I am a *necessary* postulate for you, and you for me. We shall quote just two intriguing and relevant cases below. But first, having seen (as did Dingle and others seventy years ago) how limited and limiting science is, we need to take a hard look at science itself, and ask some questions about its methods and prospects. Hence we must take another circular detour to survey the territory.

Is Science Adequate for Its New Task?
Taking Stock of the Problem Ahead

If we think back to the beginning of this chapter we shall recall that science itself and other subjects, too,

need to change their outlooks, their boundaries, and their "word games" if any search for a truth encompassing them all is to succeed. As currently constituted, the various areas of human study and even of our everyday concerns have divided the contents of human consciousness into sections that cannot survive alone, and have divided humans themselves into factions, which have caused social division and linguistic Babel. That situation must change if anything more than partisan truth is ever to be found and shared. We must achieve this communion if we, as a race, are to survive, or even to gain conscious possession of a more comprehensive view of ourselves and our place in the universe. Even political peace ultimately depends upon personal openness and honesty, so it is unsurprising that it has never succeeded for any length of time. Physics, and all those "hard sciences" that are grounded in physics, are too limited to fulfill the need. However, as our perspective upon ourselves grows to transcend perspective itself, the new, more comprehensive, aperspectival consciousness will aid and accelerate the search. It will *itself* evolve and it will evolve *its own* "hard science."

We have seen that physics excluded the spiritual (whatever its nature) but future science must be greater than mere physics and must, by some legitimate means, and despite the difficulties, either include or allow those experiences we call "spiritual." We must have a spiritual science, as, in their various ways of expressing it, Jung, Dingle, Pauli, Steiner, and many others have asserted. Roger Penrose, whom we shall later quote at some length, believes the hugely successful quantum physics of today is incomplete, and that its lack of a full account of consciousness is among its chief inadequacies.[23] To gain scientific knowledge of our spirituality we must have spiritual experiences, whatever they are, however understood (or currently misunderstood), and we must ponder those experiences if the proper testable hypotheses are to dawn. This is what we have done for millennia with our *physical* experiences, and the resulting science has certainly succeeded as the science *of the physical.* Now it must extend. Further, we shall inevitably be faced with the venerable and hoary problem of the various dualities, between conscious and nonconscious, between living and nonliving, spirit and matter, matter and energy, immanent and transcendent, wave and particle, a priori truth (which may well be what mathematics is) and spontaneous, unaccountable, but marvelous human creativity, between computable and algorismic* processing on the one hand, and the intuitive *seeing-straight-through to the answer* of "genius" on the other.

There are questions. Have our erstwhile misunderstandings invented dualities where correct concepts and percepts would have seen an undivided reality? Do we, in fact, have real dualities in our cosmos, or are they all illusory? Are they real in one domain but unreal in another? What does the word *real* mean? Can we cope, intellectually, with the duality (undoubtedly produced in part by the limitations of our understanding of the world-about) between our concepts of "realness" on the one hand and "illusion" on the other? Is "illusion" a reality and "reality" an illusion? Is reality real and illusion an illusion? Note how quickly these questions about *reality* slide into the abyss of blather about *the meanings of words*. Science must, as we have seen so often, be careful about meanings, but this degradation is something it must avoid *at any cost*. Of course, the last question, whether reality is real and illusion illusory, resolves itself if exhaustive knowledge is finally obtained, for it then becomes merely a question of allocating the available words to the distinct meanings, the clearly different understandings, that have become known. If we were to achieve a full understanding of the world we would reallocate "illusions" to a category containing simply a different kind of reality—the illusory kind. We might then regard illusions as pictures of reality, as we now regard paintings or photographs, telling truth, but not facsimile truth or complete truth. Ipso facto, the very concept of an illusion would cease and many current words would be redefined or become head-shaking puzzles for the new mind visiting the museums of the future and pondering the archaic oddities from our age there on display. Please bear these thoughts in mind as we proceed, for they point to notions we wish to draw out in due time, not least the fact of our own lack of knowledge even of our immediate world-about. Why do we, natural knowers and learners, have so little knowledge of the physical world, and why does its discovery require work? More follows from these questions than we normally recognize.

Let us come back to questions we can and should tackle now: Are what we now call illusions real (if uncommon) *levels* of reality, rather than real, if uncommon, *perceptions* of reality? Are the constituents of the many dualities merely at different points on continua, showing mere differences of degree (as in all hylic-pluralistic world-views), or are there substantive differences, differences of kind, between them, as in vitalist/dualist views? The good advice to avoid *unnecessary* multiplication of entities (Occam's Razor) will retain its force for both science and philosophy, for the very quest upon which we are engaged is to find a Grand Unity, *if we can*. That is what any search for what we conceive as "wholeness" must be about, the happy resolution of seeming inconsistencies.* So we seek wholeness, harmony, unity, but even as we pursue this goal nothing could be more foolish than to refuse to maintain an old or conceive a new category when explanation via two categories is clearly more successful than it is via only one. Only *extremely* simple things, such as clouds, are automatically whole, indeed whole *at any size*. No "thing" would be in need of finding wholeness if there were not complexity within it. Our Being exists in such a complex world and is *itself* inwardly complex, despite also having an essential self-inclusive self-enveloping unity-of-being.

There is always the hope that, as in physics, a duality unavoidable at one level of understanding will give way, easily and naturally, to unification at a higher level. Thus, to give a very mundane illustration at the level of their practical use, it would be plain silly to class cars with boats, even though both carry Beings-in-the-world and are directed by Beings-in-the-world. They have much in common, but their difference is too gross to ignore. One

---

*The more common usage is *algorithm,* but this is incorrect, and can give the false impression that an algorism is *one particular* simple arithmetical formula. The word *algorismic* in fact denotes *any* procedure for carrying out a formal, mathematical calculation, mechanically, step by step, often the same step infinitely repeated. The word derives from the name of the Arab mathematician of the ninth century CE, al-Khuwarizmi, which provides the fundamental reason for respecting the correct spelling.

*One example is the disharmony that still plagues all human societies regarding the erotic and the spiritual. Why should these faculties of humanness ever have been in conflict? But they are, to a greater or lesser extent, in every society on the planet! A more technical disharmony is that between quantum physics and relativistic physics. Both are correct, but even today their incompatibility persists and wholeness has not been achieved.

would simply have to conceive the minority of amphibian vehicles as belonging in the overlap of two sets, a notion well within the grasp of any amateur mathematician. This being so obvious a truth, the most surprising and perhaps also the grossest of all category errors is the common assertion by recent philosophers that the whole of our being can be explained within the category of present-day physics. Dingle's view was that physics is a *narrow* category incapable even of encompassing all motions. Indeed, *all* those motions we call "living" are excluded from physics as currently defined. It copes only with *dead* flies. We have already seen a dipole—a duality—between living entities and that of which living entities are aware, namely their world-about. This duality, among the many we recognize, seems the most resistant to unification, the fierce opposition of reductionist science and allied philosophy notwithstanding. And it is precisely this duality that most concerns the quest for the subtle body, scientifically understood and described for the modern world. How would we define, or, for that matter, discover, the difference between a dead fly and a living one?

Only by open-mindedness will any change of paradigm prove viable, and meanwhile claims that livingness, whatever it is, exists outside physics, or the opposing claim that it is totally within physics, would prove nothing about reality if they merely evince the prior definition of physics. So our search is for reality, not for the politics of physics or for verbal analysis of an existing situation that arose from a merely social exclusion by scientists of the past, which was convenient for their time. Please note where we now stand. Simplifying the situation much less than one might think, we see that we must open up science to honest questions it has never yet addressed, and do so despite the fact that philosophers claim that the scientific questions have long been settled in favor of materialistic explanations, and want both to prevent this expansion of science and to divert intelligent attention into questions of verbal meaning. This being our analysis of the situation, in admittedly very broad terms, we persevere and ask whether, as with the boats and cars, the one at home on water, the other on land, the physical body might not be in one "set" of the Venn diagram, the "soul" in the other, as vast numbers of humans have believed, and the overlap of the two sets be seen in the phenomenon of embodied life? It is merely a picture, and the analogy is poor, of course, that of vehicle and driver being much better, but we shall not argue from analogy, good or bad. We point out, instead, that the concept brings with it a simple and convincing account of living and dying, which monist views fail dismally to explain. The ancient hypothesis has always been worthy of Popperian testing, though the necessary veridical tests would be difficult to devise. The examination of spontaneous cases may have to suffice. An unfashionable truth we must espouse is that you should never use Occam's Razor to cut your own throat. If you really need another entity to explain the facts, postulate it without fear, especially as entities that seem separate at our present everyday level may be already a unity at another unseen level, like the physicists' four forces, which, as mentioned earlier, were all one under the very different conditions of the first instants after the big bang. Science has been successful, and all science is based on daring postulates. So, is the "soul" (by whatever name) real and independent, real in its own unique right and in its own, its very *ownmost,* individually personal way? To be a Being or merely to be, that is the question.

Indeed, that was the question, posed in other words, which we left unanswered earlier, the question whether any "part" of us, such as consciousness, intention, or will, could act *alone,* as if *itself* an autonomous, active or receptive *agent.* Another way of putting this would be to inquire whether the human being, not using either its sense organs or its muscular organs of action, such as hands or voice, can alter the "external" world. We do not see how any evidence other than *empirical observation of events that are currently inexplicable in the absence of the physical body* could answer this question. The origin of any nonphysical "causes and effects" would be difficult to discover because, being necessarily "beyond the body," they must nonetheless provide evidence of themselves *within* the body's physical world, for that is the only place we could observe or measure them. Accordingly, the evidence we shall give is of this empirical but indirect sort. We have space for only two examples, of different types, one revealing objective empirically verifiable facts, the other concerning personal Being, but we believe each to be among the most impressive and evidentially reliable examples one could hope to find.

Harold Puthoff and Russell Targ, writing in 1976, began their paper delivered before the IEEE[24] with a précis, then provided details we regard as evidence that, either moving and acting autonomously or sensing at a distance by means of paranormal communications available to it, consciousness shows itself either *free to move itself in its entirety far away from the body* or to be *not co-extensive with the body but able to extend itself out beyond the body, as if to be in many places at once, so extending over a larger area than the body's normal purview.* Such events cannot be accommodated within any understanding that is *both* strongly monist and strongly physicalist, as emergentist interpretations necessarily are. It is only by relinquishing at least one, and probably both, of these positions that the events can be explained. Puthoff and Targ's account has been slightly and unimportantly abridged but the remaining words are unedited.

In 1974 Puthoff and I were conducting viewing experiments at SRI, supported largely by the CIA. One assignment was to describe a Soviet research and development laboratory at a particular latitude and longitude in the USSR. The psychic description that we and our viewer provided to our sponsor was so outstanding that it assured our funding for several years. The results were classified *because our drawings and descriptions were verified by satellite photography.* Pat Price and Ingo Swann had already demonstrated that they could describe distant locations where someone was hiding, and we had just started carrying out experiments to describe distant sites, given only their geographical latitude and longitude. Our contract monitor, a physicist from the CIA, had brought us coordinates from what he described as a "Soviet site of great interest to the analysts." They wanted any information we could give them, and they were eager to find out if we could describe a target ten thousand miles away, with only coordinates to work from. Price and I climbed to the small electrically shielded room which we had been using for our experiments. As always, I began our little ritual of starting the tape recorder, giving the time and date, and describing who we were and what we were doing. I then read the coordinates. Again, as was Pat's custom he . . . leaned back in his chair and closed his eyes . . . then began his description: "I am lying on my back on the roof of a two or three storey brick building. It's a sunny day. The sun feels good. There's the most amazing thing. There's a giant gantry crane moving back and forth over my head . . . As I drift up in the air and look down, it seems to be riding on a track with one rail on each side of the building. I've never seen anything like that." Pat then made a little sketch of the layout of the buildings, and the crane, which he labeled as a "gantry." Later on, he again drew the crane as we show it.

Targ himself adds, "The accuracy of Price's drawing is the sort of thing that I, as a physicist, would never have believed, if I had not seen it for myself."[25]

At present physics has no explanation of such events, *unless* by resort to the concept of "quantum interconnection," or a *hidden* underlying field of some kind that

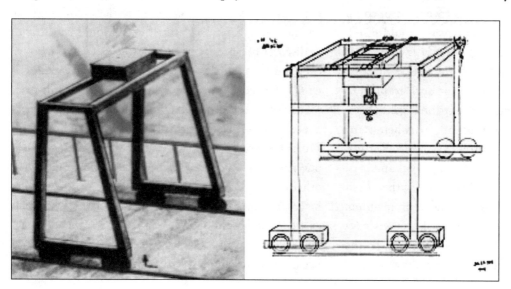

Fig. 15.8. A tracing made from the CIA's satellite photograph of the Soviet site (left side) and the drawing Pat Price made, without knowledge of the CIA's discoveries, after remotely viewing the site (right side). Better images were not available, but these still show the astonishing success of the remote viewing.

what we call consciousness can tap. That connectedness appears to operate in some sense "behind" the physical world as we normally experience it. The connection is *invisible* to us. We do not *experience* it directly, or in any way that is traceable by our senses. Price, Puthoff, and Targ showed impressively that the information-gathering, or distant observation, does happen, but the means of its happening was not apparent to them and is still not apparent. All attempts to find *ordinarily physical* means of viewing-at-a-distance have failed, like the quest for *physical* proof of the reality of ghosts. Why?

We believe the answer is as obvious as the answer to any deeply important question could ever be permitted to be. There is a serious category error, not an irrelevant merely verbal one like those dragged into service by Ryle to prove the dualist view erroneous, but an error of *real* categories, which, once understood, will show dualism correct. Prejudice has conflated a physical and a nonphysical level that truly are real and distinguishable, the distinction hidden by a stubborn refusal to postulate a "new" entity even when it is required by the facts. Instead of granting the necessity of the nonmaterial level of reality even serious philosophers speak of "eyes on stalks" when discussing distant viewing. This bespeaks, and itself perpetuates, the erroneous conflation of levels. Such words bewitch. "Eyes on stalks" is an impossibly silly, physicalist notion, showing a confusion of "levels" that should never occur in the modern mind, and, but for the current prejudice against dualistic views, never would. We do not yet know how it is done, but distant viewing is *certainly* done *without* eyes. Should we not, therefore, be postulating a duality of levels within the wholeness of human Beingness, the physical level (the science revealed when we use our ordinary sense organs and their prosthetic, physical extensions) and an extraphysical one, or *at least* a more *subtly* physical one?

These considerations raise the very same questions as the quest for the subtle body. When we build automata, such as the singing Father Christmases that appear in supermarkets around Christmastime, we know them to be such, knowing their "singing" to be the product of relatively simple technology aping the real outputs of a real human, not the living result of an inner complexity like our own. Even children who find these plastic automata "spooky" do not believe them alive. Indeed, it is precisely the knowledge that it is *not* alive, the *unbelievableness* of

the *intrusive pretence* of its own livingness by the plastic figure, the *pretended* conflation of nonliving with living, that produces the disquieting ambivalence in the young observer.* Furthermore, we know how tables and chairs and plastic Father Christmases come into being, but our own morphogenesis, and that of all organisms, is still a mystery, perhaps *describable,* but as yet not at all *explained* except by *non*physical or very *subtly* physical postulated entities such as morphogenetic fields. The postulate, very briefly, is that a morphogenetic field is, in effect, the *pattern* of a Being, something present before the Being comes into being-in-the-world, and it *oversees the development* of that Being. The notion was mentioned earlier, and will become clearer in a very natural way if the reader will have patience with the slow development of this chapter's full integral understanding.

These considerations, we suggest, strongly oppose the notion that our consciousness and self-direction is immanent, an emergent product of mere physical complexity, without influence from an "above," from the realm of the morphogenetic pattern. It is our livingness that requires physical complexity, not physical complexity that mechanistically produces livingness, the main evidence for this interpretation being that a dead body, while it remains recognizable as a body, is just as complex as a living one. Please ponder this, and its rational implications, before continuing. The argument can be run the other way, with equal force, for even within the brain there are large components having great complexity, which never evince consciousness at all, such as the cerebellum. Complexity does *not* automatically *produce* consciousness. Consciousness is, therefore, in at least two real senses, independent of biological complexity, perhaps even of biology itself.

Questions about executive actions by *independent* consciousness still have to be approached via the physical world, so our next possibility of understanding may lie in a study of the related matter of healing-at-a-distance. If quantum indeterminacy and interconnection are not sufficient for self-willed distant action, how do distant viewing and distant influence such as healing take place?

---

*Note how the child accepts television programs in which absent humans are seen to be singing, yet shrinks from plastic Father Christmases who also sing. Cats and dogs seem usually to be puzzled by both phenomena, or indifferent to both.

As we said earlier, it is not a matter of "eyes on stalks" or of healing hands on hugely extensible arms. Such physicalistic notions naïvely prejudge the very matter to be discovered, making the *presumption,* indeed, the *dogma,* that the explanation *must* be *ordinarily* physical, without extension of our present understanding of physics. Aspect's own view of his own experiment refutes this belief for he says emphatically that no *message-content* can be transmitted via the quantum interconnection. Its only content is itself. The question is, therefore, how any distant effect of consciousness or will can be physical at all. On any understanding including knowledge of Aspect's experiment it is either delusive or nonphysical. The naïve and arrogant dogma that any such process *is and must be* physical gives rise to chimerical strange loops, and is effectively this: "We all know by experience that eyes are necessary for sight. Therefore, if distant viewing occurs it must be by means of eyes, which must therefore be extended on stalks to the site concerned." We might immediately ask why we do not see the eyes on stalks of anyone nearby who is indulging in a little distant viewing, for, their eyes-on-stalks being purportedly physical, we *would* expect to see them by using our own eyes in the ordinary way (whether ours are on stalks or not). To speak frankly, this level of "reasoning" shows not only a prejudgment of the answer but also an immature and atavistic conflation of the ordinarily physical with phenomena so obviously *not* ordinarily physical that we *must* relinquish the belief that perception and action can only be via the bodily physical organs, on ten-thousand-mile-long stalks when necessary. Such *anthropomorphic* thinking invented the old gods, and the same *atavistic* confusion of levels has blighted human discovery of the facts of the cosmos throughout the history of the species. It is precisely such imprisoned perspectives that Gebser's foresight predicts we shall eventually transcend.

It was precisely the fact that we do *not,* indeed, cannot, in our normal bodily experience, extend ourselves thousands of miles to observe happenings in a foreign country that brought about Puthoff and Targ's investigation. Now that we have their evidence it would be foolish in the extreme to deny that some kind of nonnormal, or at least extremely *unfamiliar,* communication over great distance takes place. The quantum interconnection that so greatly extends classical physics exists, of course, but it

does not, on its own, explain distant viewing. The clairvoyance is tentatively explicable, in our present state of knowledge, by resort to the notion of the "teleportation" from the distant site, not of any particles themselves but of the *changes in quantum state* of particles involved in the perception process, which might correlate with or cause or even constitute the changes in the eye-brain system of the distant viewer that *would* occur if normal vision using the eyes were occurring. It still remains, of course, to elucidate the process by which this might occur. The suggestion is scarcely above the level of a postulate, certainly not yet to be accepted as theory.

Returning from speculation to witnessed narrative we note that Pat Price does not say that his normal sensing ceased when he sensed things ten thousand miles away. Neither does he say that as he sat in the shielded room he saw the gantry crane in exactly the everyday way, but he did feel the everyday Russian sun on his face, and the ordinary counter-pressure of the roof against his back, in just as real a way as if he had been there in his body and gravity had been pressing him to the roof in exactly that familiar way. These necessary quantum effects within his body's sensory systems *might* be performed by "teleportation" of quantum changes. But how? And why? Any teleportation of physical effects would have needed to be not only of the quantum states necessary for sight but also of the huge complex of simultaneous physical awareness that constitutes our normal waking range of bodily sense-experiences, and so gives us our normal operational definition of reality. Perhaps, had he tried, Price might have lifted some Russian industrial dust from the roof with his fingertips and rolled it between them to sense its grittiness, to "prove" it "real." Reality, as I saw just half a century ago, informally beginning to study philosophy and to think for myself, consists in and actually *is* a "complete set of sensory coincidences," by which I meant a complete set of the sensations produced by the five senses. If you provide the normal organs of perception with a set of perceptions that are fully consistent with past experience, you are content to say that it is reality that you have before you. If the body-mind receives the same full set of stimuli, it does not matter that they are, for the sake of argument, electronically or chemically generated in the absence of the usual reality. We still seem to see that reality.

We invite readers to ponder at length this possibility

of *virtual* reality and to picture how it might fit with our questions about reality and illusion. Reality as we experience it seems very unlikely to be the whole of reality. Perhaps there is even a "squalification" going on beyond our view, though what it *is* remains utterly unknowable. We probably *experience* only the flimsiest mirage of deep reality. Even our normal experience is to some degree indirect, "virtual," as Berkeley realized. Unfortunately, we do not have space in this book to pursue a philosophical analysis of such matters and must be content to say that a process of quantum teleportation, if verified, would bring clairvoyance into an extended physics, though "mind" and "will" are evidently still required, for, if not, how is the choice made to navigate to a distant viewing point that has been *specifically requested?* In this instance the direction to the site consisted in nothing more than highly abstract data Price could not have been holding in memory, the previously unrevealed coordinates of latitude and longitude. Of course, CIA staff knew where the factory was when they quoted only those coordinates. Perhaps Price also knew, unconsciously, by telepathy from the minds of the CIA staff. However the *direction* was achieved so reliably that a simple dualistic interpretation of a very traditional kind seems to offer the best explanation of the whole sensory experience per se, and the completeness of the range of sensations received while "at the site" also suggests a strongly dualist way of being *outside* the body, for Price did not disappear from Puthoff's view when he "visited" Semipalatinsk. He did not even seem absent from the room at Stanford in any other way, yet in some sense he nonetheless "took his senses with him." What he did not take was his *bodily* sense *organs.* Neither, so far as we know, did he enter the body and use the sense organs of some person who, at the very time required, was conveniently lying on the factory roof. Indeed, Price was able to float up from the roof *and still see.* Nonetheless, he gained the same kind of impressions and information as he would have done if observing in the everyday manner. No present-day physics quite succeeds in explaining this, but we have a suggestion. There could be *nonphysical* eyes that work in parallel with the physical eyes. This notion is simplistically stated, and without dogmatism. It is just a mind-opening idea to hold before our view, but we shall return to it, though in another guise. Now we must sum up before moving forward.

As we have just seen, our senses, however they work, *define, indeed, confine, reality as experienced by humans.* Thus the remote viewer, while apparently in the physical world, has an experience that cannot be wholly *explained as* taking place in that normal physical world, even though in some sense it *does* give what seems to him a normal awareness (a fact that supports our brand of *parallel* duality) since it cannot occur by any known mechanism of physical communication. Keep in mind that quantum interconnection of the kind demonstrated by Aspect does *not,* despite the popular misconception, allow faster-than-light messaging, nor any other *informational content* to be sent or received by us. Such information would have to travel by an additional normal, classical, channel. Discovering the interconnection has merely revealed to us the fact that *strong,* even *quasi-causal* links persist between particles that already have a joint history, and suggests that a quantum state *might* be "observable" or "experienceable" elsewhere than the place at which it came into being. Only in this special sense could information be considered to have been "transmitted." The Russian plant at Semipalatinsk did not come crashing, or even *seem to* come crashing, into the electromagnetically shielded room in which Price sat, nor did his body go to Semipalatinsk, but, at the most, only his sensing of the factory traveled there. The teleportation, whether *to* Semipalatinsk or *from* Semipalatinsk, of a *whole suite* of ordinarily physical quantum states effectively constituting a *full set* of bodily senses seems unlikely in the extreme. Occam's Razor seems better respected by the hypothesis that Pat Price showed a (nonharmful) dividedness into two than by the denial of dualism, which would require us to accept and explain all monism's mind-befuddling conceptual anomalies. At the least, Price's sensing ability went to Semipalatinsk quite outside of normal space and time, so *nothing physical* moved—and the Seer saw, so accurately that the CIA funded several more years of research on the ground of his achievement. That, as people are wont to say, is hard to argue against.

Widening the Exploration of Self and World-About

Will It Show Us the Seer?

We still face the question of how a human, normally thought of by most people today as a *merely physical* being, limited *in* and limited *to* space and time, has distant-viewing experiences. Shall we accept the notion that *in some sense, which overcomes the impossibility of transmitting messages via Aspect's interconnection,* the subtle body *is* the instantly everywhere quantum connection he has proved, effectively suggesting that the connection *itself* is an *entity,* even a kind of *living* entity (perhaps containing us all), and *so* the means by which we sometimes see at a distance? If such a scheme should prove correct, each of us would seem to participate in a single wholeness at a "higher" or more fundamental level than the everyday world-about. It would be as if the outermost kośa, in one of the Indic schemata, were so large as to unite us all within what physicists might term a universal single field. But many recoil, emotionally affronted, from a notion that both makes a physical field a conscious Being and, at the same time, forces all Beings within it to recognize their existential unity. Moreover, it demands an extension of physics into realms of what has traditionally been seen as rather nonphysical behavior (taking the word *physical* in the restricted sense to which Dingle objected, of course).

Should we prefer the alternative perspective that *we* in our *essential* Being are *separable from* the world-about but in a stronger version of the sense we saw earlier, the sense of a part-to-whole duality, which, in this "strong" version, sees each of us as a part, indeed, as the *essential* part, of what might be postulated to be a nonspatial, and perhaps nontemporal, "Seer"? In this scenario, too, each of us would be in some sense more extensive than the body. It is precisely this spread of our "presence," with its capacity for conscious intentionality, in the one part, and its total absence from the other part, which justifies the characterization of the whole as a duality. This view also explains both the evident purposiveness of Being, and its cessation at the transition we call "dying." This interpretation does not demand an extension of present physics, for if the view is correct the subtle body is *already* outside current physics and needs only an interface of some sort with the physical world in order to inhabit physical bodies and show its intentionality in the world by its various doings and makings.

The question of what it *is* that the subtle body *is* remains the one we posed before. Put too simply, no doubt, it is this: Is our essential Being a hitherto-unsuspected (or at least unexplained) extension of the physical world, or is it a distinct *non*physical entity, merely cohabiting with our physical components? Since even quantum interconnection is unable to explain fully the phenomena of distant viewing and intentional action at a distance, the opinion that our essential Being is nonphysical surely now seems far the more likely. Physicists and neuroscientists are entitled to criticize our beliefs, but if they choose to do so they will also have to defend their own. Meanwhile, our view is that vitalist and dualist explanations of our Being are as viable in today's science as they have ever seemed to earlier scientific and prescientific consciousness.

Are any tentative conclusions possible at this stage? As things stand, "spirit" might still be outside physics, and a part of us might be a part of that spaceless and distanceless "spirit," even a part of a "Great Spirit." If that were so, no empirical physical investigation could decide between extended but normal physics and *nonspatial and nontemporal* presence "simultaneously" "there" as well as "here." The physical and any spiritual entity beyond it would then simply be in the same line of view of the physical world outward from our apparatus, never to be distinguished when so viewed. We mentioned this before, but repeat it now because it is extremely important. We cannot ever see the spiritual out beyond the physical, for the physical itself obscures the view by interposing itself. Consider the simple illustration, wholly within the physical world, of a total eclipse of the sun, during which it is not possible to see beyond the moon; another is that of a line of pillars viewed from one end, which obscures the living person standing beyond the last of them, or even between them.

Nevertheless, our conscious seeing *of the physical* can rationally be described as a function of a *spiritual* Being, for, we believe, only a Being can see, whether with or without eyes. It is perfectly clear that the eyes of a dead body do not see. Livingness and seeing are inextricably conjoined. Being and thing, we believe, are different in precisely the required way, the way that justifies our concept of a part-to-whole duality. Beings are conceived to be entities that have consciousness and senses, while things are precisely those entities that do not, and are so defined, antithetically. The word *spiritual* came into being to point toward something yet "higher," yet more subtle than the being of Beings, a third level. We would need somehow to step aside and look *around* physics to see spiritual entities, if they exist. It follows that if we find we *can* step sideward and look around physics it will be *because* we are in some sense nonphysical. The spiritual that is *inside* us would then resonate with the spiritual that lies beyond the physical, *outside* us. Is not this what Pat Price experienced? Our science, on its own, could *never* discover whether there were some spiritual entity, ipso facto unobservable, in line with and beyond, and therefore obscured by, what it could and did observe.

The body's limits are (apart from instrumental extensions) the same as the limits of our physics. When consciousness is in the physical body the view-about is limited to the physical view, and the nonphysical, the supraphysical, the spiritual, can never be proven real in a manner that can satisfy *physics* from where we stand, looking out upon the physical world-about from our physical bodies in the physical world, using our physical senses. To put it rather tastelessly, to ask physics to prove to us the reality of the spiritual would be analogous to asking a dead body to answer our questions as to what life is. That physics is unable to handle nonphysical matters, such as its failure to explain the movements of living beings, should cause us no surprise for it perpetually finds inadequate its own explanations even of the merely physical. Even within its own realm as presently defined it has had to make continual revisions. Newton's physics will no longer serve all our needs, and Einstein's physics is not yet fully integrated with quantum physics, though both are far beyond rational doubt of their truth. Science must forever move on, so even now, as the twenty-first century progresses, the postulation of an essence beyond current physics may be unavoidable if we are to understand our Being; and many physicists agree.

Evidence from Paranormal Experience

So, as we have been forced to say too often, the central question remains that of whether we have to postulate something outside physics, or whether a modern version of hylic pluralism that extends present physics will explain everything about our essence and manner of being. Recent mathematics and physics have provided a new candidate to stand alongside Aspect's quantum entanglement on the one hand and the alternative postulate, an extra-physical living entity, on the other. In this, the penultimate "epicycle" of this chapter, we

need to look at the new candidate, in particular to see whether it offers the distant viewing and distant acting capability that quantum interconnectedness alone does not seem to give. To do this we shall have to return to the concept of waves and fields. After that, as we conclude, we shall make a tentative choice among the candidates, but first of all we must augment the evidence from Puthoff and Targ, presented a few pages back, for if we find, in addition to theirs, evidence of the *separability* of an *experiencing being that is normally conjoined with a body* and evidence of its *acting as an entity entirely independent of that body,* the corroboration of what we might term "duality, or even multiplexity, of body" will be even stronger.

With regard to this quest, we offer the following account, placed in 2008 in the archives of the Society for Psychical Research (SPR). We give the whole text of the subject's own account of his experience, and even a sketch he made himself, without alteration of any kind.

On 28 November 2007 I ate a meal while watching the 6 o'clock news on BBC television. Later, as I sat in an armchair, the BBC news was again beginning. The time was therefore 10 pm. At the moment the news began I began to feel very dizzy. I had felt dizzy *in this way* only a very few times in my life. I felt I had to sit stock still to try to control the dizziness, and that I would not be able to get up without falling over. I felt two completely distinct and separate sets of sensations. There was the feeling of sitting very still in the armchair, but in addition I experienced a *completely separate* sensation, as the dizziness rapidly increased to a state of disorientation *far* worse than I had *ever* felt in my life. I felt as if "I" was sitting in the armchair, completely still, but *at the same time* "I" was also being swung around from my waist upward. I felt very definitely divided into two absolutely, perceptibly, distinct beings from the waist upward. The "self" which was being swung around was completely diffuse. It *was* a swirling, *not* a body-shaped thing being "swirled," but the "swirlingness" was of the same volume and general shape as my physical body, yet completely stirred up inside itself, without internal features or character other than the extreme dizziness itself, and without external sense organs such as ears or eyes. I did not "see" out of the swirled self at all, for it had absolutely no external senses, but I suffered its intense interior dizziness.

The normal external sense organs remained sitting in the chair, and sensed the world from there, absolutely as they normally did, but with the overwhelming dizziness felt within the swirled self "superimposed" upon the normal sensing. The swinging self had no sensible head or face, but was stirred to a complete internal featurelessness. It was a "muzzy brown dizziness," swung hither and thither, and it felt extremely sick. This feeling was in itself, not in the body sitting in the chair. Furthermore, the extent of the swirling was precisely the same extent as the movement would have been if my physical body had been swinging about while I was sitting in the chair, but I repeat that I was ALSO independently totally aware of my body, stock still, sitting in the chair. I could still see the room, and saw it rock steady from my body's position in the chair. I heard normally. I believe I spoke normally. Despite the lack of internal features in the "swirlingness" it felt as strongly "me," "myself," as the self who was holding onto the chair felt itself to be the normal "me." The self in the chair felt no dizziness whatever. The amplitude of the swinging movement was as wide as the physical body itself could have covered without being thrown out of the chair, and for perhaps a minute the dual sensations continued, the physical body stock still while the swirling continued with great violence, describing figures of eight and other swinging movements over which I had no control whatsoever. It was as if I was literally being violently, urgently, pushed around and around and around, though not in my body, which was quite motionless. I had begun to feel sick and the feeling increased until I had no control of it. I called for a bowl to be brought quickly because I felt that if I had got up from the chair I would have fallen over and not reached the kitchen sink before vomiting. I was able to think quite cogently that I did not want to vomit on the new chair or on the new carpet as they would be difficult to clean. A bowl was brought just in time and I vomited up the whole of the meal I had eaten at 6 pm, and, strangely, experienced none of the pain usually suffered during vomiting. Then the swinging around quickly ceased, and I sensed myself as "in one body" once more, but a strong residual dizziness remained. I did not immediately attempt to rise from the chair, and after some time, perhaps between a quarter and half an hour, I felt almost normal again.

The next day one of my brothers telephoned to say that another brother had felt unwell, and, rising from his chair, had cried out in pain and collapsed to the floor, about 9 pm the previous evening. He had soon ceased to breathe. His wife had telephoned for an ambulance, which had arrived quickly, but my brother was clearly no longer alive, and the body was removed from his house at around 9.45 to 10 pm.

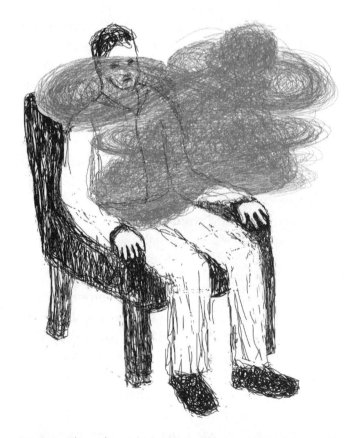

Fig. 15.9. The subject himself provided us with this rough sketch, which is his attempt to convey to hearers and viewers some sense of his experience. We print it with his permission, but allow him to remain anonymous.

I must supply further information as background. My brothers and I were brought up by a Christian sect whose members deny the existence of an immortal soul and believe that death is total annihilation. They expect instead that Jesus Christ will return to the earth and that "the dead in Christ will rise first" and will appear before him, probably near Mount Sinai, to be "judged according to their deeds." All who had heard the Gospel and so become responsible would also be resurrected from their graves, to be judged. Those judged worthy would then be immortalized and would rule over the earth under Jesus Christ, who would be king for a thousand years. None of us (four brothers) remained members of the sect, and I ceased to be a Christian of any complexion over 25 years ago. As early as the 1960s my eldest brother had left the sect and probably has no belief now. Two brothers including the one who has recently died eventually became Christians of another persuasion. In recent decades both have been rather fervent in their Christian beliefs and have viewed me with distrust.

However, one night during the 1970s, when I was myself still a very fervent Christian, there was a knock on my front door in the middle of the night. The brother who has recently died and his wife asked to come in. They were very frightened. At that date they were not yet Christians, and had for some time experienced supernatural appearances of "a little Chinaman" whom the wife thought a very lovely fellow. What had happened I never learned with any accuracy, but the spiritual or nonphysical manifestation, whatever it was, had become menacing and they had fled to me for help. Not long after this my then wife, having met another Christian, sued for the divorce she (and I) had long wished for, and this produced the typical polarization in the family. I was now the proven enemy, the devil masquerading as an angel of light, and when I ceased to believe Christian doctrine and set out instead on a serious quest for spiritual truth the distrust of me among the Christian members of the family intensified.

Thus, from the 1970s onward my brother who

has now died had never discussed doctrinal matters with me, but the other Christian brother had come to value me as an adviser and confidant. On a few occasions the brother who has now died did telephone me to share his employment problems, and once telephoned about religious questions and his lack of religious fellowship. He acknowledged that he had, at that time, no one else to turn to, but a little later he had found concord with a pro-Israel Christian group. I believe he probably still accepted the doctrine that death is absolute cessation of being until the resurrection of the body, but the belief was that one would not be conscious of that intervening period. One can therefore imagine that if he found himself still conscious yet had watched his body being removed from his house he would have been at least puzzled, perhaps terrified. Other people's accounts of out-of-body and near-death experiences suggest that he might also have found himself transported to the physical presence of any person of whom he thought. If he found that his own belief concerning the dead had been incorrect it would be natural for him to think of the close relative who had most spectacularly, in his experience, adopted the view that something of us does survive. He would have thought of me, as he did that night in the 1970s, and, having thought of me while out of his body, he would have been instantly present wherever I was, since I was limited to the physical world of "places," while he was limited in this way no longer.

A brief analysis of this account provides the following main points of evidence:

1. Consciousness can be experienced by one "person" in two modes at once, and with a sense of complete separateness between the two consciousnesses themselves and a direct sensation of a complete separateness between their content and their loci, yet without violating the person's sense of being one person. The two "I"s were both experienced as single selves, *completely* distinguished from each other, yet remaining one, and each was experienced, despite the separation,

as still a *complete* self. This strongly suggests that duality of being is the normal, continuing situation of a living person, but that exceptional conditions can bring about the dividing of the consciousness, which is then experienced as a simultaneous separateness and differentness, indeed, of two ways of being in two different loci.

2. This can occur, or be caused to occur, with no perceptible materially physical cause in the situation of the one who has and survives the experience.

3. There is no rational ground for rejecting the evidence of causation (in the everyday sense of that word), which is inherent in the fact of the simultaneity of the death of another with the experience of the survivor. In the present instance, the one who died seems to have been the invisible cause of the experience of the other. No other explanation presents itself, and the temporal coincidence cannot be ignored.

4. Such experience can apparently be caused (since there is no rational ground for rejecting the evidence of such causation) by a nonmaterial (or nonphysical or nonembodiedly biological) part of the person who dies having a direct, strong effect upon an equally nonmaterial part of the survivor, which part is revealed as distinct only in and during the experience, normality resuming shortly afterward. Further, this experience, apparently caused nonphysically, may produce absolutely no sensation in most faculties of the normal physical body-consciousness of the survivor, but may nonetheless include strong perturbation of the person's involuntary bodily processes.

5. There is a strong link between the sensations of the less-physical part of the divided consciousness with the metabolic state of the physical body, but no coincidence whatever with the five senses of the physical body, at least in the present instance, in which the lower part of the body-consciousness did not divide.

6. There is ground to associate the death of one person with the experience of another in such a way as to render rationally credible the survival of a nonmaterial part of the one who has died on account of its apparent communication with a similar less material-seeming part of the survivor. While unambiguous person-to-person communication such as in normal life was not experienced by the survivor in this case, no one could expect this to occur, for this was an occurrence *after* the end of one of the lives, but the coincidence in time is impressive, a unique experience in the life of the survivor at a unique crisis in the life of the other. The mathematical probability of this coincidence of time occurring without the event containing causality in the normal sense, or meaningful relations, is vanishingly small. The case therefore appears to give evidence of the continued existence after death of a nonphysical part of a person, which is of similar nonphysical kind to a part of another with whom it communicates, who, sensing that the communication is indeed with that similarly nonphysical part of himself, not with his body, then survives. It is simpler to accept this as veridical evidence of our dual nature than to deny both the duality of being of living persons and the survival of an other-than-physical part of a person beyond death. Moreover, the two brothers lived over two hundred miles apart, so a communication of a nonphysical kind is what one would expect, neither physical part of either person being able to move so quickly into the physical presence of the other, and the one having died having no means of achieving this at all.

Does the evidence in these two examples, Puthoff and Targ's and the SPR account, allow us to build a cogent and probable picture of our Being, or at least of our *way of* being? We believe that in an area of inquiry in which there can be no direct evidence such as we have for most physical phenomena we do have strong clues. For example, we seem to be confirming the reality of a consciousness with a *self-knowing* feeling of *interior* structure. Despite being "interior" to its own sense of its own selfhood, it can in some circumstances act as if extended outward beyond the normal, customary, habitual locus of that "interiority," which is, of course, the location of the physical body. This consciousness reacts with what we already know as "the physical world," the phenomenal "world-about." However, when it does extend or travel beyond the body, as Pat Price's consciousness seems to have done to view a factory ten thousand miles away, the consciousness still stands back from that distant part of the world-about in just the same way as when, in normal circumstances, it is conscious of the world immediately around the body by means of the bodily senses. What we think of as "the five senses" are therefore not merely, necessarily, and solely the senses *of the body,* but are a *limiting* range of senses that the Self, or Being, *itself* has, and that sometimes work without and outside the body in a similar manner to the way they habitually work *within* the body.

This suggests that the extensible (or traveling) Being is no more of one substance with the physical body than it is of one substance with the physical world as a whole, though its observational and other faculties are similar. While still acting *in parallel with,* or *as if* using, the bodily senses it does not use their sense organs when "away from" the body. Pat Price did not see at a distance using eyes on stalks. He did not only *see* in the *normal* way (despite being away from his body) but also *felt* the sun on his face in the *normal* way. Yet he experienced these awarenesses without using bodily organs of sense. Was he not, then, a seer and feeler *whether in his body or not*? Consider the implications of this. The Being sees and feels, whatever the circumstances; the body makes no difference. We might postulate, therefore, a *Being having a sensorily limited way of being* preexisting the sensorily equipped body that it then uses, as if the two had been designed for mutual fit, or even as if the preexisting *Being-that-has-a-sensory-way-of-being* manufactured the body, with its sense organs, in the womb by acting as its morphogenetic field, *not the other way round*. Accordingly, we repeat our suggestion that it is spiritual evolution that brings about organic evolution, *not the other way round*. Everything that is, here in our everyday world-about, is generated by a preexisting morphogenetic field. Every reality stands forth from its pattern.

The Subtle Reality of the Ghost

This antiemergentist view differs from that of both Feuerstein and Jung, of course, both of whom were too deferential toward the old, exclusive physics. It also places the Eastern notion of karma firmly within the world of Western science, to be evicted only on the ground of incontrovertible disproof, which we believe will never be found. Instead, we believe, physics itself must change as Dingle and the misled Jung himself required. Extensible being exists in a "place," or exists in a "state," that differs from the world-about and the physical body, which seem to be parts of one and the same *merely* physical world that is *wholly external* to the mobile component of the sensing Being. Even if capable of being *generated by* the physical (which we deny), this mobile component of Being has an ability to *act* independently of the body, sensing objects, bringing messages *having independent content* (which quantum interconnection alone cannot do), and forming reportable *memories* even from ten thousand miles away, a fact that is quite impossible to explain by classical or even recent physics.

We therefore agree with Popper, the philosopher of science, and Eccles, the neuroscientist, that there is a ghost in the machine, and contemptuously reject the view of Ryle, who was not a scientist of any description, not merely as irrelevant, though it is certainly that, but as the arrogant and foundationless opinion of a graduate of the Modern Greats School of Philosophy, Politics, and Economics. Ryle's opposition to any idea that resembled the old doctrine of the immortal soul seems to go hand in hand with an emotional rejection of the Church, a skepticism with which, so long as it is shorn of emotional irrationality, we strongly concur. But did he not even consider that some kind of immortal soul could be a *scientific* fact, long predating, though later usurped by, the Church, and that belief in some undying essence was not necessarily besmirched with the ecclesiastical hypocrisies and cant that accrued around it over the centuries? If there is a part of us that is not bounded by the "timespan" or "history" of the livingness of *the body,* this was surely the case long before humans began to invent gods in their own image, let alone to found churches and impose dogmas upon their fellows, and if this is indeed the case it is a fact arising not merely prior to, independently of, and untouched by all religious questions, but, discovered already or not yet discovered, was always and still remains a *scientific* fact with which only a real god preexisting all humankind's invented gods could interfere.

We remain uncertain what it *is* that the ghost in the

machine is, but, while it does not yet appear* *what* it is, it *is* ourselves, in some deeply real sense. In Heideggerian terms it is the *Being* that is *There* (in the sense assertive of its reality, not the topological sense, though, of course, it is *also* there-in-the-world-about). No alternative "map" of our way of being explains the facts. As we have said before, the simplest and most striking demonstration of the explanatory power of our view is the understanding of dying, which is, of course, precisely where we might expect to find real proof of our duality. No physical science has succeeded in defining death, while the view that the *living* Being is not physical offers a simple explanation. The "ghost," invisible even in life, leaves, and the evidence of its leaving is just as certain, yet just as indirect, as the evidence of its presence had been during embodied life. If it is *not* a physical entity this invisibility to *physical* means of seeing (such as eyes) is precisely what we would expect. In what manner it survives independently after death, and, if it does so, for how long, or whether it "survives" *timelessly* after death just as it already existed before birth, or whether it ever returns to the physical world, are further questions.

Every Man His Own Solipsist

Let us take stock once more. The world-about contains other beings *outwardly* appearing much like ourselves, inferably, therefore, *essentially* beings of the same kind. I am aware of myself, and aware even of my awareness of myself, which some accept as a sound definition or proof of consciousness, yet my own I is invisible to me. Indeed, it is just as invisible to me as it is to you. No I can ever be seen. However, this, too, is exactly as we would expect, for the I is the Seer, not the seen, and the "I-ness" of others is similarly hidden from my *physical* view via my sense organs, which is, again, precisely as we would expect. The whole schema is self-consistent, no matter what abstruse intellectual objections may be raised against it. Each of us can therefore perceive ourselves as the solipsistic "I" of his or her own world. Each of us is a "Being-in-the-world," and each of us experiences our own "I-ness" directly, which is why we can

*The use of John the Divine's phraseology is deliberate. Our readers might like to ponder all the allusions to, parallels between, and consequences of the ideas we are here describing and John's words in his first Epistle, 3.2 in the King James Version. The Hindu "Tat twam asi" is also in mind as this is written.

accept that we each have a *limited* solipsistic status, but our sense of "I-ness" is too strong to withhold the recognition of an *essentially* similar "I-ness" from each other. We do not have each other's experience, but we do know the Other is here, living alongside us. There is absolutely no reason to doubt the similarity in the nature of our being. You are *"other I"* to me and I am *"other I"* to you. With inner arms and smiles we reach out toward each other, in recognition and care, but invisibly, sometimes sensibly, but even then not necessarily using the bodily organs of sense but, rather, an intuitive inner sense that seems real yet is hard to define and impossible to observe as a thing-in-itself. Neither you nor I insult the other by claiming "it" is nothing but an automaton moving around the physical world. Even Dingle's fly, while living, knows another fly when they meet, and neither you nor I are plastic Father Christmases singing in the supermarket. So in what kind of world do we live and move and have our Being of solipsistic I-ness?

An Even More Deeply Hidden Wave-World

To assess the tentative answer of recent science we need to look at the possible third candidate, mentioned above. We cast doubt, *grounded in the physics itself,* on the notion that Alain Aspect's quantum entanglement is a *sufficient* explanation of human knowledge of, or conscious control of, events at a distance, preferring an understanding much closer to the ancient belief that we are at least duplex beings, one part perishable, the other not, and are perhaps even more multiplex than that. The third candidate, like Aspect's quantum interconnectedness, seems to be an entirely physical phenomenon since detection of it is physical (though very indirect, as we shall see). It has raised puzzling questions for both physicists and biologists, between whom it has engendered violent debate, and it stands in the same relation to what we might call our everyday experience of physical phenomena as Aspect's quantum entanglement.

Like the phenomenon he confirmed, the seemingly physical reality we shall now describe is unobservable for our five external bodily senses, and it may not be available to us for use in transmitting or receiving messages. As far as our experience is concerned it seems to teeter on the very edge of physicality. It makes no intelligible images within our consciousness, yet (again like Aspect's interconnection) it is claimed to underlie more accessible phenomena the evidence from which allows us to *infer* that, despite its nonsensibility for us, it is *real*. We *can* make observations *that depend upon its being a physical reality* by using *real, physical* prostheses similar to those used in Aspect's experiment and other physical research, such as magnetometers and interferometers, and (anticipating our story a little) their use in the experiments confirms the *reality* of the postulated invisible entity.

Again like quantum interconnectedness and entanglement, it is a reality that permeates vast volumes of space. Some who have studied the evidence for it also believe it to be an instant communicator across that space, essentially timeless, static, everywhere-present, but, as we said, without imparting *to us as large-scale physical beings* any ability to use it for carrying our messages as opposed to its own "message." This further similarity to Aspect's quantum interconnectedness leads us immediately to ask whether it might not be the same entity of spaceless, timeless, static (yet also active) connectedness that we already know Aspect's "entanglement" to be, but viewed via different apparatus and presenting, therefore, a somewhat different aspect to our view.* This may be the case, but for the moment, let us suppose that it is a different entity and try to unravel, stage by stage, what science has, thus far, discovered about it.

What is postulated is that uncoordinated energy, which, as waves interact with each other, neutralizes itself *in our world,* remains physical, but as a field of what are known as scalar and vector *potential waves.* For our purpose, the search for the subtle body, we need not give detailed definitions of such waves now, though a little more will be said, in a suitable place. This postulated field of potential waves lies outside our everyday view, forming what we might picture as a huge underlying vat of *substantive and real* potentiality out from (the sense is that of the Greek ἐκ again) which all those things we, in our limitedness, call physical realities can emerge, or reemerge. Such words will instantly remind us of Neo-Platonic notions of emanation, but before we can consider them we must explain the present-day physics that underlies them.

To achieve this understanding we must, as so often, look back at the history of science, starting again

with electromagnetic waves, and this time watch not the "solidification" of a single "real" particle out of a group of strongly related "superposed" *possibilities*—the process described by Schrödinger's "mathematics of alternative futures"—but the uncoordinated crowd behavior of waves that are *already* real, already here-in-the-physical-world, and are therefore behaving as Maxwell's mathematics had described, many decades before Schrödinger. Again, we do not need exact definitions. Maxwellian waves are simply the electromagnetic energy waves of the world-about of our everyday experience, apart from gravity the only force that directly affects us as embodied Beings-in-the-world. The sun's rays are an example of "ordinary" Maxwellian waves. Electricity flowing in circuits is another manifestation. These waves, according to circumstance, meet as we earlier described, adding when in phase, cancelling when out of phase. It may be useful to look again at figures 15.3, 15.4, and 15.5, but in particular 15.3 diagrams 2, 2a, and 3.

It is no wonder that Maxwell's electromagnetic theory preceded Schrödinger's wave mechanics, for Maxwell dealt with phenomena that were, in some sense, *readily accessible,* such as solenoids and their actions, while Schrödinger dealt with *mathematical prediction* of prematerial *occult* processes, the propagation of waves. This distinction is not absolute, of course, but one of degree, for all physics is hidden to some extent from our view, needing our contemplation and imagination to reveal it to our understanding. Since Newton postulated a force of universal gravitation that was *invisible* in that the means of its pulling objects down to the planet's surface could not be seen (while a shove against a stone with the foot could, in an everyday sense, be watched), the progress of science has been ever further into the occult, *using the technological prostheses that the discovery of what was hidden would require.* The scalar and vector potential fields, which we are calling the possible third candidate for the subtle body, are "occult" in this sense, which is, of course, precisely why we might want to use the word *subtle* to describe them.

Already, an entity of this deeply hidden kind has entered the intelligent public's consciousness and has acquired names. Some, stressing the absence of heat or other radiant energy in this field of *potential only,* call it the zero-point field. Others, mindful of its potential

---

*No pun upon Alain Aspect's name is intended, of course, either here or by other chance juxtapositions of the word and the name.

to produce what we call "reality," conceive of it as a "quantum foam," from which particle-antiparticle pairs constantly appear, the particles sometimes becoming material in our world. They become material if, but only if, particle meets particle in such a way as to produce a more permanent entity, such as an atom, too "solid" to disintegrate and so fall back into the foam from whence its components recently appeared. Others again, recognizing that the postulated reservoir of scalar and vector potentials can contain no *matter* as we understand that term, call it the "quantum *vacuum*," but recognize that it is empty only of *realized* matter, for the quantum vacuum is seen as once having contained all the "protomatter" from which our sensible world-about came. It is also claimed that the vacuum still contains, as a vast supply of "realizable potential," *almost* all the matter and *almost* all the energy of our whole physical universe.

As always, the attempt to devise verbal descriptions fails, and we shall give no further excuse than this for the utter inadequacy of these forms of words. We invite the reader to do what Einstein did, and contemplate the ideas as pictures. Note, however, that we are not asserting that a zero-point field, a quantum vacuum, Aspect's interconnectedness, and a huge vat of scalar and vector potentials are necessarily one and the same entity. That may or may not be the case, but the *concepts* certainly seem closely related. Meanwhile, relevant research is still ongoing. We must now return to Maxwell, to complete the picture we are attempting to draw.

The world is full of Maxwellian waves, "unrelated" to each other, and "real," issuing from a myriad seemingly *independent* sources and rushing hither and thither, struggling amid matter, escaping from matter only to collide with it again and be absorbed, meeting each other head on, or traveling alongside, or across each other's paths.* We recall that waves are postulated to consist of what we call "energy." There is unimaginably huge energy "out there," but much of it is uncoordinated, counterbalanced, mutually opposed, and therefore self-nullifying.

This usual state of affairs is like a crowd in the marketplace, each person going his own way, vying and

veering, weaving and waiting, pushing and pausing, the crowd as a whole making no *coordinated* movement, despite its huge energy and chaotic inner "vibration." In a laser beam, by contrast, the energy waves advance like an army marching in step. Only when waves are brought into phase with each other and travel in parallel do we gain a *sensible* first impression of the sheer quantity of energy around us in the physical world. Even a tiny laser, no more *powerful* than an indicator light on an item of household electrical equipment, gives a beam so *intense* that it is seriously damaging to the physical eye to look into the beam.

The average level of chaotically moving energy around us seems low, in everyday experience, but the laser beam's *coordinated, directional pressure* reveals the sea of ambient and available energy to be huge. The relevance of this will be apparent if we now recall that, in normal physical interactions, energy is neither created nor destroyed, but only rearranged. Sometimes, two or more waves will happen to come into phase, and their energy will then add together. This is like the first step toward the laser's coherent intensity, after it has been switched on and its coherence is building up, yet the sum of energy in the whole system has always been, and still remains, the same. Only some such process of coordination or synergy brings the huge volume of ambient energy to our attention. However, what intrigues us here is the utterly unobtrusive opposite effect, as if the energy were infinitely dissipated, when two waves are precisely opposed in phase, the "push" of the one totally cancelling the other's "pull" so that the net energy *at that specific point in our familiar space* drops to zero. The question is, bearing in mind the principle of *conservation* of energy, where or how the energy *known to be present* in the system as a whole "hides" from our view in what we might call this "antilaser" situation, when the waves are out of phase with each other and mutual cancellation of wave energy is occurring. Many a bright school student has asked this question, and received no convincing reply from the teacher.

Teachers of school-level physics have for a century or more resorted to unconvincing talk of "potential" as a cover for their misunderstanding of the actively dynamic yet hidden physics of our everyday world, and, curiously, physicists themselves have only supplied a satisfactory answer within the past half century. Even more surpris-

---

*The hint, here, at Neo-Platonic and Kabbalistic views of our relationship with the Above is deliberate, and the reader is invited to explore this "picture" of our way of being, using the rest of this book and others listed in the bibliography.

ing is the fact that the answer had been discerned by a few, decades before, yet for many years thereafter was rejected by most theorists. Such surprise may be misplaced, of course, for even Maxwell's correlation of electricity with magnetism, now taken as proven beyond all doubt, was similarly resisted when first published in the nineteenth century. However, the human mind is self-observant enough to have understood its own foibles and so invented the word *stolid,* which we now use, for many, even among scientists, stolidly maintained a huge skepticism regarding the reality of the postulated underlying scalar and vector potential standing waves, as though it were a valid principle that "If I can't see it directly it doesn't exist." Everyone, scientist or not, knows that this is not the case.

The Imagination of Mathematicians Yet Again . . .

The answer had been anticipated, and the calculations made, by mathematicians long before the corresponding physical phenomenon was shown to be real by the experimental physicist Akira Tonomura and others. As so often, mathematicians had foreseen much better than others the real-world correlates of their theoretical discoveries. A famous instance was the English mathematical physicist Paul Dirac's confident prediction of the existence of antimatter on the purely mathematical ground that in one of his equations the result remained invariant regardless of whether one of its terms were positive or negative. He was right, for antimatter was duly discovered. Similarly, as we saw, John Bell predicted by means of mathematics that there would be an observable *difference* for experimentalists such as Alain Aspect to measure (if sufficiently sensitive prostheses could be devised) between the predictions of quantum physics and those of deterministic physics. It is not to be wondered at, then, that many mathematicians are Platonists, believing that our "lower world" of physics embodies the truths of a higher and prior world of forms, namely eternal mathematical truths. Our world is governed by mathematical fact as if the principle "As above, so below" applies.

The postulated explanation of the fact that the energy of "real," propagating waves, when opposed in phase, disappears from the purview of our usual measuring instruments is not that it mutually destroys itself but that it "subsides" into what we might think of as a "sink" or "vat" full of a different, seemingly more fundamental, kind of wave. These different waves would be less easily observed than Maxwellian waves, and, for mathematical reasons lying far beyond the scope of any book such as this, they were postulated to be longitudinal rather than transverse, and to be static, in a certain sense of the word, rather than traveling. The waves would roll to and fro without overall directional progress, as if like the waves in a violin string. They were described as *standing* waves for this reason. Here, we interpose the hint that such invisibly present waves might be conceived to be an all-enveloping "mobile stillness" of Platonic *just-being-there-behind-the-scenes* within which a whole cosmos might be gestated and might thereafter subsist as the more readily visible world in which we live and have our conscious experience. Indeed, in the minds of many mathematicians and scientists, the postulated "standing waves" are conceived to be the "progenitors" of the transverse electromagnetic waves of Maxwellian physics, since it appears that *interactions between pairs of* the potential, or *standing,* waves generate the Maxwellian *propagating* waves of our more tangible world. Hence the use of the word *potential* in naming the underlying non-Maxwellian waves. They contain the potential for the Maxwellian level of reality, that of our everyday electromagnetic bodily sensing and acting.

Standing potential waves are very difficult to detect, not only because the ubiquitous "real" Maxwellian waves mask any *indirect* effects that potential waves *might* have upon all the *usual* detectors of Maxwellian waves (please note carefully the phrasing we use), but their different nature itself means that equipment to interact with and thereby measure them might be difficult, perhaps impossible, for us to devise. While we should not think of the problem as precisely the same—for it is not—it is certainly close to the problem we posed in our thought experiment about the fictional "squalification coefficient." The "world" of standing potential waves, while *imaginable,* is *totally* unknown to our *everyday conscious awareness,* and all the detectors we *do* have exist within our *familiar* world (where, and for the purposes of which, we invented them), not in a strange and invisible foundation layer or all-encompassing envelope-of-the-cosmos that, relative to the world we call real, is "only" potential. We can only conceive and make "real-world" instruments. In our world of *matter-and-real-waves* it might be forever impossible to devise means of detecting the postulated potential standing waves *directly*. Again, please note our phrasing. It cannot be taken for granted that instruments that *can* sense "real" waves will *also* be able to sense the postulated very different potential waves. However, starting from Dirac's mathematics, the physicists Yakir Aharonov and David Böhm predicted that the potential waves would be proved to exist by their *effects*, for example, upon the propagation of electron waves; they claimed that these effects *would* be observable using *our* instruments. Again, there is a close relation between the apparatus and methods of the double slit experiment and Tonomura's experiment.

Tonomura's experiment, which we shall now briefly outline, has indeed shown convincingly that there *is* "something there," his result being an *inference* from the *our-world data* he collected, not a *direct observation or measuring or sensing* of the potential waves themselves. As we have noted, our capacity for direct observation is limited to what our bodily senses convey to us, extended by instruments that are essentially similar in their means of sensing. Thus the world of the "standing potential waves" themselves is no more *knowable* by us than the *completely imaginary*, indeed, *pretended* "squalification coefficient," which perhaps entertained, or more probably annoyed, us earlier. Perhaps, then, it is not to be wondered at that, as we remarked earlier, nineteenth-century predictions of "scalar and vector potentials" by mathematicians and a very few physicists were, for several generations, ignored or even scorned. However, a few, including Maxwell himself and Tesla, Poynting, and Heaviside whom, though important to science, we have no space to discuss, may have foreseen the *subtle* reality that Tonomura has now confirmed by experiment.

If potential waves cannot be directly sensed, we have reason to question whether they should be considered parts of the physical world at all. Alternatively, since Tonomura has shown that they *are* reliably *inferable* from "real-world" data, excluding them from physics might seem unjustified, in which case we should rescue them from their precarious teetering on the edge of the erstwhile *extra*-physical *by redefining physics*, however slightly. If we do that, physics itself extends outward, receding from us into an even more remote region we might call the "inferable occult." The cosmos, *our* cos-

mos, that in which our very livingness *is*, now has yet another invisible layer of even finer "subtlety" than electromagnetic waves. It seems that the cosmos itself may have kośas just as we, within it, have kośas.

Note how the meaning of the word *real* is beginning to slide. Perhaps we now glimpse something of the ever-shifting complexity of the cycle of observation, thinking, interpretation, and (not the least of the difficulties) verbal recording of observations of the world, for any scientist working near the frontier with the unknown and having only our existing words, *the language of our ignorant past,* to work with. As we have said before, only an experiment yielding results *within our sensible world* can prove *to us* whether or not mathematically described "waves of fundamental potentiality" are "real." Mathematics itself convinced humans that Schrödinger and Heisenberg were each describing a reality, but a reality we might call "subtle" because (though only because) it is impossible for us to "see" it directly. The double slit experiment then gave us observables, results we *could* see, which seemed to constitute *sufficient reason* for us to believe that the physical states and processes the mathematicians had described warranted our acceptance as "real" rather than as "subtle." Later, Alain Aspect made the experiment described earlier, which revealed the "subtle" and invisible quantum interconnection underlying "things" within our everyday world-about, and—though we still could not "see" or "sense" it *directly* using the body or even its technical extensions—we began to conceive of quantum interconnectedness as "real." Tonomura and others have now done the same for potential waves. Meanwhile, the verbal slippage continues, and entities formerly in the "subtle" category are now conceived to be "real." Thus does physics become more and more occult, yet more and more credible, more and more real-for-us. Let us get to the experiment itself.

The Technical Challenge of Tonomura's Experiment

The questions facing experimental physicists such as Tonomura might be put like this: What has happened to wave energy when it cancels itself out and therefore might seem to have been destroyed? Has the energy really been destroyed or has it merely disappeared from our view? If it has merely disappeared, where has it gone, why can we no longer "see" or detect it, in what form does it still exist, and how might it reappear before our body-based five-sensed science, using instrumental extensions if and when necessary?

If the principle of conservation of energy is to stand we must postulate a field, of a different type from the Maxwellian, in which we shall find the energy that has been "lost" from the Maxwellian field. Crucially, since the energy cannot have *disappeared* from us unless into a *place beyond our sensing and measuring* (for that is what "disappearing" would necessarily be, in this context), with what equipment shall we be able to find it *in its hiding place*? It is essential to find it *there,* not in the already-known physical world, for if it reenters the everyday world it will be as the familiar "real" waves of the everyday world, not as potential waves, and we shall not be able to prove either that it was ever in the postulated potential world or even whether that world of potential actually exists. So Tonomura's practical task was to devise an elegant and *fault-free* experiment that would *truly* test and measure *what needed to be tested and measured.* Yet no one could invent means of detecting or measuring the postulated entity *directly,* for that interaction would *bring the potential waves back into the everyday world,* so defeating the whole purpose of the experiment.

The entity sought, then, was far more elusive than anything in the everyday world of our senses, yet, as always, only the instruments of the everyday world were available to make the sensings and measurings required. With regard to the *practicalities,* therefore, researchers saw that the postulated potential waves would be detectable only if all other wave fields within or around the detector were first removed, so leaving intact and unobscured an observable *effect* on our everyday world by the postulated but totally invisible underlying field. But the very nature of wave fields, which permeate the whole of space, makes their removal difficult. *If we can* remove all vestiges of electromagnetic radiation from a volume of space we might try to look into that volume of space to see if anything is still present. But how, and with what, could we look? Already, there are two kinds of technical problem.

However, a far greater problem now looms for this plausible-sounding procedure is impossible or unserviceable on at least two counts. First, the sensing equipment could not be relied upon to register a postulated "new"

wave of a different type without introducing precisely the kind of wave it was necessary to exclude in order to isolate the postulated waves. (For the present, we ignore the gravitational field because, unlike the myriad intercrossing electromagnetic fields, terrestrial gravity is very nearly constant.) Second, following directly from the first problem, if one were to probe the volume of space supposedly emptied of electromagnetic waves by using an electromagnetic wave, seeking its interaction with whatever remained within the "empty" space, it would no longer be empty of electromagnetic waves, for we should ourselves have flooded it with precisely that kind of wave.

Even this does not exhaust the problems, for how would we clear the volume of all electromagnetic waves *except* those we wanted to introduce as a probe? To do this would violate the very nature of our world, in which an infinite variety of electromagnetic radiations fly hither and thither perpetually, reinforcing and canceling chaotically. There would be no way to permit entry of just one probing wave into any lacuna that had been *successfully* shielded from *any and all* such waves. If we had succeeded in removing all electromagnetic waves, what waves would there be to find? Was it not these very same electromagnetic waves that would have to be excluded *totally* if we were to discover any *dissimilar* entity, such as potential waves, "hidden behind" them? Yet further, if, as we would be expecting, the postulated waves were *non*electromagnetic, an electromagnetic probe *might* not interact with them at all. Was not the postulate to be tested the belief that the hidden waves had in some sense "collapsed out of" the electromagnetic world and so disappeared from the view of observers with electromagnetic bodies, electromagnetic senses, and electromagnetic instruments, who lived in that world? The strange waves might stay hidden, once isolated from our everyday world. The experimenters could expect no valid result from use of an electromagnetic probe, yet if the postulated, strangely *non*electromagnetic, field were real they would probably still be unable to detect it by any kind of *direct* probing *unless they could create strange equipment we are incapable even of imagining. That would be possible only if we already knew what the field was, and perhaps not even then.*

This brief survey shows how great the problems of experimental design can be, and why we remarked earlier that any experiment must measure *what it is necessary to measure,* not something else. Now, too, our thought experiment about the "squalification coefficient" seems less silly, for it showed we could *never* devise measuring tools for entities beyond our realm of direct, indeed, personal, senses (their range, as always, extended by prostheses when necessary). As we remarked many pages ago, science is not what the layperson thinks, and even for the professional experimenter it is always past experience that sets the present imaginative and technical limits, while the technical and even conceptual difficulties in designing the experiment can be almost insurmountable. All the experimenters would be able to do was to "invite" the postulated field to show itself, not *within* the radiation-shielded lacuna they hoped to set up, into which no one could "see" at all, but outside it, in our familiar electromagnetic world. This would take great ingenuity, for even there, only the *effect* (if any) of the hidden potential waves would be perceptible, never the waves *themselves,* which, while present, would remain hidden from *our* natural way of sensing by *their* different nature. *We* are electromagnetic beings, the potential waves were postulated to be *non*electromagnetic. Even if it were still *within* physics, the postulated field must be at least "once removed" from *our way of seeing and being* into some more "subtle" layer of physics. Our normal experience comes to us from a world-about produced by a varying electromagnetic and a more or less constant gravitational field. Tonomura was looking for an entity that, on the ground of the principle of the conservation of energy, we *can* pronounce to be a *necessary* postulate, but one that we cannot *imagine,* cannot *sense,* and cannot *directly* interact with using *any* of the instruments we *can* imagine. Our only clues to the nature and facticity of this field are the conservation of energy, leading us to believe that the canceled energy of electromagnetic waves still exists in another form (though that principle *might* even be false in the *world-beyond* of the postulated "new" entity) and certain mathematical patterns that had predicted the form of the "new" waves. We might, if we were sufficiently ingenious, observe the waves *by their effects* (not directly) in the world of everyday experience to which we are restricted. The predicted potential waves themselves *might* show, *indirectly,* that is by their *effects,* evidence of their presence and reality. We consider ourselves entitled to use the word *subtle*

of so elusive an entity, though it might be a very "real" subtlety, the postulated level utterly fundamental to our *physical* being. And, our use of the word proving nothing by itself, the entity might, or might not, be conceivable as a subtle *body,* though if so it would be a "nonmaterial body," or way of being, in which, in some unfamiliar way, we *all* share.

The inability to probe any shielded lacuna wherein only the postulated new field would exist seemed an impasse, but Tonomura's method of overcoming this was both ingenious and elegant. He arranged for the postulated field itself, if it existed, to *be* the necessary probe, and to deliver its "findings," if any, back "here" in our everyday world, to be sensed with familiar instruments. Thus his conclusion would be not a "direct" observation, but an *inference from* observations (though this, as careful consideration by the reader will show, is true of all experiment). He based his apparatus on an experiment of 1932 that itself had already convinced some physicists of the reality of the potential wave field, but he incorporated refinements that met certain objections that had been raised against the earlier experiment. Tonomura's improved system used the chemical element niobium in a superconductive state to encase *completely* a more-or-less ordinary *annular* ferromagnet. The superconducting niobium served a double purpose. It absorbed all magnetic and electric fields that impinged upon its surface from *outside,* thus preventing those fields from reaching the totally encapsulated annular magnet. It also confined the magnet's own magnetic and electric fields *inside the magnet itself,* preventing them from spreading either inward into the space *inside* the central hole of the annular magnet or *outside* the outer circumference of the niobium capsule. Electron waves would be projected both through and outside the annular space in the center of the magnet, and these areas would be observed to detect any changes. The system would thus consist of a magnetic field and an electron wave field that, on account of the superconducting niobium between them, could not interact *directly* in any way that could affect the observations. Diagram 1 of figure 15.10 shows this schematically.

Tonomura then projected electron waves toward the annular magnet, perpendicular to its plane, so that they produced interference patterns similar to those produced in the double slit experiment. The interference patterns

Fig. 15.10. Diagram 1 shows the fundamental principle of Tonomura's experiment, represented schematically. Diagram 2 shows what is typically observed as the interference pattern made by electron waves passing around and through the annular magnet as recorded from beyond the magnet. Diagram 3 shows the sudden deflection produced when the gradually increasing magnetic flux reaches a level at which a quantized change is imposed upon the electrons passing through the magnet's central hole. The effect is to alter their phase, which causes a displacement of the pattern of light and dark interference fringes. Careful comparison of the pattern of light inside the magnet in diagrams 2 and 3 shows that in diagram 3, showing the effect when the magnetic flux is sufficiently greater than in diagram 2, the electron waves have been deflected from the path followed by the waves passing outside the magnet. The effect could only occur if there is a field that is immune to the superconducting screening-off of the magnetic flux and is transmitting to the screened-off electron waves passing through the magnet's annular hole an effect imposed upon it by the magnet (through which it permeates). The magnet, its field being contained entirely within itself by its superconducting coating, could have no *direct* effect upon the electrons passing through its central hole. The effect observed can only result from mediation via the postulated all-pervading potential field. Thus, by observation at *our* level of the physical world of an effect *inferrable* as mediated via a *more fundamental* "source-field," the reality of that field is confirmed.

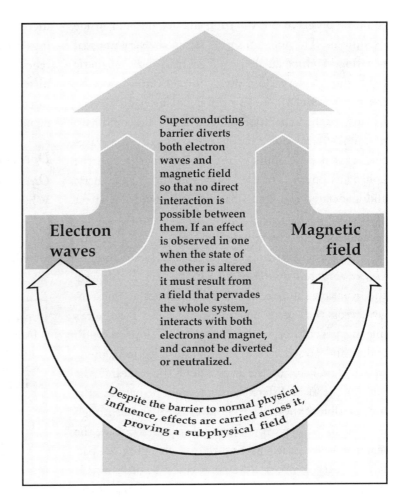

Diagram 1

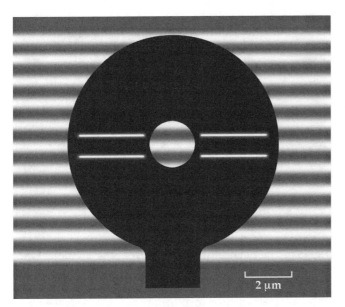

Diagram 2

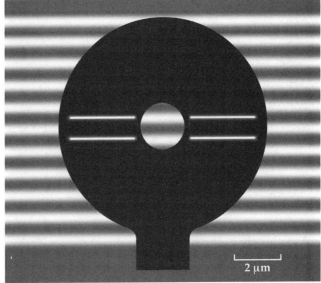

Diagram 3

could be observed both outside the magnet and inside its annulus. The apparatus thus set up the very unusual situation in which an electron wave field and a magnetic field, though very close, were both diverted away by the superconductor, and so could not meet or overlap. Because of this separation the magnetic field could have no *direct* effect upon the flight of those electron waves that passed either outside the magnet or through the hole at its center. The electron waves and the magnetic and associated electric fields therefore could not affect each other *unless, first, the postulated potential field was in fact present, and second, the "insulator" of superconducting niobium notwithstanding, the potential field also permeated unimpeded through the whole system.* If this were the situation the potential field would act as "messenger" across the superconducting barrier, and Tonomura's ingenuity would betray the "subphysical" hidden field's reality and presence to us, here in our electromagnetic world. The crux of the experiment thus became the question of what difference there might be between the propagation of those electron waves that passed through the hole in the magnet and those that passed outside the magnet. Would their paths differ, so changing the pattern of interference in a way that could be observed? If so, the difference would be *caused* by the magnet's field, but it would have been *transmitted to* the electron waves by the postulated underlying field.

Naturally, the experiment was run many times, and Tonomura used magnets of different strengths. The result of the experiment was that when the gradually increased strength of the magnet reached a specific value, there was a sudden clear shift in the phase of those electron waves that passed through the hole in it. A *sudden* change as the magnetic flux was increased by very small steps accords with the requirements of *quantum* theory. All changes in our physical universe are *quantized*. There are no smooth and continuous transitions in our physical world. A very crude macro-world illustration of the quantum jump would be the way a heavy piece of furniture at first refuses to move when pushed, then, as the force increases, suddenly jumps a little way, but then sticks again. All changes in the physical world are of this intermittent nature, and there are no intermediate states between the possible quantized states. The jump itself is, in effect, an instant of nonexistence. The evidence that the effect of the magnet is quantized

increased the mutual corroboration of the new findings with the whole body of quantum theory. The existence of an underlying or "background" field of a type different from the familiar electromagnetic field, but interacting with it, had been indirectly, but irrefutably, demonstrated.

Does the Potential Field Relate to the Quest for the Subtle Body?

What conclusions can we draw relating to our quest for the subtle body? The potential field, evidently present but invisible throughout our world, might be a substrate for what we call physical reality. It might be a greater

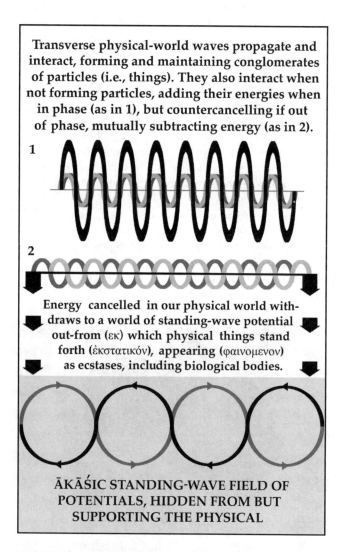

Fig. 15.11. The physical world arises from the potential field, to which energy subsides when mutual cancellation occurs in the physical world. Where other interactions occur, particles are formed, hold together as "things," and move when energy quanta are "trapped" in matter.

world *inside* which our whole physical and familiar world exists and has its being. Notwithstanding its complete ineffability in *our* normal *sensory* experience, which is classical-world experience of chunky solid objects of handleable size that push and pull each other around, the potential field appears to be *the very ground of our physical existence.* Without it, we can no more exist as *physical* beings than can stones. It affects our physical world at the most fundamental, most subtle, most occult level of it that we have yet been able to detect. Indeed, our world exists *in* this potential field. Such a picture seems Platonic and Hermetic, unexpectedly so to some, but undeniably so nonetheless. Should we regard the potential standing waves as "higher" than our visible world, or as the fundamental "lowest" ground of its possibility? Perhaps they are both, though, of course, both "high" and "low" are merely metaphorical in this context. Perhaps the very notions of metaphorical "higher" and "lower" levels are now obsolete, useful as expressions of relative position only when our thinking is restricted to our physical world-about.

Whether the notions are appropriate or not, the implication that our *individuality* might depend on something that *conjoins* us might seem to Modern Secular Man a little odd, raising the question whether we are Beings consisting only of "material," or "substance," ecstases standing out-from the world of potential waves, or Beings existing in more than one level, and depending, at least in part, on a very different world from the one we see day by day. The question is based on nothing more than our unsophisticated, unscientific everyday view of ourselves as living Beings in a nonliving physical world, but this naïveté does not itself invalidate the belief. It simply leaves it unproved. It seems at least arguable, even for some who have long been of the physicalist persuasion, for it is a very natural intuition for any of us to heed. Why is it so natural? Might it be natural because it is true? It raises the question we have faced before, whether we are single in essence or dual (or even multiple). If there is any sense in which the individually experiencing, substantively distinguishable Beings that we undeniably are constitute One World, we shall surely find it true *at the level of that foundational world of standing waves.* However, if we are all one at that level the nature of and reason for our *individuality* will need to be investigated, as will the distinction between living

and nonliving. Does that latter distinction arise from the subphysical level of potential waves, via our physical complexity, as many believe, or is it only one part of us that stands forth from the level of potential waves, our living-Beingness in its *essential* nature deriving from some other source?

If we are the individuals we feel ourselves to be, each having what seems free choice, and distinguishable *by our own assessment*—that is, each in our *own* discernment—*from one another* on account of each having *only our own* experience of consciousness, it will be as inhabitants of *this,* our familiar world, *this* human-level world-about of I and Other I, that we show such *sufficient reason* to regard ourselves as individuals. We define individuality as a description of precisely such palpable separateness from and difference from each other, even though we also see ourselves as *fellow* Beings. Whence our separateness and our individuality of character? The belief that it arises solely from physical complexity has severe problems, as we shall see, some of them, curiously, of a kind Gilbert Ryle might have pointed out had his anti-Cartesian stance not prevented him discerning where *real* distinctions could have been made instead of irrelevant distinctions within *language bearing no relation to any reality,* whether physical or "spiritual" (except, of course, the unreal reality of language itself). Might we derive our *unique* beingness from another all-pervading "field," of a "higher," nonphysical, superphysical (not subphysical) kind? We suggest that only such a picture provides a full explanation of all our observations of ourselves and others in the world. Our choice-asserting Beingness may *supervene* both the field of potential waves and *its* phenomenon, the physical world, both *as a physical entity and *also* as something "higher," which makes each of us a Being-that-is-emphatically-*There* in the world-about, not a mere thing-for in the world. Even adamant physicalists have been tempted by this intuitive self-assessment, with or without the Heideggerian terminology. Might it be *true?*

Let us explore and test this conception of ourselves as Beings of dual origin and nature. The potential field seems no more able than Aspect's quantum interconnection to provide us with even the smallest degree of personal autonomy or free will, but only with what we might picture as "the being of stones in the soft machine of the body" yet *we* exist *each as an individual I* in that physical world, which itself seems only one level "above" that potential field. Our very Being as individuals, our *essential* essence (the reader will understand and excuse this *intensifying* or *emphatic* tautology), may lie *elsewhere than all the physics that underlies our being-here.* Do we appear out-from *both* a higher, supraphysical level *and* a fundamental infraphysical level, meeting as dual Beings in the physical realm between them? If so, the perspective would be that our *being-here*ness depends on what the physical world emerges from, namely the potential field, but our *true self*ness is some*where* else and *consists of* some*thing* else. Of course, this view is unfashionable among most philosophers and biologists, more acceptable to some mathematicians and physicists, but no one could rationally disagree that it would be a gross mistake, and an immense arrogance, to believe that nothing exists but the world of the *visible-to-us,* not least because that world *itself* (physics) is *already* largely occult (no one has ever seen gravity, or a potential wave, or even a photon or electron *as such,* nor heard, smelt, felt, or tasted them), and, moreover, *itself* leads us to postulate another, higher world, as we shall see.

Even *in* our everyday world, almost every level of the totally *this*-world study we call physics is occult. Humans are unable to think in other ways than human ways. We cannot find out what is beyond us, but only discern, from outside, its *necessity-to-be,* and picture it in a human way. Tonomura did this to confirm the reality of the potential wave field. Aspect did it to confirm quantum interconnection over large distance. We cannot find out what is beyond us, and can think only as humans think. Hence the repetition of anthropomorphic images in the Ripley Scroll (shown in plate 28), in which a higher world is depicted using the same human polar forms of female and male as are used to depict the lower level. What else could a fifteenth-century illustrator have done? Even in Ripley's own day artists were beginning to visualize their subject matter more abstractly. Mantegna's painting, shown in plate 34, is a view-from-below upward to the sky, dating from around 1470, and shows the vault of heaven as a *trompe l'oeil* effect, which was exploited by later artists attempting to depict the World-Above. As consciousness developed still further, artists gradually ceased to show cherubs and other beings floating in the firmament of heaven, and eventually showed only great vaults of blue surrounded by cumulus clouds, still a terrestrial reality attempting to depict the undefinable "spiritual" world, but without the obvious anthropomorphism of earlier and more naïve minds. Even today we can go no further except, perhaps, by painting some nondescript maelstrom of color, or a black starry sky, in an attempt to indicate the above. Nonetheless, despite our smallness, it is easy for us to imagine *that* other worlds and ways of being exist, for even *within* physics we have to postulate "dark energy" and "dark matter," and find no difficulty with these notions of *invisible* entities and essences, but it is impossible to imagine *what* the content of other worlds might be, just as it is impossible to *depict* them. That very unknownness *is* their *other*ness as "seen" by our kind of Being. The thinking that understood the principle "As above, so below" gave us both an insight and an awareness of our gross incapacity.

Now, we need a Gebserian freedom to look *around* or *past* all perspectives to a global just-seeing of what will then be a greater world. Perhaps some such further-seeing "hologram" will construct itself within our "minds"— whatever it is that our minds are. We can perhaps begin to view our own nature as we viewed other matters dealt with earlier, seeing ourselves as one when viewing in top-down mode, as individual selves in the everyday view of our world-about, and again as one, but physical, in the bottom-up mode that recognizes the underlying potential field. Such a concept should not be difficult to grasp, whether factually "true" or not. After all, physics itself has a similar multiplex structure, with its four forces, not just one, and its matter-energy dichotomy, "down here" at the level of our everyday experience. Physics also has its arcane, perhaps "lower," level of potential waves, as we have seen. So, then, do we, for our physical matter is part of the physical, sensible, world (even the most inane truisms sometimes need to be stated), while our consciousnesses are invisible, only inferable from physical movements of particular kinds, which only those things we describe as "living" evince. Living and nonliving are not the same.

There is, as we pointed out before, a difference in "mode of being" between a living human and one whose life has ceased. That difference might parallel the inferable but invisible division within the physical that exists between the everyday obvious and the hidden potential that underlies it. There are, it seems, levels among levels, and the words *gross* and *subtle, real* and *potential,* no matter that they shift, are not meaningless, but simply Janus-faced and perspectival, describing matters of viewpoint, of degree, or of small steps of difference; and, in harmony with this, Gebser predicts we shall in due time be able to see ourselves in two ways at once, top-down and bottom-up, aperspectivally. We believe parallel statements could, in principle, be made about the higher world that we are bound to postulate if any cogent explanation of our being is to be made. That world, too, might have its levels, and at least one of our levels might be, in its true essence, within that higher world. Tat twam asi. But for evidence of this we must await our last "epicycle," this chapter's final turning, reviewing the matter provided thus far, and moving to its conclusion.

As we have said, dualism of any complexion is currently unfashionable. Penrose, indisputably a leading scientist and mathematician, acknowledges it, but, seeming to recognize its mysteriousness, chooses not to write about it. Popper, too, understood physics with unusual depth, but also declines to answer the question as we have posed it, "What *is* it that we are?" Yet it is surely a question for an unprejudiced and expanded science, so we ask why philosophy regarding matters of our essence from graduates in languages, and philosophy, politics, and economics (PPE), who have no grasp of science or mathematics, has so powerfully cowed the opinions of people vastly more knowledgeable and less prejudiced in the relevant matters than themselves.* Fools have stepped in where those far better informed have hesitated, and the fools have been believed.

Returning to physics, and acknowledging that everyday-physical realm in which our *non*duality, our Being-in-the-world, supervenes, we now meet a surprise, an anomaly. Indeed, it is a double anomaly, for it occurs precisely where, given the facts, we would expect it to be impossible. It is anomalous for this anomaly to occur where it—apparently—does, *wholly within normal, accepted linear-logical physics.* The anomalous anomaly is this: Recent research shows that living organisms do

not react to electromagnetic influences (which are *physical* matters giving rise to *physical* measurements) in the formulaic, measurable, calculable, law-evincing way that physics would predict. This reminds us at once of Dingle's living fly, but now the facts are established by precise measurement, the physicist's very own favorite tool. Amplitude of response by living organisms is *not* proportional to intensity of stimulus. A very weak electric field can have an effect on a living organism when a much stronger field has no effect at all.* Further, organisms have an ability, unexplained by physics, to sense and react to small stimuli amid cacophonous electromagnetic noise from the environment. Waves of all lengths form a morass of canceling and reinforcing energy, yet organisms seem to filter out and respond to receipt of just those few radiations within the noise that are important for life, even when other ambient fields might be expected to interfere with, or even swamp, the weakest signals. Of course, as physics predicts, intense fluxes of radiation, even of the "acceptable and necessary" wavelengths, can eventually override the natural small signals, and may, at least normally, damage the organism, but they do not seem to do so deterministically. Physics, the very system within which the measurements are made, seems unable to explain the exquisite *selective* sensitivity shown by organisms. By the *anomalous* measurements it obtains, physics itself points unwaveringly to the reality of something *outside* itself, at least as presently constituted, something, moreover, that is central to our being as *living* beings, able to influence the expected mechanistic evolution of the physical world.† Somewhere on the same spectrum of the living organism's "escape" from mechanistic physics we may find the phenomena of fire-walking, telepathy, and clairvoyance.

Dingle must have been aware of a possibility, however remote, of such an anomaly, for he saw *prima facie* evidence in the movements of the humble fly, and what we want to add is that this *utterly unphysical* result *within* the realm-apparent of *physics* suggests that we, as Beings-in-this-*physical*-world, do *not* exist *wholly* within the physical world, but have at least a little independence from, and perhaps even some control over, it. The concept

---

The New Oxford American Dictionary gives: **cow** verb [trans.] (usu. **be cowed**); cause (someone) to submit to one's wishes by intimidation: *the intellectuals had been* **cowed into** *silence.* ORIGIN late 16th cent.: probably from Old Norse *kúga,* **"oppress."**

---

*Robert Becker's book *The Body Electric* teems with examples.
†Readers may like to consult David Böhm's *Wholeness and the Implicate Order,* which lack of space forces us to pass by.

of willpower may not be delusive, after all, and the fact that consciousness can be *experienced* by its "owner" but only *inferred* by *other* Beings-in-the-world strengthens the conviction. Whether "absolute proof" can be found of such a dual process, physically determined on the one hand, free-for-intentionality on the other, is almost irrelevant, for physics *itself* is not "absolutely proven," as Dingle knew and all physicists have always known. Only the naïve layperson thinks, of any matter, that "Science has proved it." Physics is scarcely even *its own* judge, though to some its *self-consistency* might suggest its truth. But most mathematicians would deny even that, as we shall see. How, then, could physics be appointed judge of matters that *might* transcend it? Does physics *itself* prove every claim made by physics *itself*? What we contend is that the evidence that there is something beyond physics is of a different order from physical proof, since its witness is within our Being. We suggest that only the kind of overall picture we are painting carries *conviction* as a description of a global truth, and the kind of "just seeing" that we advocate, and by which we are led to postulate a multi-leveled reality, is also the ground of the physics we all accept as veridical. We made physics. It did not make us. The Whole is greater than physics, and the discovery that physics points outside itself causes no surprise. We conclude that we are *alive,* and that, now almost by definition, by its distinguishability from physics, *our aliveness itself is outside physics.*

Of course, "unphysical" behavior such as large responses to small stimuli reminds us immediately of homeopathy, and, just as they have reacted against claims by homeopaths and researchers into homeopathy, many scientists, including some physicists and most biologists, reject the discovery of nonlinear response in living organisms as incredible "unphysical behavior," and therefore untrue.* But, we say again, we made physics, so it can no more be the final arbiter than we ourselves can claim to know all truth. Physics, our product, is not big enough to forbid unphysical behavior. It has insufficient authority, insufficient scope, insufficient certainty. Further, physicists' incredulity merely reveals as an underlying *presumption* their tenet of faith that their

narrow science, having excluded all *living* motions, is final arbiter on matters of *life*. This is no strange loop, possibly true (though probably not) but merely a logical circularity, a fundamental, if naïve, sin of thought. All physicalism assumes, in some such way, what it claims to prove, when it ought to be acknowledged that the only truly scientific question concerning any claim is not whether it is *credible* but whether it is *true*. Once upon a time, before the wheel was, the wheel was incredible.

The a priori pronouncement that a claim is incredible is irrational, but it has many precedents, ancient and modern. As we see from Acts 17.16–34, the "very religious" men of Athens were, nonetheless, philosopher-scientists of a kind. Many were Epicureans and Stoics, and all were keen to listen to word of "new gods," yet they showed their skeptical prejudice as soon as the unphysical notion of nonphysical life assailed their ears. Likewise, we read in Acts 19.23–41 of the good citizens of Ephesus, physicalists to a man (though showing thereby their ignorance of at least some of the philosophers of their age), who refused to hear of nonphysical gods, proclaiming of their notably physical goddess (she of the overdeveloped milk lines) "Great is Artemis of the Ephesians" in order to shout down the opposition. They were, of course, encouraged in this by those who trade truth for trade. Tin gods and silver goddesses were economically important, and economics, as we know, is always final arbiter in decisions as to what the unthinking members of any society regard as true.

Some of their descendants are half as ignorant and just as active. In the notorious case of the French researcher Jacques Benveniste, the editor of *Nature,* John Maddox, arranged for Benveniste's laboratory procedures to be observed by a conjuror in order to detect the fraudulent practice and misrepresentation of results that, according to Maddox, *must have been* going on. The ensuing persecution of Benveniste was severe, yet at least four other research teams have confirmed his findings. Homeopathy is still puzzling to scientists incapable of following to its proper conclusion Dingle's recognition that *living* organisms do *not* obey the laws of motion. However, it is beginning to be recognized as a phenomenon that science should humbly observe and attempt to explain, rather than dismiss as "Hooey," which was Maddox's one-word verdict on it, broadcast to the ears of the world in a BBC radio program at the time. Maddox

---

*James Oschman's *Energy Medicine: The Scientific Basis* provides much interesting and important information, topically on pages 203 to 206.

the scientist's atavism is as outdated as that of the linguist Ryle, and knows nothing yet of Gebser.

Living We-ness

James Oschman's *Energy Medicine: The Scientific Basis,* cited earlier, concerns itself *solely* with the physical, and is an excellent introduction to a rich field of research that, despite its never advocating belief in nonphysical entities, many scientists still sweep aside, slandering the findings with their unjustified skepticism. However, neither physicists nor biologists have any such right to demand that empirical facts *of the very same physical kind that they themselves purport to be the only valid evidence* be swept aside merely so that their claims to intellectual territory and a despotic right to impose dogma shall not come into question. Oschman gives factual examples, and explains that we seem to have evolved to live among pervasive pulsing electromagnetic fields that are beneficial to us, while other such fields are damaging.

Particularly interesting to us is the fact that the extra-low frequency pulsating magnetic field known as the Schumann resonance, which envelops the whole earth with standing waves that bathe us throughout our lives, is remarkably similar to the varying magnetic field detectable near a healer's hands; it pulses at around the same mean frequency, between seven and ten cycles per second. The Schumann resonance is set in motion and maintained by lightning, so, here, inanimate physics and living beings seem to find an interface. Our *Being-in-the-world* is *Being-in-the-vast-sea-of-the-Schumann-resonance.* The question, put elsewhere in other words, is whether conscious livingness is more than physics or less than physics, a mere excrescence of it, an oddity in the physical world, or its independently appointed director. We may help ourselves decide by repeating that we made physics, it has always been narrow by design, and Dingle, Jung, and Pauli wish us to extend it.

We have given evidence, *from within physics itself,* that can be rationally interpreted in only one way: we in our "we-ness," as distinguished from our "physical-thingness," do *not* live and move and have our very being *entirely* within the world studied and explained by physics. If "we" were ever to find a complete physical explanation of every facet of what "we" are, we would not have explained our "we-ness" itself. There seem to be several reasons for this, including the fact that physics is

our invention, yet the argument of most *biologists* would be that *physics* explains *us,* and does so *completely* and *consistently.* But even allowing for some kind of mutual interdependency of being between us and physics, such "tight" circularity, put forward as a *complete* and *consistent* explanation, does not appeal to us either intuitively or logically. The circularity is too small even to permit us to postulate the presence of that suspect entity the strange loop, so small it violates the manner in which thoughtful human beings think.

The notion that physics explains us *completely* and *consistently* also violates its own claim to constitute proof, for physics *depends on* us. Being our creation, physics "lives" and moves and has its very being *in us in our us-ness, not in our physicality.* It was only to explain physicality that we devised physics, and without us there would be no physics capable of arrogantly calling into question matters beyond its own purview, such as our nature as Beings. When the hard factual evidence of physics itself thus points back toward an interpretation that lies outside physics-as-constituted the only reasonable response is to extend physics or to postulate an additional, nonphysical entity, as we saw many pages ago. The question, then, remains whether physics explains us completely and consistently, and we have seen that it does not. Either our we-ness (as opposed to it-ness) is *at least* an emergent higher-level reality arising out-from the lower realities physics investigates—and we have argued against this view—or our own invention (physics) is, as we would expect, too small, *itself requiring us to postulate the independence from it of our we-ness,* the independence from physics of our own existence *as Beings.* Our living we-ness seems to survive the limits of our physics.

Our next task, having given some of the evidence for a real duality of being discernible even *at* (though not *in*) our everyday-physical level, will be to find where, within ourselves, the interface lies between the physically lawful and merely mechanistic and our "ownmost" self-willed livingness. But before moving on we must remind ourselves that our thinking on this subject, as on any other, is human-shaped, and limited, a fact that gives rise to another meaningful truism: our Being *as humans* is indeed *Being-in-this-one-and-only-world-about-that-we-can-imagine.* We are one with our world and it is one with us. We are in a part-to-whole mutuality with the world, and that duality exists in virtue of the fact that we *sense* it. It is our capacity to *sense* that itself constitutes our *polar-duality* with our world-about. Our sensing we-ness is more real than the world-about within us, for that world-about, itself a part of Being-in-the-world, is *constituted by* our sensings. Sensing is not merely a feature of our being that is not shared by tables and chairs. Sensing *is* what we might term our *polarity from* tables and chairs. We are *Sensors-in-the-world,* and our sense is not of the world sensing us (which it may or may not do) but of *our* sensing *it*.

Now, we remind readers of our two case studies. Pat Price saw without his eyes and felt without the nerve-endings beneath his skin. The Society for Psychical Research's contributor felt his being divided into two Beings, both affected, though very differently, by *feeling*. Feelings are experiences that Beings have, and tables and chairs do not. The immediate feeling of this man, his overwhelming dizziness, was, moreover, in his non-physical part, not in his physical body, which remained almost inertly undisturbed. There seems, therefore, to be an interface between a physical, lower sensoriness and an upper, subtler sensoriness that dominates, maps onto, and uses it, in large measure by *overriding* its physical laws by will, yet also allowing those physical laws their sway in the fulfillment of the will's demands.

It is clear that, whatever its nature, whatever the details of the process, consciousness can and does operate the physical body. It would be doing so even in one who now rose to shout this idea down. If physical reality is the manifestation of all those qualities that physicists measure (in principle, what the five bodily senses sense, and nothing beyond), then consciousness escapes physics, both by definition and in reality. Physicists will therefore be qualified to comment on consciousness only if they *succeed* in extending physics to include it in a proper, respectful manner, its failure to evince even a single physical *property* (as opposed to physical *effect*) notwithstanding. We believe this will prove impossible, and have given evidence for our view. It is physics, long ago *defined* in such a way as to exclude consciousness, not consciousness itself, that must make the accommodation (if it can), for *consciousness is primary* for Beings, and physics, an invention of Beings, is only secondary. Our sense of being Beings is precisely what it is that our consciousness is conscious of. And consciousness even has temporal and other priority, for it was consciousness

itself, already present and working, that invented physics, *not the other way round.*

Roger Penrose's Quest for the Nature and Locus of Consciousness

One highly qualified, highly perceptive scientist-mathematician whose view we value greatly is Roger Penrose. His book *Shadows of the Mind* provides a survey of the relevant physics and mathematics at the highest level that most nonprofessionals can assimilate. Part one of the book is mainly concerned with physics, and in part two his major quest is to discover where in the body, and by what means, consciousness appears and operates. On account of the technical nature of the book it is difficult to summarize. It is also important not to misrepresent Penrose's position, especially as he would be less willing than we are to espouse a strong dualist position. He chooses to avoid the vexed topics of dualism and vitalism, and leaves the question open. We shall therefore be content to give the briefest possible outline of his view and suggest that our readers read him for themselves.*

He seeks a locus within the physical organism where consciousness might arise in (or, if it should be any kind of separate entity, interact with) the body *by means of quantum coherence,* the process of arranging "wavicles" as coherent groups, not as randomly acting individual waves. This is the process that occurs in lasers, a special kind of *resonance*. He suggests that organelles called "microtubules" in the brain and elsewhere are probably that site. Accordingly, we must state, as briefly as possible, what microtubules are. Microtubules are very small hollow intracellular structures, containing pure water, which perform many tasks within the body. One of the most important is their part in the operation of neurons, additional to the neurons' long-recognized function of transmitting electric charge by movement of sodium and potassium ions through cell walls and back. Some microtubules lie along the axons of nerve cells.

Penrose believes that the teamed-up common flow

---

*Full details of Penrose's *Shadows of the Mind* are contained in the bibliography. We believe readers will be particularly interested in sections 2 and 3 of chapter 4, section 17 of chapter 5 (which goes much further in explaining quantum entanglement than we can in this book), parts of chapter 6 and most of chapter 7, and sections 6 and 7 of chapter 8 (which include description of the Platonic world of mathematical ideas).

of quantum-level particles in and around the microtubules is essential if consciousness is to appear *in or via the body*. Perhaps, he suggests, the coherence itself *is* consciousness, perhaps consciousness is a separate, or separable, entity that uses the coherent volume as an interface with the body as a whole. But microtubules are unlikely to be the whole story, he says, for "Large scale quantum coherence does *not,* in itself, imply consciousness of course—otherwise superconductors would be conscious! Yet it is quite possible that such coherence could be *part* of what is needed for consciousness."[26] Penrose believes that consciousness, if it is to find physical manifestation, will be, or will at least require, a modification of the normally physical realm of particle chaos into the coherently physical realm of large-scale, high-temperature, quantum coherence, apparently a rare state but present in microtubules.

But since even that rare coherent state seems, on its own, less than sufficient for consciousness, and not necessarily or automatically conscious *itself,* there must be *some sense in which* consciousness is a different entity communicating with the normally physical via the sites of quantum coherence. This is consistent with Penrose's rejection of Dennett's and similar views on the nature and origin of consciousness as nothing more than a *state* of the physical world arising automatically and without will, as an epiphenomenon of complexity.[27] We, too, reject Dennett's and similar views. It is interesting that Dennett was at one time a student of Ryle, the exponent of ordinary-language philosophy without knowledge of science. Wittgenstein, a philosopher with similar interests, always avoided the pitfalls, which trapped others less wary, neither becoming a logical positivist nor joining the school of ordinary-language philosophers. A full examination of these philosophers' work is far outside the proper concerns of this book, and, as we have pointed out, utterly irrelevant to the questions of properly weighed empirical fact, which do concern us.

Penrose's Questions
Penrose asks why it is that consciousness appears, as far as present science knows, only in or in relation to brains, but does not rule out the possibility that consciousness might be present in some other physical systems. Again, we would agree. Then he asks how an ingredient as important as the unpredictable, noncalculating, nonal-

gorismic character that consciousness seems to have (we, too, remarked upon it earlier) somehow entirely escaped the notice of earlier physicists and is still ignored by many of them. We think he shows a certain pro-physics bias with regard to both questions. Mind is acknowledged to be elusive, consciousness not even permanently present "in" the body. He makes this point himself, and with some force, in the passage just noted. Why, then, should he not allow at least the logical possibility that mind might exist and function without being present in brains or in *any* physical system, whether of the required structure or not? Perhaps unwittingly, he seems, here, to *presume,* as do countless others, that the only way mind or consciousness exists is in or via the brain, an ungrounded assumption for which humans have not the slightest evidence, and one that he has himself questioned, at least tentatively. Our two case histories, dealt with in detail earlier, strongly suggest that conscious mind can exist and function in a manner that is radically independent of, yet powerfully influential over, matter, including especially an influence over and within the physical body. The presumption in favor of the view that only *physical* proof of the presence of mind would be valid is therefore completely without ground. Physics is the laws of matter. Consciousness, livingness and mind are *essentially* law*less,* at least within the matter-world of physics.

We have no reason to believe there can be no mind or consciousness if there is no physical brain for it to arise in, or through which it might make itself known to other Beings-in-the-physical-world, especially as mind *itself* is *never* visible, even when most people would claim it was present in a brain. All we ever have, even among ourselves, the embodied living, is indirect evidence of its presence. We therefore cannot *know* that it is *not* an invisible *substance.* Minds may be alive and in communication *with each other* outside bodies and *we,* the embodied, would not know of it *because no evidence would be visible to our all-too-obviously limited five bodily senses, which are the sole basis of all science, including physics.* Invoking the notion of a *strange* loop to explain the structure in which life, consciousness, and mind appear in brains simply invites the suspicion that the asserted strangeness is an ad hoc invention, a means of escaping a difficulty imposed by preexisting wrong hypotheses, a tempting ploy of which wise scientists have always, and rightly, been wary. Why should consciousness, itself of elusive, evanescent nature, or livingness be so limited that they could exist *only* in "solid" physical bodies and why should it be *only* in or via "solid" physical bodies that one consciousness could become known to another? If you are awake and I am asleep (and therefore, as most would claim, not in communication), does that fact make either of us nonexistent? Logically, such a claim would be risible nonsense, while empirical investigation is simply irrelevant here since it could only discover *physical* entities, so perpetuating the very assumption it should be our aim to test. *Of course* I can only communicate with you *via the physical world* when both of us are awake in the physical world. But nothing is proved by this against either dualism or vitalism. Why do we not more easily realize this? One does not have to have made the error of reifying consciousness as "a Consciousness," mind as "a Mind," or life as "a Living Being" to perceive the power of the argument. The reification might *follow* the perception of the true picture, but the veridicality of the picture certainly does not depend on the reification.

Fortunately, Penrose is not so prejudiced as many philosophers and scientists, indeed he has admirable openness and intellectual humility, but we believe he does not give sufficient weight to a possibility, which he does acknowledge, that mind might exist elsewhere than in brains, and might inhabit brains only as one of its possible modes of being, the *only* mode that would be evident *to other brain-bound minds,* namely *those in the physical world.* We believe the evidence is that conscious mind is *nonphysical in a deeper sense than that in which physics is occult,* for no one has ever seen it, touched it, and so on, yet, acknowledging the frequently seen error of reifying what might not be a "thing" of any kind, we argue that this very precaution of avoiding the reifying or physicalizing of an entity that may not be physical *supports the dualist position that both physical and nonphysical entities exist.* Mind may indeed be a *totally nonphysical* thing, in other words it may be a *spiritual* thing, a spiritual *re*-ality, a thing having the spiritual kind of thingness. So we still have no warrant to claim that we can seek consciousness and mind *only* in physical bodies. Even if mind were to have the nature of a pattern, such as a morphogenetic field might be or have, we could legitimately regard it as a substance or thing *of that kind.*

Regarding Penrose's second question we have to respond with another: Why should physicists be thought likely to perceive every entity that exists? Physicists see physical things. If there are *nonphysical* entities we would think *physicists* very likely indeed to fail to perceive them. If I survey a landscape I cannot see what a geologist sees, inferring the substrata from the vegetation, for example. Does my ignorance make him or her wrong? Part of the proper response to Penrose's surprise is, therefore, to point out that, as Dingle showed, the referential world of physics is narrow *by intent.* Physics as a formal study came into being by a deliberate act of consciousness itself, namely the deliberate exclusion of precisely those noncomputable, unpredictable, and elusive entities or processes, which it knew it would fail to describe by "physical law." *But these unpredictable elusivenesses are precisely the imputed characteristics of consciousness!* Consciousness *excluded itself* from physics, in order to bring modern physics into being, detaching its study of *the world-about, in itself and as it is* (that is, the study of only one part of the part-to-whole dipole of Being-in-the-world), from the stranglehold of magical and mythic consciousness and their irrational paradigms. This being so, it is entirely as we would expect that physicists did not notice the noncomputable operation of consciousness, for they had *thrust it out of their field* (though they used it as their chief tool). The very hallmark of consciousness *must* therefore be its *unpredictability,* its *lawlessness* when judged by the laws of physics, for, as we asked many pages back, if consciousness is physical *in the same sense in which the world-about is physical* why was there a need to exclude it?

In Penrose's own description, consciousness operates in a *non*algorismic way. It is *not* like the automatic and predictable operations of a computer. It is *non*computational. Recall Dingle's fly. Inevitably, physics, *as we have known it,* cannot even begin to look for consciousness, the main reason being that consciousness *itself* cannot be sensed with our *external* sense organs, which (with a few extensions) are the *only* tools physics has. So, regarding this same question, we would also say that it was unlikely that physicists would find noncomputability until the appearance of Turing's mathematics. (For context, we explain that all computers work by operating algorisms of a kind defined by Turing.) However, as soon as Turing's mathematics *did* appear physicists would be aware of its implications and might even expect to find noncomputability in their world. They would look for it. But is not this precisely what happened? Penrose himself tells us how, beginning with the Diophantine equations, which lay, intriguing but little understood, for many centuries, and recounting something of the contributions of Hilbert, Church, and others, which culminated in the more comprehensive ideas of Turing, humans devised, in due course, the general purpose computers we all now use.[28] What Penrose sees as surprising is, we suggest, exactly what one would expect.

Consciousness escaped the notice of physicists for several reasons, not least that until recently, and *by their own definition of their universe of discourse,* it lay outside their field. But much more can be said. The present evidence seems to be that this exclusion was rational, after all, for consciousness has shown itself lawless and noncomputable, indeed completely unphysical, though able to communicate with other consciousnesses *via* the physical. If *nonphysical* in *essence,* it follows that consciousness, mind, livingness, all need *a bridge to the body* if they are to be seen to be *present in* the body. We have already made this point in other ways, and it was one of Jung's points (though he overstates it) in the epigraph with which this chapter begins.

Finally, among our allusions to Penrose's valuable and welcome thoughts we note the contrast he points out between the quantum-level behavior of small things, even over large separations* and the familiar behavior of larger things, the entities of classical physics, which interact more crudely, simply pushing and pulling each other around. He asks whether it can really be the case that there are two kinds of physical law, one operating at one level of phenomena while the other operates at another. This notion is quite alien to the traditions of practical physics, but, whether or not differing sets of laws operate in the classical range and the quantum range of the physics of the world, the *possibility in principle* of a duality of action does not surprise us, familiar as we are with the Hermetic notion "As above, so below," but *also* with the notion that the below is a *limited* version of an *unlimited* Above. The limited and the unlim-

ited, another part-to-whole duality, might rationally be expected to reveal different laws, and the idea of two kinds of law would be much less surprising to physicists, too, if they came to believe that the physical cosmos is home to a *self-directing* consciousness, such as the consciousness we all normally experience within ourselves, for that, too, would form a duality, the conscious Being being free to make choices, the mechanical world in which it lived evincing rigid law. Of course, such a duality is not what Penrose has in mind, nor Dingle, both of whom are thinking in terms of changes needed in the physical theory of their times.

But the matter to which we have drawn attention is highly relevant, for it remains to be explained how Dingle's fly seeks and consumes food when and wherever it wishes, no matter that the wish is dictated by physical need, for the need to fly off instantly supervenes if an enemy comes into sight. The fly has consciousness and self-determination sufficient to perform at least that act of choice among choices, allowing one priority over another. Something frees it from automatic eating when a predator appears. *Of course,* this alone does not *prove* that Dingle's fly has a consciousness *like ours,* or a soul, nor that we are souls, but at least we, like the fly, do *not* experience *ourselves* as totally helpless, like tables and chairs, nor *in that helplessness* nonetheless *conscious* of coercions the universe is thrusting upon us. On the contrary, consciousness is *not* totally helpless and, while consciously suffering certain constraints, does not *feel* itself to be totally helpless. Our consciousness tells us that it, itself, *is* able to make at least a very large range of decisions without any sense of being prevented by *physical* forces majeures. We are aware of bounds set by physical law, but do *not* feel *totally* coerced. So perhaps via the quantum world of the very small operating via microtubules we do indeed navigate a measure of freedom afforded us by a *different* set of physical *or nonphysical* laws, those of our own free will to act, within bounds, but choicefully, using a range of indeterminacy allowed us by the physical world. This would not be quite what Penrose has in mind, of course. It would be a law of our *mind,* not a different *physical* law, but to find two laws, one rigid and physical, one allowing the flexibility we intuitively feel in our mental life, cannot cause surprise to dualists or vitalists.

The quest is, then, to find the source within the

---

*This is a reference to the results of experiments such as Alain Aspect's and the infinitely delicate waves and particles in the double slit experiment.

physical world-about of our freedom to act choicefully within it. We have ourselves, earlier in this chapter, laid a foundation for this, and also quoted Penrose with reference to the Schrödinger wave evolution, so here we shall allow another writer to carry our thinking to its next step. We are not sure the interpretation of Aspect is correct, and in any case consider Schrödinger and Heisenberg more relevant to this particular matter, but the passage seems otherwise both pertinent and correct. The unknown writer says,

> As science progresses, the infamous wave-particle dualism may be resolved into a single theory, but, as the work of Aspect and others shows, without removing willed control over distance or indeterminacy from physics. It may be that as one determination of a wavelike action, that is one 'choice' from the many superposed Schrödinger states, is made, it sets the other (the particle-like) action free, perhaps for only an instant, but nonetheless free, to be influenced by animate will. Thus, the wave-particle duality, whatever its theoretical status and whatever the real essence underlying it, may be the locus of free will. It may be that the Creator, setting the world in motion, allowed an infinity of moments in which its evolution would be influenced by lesser beings.

We quote this writing of unknown provenance because it is at least largely correct, perhaps wholly so, and because its context may well overlap with Penrose's search for the locus of consciousness within the physical organism. What, then, would dualists or vitalists want to call the microtubular interface? Is it an *entity* at all or is it, as we suggested earlier, merely the joint-face between the physical being and a nonphysical living Being? Perhaps the best related paradigm from another culture is the kośa-body, containing a cascade of interfaces between the layers of a body itself less material as one moves "higher" within it. An extended biophysics might find much scope for research into such ideas, though Western science might wish to change the Sanskrit terminology for something more familiar. An interpretation of this type allows for loss of in-body consciousness when the quantum coherence in microtubules lapses, as in sleep, and in death.

Puzzles remain, of course. Why are we not aware of being conscious while the body sleeps? But, *to some degree,* we *are* conscious when sleeping, as dreaming shows us, and some witnesses assure us a consciousness resembling that of waking life occurs in lucid dreams. Consciousness *itself* is already known to have its layers, or levels, or modes. We experience them, and Gebser believes they are increasing in number as we evolve. So the need is first to be sure what all the types of consciousness are. Perhaps even in deep sleep we *are* conscious, faintly conscious of being very slightly conscious. Perhaps this is somewhat like, or on a par with, the waking consciousness of the fly. We are sometimes aware of a *stepwise* increase of consciousness as we awaken, moment by moment, from sleep. Do the steps match the levels of some kind of layered multiple composition, one part being what we call material, other parts not, with at least two layers in contact, in unimpeded communication, interfacing the physical with the nonphysical? It is very difficult, in fact, to imagine why the body, a physical system, ever needs to sleep, even more difficult to understand how, *if that is all there is,* it even *could* sleep and *then awaken to tell the tale.* How could consciousness survive sleep if the body were *all* there is? Why does it not do what many other physical processing systems do, that is run continuously? In some respects it does, of course, but consciousness is variable and full consciousness intermittent. Perhaps, then, it is some nonphysical part of us that needs intermittently to rest, not the body-machine itself. Wherever it is within our complex being that the discontinuities of consciousness and rest occur we remain aware of our own continuity as persons before and into, through, and after those periods. A merely physical system could not do that, for it could have no long-term memory. We see this in ongoing natural or physical or, therefore, chemical processes. Whatever the *substance* of that memory, whether the material relics of physical processes (including chemical and biochemical processes, of course) or some kind of abstracted energetic state recording what had once been, it would, in *any* case, be continuously eroded, consuming and changing the very matter that was to be remembered, and so destroying even the capacity for the keeping of any record. Putting it another way, in the physical world, alone and in itself, what might, in principle, be remembered is part of the very mechanism required to make and maintain the memory, so the system's own ongoing

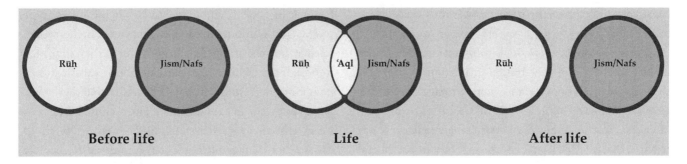

Fig. 15.12. The Sufi view of life, embodied and disembodied. Embodied life is shown using the device of the Venn diagram to map the overlap of two distinct and separable sets, illustrating a strongly dualist interpretation of our Being. The terms used in this diagram, which is based on Richard Kurin's presentation of it, are explained in chapter 6.

changes can never record all its own history, and will in fact inevitably destroy it. Memory can only be maintained indefinitely by something entirely outside the whole system of that which is to be remembered. Here, as before, the reader may see a reminder of the ākāśa and a foreshadowing of our final section. Perhaps, then, a suggestion some would find extremely strange might after all be true, that during periods of unconsciousness (and in some measure even when conscious) we are being lived from outside, rather than living as autonomous selves, and in some way it is this that produces temporary cessations of consciousness-to-ourselves such as occur in sleep. Perhaps we are indeed, as Indic belief has it, Brahman; perhaps the overlap with higher levels of being has itself a steplike structure over which conscious self-awareness distributes itself like a Boolean operator in electronic equipment, unifying a range of subsidiary and independent processes, of which the person may or need not be conscious, into a Being. Perhaps it is from within such complexities that disparate interpretations such as Sankara's Advaita and Madhva's dualism arose, and perhaps they are all correct, their difference being merely that each observer perceives divisibility in the nature of embodied (that is complete) humans at different points on a range of quite small steps. We remind the reader that we cast doubt, almost scorn, on the reality of the monist-dualist distinction, considering it a matter for narrow minds not yet aware of the possibility of a higher integration of mind and body as Being. Ultimately the monist-dualist pseudo-problem is a fiction of our limitedness of view. It is perspectival. Our interpretation is that the physical-to-nonphysical interface *itself* seems to span a number of parts or layers, allowing *different* dissocia-

tions of Being from body for different *purposes* and with different resulting *experience*. The independence of the spatial extent of consciousness of the *world-about* from bodily extent, of which clear evidence has been given, may be in the quantum interconnectedness of the physical universe, confirmed by Alain Aspect, or in the scalar and vector potential wave field, confirmed by Tonomura, or, as we pointed out, these postulated separate entities might simply be narrow perspectives upon the same superhuman level of the Universe's own Being. Other divisibilities may be outside the quantum world, in an unchartable placeless and timeless just-beingness above and beyond all physics, howsoever extended. If so, they are among those entities of which nothing can be said *because,* while we do, apparently, *experience* them, since they are part of what we *are,* nothing of them can be beheld by our attention and so *analyzed, distinguished, or identified* in experience. These constituent entities, if they exist as postulated, may be the Being who, on account of being the Seer, cannot be seen. Perhaps we are more complex, and, in our minuscule negligibility, far, far larger, than we have ever thought.

Returning from such wide-ranging speculations to Penrose's concerns, if we reach a conclusion it must be that the quantum coherence, which he believes exists in the microtubules of the physical body, is an *interface* between a *multiplex* consciousness and the physical body. This, while more complex, nonetheless resembles the very simple Sufi view, illustrated above.

The Resurrection of Descartes

Whatever the language describing it, and whatever the ultimate analysis into levels or layers or parts, the view we advocate of our *Being-in-the-world* when seen (as we must see it) *from its own level,* is a *strongly* dualistic and even more strongly *vitalistic* interpretation. The main duality, the dualism that resists unification, is precisely that between livingness and mere physicalness. This view is remarkably close to that of Descartes, expressed, of course, in the language of crude seventeenth-century science, that the soul attaches to the body in the pineal gland, the third eye of the mystics, *itself an organ having microtubules.* As we look back at him, we see that Descartes made mistakes, but so does modern science. Moreover, even modern science is unable to move far, at least during any one of Gebser's eras of consciousness, from certain fundamental patterns of thought, which are distinctively, and limitingly, human. Descartes' thought was limited in this way, but so is ours. Nonetheless, great changes do evolve from small shifts of perception. Just as the very small changes made to classical physics by Einstein's theory of special relativity wrought huge changes in understanding of the physical *world-about* so the interiorization of the world explained by Heidegger, which might seem a small change from Descartes' view, entails a huge enlargement in our perspective upon ourselves and our way of being-Beings-here-in-the-world. The old dualisms and monisms all give way to a comprehensiveness of view that outdates them all, and we attempt what must be a gross caricature of it in our diagram, figure 15.13.

Science since Descartes has served us well enough, by removing fantasies of the magical and mythic mind, which had no ground in *fact-in-the-observable-world,* by narrowing its focus and by establishing increasingly sound theory within the remaining narrower field. Now, it must reexpand, but into truth, much of it old truth, but cleared, now, of prescientific distortions. The *interior* connections within science will now be very different, nearer to a truly geodesic, truly physical structure than the ramshackle ropings-together and strangely looping fanciful conflations, which were alchemy's messy mix of mind and matter, and which included anything from poisons posing as panaceas to a veritable zoo of fantastical beasts. Physics, as *Being-in-the-world* studies it, and all the physical sciences with it, will become more truly themselves than was ever possible before. They must not, and never need, return to mythopoetic elaborations born of awe, of the ennui of an ignorance helplessly stranded

for lack of tools of thought, and so bereft of concepts to test and equipment to test them, which the meager science and the meager technology of earlier times had imposed, and which had therefore been substituted by imaginary correspondences with neither facts to justify nor hypotheses to explain them, and were in reality barriers against true science struggling to come to birth. Of course, our own hypotheses are, for very different reasons, still only partially correct, but, as Jung believed, they are on the right lines. There are now more of the correlations for which Dingle hoped than existed in his day, both within physics and with other sciences.

The expansion of science is supported by those who see that humankind's consciousness contains potential never yet made good, but which is now within Gebserian aperspectival grasp. But these expansions are grounded in an understanding of our Being against which some still mount violent opposition. The antagonists are not against new science, nor in every case against new spirituality, though, ironically, many of them understand neither, but against precisely those same old fruitless fictions that science long since evicted from its house. Philosophy, which rose in protest at alchemical and religious caricatures of spiritual truth, now opposes new growth in both science and spirituality by asserting perverse, groundless, and restrictive mechanistic or physicalistic dogmas of its own. Ironically, the denial that our Being involves any kind of indwelling livingness apart, this stance *perpetuates the mechanistic world-view of Descartes,* a philosopher most present-day philosophers despise, for after that denial only mechanism is left. Much of today's philosophy is thus enslaved to the old narrow physics of dead flies, which depends upon the totally unproved dogma of emergentism to explain consciousness.

A further irony is that philosophy, thus enslaved yet unaware of its captivity, turns upon scientists to refuse them what their most gifted have always allowed themselves, a free imagination and the necessary flexibility in use of existing language that mars communication only for the careless writer and the unimaginative reader. This is like insisting that Bruckner should use only the harmony and counterpoint of Bach. It is no wonder that, for fear of this fashion in philosophy, scientists often try to measure nonquantifiables such as personal experience, when truth is to be found only by using the method of observation that makes the *appropriate* assessment of *entities that have been allowed to reveal themselves-as-they-are-in-themselves,* and so to be observed *in experience.* What else would a science of *Being* be based upon than *experience*?

Those problems of picturing and communicating, which we all have to suffer at the hands of language, scientists, too, should be forgiven, but few philosophers (we have earlier seen Ryle's obsession with words) have the grace or the understanding to allow them that.* Worse, today's reductionist philosophy, like alchemy before it but for totally different reasons, is itself found wanting. What arose in alchemy out of ignorance now shows itself in philosophy in the rejection of unfashionable research findings and too much reliance on left-brained entirely verbal logic, far too sly a guide, which, usurping contemplative visual imagination, leads a great many astray. Some scientists join this conspiracy of prejudice, but philosophy's outmoded rearguard action will eventually fail. Let us turn away from these problem people, and look instead at the present status of both the notion itself and the theory of the subtle body, for this deals the *coup de grace* these backward-looking skepticisms deserve. We make no apology for presenting a *personal* viewpoint for a *personal* view of such matters is all there is, and all we need, for it is a better guide to what it *is* that *persons* are than abstract philosophical systems argued ad nauseam in words could ever be. We need a science of *ourselves,* and the subtle body is a *person,* and, moreover, a person who has *experiences* that are unique to him or her and of which that person is *aware.* Given only that it is carefully contemplative, this scientist-of-self is its own best guide.

Visualizing a Scheme of All Logic, and Its Consequences for Our Understanding of Reality

If written statements of all truths and all logical arguments were laid out on a surface so that the consequences of each argument became the premises for those that followed we would expect to find that they assembled themselves into a complete and harmonious, if also immensely complex, disc, a kind of universal

jigsaw puzzle or infinite tessellation, crisscrossed with all the logical statements that could ever be made. Our aesthetic sense, even if there were no other consideration, would lead us to expect that this body of truth, with all its internal relationships, would form a self-consistent, beautiful completeness. Many mathematicians of the early twentieth century would have agreed, at least in broad outline. Indeed, Bertrand Russell and Alfred North Whitehead set out, as the nineteenth century gave way to the twentieth, to demonstrate that all of mathematics could be derived from logic, and that a complete and self-consistent scheme would result. In effect, this was an attempt to remove what have more recently been termed strange loops, by which any body of subject matter, including logical systems themselves, reached a size and complexity at which they referred back to themselves, so destroying their logical *linearity* and vitiating their value as *proofs of their own validity.* What Whitehead and Russell were attempting was to replace all unexplained, or presumed, or self-referential (strange loop) relationships within mathematics by linear logical connections to form a *simple* self-proven hierarchy, and they hoped their work would reveal the whole of mathematics to be a complete and self-consistent body of logical truth. It is generally recognized that they did achieve a self-consistent scheme. They hoped eventually to complete their work, *Principia Mathematica,* by grounding every part of mathematics within logic. Exhausted by their efforts on volumes one to three, they delayed embarking upon the fourth, intended to treat geometry.

Let us delay a moment ourselves, making a small detour before continuing. We usually take arithmetic (or any other part of mathematics) for granted, but underlying it are principles, accepted as true since they seem so to our intuition, but in fact relied upon without proof. These are the axioms of the system. An axiom is "a self-evident truth, universally recognized to be true." Such a definition has always failed to satisfy thoughtful minds, proof of any assertion being preferred to acceptance of it as an axiom, but life becomes unlivable if we insist that everything be proved, so we have, for the most part, accepted axioms and forgotten them in order to get on with living. They are a part of the human condition, which is a realization to be pondered, for, as we shall see, it is more significant than the mere assertion of it seems.

---

*One of the worst examples we have seen is Peter Hacker's *The Philosophical Foundations of Neuroscience,* to which M. R. Bennett lends his name as coauthor, though the writing seems almost entirely Hacker's.

It points to the unseen but essential structures of our world, for axioms held as abstractions in the thoughtful mind do have parallels in the real world. We cannot prove everything, but we can sometimes be sure the unprovable is there. We noted earlier that each Dasein knows it is itself *there,* just as the thoughtful Descartes said, but Dasein cannot *prove* itself *there* even to other Dasein alongside whom it is living in the world. To doubt the *reality* of other Dasein is *possible, but insane.*

Even the apostle Paul was aware of the principle of the axiom. But perhaps this should not surprise us. He is known to have been something of a Platonist, and his statement that, in effect, we have no alternative but to embrace faith, taking some beliefs on trust, is equivalent to the mathematician's acceptance of axiomatic truths and the systems that are built upon them. Note that this situation *itself* is an example of precisely what is here being discussed, namely the bounded nature of human thinking, which imposes limits on all systems of explication. Dingle and Jung, too, seek a system to embrace *all* human knowledge within *one* schema of rationality, within one science. When in Rome one should act as the Romans do, and when a human one *will* think as humans *can* think. Again, to do otherwise will cause others to think one insane. Even the "highest" *human* thought will surely be misunderstood by the many, and will earn the thinker that reputation. The minor composer Louis Spohr, upon hearing Beethoven's seventh symphony, declared him fit for the madhouse. We need make no comment.

The thoughtful accept the consequences both of their discoveries and of the resulting logic. Thus, in 1931, before Russell and Whitehead could complete their work on geometry, Kurt Gödel's two famous theorems of incompleteness were published. Gödel's logic denied that the completeness and consistency at which Russell and Whitehead aimed was even possible. An axiomatic system might be complete, but in that case it would contain at least one unprovable, perhaps even ambivalent, or paradoxical, certainly *undecidable* proposition; or it might be totally self-consistent, but it could never then be complete. The theorems showed that, in simple verbal terms, no axiomatic system (a few very unusual and very small systems excepted) can be *both* complete and consistent. This brought the startling revelation that it is impossible to prove an axiomatic system valid at its own level or by referring only to its own content. It cannot be completed *and* made consistent by strange loops of logical self-referral *within itself.* One might, if logically possible, disentangle the strange loops, rearranging their logical cross-causations as simple linear threads, but then, after the last step of this reduction to linear logic *at least* one logical loose end, one unprovable grounding belief, one axiom, would remain unproved. Thus, a branch of mathematical logic *itself* had proved all our mathematical systems dependent upon at least one tenet (usually, in practice, there would be more) that could *not* be proved *by, or within, that system itself.* It remains true, of course, that mathematics approaches, more nearly than any branch of human learning, both consistency and completeness, for precisely those features have been its main aims, but even it shows a hierarchy of levels of what we might loosely term *logical authority.* Each subsystem of mathematics, and perhaps any entity dependent upon mathematics, *depends from** unprovable axioms greater than, or more fundamental than, itself. Only a larger system, if itself already proved, could supply the missing item of proof to the smaller system. So our humble illustration of a disc of all truth and logic, could not, after all, be complete and consistent since it would have to *depend* from a higher level.

Mathematics has often led the way for physicists to make discoveries about physical reality. Why is this, and how does mathematics, that world of abstraction, that mass of mere ideas that has so often directed the advance of physics, relate to physical reality *itself?* Why does the correspondence, often hinted at in this chapter and referred to yet again just a paragraph or two ago, exist, and how does it work? Physics, despite its occult character and the evanescence of its waves and particles, is largely down-to-earth, empirical, in its experimental methods. It therefore offers no explanations or confirmations to match the *a priori analytical certainties* bestowed by mathematics. Does our physical world, then, with its uncertainties for us who live in it, not merely *find its means of explication* in the certainties of mathematics but, beyond that mere parallel, *actually depend upon* mathematics in some *real, substantive sense?*

---

*We use the word *depend* in its root meaning. *The New Oxford American Dictionary* gives: ORIGIN late Middle English . . . from Old French **dependre,** from Latin **dependere,** from **de-** "down" + *pendere* "hang."

What would be the consequences if this were the case? At least some of what had seemed to be incomprehensible strange loops, or timeless, noncausal, mutual interdependencies of being in the *smaller* system of physics would be linearized in the simpler and more rational explanation that that system is part of a *larger* system, namely mathematics itself. Mathematics would then be a nonphysical, nonmaterial real world from which the material, physical world depends. This structure would leave the *components of* any purported strange loops intact, of course, only their *irrational strangely loopy connections* now straightened out. Instead of its inward-turned, closed-off strangeness spuriously suggesting the system's completeness-in-itself, the above from which, in truth, the system depended would now appear, as if the blue sky seen through the clouds of the *di sotto in su* painting.

Adding detail to the picture, we would suggest that the higher world acts as a Boolean operator upon our lower world, *each* of the subsidiary levels, *each* of the components, of which would now be explained by *its own* linear dependence *direct* from the above. The strange loops purported by some would be unnecessary, and we would therefore have no longer to accept their illogical strangeness. Even self-evidently true axioms and the necessary postulate of an Above are more acceptable than strange loops.

If the notion of the strange loop offends, as it surely does, it does so for good reason. How, otherwise, would such an entity ever have seemed *strange* to rational beings? Its logical offensiveness *is* its strangeness. The alternative suggestion is that *everything* we see hangs from something higher that we do *not* see, and does so *directly at every point,* so that anomalous postulates such as strange loops, which affront our logic, are unnecessary. We, *and, indeed, our logic itself,* depend in this same way, and that logic, if used with care and honesty, can be relied upon, *being consistent with that from which both our living selves and the physical world depend.* In the world of our view-about the *success of our science* is the empirical *validation of our logic.* In itself and used with honesty and care, it is reliable, though our use of it is fallible, of course. We should rely upon it rather than upon strange loops too cleverly invented to explicate *without* recourse to an Above but which fail because they affront that very same power of reason

which overcleverly brought them into being. There is no available alternative to our own logic. It is that by which we humans are bound to assess *all* our thinking (including our thoughts about strange loops). If our own invention seems strange we should invent something better. This we are trying to do, and the schema we advocate has a harmony with our intuitive sense of ourselves, a harmony that is lost if we have to accept the *strangeness of allegedly causal* yet *self-referring* loops. Perhaps the notion only came into being as a ploy to avoid the consequences of the dependence of small systems from greater ones that Gödel's theorems present. The *strangeness* of strange loops *is* our intuitive sense that something is not right, so the vertical linear-dependence structure we now suggest (along with horizontal, timeless, and noncausal interdependency of being) ought to be preferred. If we can find, test, and accept a scheme that thus eliminates any merely apparent, putative strange loops we shall have approached truth more closely than before. But we shall not hope to remove the very last unprovable, the very last loose end, the ultimate axiom, but shall joyfully accept it. The apostle Paul may have been right that we have no alternative but to trust (Greek πιστις), but it will be a trust *necessitated and predicted* by reason. And, of course, there is still a place for self-reference in any dependent system, for such inner consistency is precisely what one would expect in a system showing design, and especially a system of which one is oneself a part.

If physics depends from mathematics, we could, without our appreciation of mathematics, find no explication at all of the physical world, either as an eternal entity, an ultimate self-validating but stupefying interdependency of being, or as a system depending from a higher realm; but the human mind, whatever it is that it is, increasingly absorbs understanding from that realm of mathematics *with which the human mind itself seems, its ignorance notwithstanding, to communicate and to be naturally in tune.* Even babies, as we saw many pages ago, are born topologists, and add to their knowledge daily. It is almost as if mathematicians listen to *mathematics itself,* contemplating it in the light of their own logic, so coming to comprehend new facets of its seemingly infinite wholeness.

The world of physics thus depends from *the world of* mathematics, and we, in *parallel* dependence from above, alongside that world of physics, observe and interpret it

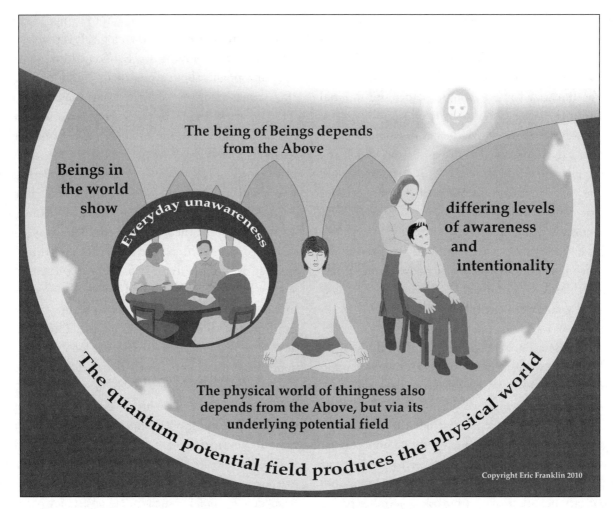

The being of Beings depends
from the Above

Beings in
the world
show

Everyday unawareness

differing levels
of awareness
and
intentionality

The physical world of thingness also
depends from the Above, but via its
underlying potential field

The quantum potential field produces the physical world

Fig. 15.13. We, as *Dasein-here-in-the-world*, live in the overlap of the world of things with the world of livingness. Recognizing this, we have naturally conceived two realms, which the Hermetic tradition designated "the above" and "the below," a useful notion, but one that, throughout history, has been unable to resist the confusion of levels in human consciousness that we see, despite the best efforts of human thinkers, in such imagery as that of the Ripley Scroll (plate 28), in transcendental art, and in myriad other manifestations on account of the unimaginable nature of the above. We have perforce seen the above as *like* our own lower level, though better, creating gods in our own image. Thus the very notion of "As above, so below" has itself often been taken too far. The fact is that we simply *cannot depict* the above. Humans show very different depths of awareness, often being naïvely ignorant of the delusions that are almost universally accepted as the axioms of everyday life. The popular misunderstandings of science arise from this somnolent semiconsciousness. Superficially different, but arising from a similar inadequacy of consciousness, is the failure of verbal philosophy to find answers to the conundrums it perpetually generates for itself, for they arise from a spiritual blindness that fails to perceive its own lack of imagination and its resulting bondage to words, and therefore fails both to escape that limitation and to perceive the nature of reality-as-it-is-for-humans-here-in-this-world. We have to include such thinkers with those mundanely unaware, engulfed in Heidegger's *they-self*, our *social* selfness, on the left of our illustration. Some healers, by contrast, are aware of guides, perhaps the latter-day descendents of gods made in man's image, who may even have names, and of whom they may hold visual images, so our illustration includes such an impression. Creative minds have their own ways of greater-than-normal awareness, known to their own consciousnesses, of course, but impossible to picture for view from outside. They can be recognized only by their outward manifestations. A portrait of Beethoven thinking his music and writing it down, somewhere within our diagram, would tell us nothing important about him, and nothing at all about his music. We must not only remain silent about matters of which nothing can be said, but must also accept the impossibility of depicting entities that cannot be depicted. They are matters for the individual conscious Experiencer, not of the bodily senses we share with each other.

as a function of our *Being-in-this-world*. Now this begins to make very good sense, though we realize at once both that we are relying upon human reasoning (we have just shown that we have no alternative, but that it is also generally reliable) and that in accepting this view we are espousing, in the early twenty-first century, essentially the view that forms the core of the Vedic understanding, of Neo-Platonism, and of Hermeticism. We might no longer show human figures at both higher and lower levels when we attempt to illustrate our schema, as George Ripley did, for we simply cannot see higher than a certain very slightly higher, imaginable level than that of our own being, but while acknowledging that any Higher Being is not, after all, likely to be much like us, and therefore should *not* be pictured as "like us but bigger, better, and more terrible," as primitive people saw Him, or Her, we do depend from that unseen and unimaginable Higher Being.

"As above, so below" now becomes simply: "The world-*about*, with us in it as *Beings-in-the-world*, depends from a World-*Above*, and, despite being *in* the *world-about*, we in our we-ness seem also to be at least partly *in* that unseeable Above, for we *are* the *living* Seers of the evidently largely nonliving world-*about*." We have heard this before, in other language, for it is Tat twam asi. Now Gebser, too, makes even better sense. We can *aspire* (please note the word) to a more comprehensive perspective, so comprehensive as to see from above all perspectives, so finding a monist top-down view within which dualist bottom-up views, at their own level and within their limited perspectives, all subsist.

So we wonder what we shall perceive if, as we aspire upward, we also look the other way, downward? Gödel's theorems prove that systems cannot be both complete-in-themselves and totally self-consistent, yet, by showing this very structure of *dependence*, they provide us with an indication of where the explanation of our evident superiority, as *Beings*-in-the-world, to mere *things*-in-the-world will be found. We suggested, for reasons having no obvious connection with Gödel's mathematical logic, that there is a doubling or interfacing at one of the levels of embodied being. Above the interface, we believe, is livingness, below it physics. Higher than physics is mathematics as a priori truth, the world of Platonic Ideas, a real world, from which the whole of our lower, physical, reality depends. And we in our we-ness also depend

from the above, but, we believe, in a different way or by different means.

Our bodies are, clearly, both by definition and by empirical observation, part of the physical world, part, indeed, of an *electromagnetic* world, but we in our embodied wholeness are *lived* bodies, our individual livingnesses also *depending*, but, we believe, doing so in a manner unconnected with the physical world's dependence. This unfashionable view is at least rational, for there does, after all, have to be a difference between being dead and being alive (or we would never have noticed the need to make that distinction), and we need to know what that difference is. The mathematician might, we believe, conceive our livingness as depending from the above, but as making only an *asymptotic* approach to the physical world-below in which it forms our complex embodied selves by existing *alongside* the physical. We are indeed *in* the physical world, but not *of* it.

The Resurrection of Vitalism

We need to make one final, brief epicyclic detour, to answer what may seem the ultimate question: What is it that makes us alive? When Franklin, Mesmer, Faraday, Maxwell, and many others had made their various contributions to our understanding of electricity, it was thought by some that electricity itself might be the elusive life force. It did, after all, re-animate the nervous systems of recently dead animals. Attempts were even made to revive the dead by subjecting the body to electric pulses. The attempts failed. In fact the excessive presence of electricity killed rather than made alive, as other experience showed. We need not tarry over this backward look, for we now see the reason why electricity can never be alive. Electricity is one of the two all-pervading forces (the other being gravity) not of living beings of any kind but only of the physical macro-world of our experience and, therefore, the physical body itself, as the later electrobiologists, finally emerging from the disdain heaped upon them by those who had seen the errors of earlier vitalisms, showed. As so often, the error had been a failure of vision, of imagination, and a confusion of levels, a failure to "see" two worlds because only one was visible. Electricity is not livingness. It is nothing more than a part of the nonliving world of matter, and therefore it is not the life force, a fact that ought to have been obvious even when electricity was excitingly new. To put the matter rather willfully, though not without point, only Livingness is livingness. We do not know *what* livingness is, so we can say very little about it, but it is that *necessarily* postulated entity that leaves the body when it dies. We have no explanation either of living or of dying without it.

So this chapter's finale, had we called it another epicycle, would have been misnamed. We should instead consider it a hyperbola, curving out far above physics, or an involute, descending directly, tangentially, to our physical *world-about,* and, unlike those cycles, which, thus far, have all turned to carry this chapter forward, the Gödelian insight shows "As above, so below" to be, in our picturing imagination, just such a *double* secure line, indeed our lifeline, stretching far out above the body, far beyond the brain, far above our minds (whatever, in their unknowableness, our minds may be), a line that never returns (as a strange loop would) for it is anchored in the invisible Above. One strand supports the physical world, explaining why that world is itself explained by mathematics. The physical world could be said to be mathematics modeled in matter. Our earlier epicycles, in constructing this chapter, lay entirely within physics, the bounds of which they very slightly stretched. One of the curves we now describe reaches upward, out of the physical into mathematical logic, its source the Platonic world, yet in its lower reaches it dictates our understanding of the physical world-below. Now we leave physics behind, for the other strand is our living Selves, conceived in some traditions as "sparks of the divine" or by use of some other material-world metaphor. We still cannot *picture* anything beyond our material world but only *infer* it as a necessary postulate. We suggest that it is by this strong duplex cord, depending from unknown higher regions, that the whole cosmos of our *Being-in-the-world,* which is *Dasein-amid-physics,* hangs.

We shall, of course, be accused of abusing Gödel's theorems to support what many would condemn as religion. What did Gödel himself believe? He was a theist,*

---

*theism |ˈθēˌizəm| noun: belief in the existence of a god or gods, esp. belief in one god as creator of the universe, intervening in it and sustaining a personal relation to his [her] creatures. Compare with **deism**. ORIGIN late 17th century: from Greek ***theos* "god"** + **-ism**. (We have added, in square brackets, the feminine "her" where the dictionary gives only "his.")

firmly rejecting the notion that God was merely an impersonal force or thing or principle that, or who, did not ever intervene in our low world. He believed there is an afterlife, writing, "I am convinced of the afterlife, independent of theology. If the world is rationally constructed, there must be an afterlife."

Much of the material of this book has not seemed to describe the subtle body *per se,* it has not told us what the subtle body *is.* It has often seemed to be description of religious practice, or of a paraphysical somatic morphology, or of the making of pictures in the physical *world-about* upon which to meditate, or information about *using* the subtle body, with its currently sporadic powers of communication and intentional action at a distance, whether to heal the physical body or as a means of clairvoyance. The subtle body has been very difficult to describe or define, but it seems at least to be a *necessary postulate.* No other explanation than that the subtle body is in some sense a real, if also nonphysical, thing offers rational explanation of a number of well-attested phenomena, not least the event of dying.

So we should ask: What is the nature of a necessary postulate? In other words, what justifies the claim that we cannot avoid postulating that there is a real thing, whether or not we know what it *is* that it is, which justifies our acceptance of the term *subtle body*? Dingle has something pertinent to say. In his chapter titled "Words," he defines a postulate. It is, he says, "a concept invented in order to interpret experiences in terms which make possible the expression of a logical connection between phenomena."[29] As examples he gives a list that will surprise most laymen in matters of science: the electron, light, physical time and space, mass, and mind. These are all unobservable and, with the exception of mind, a term we have avoided defining, even ostensively, each is *inexperienceable as itself.* Mind *is* ourself, inexperienceable by *others.* The evidence for every one of these necessary postulates is *indirect,* though mind has features the others lack—which should alert us to its difference from the other entities, which are all physical components of the physical *world-about.* Even mind, qua entity, we do not see, but rather *infer* from our use of and *direct experience* of it. What we do experience in the sense of *observe* is the *effects* of the postulated entities, and, Dingle explains, after applying reason to our observations of those effects we can make far more definite statements, called hypotheses, about the *relationships between* the postulates. Postulates can therefore be seen as analogous to the unprovable but necessary axioms of mathematics, while the hypotheses of science parallel the theorems of mathematics that follow from its axioms. Down here, it seems, everything has these two levels.

Thus, the necessarily postulated entities of physical science, *in themselves,* in their *what-it-is-that-they-are,* remain mysterious, undoubtedly *necessary,* but un*knowable, inexperienceable even by the solipsistic I,* which thus shows itself to be *not*-of-the-physical-world. That is itself an extremely important point. It is the physical world that is occult, hidden from us, rather than ourselves as Experiencers of the *experience* of experiencing. We ask the reader to pause, if this is an unfamiliar thought, to ponder its importance. But now we wish to make another, equally important. The status of the necessary postulates of physics is precisely the status of the invisible but undeniably inferable subtle body. It has precisely the same *scientific* status as the postulated fundamental entities of a very successful science, itself long-since vindicated by the equally successful pragmatic technology it has produced. The subtle body is just as real as the photon and the electron. It may be a *more* reliable real entity than they, for if it is the subtle body, or even just one layer of a subtle multiplexity, that we each *experience directly* as "my own solipsistic I," then it is, for us, and in our normal usage of the word, *more* real than any of those physical entities, all similarly postulated *by us,* of which *not a single one of us* has any direct experience; and, to prove that this is indeed the case, *each* of us has precisely such direct experience of him- or herself, and (normally) *no direct experience at all of any other person or thing.* The rightness of this view is corroborated rather than denied by the fact that sometimes persons do see into the experience of other persons, as, for example, in clairvoyance, not least because this demonstrates *their* reality alongside ours. Nothing in science is more securely proven than that the solipsistic I exists *in its own experience,* which bespeaks its *more* real existence in the world of *our* Dasein and *our* observing than that which electrons or photons can ever prove themselves to have. We cannot doubt the reality of electrons or photons (for the electromagnetic hypothesis works) but we can never observe them as we observe our own inner consciousness. Our inner consciousness is *there* and no one can deny its being-there, its Heideggerian *Da-sein.*

Science, in Dingle's definition of it, is the application of reason to experience. The solipsistic I is thus the very ground in experience, the absolute sine qua non, not merely of *all* human science but also of *all* human philosophy—*not the other way round.* And its method of working, its very way-of-being-in-the-world, is empirical. It is an observer, a discoverer, an interpreter, a hypothesizer, and, finally, it is an actor-on-the-basis-of-its-own-hypotheses. As we saw much earlier, its Being-*in-the-world* consists in such awareness and such doings and makings, as both Heidegger and Popper claim, each in his own terminological style. This solipsistic I is, from before its birth and throughout its life, a scientist and a technologist. There could be no philosophy at all without Dasein's empirically obtained thinkings about itself and its world. Even words, the sole fodder of many twentieth-century philosophers, could not exist without this self-aware consciousness to invent them. Of course, this view does not constitute quite the same statement as Descartes' "I think, therefore I am," but it is closely allied to it. Our main difference from Descartes is only in our interpretations of the world, for we agree in our recognition of our essential Being-there. Whether that Being is, by essential nature, a Being-that-thinks or whether, as most philosophers have recently insisted, the Being *is* nothing more than the thinking, a mere assertion that dismally fails to satisfy our sense of self-ness and (more importantly) lacks even one shred of *external, independent* proof, is a question that, if it is to be illuminated, let alone answered, seems to require Gödel's notion of the undecidable proposition, the axiomatic dependence from something higher, since the solipsistic self *cannot,* any more than any mathematical system, validate in a *logical* way a belief in its own reality from *within* the limited system of *itself-as-it-exists-in-the-world.* This needs to be pictured, experienced, contemplated, and its simple rationality, its economy and beauty, *seen,* for recent philosophy has done its merely verbal best to erase this view from human consciousness. To take up again a point from a few lines ago, philosophers must, if they are to find truth, return to the empirical enquiry upon which their very existence has always depended, for they will *never* find truth in words. Words encapsulate only the errors of our past, if even that. Words are not even an axiomatic system, provable except for an axiom or two, but only a clumsy *mapping* from such systems, *totally* divorced even from the substance they are purported to re-present to us.

Humankind's newest science, having a clearer, more rational view than its forebears, alchemy and ecclesiastical dogma, knows its own way forward, for now it includes the study of our Being as it phenomenalizes itself before *our own* view. Science now *includes* the science of our solipsistic selves-in-the-world. It does not need philosophy as we have had to suffer it, increasingly, for the past two centuries or more, as philosophy itself had earlier suffered and fought off the rampant medieval church on the one hand and the childish, fantasizing silliness of alchemy on the other. Philosophy, like religion and science, is entirely the product of the solipsistic I, whatever its nature, and therefore wholly dependent for its subject matter upon the solipsistic I's *empirical discoveries in the world*. As we remarked earlier, there can be no philosophy without empirical facts. Philosophy, therefore, not only depends on us (*not* the other way round), but also cannot stand against the *ongoing* empirical discoveries of science, but, as Harri Wettstein, the Wittgensteinian, advises, must itself reembrace the empirical. So we shall go far beyond Heidegger, for he would make no surmise regarding the state of Dasein before its birth or after its death, while science itself has already given us reason to believe that we may do so, after all. As it reexpands, today's science, setting aside the merely verbal dogmatizings of Ryle and his successors, will accept and explore the *empirical* evidence that the long-neglected, discredited, even despised and ridiculed invisible subtle *body* is there after all, *more real* than any entity in the physical world, for the evidence suggests, strongly, that some *invisible and unphysical* entity that is our ownmost *very essence* defines the difference between the living body and the nonliving body, and does so because it depends, independently of the physical world, direct from a World Above the *very essence* of which is *living*ness. We are justified, therefore, in reinvoking notions of *Self*, of *Dualism*, and of *Vitalism*, for the subtle body has *at least* two layers, of different depths or degrees of subtlety, and is alive and well and living in each one of us.

SIXTEEN

Consciousness and the Subtle Body

Neither science nor philosophy can even begin to explain how it is possible that mind, consciousness, or spirit could influence matter or energy (subtle or electromagnetic). Nevertheless, the evidence is there, demanding explanation.

DAVID FEINSTEIN, *SUBTLE ENERGY: PSYCHOLOGY'S MISSING LINK*

Over recent decades a radical paradigm shift has occurred in our view of ourselves and the world we live in, particularly in relation to the subtle body and the exploration and application of "subtle energy." After a century of opposition to the new ideas, perspectives on consciousness, healing, and human potential are now all changed. As one journal dedicated to the study of energies and energy medicine puts it, "There is now a widespread appreciation of the energetic component within many disciplines including quantum physics, therapeutic modalities, healing, psychology, consciousness, psi, and the understanding of our multidimensional existence."[1] Indeed there is, but we feel bound to wonder when it was that physicists did not appreciate the "energetic component" of the matters they study. Already by the middle of the nineteenth century physicists were developing the theory of electromagnetism. A hundred years earlier still mechanics and dynamics already encompassed such notions as force and acceleration, which are necessarily matters of energy, whether that word was used or not. Even half a century before that Newton had already recognized that gravity was a universal phenomenon

involving the energy of movement, which Kepler's laws of planetary motion and his own general laws of motion had revealed.

What may indeed be new today, at least in the West, is acknowledgment that conscious intentionality is *itself* a "force," and may even bring about "action at a distance" of its own as-yet-unfamiliar type, and do so by means of a *kind* of energy not described by the field theories that originated in the nineteenth century. Alternatively, of course, the energy put into action by intentionality might be one of the already-familiar forms, but *the release of it into action* takes place as if it is itself a kind of field effect at distances from the intender never before proved to be connected in such ways. As mentioned earlier, James Oschman, in his book *Energy Medicine: The Scientific Basis*, gives evidence that living organisms do seem able, in a manner described by some as "unphysical," to filter the surrounding electromagnetic noise and respond to very small signals at frequencies resonant with particular tissues or electrical pathways within the body.[2] However, this alone may not be sufficient explanation, for intentional processes involving the electromagnetic responses of our physical structure would need a means not merely of transmitting the postulated energy of intention out into all of space, but of *directing* that energy from the originator of the intention to the *particular* patient, the *target* patient, which would be an effect not easy to account for even by present-day physics. Perhaps the teleportation of quantum states (rather than long-distance transmission of particles or electromagnetic energy) acknowledged by Alain Aspect might, after a great deal of difficult research, prove itself to be the means. However, even such a physical process, if ever accepted as empirical fact, would require deeper explanation.

Where, in such a system, would matter end and spirit begin, and why? Something outside *present* physics would probably still be required, and it may, after much research, be necessary to postulate what we would call a *spiritual* faculty, which Beings would have, and physical things lack. Questions of the bounds of physics would then arise, and what Poortman terms hylic pluralism would reappear in modern garb, and, of course, be questioned by those who want to discover whether there is a single continuum of subtler and subtler levels of matter, or whether spirit is in deep reality something else, in short whether we have a genuine duality or only a continuum. This, it will be recalled, is a question raised by von Franz, though at a simplistic level that will certainly not be adequate in the future. The research required to answer these questions would involve at least the extension of physics envisaged by Dingle and Jung, and perhaps the conclusion that something entirely outside physics, no matter how far we could legitimately extend it, is at work. Such research might be characterized as the study of how *consciousness,* in the mode of *intending,* affects the *physical* body via the *subtle* body.

Some impression of the speed at which attitudes have, finally, begun to change is given by the fact that, even before the establishment of the necessary new science, public medical practice has already begun to change. Complementary and alternative medicine (CAM) provides an approach to health care that is officially recognized in some Western countries, and already "the subtle body" has become the iconographic medical model underpinning many therapies. Therapeutic Touch, Reiki, Polarity Therapy, and various types of bodywork and massage are a few of these, and some treatments evolved from Eastern traditions are also included. So far, despite great interest in these therapies, scientific research has been focused on the healing tools and little is known about what happens to the healer in the healing process. There is an assumption that what happens in the process of healing is accomplished through the application of various strategies and methods when, in fact, it is the "application" not of any technique but of the *healer as conscious person,* or, more specifically, of *the healer's energies* to the patient that really brings about the healing. It is the *intention* to heal, we are now discovering, that alters the consciousness of both healer and, ultimately, client or "healee," and so creates substantive change. Most healers and alternative medicine practitioners believe that having the sincere and conscious intention to heal is an absolute *prerequisite* of success in the healing encounter, and some even begin their session with an invocation or prayer that states that intention.

Many questions present themselves to our openness of mind: Where does healing come from? Does the healer's "attitude," using that word in a broad sense, make a difference to the outcome? How is healing influenced by our beliefs and intentions? What is it that healers experience as they work? How does the subtle body function in the healing process? Which layer or layers of the subtle structure are involved?

The Subtle Body in Healing

Let us look briefly at some healers' perceptions of how the subtle body is involved in the process of healing, beginning with the "etheric body," the subtle body-layer believed by many practitioners to be in some sense the "closest" to the physical body, and to be involved in healing as a whole, which, of course, includes physical healing. While no precise equivalent of Leadbeater's term *etheric body* is found in the Eastern traditions, we have seen already that precise interpretation of ancient terminology is difficult, and rejection of unfamiliar notions is unwise. We must overcome ambiguities of language and discern the realities beneath, for, as we have seen, the general outlines of theory from other cultures are similar. Following Leadbeater, many Western healers believe his postulated etheric body is involved in the process of physical healing and it appears to correlate with the "body of energy," the prāna-maya-kośa, composed of the life force, the energy field that links body and mind and sustains all the physical functions. It is thought that the etheric body first forms, then sustains and maintains, the form of the physical body, and it is accordingly considered to be an "energetic blueprint" for which another Western term, the "morphogenetic field," might be used. The etheric body is also associated with the emotions, already known from other studies to have profound physical effects, and with matters of identity, sexuality, and relationship. Clearly, if real, the etheric body is an important entity, and the attempt to understand the matter will be worthwhile.

As always, there are verbal uncertainties with semantic consequences to resolve, for the English word *ether* is usually regarded by most yoga practitioners and scholars of Indian philosophy, and by some scientists, such as Ervin Laszlo, as the correct translation of the Sanskrit word *ākāśa,* meaning "all-pervasive space," the first and most fundamental element from which all the other elements, air, fire, water, and earth, devolve.[3] (See chapter 3.) "Akash embraces the properties of all five elements: it is the womb from which everything we perceive with our senses has emerged and into which everything will ultimately re-descend."[4] This reminds us of the potential field confirmed to exist by Tonomura. Here, as we hinted in chapter 15, we might have a fruitful notion of the oneness of all life, or, of course, merely a misleading verbal conflation without analog in the world of human experience. Interpretation of the term *etheric body* as "akashic" would accord it a far larger role than an interpretation in which it is thought to be only one of many layers. We shall not prematurely foreclose this discussion, for the subtle body, whether multilayered or simple, is the quest of the whole of this book. For the moment we shall assume many layers, as Indic tradition has done, and look forward with open mind to the *possibility* of simplification only much later.

Since most healers seem to believe that healing involves some form of higher intelligence or intuition than our own, it would appear that another subtle body kośa or sheath, the vijñāna-maya-kośa (the body of intelligence), is also at work. The vijñāna-maya-kośa is a higher form of cognition and understanding, which includes intuition, and discerns what is real and unreal. In fact, the general consensus is that most of the layers or levels of the subtle body are engaged in the healing

experience since the process of healing is *itself* thought to take place *holistically,* as, of course, the word "healing" itself suggests.

The experience of mystics and yogis attempting to unite the individual self with the cosmic Self in samādhi may be similar to the healer's experience of what we call "cosmic consciousness." In deeply altered states of consciousness, many people experience a kind of heightened awareness that appears to be a direct "presentation" to the meditator of the universe *itself.* The experience recounted by Christopher Bache, a professor of religious studies, after practicing holotropic breathing,* is a good example. He reports that "the unified field underlying physical existence completely dissolved all boundaries. As I moved deeper into it, all borders fell away, all appearances of division were ultimately illusory. No boundaries between incarnations, between human beings, between species, even between matter and spirit. The world of individuated existence . . . was revealing itself to be an exquisitely diversified manifestation of a single entity."[5]

There are similarities between Professor Bache's experience and that of Olga Worrall, one of America's most studied healers. Her description of her own experience suggests that healers should seek a state of consciousness that transcends a boundary that normally impedes us. They will then find that the healing power flows, but not from or even through the healer herself, for it *flows from elsewhere and directly to the patient.* "Spiritual healing," she believes, "is the channeling of energy into a recipient from the universal field of energy which is common to all creation and which stems from the universal source of all intelligence and power (which some people call God)."[6] Her experience is that the energy becomes available to the healer through tuning her personal energy field to a harmonious relationship with the universal energy field so that she acts as a conductor, or rather as a transistor, merely switching on the flow from universal field to patient. Within this transcendent state, is the healer "above" the physical because the healing power comes from the "above"? In what sense is the healer "there"? Can we read "As above, so below" as meaning "As in the *mind,* so in the *body*"? We said something about top-down views and bottom-up

---

*Holotropic breathing is a technique similar to the Yogic practice of *bhastrika* (the bellows) referred to in chapter 5.

views of the cosmos in chapter 15, and here we have an example of multiple levels and of the two directions of view, toward the body and toward the "above," whatever its nature.

Olga's husband, Ambrose Worrall, who is both a scientist and a healer, states a view similar to hers but adds something further that helps us understand this. He believes that "Although I am *instrumental* in creating the conditions which permit the force to flow, actually I have no control of it whatsoever."[7] So while a healer *initiates* the healing by his or her *own* compassionate *intentionality,* that is, holding in mind or heart the wish for another's well-being, and opening up to a spiritual or energetic healing force, it arrives (and leaves) without the healer being able to control it in any way.

Our next step in forming an understanding is to discover what Ambrose Worrall means by "creating the conditions." Perhaps Dr. Daniel Benor, an advisor to the British government on Complementary Medicine, who has studied healers for several decades, can throw some light on this. He reports that an article on experiments in the relief of pain was published in the Journal of the Society for Psychical Research as long ago as 1946. In the article, Frederick Knowles, a healer who, to gain a deeper understanding of his own practice, studied both healing in India and Western medicine, states that an important factor in what he calls psychic healing is the healer's mental concentration upon the process of recovery that he wishes to promote. He found that his results depended very largely on the amount of concentrated effort of thought that he put into the treatment. He says, "In a few whom I treated many times and where this treatment produced complete but only temporary relief from severe pain . . . I had the opportunity to omit this mental concentration upon occasion, behaving otherwise outwardly in my usual manner during the treatment. . . . After such a failed treatment, I then applied the concentration process and relief occurred as rapidly as usual."[8] Clearly, Knowles believed that the healer must bring a strong intentionality of his own to bear, an intensely focused willing forward of the healing process. This seems a perfect example of what it is, including the capacity to care and to intend, that shows that we are Beings rather than merely material machines. Note, too, that Knowles had the experience of allowing himself to lose intention, with the result of failing to

heal, and the experience of bringing back the power by renewed concentration upon his purpose. Clearly, his own intention was necessary if the healing was to work.

Further questions immediately arise: Is human intentionality all that is required, or is there a higher agent at work in all successful healings? How does healing intentionality work? Can we increase our ability to use it? What is it that healers are describing when they talk about the energy becoming available to the healer through "tuning her personal energy field to a harmonious relationship with the universal field of energy," as Olga Worrall puts it, so that she acts as a conductor between the universal field of energy and the patient?

In attempting an answer we need first to decide, at least roughly, what we believe we should mean when we refer to a process of *healing.* Then our observations will act as a test of that hypothesis, confirming or denying it. What seems, from the observations, to be essentially *one* process of restoring well-being, that is, wholeness, operates nonetheless in a range of ways reflecting the terminologies of different traditions of practice. Thus we have the terms *energy healing, psychic healing,* and *spiritual healing,* but, doubtless because one central process appears to be present, these have become more or less interchangeable. Daniel Benor defines *spiritual* healing as "the systematic, purposeful intervention by one or more persons aiming to help another living being (person, plant, or animal) by means of *focused intention* . . . and without the use of conventional energetic, mechanical or chemical interventions."[9] The last part of the definition is particularly important.

Consciousness and Energy Fields

The study of energy fields, both human and universal, is an exciting new development in our understanding of what happens during the healing process, and it has become an important concern of consciousness studies. Although this research began decades ago with the study of brainwaves (see chapter 3) and altered states of consciousness during meditation, there seems to have been a long interval when there was a lack of interest in what present-day consciousness researcher Marilyn Schlitz calls our "interiority."[10] She states that it is a peculiarity of modern science that it allows some kinds of metaphors and disallows others. For example, she says, it has become acceptable to use more holistic and nonquantifiable metaphors such as *organism, personality, ecological community,* or even *universe,* but it is taboo to use non-sensory "metaphors of mind" that tap into images and experiences familiar from our own inner awareness. It is not yet acceptable to assert that if distant intentionality (as in distant healing) were empirically proved it might indicate the involvement of a supraindividual, nonphysical mind, which would in turn suggest that *a whole system* was evolving, and that the mind at work in the situation might be part of "another order of reality." Yet this dualistic interpretation is clearly compatible with the testimony of Christopher Bache and the Worralls. But, Schlitz says, even this antagonism is now changing. There is now great interest among frontier scientists in the nature of "embodiment," in the question of how our consciousness, as expressed through the layers of the subtle body, the aura or field of energy, determines our reality.

Emerging from its focus on the physical world of Newtonian physics, the present scientific view of reality, underpinned by relativity theory and (more relevant for us) field theory and quantum theory, supports the idea that we are composed of energy fields, and presents a view of the universe as a single entity in which all things are interconnected. We are living within Indra's Net. Professor Ervin Laszlo explains this view in detail in *Science and the Akashic Field,* in which he observes that in the world of mainstream science a new concept is emerging, rooted in the rediscovery of ancient tradition's Akashic field in the "new" notion of what he calls the "vacuum-based holofield."[11] The expectation is that this field is probably one and the same as the quantum vacuum, which is itself perhaps one and the same as the scalar and vector potential fields, perhaps also the medium of the interconnectedness confirmed by Aspect, but perhaps an even more fundamental substrate of the Whole. The frontier of science is always a place of uncertainty, always the borderland between ourselves and our ignorance.

According to the A-field concept, the universe is a highly integrated, interconnected, and coherent system, much like a living organism. On reading this we immediately make a mental connection across Indra's Net to the principle so often mentioned in this book: "As above, so below." Returning to today's scientific metaphors we see that the pervasive feature is "information,"

not in its everyday sense but something more substantial and causal that in-forms or "prepatterns," then actively generates and conserves, reality itself, and is present within reality as all-pervading pattern. The notion is not new, for something much akin to it underlies Plato's, Aristotle's, and the Hermetic and Neo-Platonic views of the *leveled* structure of reality's Whole. There is a "perennial intuition" in many traditional cosmologies and systems of metaphysics of a meta-world of timeless ever-presence containing the familiar world of space and time. The ancients knew that space is not empty; it is the origin and memory of all things that exist and have ever existed, but they came to this knowledge through personal insight and mystical experience. As Laszlo puts it, "The current rediscovery of the Akashic field reinforces qualitative human experience with quantitative data generated by science's experimental method. . . . [A]s sustained research deepens and specifies the theory of the A-field . . . this will profoundly change our concept of ourselves and of the world itself."[12] In our own view, the subtle body extends, as if itself a "field," into the ākāśa, which itself extends without limit, pervading everything. This effectively expands the subtle body far beyond the "immortal soul" as traditionally conceived.*

Professor Laszlo believes that as people learn to work with the A-field, ways that as yet are undefinable and only vaguely imaginable will be discovered to beam active and effective information from one place to another, instantly and without the expenditure of physical energy. He believes that in the future we may learn to teleport not just the *quantum states* of atoms and molecules but, eventually, even living cells themselves, organs, and the elements of consciousness.[13] We think the first stage of this is already happening, for in spiritual healing, distant healing, and prayer-for-healing, which seem to be the same transcending and fundamental process, intentionality as motive "force" seems to influence the quantum states, and thereby the chemical-level interrelations between them, of atoms, molecules, and whole cells. In what else would healing consist at the level at

---

*To deal with the speculative physics in detail would expand this already quite large book, so we have not done so. Those who would like to study the matter further should read Fritjof Capra's *The Tao of Physics,* and Laszlo's *Science and the Akashic Field,* among many other works, some of which are listed in the bibliography.

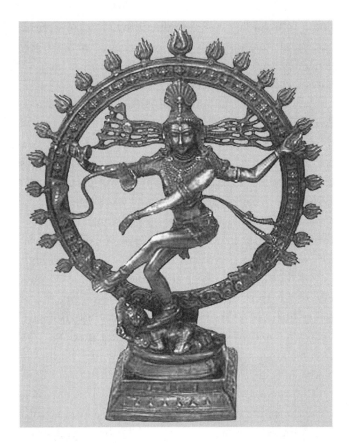

Fig. 16.1. Siva in his dynamic form as Nataraj, Lord of the Cosmic Dance, conveys to Hindus the same idea of ākāśa as quantum field theory does to the physicist. Both are intuitions of reality that, while amenable to imagination, are difficult to express verbally due to the limitations of language and linear-logical thought. (Photo of art from the author's personal collection.)

which the need for healing had been perceived, namely that of the biological body? If distant healing happens, at least the first stage of the process of which Laszlo speaks is already occurring.

Healers have known how to influence the conscious awareness-of-self and the physical bodies of others for centuries. What has not been known until recently—until the quantum theory dawned and Alain Aspect, Akira Tonomura, and others made empirical tests of entanglement and potential fields, and yet other research was done, which Professor Laszlo reports in some detail in his book—is *how* it happens. We now begin to understand at a level at which, before, we could only believe, imagine, and fantasize. Alchemy and its sprawling, floundering fantasy were, at one time, all we had, but these human functions, on their own, are not now felt to be sufficient. We ask for intelligible explanation of

the kind we call "scientific." Now, spiritual aliveness, coupled with science, will make much greater progress toward truth.

One of the world's leading specialists in the structure of matter, Dr. William Tiller, presents a model of the subtle body from a scientific perspective.[14] We remind the reader, before proceeding, that scientific models are tentative, involving postulated entities and a hypothesis, as yet unproven, to explain them and their relations, the whole body of conjecture capable of, and eventually actually subjected to, rigorous testing, as we were at great pains to explain in chapter 15.

Tiller postulates *subtle* levels of substance existing in the body, each of which emits radiation in much the same manner as *physical* substance generates electromagnetic radiation. He explains that just as the physical body has a radiation field—which, like all fields, extends throughout space and is the means of *electromagnetic* interaction with other particles or waves, whether singly or as aggregates, and which therefore acts, within its own range and type of radiation, like the familiar radio or television antenna—so the etheric body and the even more subtle bodies will each have their own characteristic radiation field, functioning similarly as a receiving and transmitting antenna system. Each of these postulated antenna systems is expected to show effects at the physical level that, just as in Tonomura's experiment, are transmitted to and from the underlying potential field (thought to be the A-field itself) and, via that potential field, from the other subtle-body fields of all the other types. Tiller believes each field is sensitive to radiations from all the other fields, and therefore carries the effects of changes from one field to another. All produce change in the fields of ordinary everyday physics, the Heideggerian world-about, which we sense directly in the body and via the body's external sense organs. To detect the many subtle fields now postulated, sophisticated equipment will be needed (for reasons analogous to those given regarding Tonomura's experiment). However, if the quest is successful fields beyond the senses of our bodies and beyond our conscious knowledge will become known to us, just as quantum interconnection and an underlying field of standing waves have been confirmed by Tonomura.

Our minds, containing these new awarenesses, albeit indirectly, will change accordingly, and become more powerful by their enhanced knowledge. In this way, Indra's Net, the "universal communicator," will show itself not only to range across the space and time of our *sensible* (visible) world, but to communicate between invisible fields existing at different depths of the occult parts of reality, so enlarging the *intelligible* world, the world we cannot see, in any sense, but can know about. The Vedic Axis might, then, seem to arise from even deeper, invisible roots of the whole physical cosmos, "up" through the physical earth, the physical body, with its own interior levels, and up toward the gods, perhaps "higher" than even the higher chakras above our heads are intuited to do. If science can demonstrate the reality of such fields, the totally occult would have entered the intelligible, if not yet the sensible, and the human mind would expand to encompass "perspectives" unimaginable only a few decades in the past. This schema, if confirmed, would be ground for a hylic pluralistic understanding of our Being-in-the-*world-as-such* and our Being-in-*physical-bodies*-in-the-world that is deeper, or higher, than anything imagined by the ancients.

If Tiller is right, just as in what might be called everyday-world (gross-matter) physics every particle has a surrounding radiation field, so an auric sheath or *kośa* will be present as a field of radiation around each of the subtle bodies that constitute the complete human. Tiller goes on to say that what this implies is that if we have materials that interact with or resonate with a specific level of *subtle* substance, and if one or more of these substances is placed in the appropriate auric sheath, a response to this disturbance of the particular standing wave field will manifest both in that subtle body and also in the physical body. "If this response can be detected," he believes, "it would make a useful diagnostic tool."[15] No doubt much work has to be done before the hypothesis can be accepted as theory.

So we have, now, at least a possible explanation of how healers scan another person's aura, sensing changes in its temperature and density. In this way, impossible to describe since it is the healer's inward personal experience, she or he "reads" the patient's emotional and mental states. But the question posed earlier remains. What makes it possible for the healer to introduce changes into these patterns of emanations? What changes go on within the healer's energy field that makes it possible to "send" intentions, that is, directives to heal the other

person's body? *How* does the *mind*ful, focused intention of healing create change in the other's *physical* body? Or, to put it another way, how, as a matter of science, is the gap bridged between the healer's intention and the patient's belief on the one hand, and the patient's biochemistry on the other?

Information Molecules

We do not have the whole answer, but we may already have the major component of the *physical* part of the answer. Dr. Candace Pert's research on the role of neuropeptides in the immune system led to her discovery of endorphins (endogenous morphines), the body's natural painkillers, popularly known as the "feel-good hormones." She realized that "Your subconscious mind is really your body. Peptides are the biochemical correlate of emotion. . . . They provide our body's most basic communication network. . . . This means that emotional *memory* is stored throughout the body . . . and you can access emotional memory anywhere in the network."[16] Pert discovered that the body-mind uses a network of *information molecules* to control our health and physiology. These are small proteins or components of proteins, and they react with other proteins in the body, with a wide range of effects. They turn genes on or off, and they correlate *causally* with changes in our moods.

Pert's view is that emotions, from anger to fear, sadness, joy, contentment, courage, pleasure, pain, awe, and bliss, *consist in* a wide range of states of body chemistry, and therefore, since we *feel* these states, the body chemistry *is* our subconscious mind. As all alternative practitioners know, emotional residues are indeed among the most potent causes of dis-ease, and Pert confirms what many healers have long believed, that "Repressed emotions and memories might actually be stored in receptors throughout the body."[17]

Biochemistry is very complex and we can illustrate it only in principle. The general pattern of the reactions Pert discovered is that a smaller molecule, such as a peptide, approaches the usually larger receptor protein molecule and attaches itself, so changing the chemical reactions of the receptor protein (see plate 33). This attachment affects metabolism in some way, sometimes altering emotions fairly directly, sometimes ensuring that other reactions, whether sensed or not, proceed as they should. This is, of course, the chemical level of bodily illness, but the root cause level may be emotional, an effect of an experience.* Fortunately, the causal route can often be reversed, not least by positive thoughts and healing intention.

Sometimes the wrong molecule gets attached. Stress, for example, might cause a change in the acidity of the surrounding fluid and a molecule that will have a damaging effect might then attach itself at a relevant site more readily than the health-conserving correct molecule, perhaps causing a more-or-less permanent deterioration. Alternatively, a foreign molecule, finding its way into the body, might be similar enough to the correct molecule to attach itself, excluding the correct molecule. We classify such invaders and usurpers as "toxins." They disrupt the correct progress of body chemistry, with greater or lesser damaging effect. Viruses also can invade and attach themselves in this way if they mimic the proper molecule. Sometimes such wrong attachments become permanent. However, this description at the chemical level of molecular combination is not the whole story and a physical explanation involving energy fields may be more closely analogous to actual events in the physical body, whether brought about by intentionality or not. Plate 33 illustrates both levels of description.

Beyond Biochemistry

Pert's work provides, as we said, the physical and chemical part of the description, but, again, our main question concerned conscious intentionality, and remains unanswered. Since body chemistry controls feelings, might we not change our moods by mindful control of those body chemicals, as an act of intentional self-healing? Is Pert's biochemistry (whether described at chemical level or field level) reversible by human will? If, as we think, "mind" is in some sense "higher" than body, can we not apply the principle "As above, so below" and impose beneficial change upon the body by top-down causation originating in the will? Is there any evidence for the existence and living operation of a mind that is not the victim of body chemistry, but may even be master of it? It might be expected that since the energy-field description of the processes is more fundamentally correct than the chemical one, this might indeed be the case. Human will, not to mention the evidently superhuman Will, attested by the Worralls and many others, that operates in healings, might, perhaps, be perceived as closer to, and therefore more influential upon, physical fields than upon molecules of "gross chemical matter."

Pert herself is not as extreme a physicalist as our presentation of her basic ideas may have made her appear. She acknowledges the human capacity for willed action, for she says that even the simple act of breathing deeply, as recommended in yoga and meditation, alters the flow of peptides. "There's a wealth of data showing that changes in the rate and depth of breathing produce changes in the kind of peptides that are released from the brain stem."[18] We all believe we can breathe more deeply simply by choosing to do so. This requires a choice-making self, an intentional self, which is not the helpless puppet of biochemistry. Mind and body are clearly closely connected, and an unhealthy body can certainly impair the working of the mind, but other areas of science show that the energy fields, far more important than they were once thought to be, may be an arena of mindful control. The crucial factor, we suggest, is the reality of *choice*. To choose, or to be unable to choose—that is the question. Notwithstanding the skepticism of many biologists, even today, and many philosophers, our *experience* is of a *real* (if finite) capacity for choice.

The British biologist David Hamilton extends the realm of the psychosomatic even further than Pert, and, we think correctly, draws attention to human choice, will, and intentionality in doing so.[19] He brings us back to the ancient question of the independence of mind from body. He believes that our beliefs and intentions can actually create matter. He says that "intentions can influence the creation process in two ways . . . they produce neuropeptides which circulate around the body and fit into receptors where they bring about changes including switching genes on and off," but, at a deeper level, they also influence the point at which consciousness condenses into subatomic particles. Note the word *condense*, for this recenters his position, drawing it back from what might seem an extreme dualism. While asserting the large extent of mind's independence from body, he shows that he also accepts a balancing view reminiscent of Pauli's and of others that mind and matter are,

---

*Conversely, as we know, some chemicals, when taken into the body, produce certain feelings without any of the usual causes of such feelings being present in the life of the person. Among these are hallucinogenic drugs, so named precisely because they induce feelings that are not grounded in our normal reality.

like matter and energy, ultimately intermutable. He thus reaches toward all those who believe there is a degree of consciousness in the "grossest" matter.

This is a more important point, here in this chapter as well as throughout this book, than might at first appear, for our chapter title lays stress on consciousness, not on chemistry, on subtlety, not on mundane physics, and the whole book is about Holism in the broadest sense we can give it at this epoch in the history of our Being-in-the-world. We believe the seemingly opposed views of those who stress the physics and chemistry of the body-mind and those who stress the freedom of human will are ultimately only true-but-partial *perspectives* upon the great Wholeness that is the All, and those perspectives are therefore ultimately compatible. Argument has long raged between dualists and monists, but it dissolves into the realization that dualisms are simply bottom-up interpretations, monisms top-down views. Each of these, and many other interpretations, simply need to broaden a little for their compatibility and mutual necessity, indeed, their *interdependency of being,* to show.

Accordingly, we see Hamilton's view within this global compass. He continues, "your intentions influence the creation process, sending pictures to the place and moment when vibrations become particles and so influence the nature of the particles . . . the more you visualize new healthy cells, the more new healthy cells are created."[20] His idea follows from the physicists' belief that the whole of space is filled with an entity they have called the quantum vacuum. It is indeed a vacuum in that there is no everyday-world matter in it, but it is not empty. The quantum vacuum is *potential* being, the source of all the matter in our world. Particles pop into the universe of our being from the quantum vacuum, and return there, seemingly spontaneously. Hamilton is telling us that we can imagine, and so achieve, the reversal of damaging changes in our bodies by the influence of conscious will over what comes to us across the interface between the quantum vacuum and our world.

The concept of the Void, the vacuum, is not new, of course. We find this same idea of continual creation, dissolution, and re-creation of entities in Hinduism. Faced with our perceivable, *sensible,* world, we humans interpret it in the manner inherent within us, and we see facing us the kind of world we are constituted to see. Our Being *is* being-in-*that*-world. As we develop our perceivable world, using imagination and foresight and bringing entities to realization, we naturally produce a world about us that we understand, for we could produce no other. This is the whole project of science. Physicist Fritjof Capra draws attention to the symbolism of Nataraj, Siva in his aspect of Lord of the Dance (see fig. 16.1), and to a correspondence between the creative-destructive Dance of Siva and the contemporary scientific image of the dance of quantum particles out of and back into the vacuum.[21] The Void, the quantum vacuum, is misnamed, being full, but we misnamed it because, while it is a *necessary, inferable* postulate, it is entirely beyond the view of our senses, and therefore at first seemed empty. The inferred Void itself is, for us, unobservable, nonmeasurable, nonmaterial in our sense of that word, yet seething with minute activity and, its activity notwithstanding, it is also timeless, the womb of the world in which we have our Being, the world of measure, of matter, of processes of change (which is what time is, of course), and of the limiting fictions we call "space" and "time."

Distant Intentionality

Some of our earlier discussion foreshadowed the conclusion that since *we* have consciousness in some degree, it is not unlikely that consciousness—a greater consciousness than ours, of course—is everywhere. The question arising, therefore, is whether we have *evidence* for the anticipated nonphysical, *extra*physical, *pre*physical component or process or even *entity* at work in our world. Telepathy is suggestive, but difficult to prove convincingly, so perhaps does not provide sufficiently strong evidence taken on its own. Distant healing, on the other hand, if demonstrated sufficiently often, would convince us that intentions are effectual at distances from the intender that preclude the normal action of any of the four acknowledged physical forces, which, as we have mentioned earlier, reduce in strength with distance.

The next step, then, must be to test for evidence via experiment. Experiments already performed range widely from attempts to increase or inhibit the growth of fungus cultures by "intention-at-a-distance" to the search for a correlation of positive mental intent with physiological effect in human "targets" distant from the intender. Recent studies, which include investigations of consciousness, our present topic, support the belief that minds can interact through telepathy and remote viewing, a method of obtaining information about distant places and objects of which a strong instance was described in chapter 15. We shall investigate these and related matters further.

However, before proceeding, we must make a short, but very important, detour. Clearly, taking the rational probability that there is a greater consciousness and the doubt as to the efficacy of distance-limited forces together with the experiential fact of our own consciousness and will, we are entitled to posit a Great Being hidden from us behind the visible scenery of our world-about. The question then arising is whether the Void is *itself,* in some sense, just such a Living Being, greater by far than us. Equally clearly, we cannot address such a question, let alone answer it, but to leave it unmentioned would be a gross mistake, even a supreme insolence toward any such Being. We recognize ourselves as Beings; how much more must we recognize the probability that there exists a far greater Being. As we said in chapter 15, even our own beingness, as such, is unobservable, so it can hardly be objected that no Great Being is observable. Our senses and our science are limited, and even within our familiar world-about, we do not see the forest *as such, or as if from outside it,* when surrounded by the trees. However, since nothing more can be said here on this question, no matter that it is crucially relevant to everything, we return to the mundane level and argue upward from there.

Among the four forces of mundane physics the only contender for acceptance as the means of healing is electromagnetic transmission from the human brain via the healer's hand, but this field reaches no more than an inch or two from the hand before attenuating to a very low density and becoming totally swamped by other electromagnetic waves. So something more is at work, at the very least an interconnection of some other kind, between the healer's mind and the patient's body. Quantum interconnectedness, demonstrated by Alain Aspect, will not *fully* explain the success of the *targeted* intention, which distant healing of a *particular person* requires us to postulate. What any hypothesis would require, whether grounded in current physics or not, would be a new kind of "ether," a background Great Consciousness, perhaps, which (or Who) transmits the intention, or the intended effect *itself,* to the *chosen* recipient. These postulated essences and communication channels might, of course, be *meta*physical (we have tentatively used the word "spiritual" elsewhere), rather than *extended*-physical, in which case they could not be detected by physical means. But our minds can imagine them, and *indirect* physical evidence of their presence might be gleaned. They may be not mere postulates but *necessary* postulates.

We mentioned experiments. Dr. Larry Dossey has made a special study of these experiments, and finds that they support the belief that minds can interact through telepathy and remote viewing to influence the well-being of humans suffering a broad range of physical, emotional, and mental conditions.[22] Among the studies that Dr. Dossey reviewed, the most relevant to the questions of distant intentionality (and also to prayer) in healing seem to be experiments conducted by William Braud and Marilyn Schlitz, two of the foremost researchers in the field of intentionality, healing, and consciousness. In the reports of a group of 13 experiments with 62 people attempting to influence 271 distant subjects, Dossey found evidence for the following conclusions:

1. The distant effects of mental imagery compare favorably with the magnitude of effects of an individual's own thoughts, feelings, and emotions on his or her own physiology.
2. The ability to use positive imagery to achieve distant effects is apparently widespread in the human population.
3. These effects can occur at distances up to sixty-five feet (twenty meters). (Greater distances were not tested in these experiments.)
4. Subjects with a need to be influenced by positive mental intent, that is, those for whom the influence would be beneficial, seem more susceptible than others.
5. The distant effects of intentionality can occur without the recipients' knowledge of the time of the transmission of healing thoughts to them.
6. None of the participants used the effect to engender harm.
7. Subjects appear to be able to prevent the effect if it is unwanted.[23]

Daniel Benor noted that in nearly 200 studies that he reviewed "distance, *even thousands of miles,* doesn't appear to limit the effects of healing."[24] Given that the four *physical* forces diminish with distance, *distant* healing cannot be performed by any of the four physical forces acting normally and unaided. The data therefore confirm the need to postulate a force the full nature of which we do not yet know.

This unknown force would have to be either a function of the vacuum as it allows particles into being, ensuring that the right particles arise at the right places for healing to occur—Tiller, Dibble, and Kohane suggest this—or a completely separate force, higher still (or more fundamental still) than the vacuum. Perhaps, as suggested, a paragraph or two ago, this force is personal, since some research supports belief that prayer, an intentional address to a Person, is effective in healing.

If our human, limited intentionality is effectual in healing *at any distance,* it seems that the part played by our intention must be to set up conditions in the physical world in which a "higher" force, will, or consciousness performs the healing. We already have some corroboration for this hypothesis, for is not this what Knowles, the Worralls, and Benor concluded was happening in healing? That it happens at a distance simply confirms the additional contention that it cannot be the result of the currently known *physical*-world forces *alone.* If we generalize our expectation of what follows from this to all experience, not just healing experience, we shall postulate that, by means that are as yet uncertain, *consciousness in a human being does have available to it connections as both transmitter and receiver to other human beings (and probably to animals and plants, and perhaps even to stones), via quantum interconnection in the physical world and by another means as yet beyond analysis and description.*

This seems to be the kind of total interconnectedness and oneness of Being that allows a meditator to perceive by experience the truth of the claim "Tat twam asi." We postulate such All-Being (known, as we have seen, in Indic thought, as Brahman) because we begin to see evidence in the physical *world-of-our-everyday-mode-of-Being* (a quasi-Heideggerian concept) both of a connection via that physical world-about and of *another* via a "higher" connectedness. Note from our phrasing that our own part in this scenario could have nothing of the

miraculous in it. We merely cooperate with something higher that, for the very reason that it is higher and far more capable, might properly be thought a worker of miracles. This is the "picture" that seems to fit, and it is a dualism that refuses to be denied. It also fits what we believe to be the most rational picture of ourselves. We, as Beings, are ourselves a part of the same world in which healing takes place. We, down here, walking the earth, are interconnected, not visibly or at our everyday level, but via our own invisible consciousness. This is a picture of "layers" of being, and a modern version of "As above, so below," the perennial philosophy, its validity corroborated, not denied, by today's science; and it is the case because we humans are what we humans are: limited, but with the relatively great imaginative and conceptual power to picture precisely *this* structure because our living-Beingness is "elsewhere" but our physical presence is "here." We see the physical world as if from outside it (and are able to *imagine ourselves having powers beyond its limits*) for the Seer *is* outside it.

As we have seen, the idea of the connectedness of all entities is present in the myths of many cultures. In chapter 11 we described the myth of Indra's Net, in which each jewel in the net reflects all the others. This thought experiment—for that, in another milieu, is what it would be called—rightly scorns philosophical criticism, for it is a concept of the imagination, flying free of any obligation to justify itself apart from the question of whether it rings true as an intuition about reality. Nonetheless it is rational in its own way. We know perfectly well what is being represented, and no representation, being merely that, merely a kind of aesthetically experienced mnemonic, has the duty to equal what it represents or to prove *itself* a real entity, or to show rigorous logic. It merely *refers to and illustrates* a greater real entity. Gebser's magical consciousness and its creative possibilities are still available to some of us in this era of the common person's materialistic torpor and the philosopher's left-brained intellectual and verbal criticism, which will forever miss the whole-brained mark.

Do we have evidence, down here in the physical world, of the interconnectedness of which we speak? Some healers believe that the very fact of distant healing is itself evidence of a distance*less* spiritual "space." Telepathy, clairvoyance, and clairaudience also seem to appear out-from (Greek εκ) the same source. The quantum physicists believe that, despite the undeniable falling off of the four forces with distance, even the physical world, considered alone, is interconnected through and through in some way that is still mysterious. A world of potential underlies what we call the real world. We gave some space to this in chapter 15. Perhaps distant healing occurs through such an interconnectedness, by an "entanglement" brought about not by the merely automatic physical-world process of generating "spin pairs" of particles (which is happening all the time whether we intervene or not) but by intentionality or prayer, by an intervention of *mind per se* without *any physical* means. It would take place either as an instance of quantum interconnectedness, via the quantum vacuum, or by a distanceless "space" entirely outside the physical world, beyond even the "zero point field," as the vacuum is often now termed. It is possible that discoveries in quantum physics have vindicated some earlier Eastern claims to "magical powers," the siddhis, the different accounts of which demonstrate the basic unity of human experience and our interconnectedness with "all that is." But perhaps consciousness *itself* is in some valid sense that spaceless space, experienced as the natural outcome of meditation's attempt to connect with the beyond. The very difficult research into such matters has only just begun.

Prayer as an Act of Consciousness

Benor, Dossey, Braud, and Schlitz have been studying the role of intention, prayer, and meditation for several decades. For millennia many have held that consciousness is itself an efficacious "force" and that it is by nature *un*physical, that is *un*spatial and *un*timely. From these grounds Dossey argues that since prayer is an *act of consciousness,* and therefore does not originate in the physical world, the manner of its operation must also be nonphysical, and that, being nonphysical, it will also be nonlocal, not limited by the space in which we have our embodied Being-in-the-world.[25] The next question for science would therefore be: Is there evidence that consciousness—the prayerful *intender itself*—does *not* have its being in our everyday world of distance and time-lapse, but is *in and of itself* already in an "elsewhere that is not *any*where," and that does not "suffer" from

distance? This, of course, is a modern formulation of an ancient question, that of whether such postulated entities as mind are material or nonmaterial. Most cultures have wavered between the view that mind, spirit, soul, and other entities are matter, but of a very "fine" or "subtle" kind, and the view that one of them, at least, is something radically different.

We shall first have to glance back at physics, *and be sure we understand it,* before we can go forward in search of the answer. For the layperson trying for the first time to grasp the idea accurately, the linguistic and conceptual problems are almost insuperable, for notions based on our everyday experience are violated at every step while the explanation *must* use familiar words, and must introduce one at a time concepts that in reality are linked and simultaneous.

Let us first be clear what we are looking for. We are looking for a *difference* between *our* way of being and the way of being of the *physical world,* the way the physical world *works*. If we can find no such difference we might be merely parts of the physical world, and probably automatons, our consciousness a delusion or, at most, a mere byproduct of our physical constitution. You will recall that we gave some space to this question in chapter 15.

What, then, is the character of the physical world? The physical world is *discontinuous*. It is here one moment, gone the next, and back again, slightly changed, a moment later still. It changes by tiny steps, by what we term "quantum jumps," quantum jump after quantum jump after quantum jump, quadrillions of extremely tiny jumps in every second, and the whole physical world is perpetually changing in this way. There is no intermediate stage within each quantum jump, no smooth transition from one state to the next. A particle is in one quantum state or another. There is no state between. The physical universe is therefore discontinuous, changing by a procession of quite distinct states or moments, an infinite sequence of *discrete* "nows."

We are now ready for the question posed earlier. It is a question for science, not for philosophy, for empirical investigation, not for armchair semantics or analytical logic. Nor is it a question of language. Here it is again: Is there evidence that the conscious prayerful *intender* does *not* have its being in our everyday world of distance and time-lapse, but is *in and of itself* of a truly different

Fig. 16.2. This diagram attempts to illustrate two notions, the quantum physicist's view of the passage of "time"—the physical universe evolving by a perpetual series of quite distinct states, a succession of discrete, disconnected, unmerged "nows," not as a continuous flow—and the relationship between our conscious selves and the cosmos.

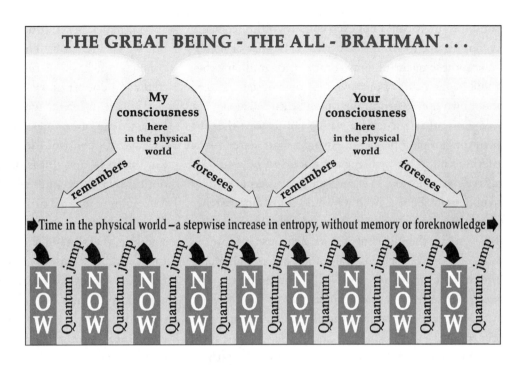

nature, and therefore already *in* an "elsewhere that is not *any*where," and that does not "suffer" from distance?

Our first step in answering it is to ask a further question. How could any part of a system such as we have described, all of which is perpetually changing, quantum jump by quantum jump, remember any past state of the whole system, any past state of *itself*? It is at every quantum step no longer what it was, and it departs further and further from any state from which (hypothetically!) we might start to survey it. If it set some part of itself aside for the purpose of being the memory of the whole it would, in that very act, already have failed on every count. The part set aside would have to record its own setting aside, as well as everything else, yet the smaller cannot fully record the greater. Furthermore, at every change some part of any (hypothetical!) *record of* change would be lost. Even if the whole system were to return to a state identical with some past state it would, as we conceive matters, still not be the selfsame self that it had been before. You cannot step into the same river twice, even though the hydrological cycle will bring back the same water molecules time and time again. Our consciousness would protest that a circular sequence of changes had occurred that meant that even though the system showed itself to be in the same state as it had once been it was not in reality the same. How would we know this? By *our* having *remembered* at least some of

the former states, something the system itself could not record, being too small. *It* has no memory of itself, yet *we* remember it as it was. The system itself could not even *know* that it had returned to a past state. We need not argue this exhaustively, for the conclusion is already clear. Here, we suggest, is the main clue, and we present it as another question. How can our consciousness alert us to the limitations of a physical system if our consciousness is itself even *a part of* that physical system? The Seer is outside the seen.

Any entity who can raise such objections as these, objections grounded in psychological self-awareness (which includes memory, of course), has, by that act alone, already proved itself different from the physical. This is what we set out to prove. Philosophers might raise objections, but empirical science acknowledges the probability that our argument parallels the facts.

A little more can be said, to fill out the picture. There is no psychology of chairs and tables, or even of the most complex machines. We, by contrast, are Beings with a consciousness that remembers, who can protest that the restoration of a past state of a physical system does not genuinely prove either the self-identity or the continuity-of-being of that system but only of our own as rememberers. We have even discovered that it processes by discrete states separated by quantum jumps. If we were, in our inmost essence, just parts of that quantum-stepping world, we surely could not even conceive of *real* continuity, nor be able to sense whether those lacunae of nonexistence, those quantum jumps, took place at all, for they would be moments of our own nonconsciousness, indeed of our own nonexistence. We would be carried along, not even aware that our nature was to fail to see either the quantum-jumping process itself or its past states, or its intermittency. Our own gaps of nonexistence would be gaps of consciousness, so even a lacuna of a century would be undetectable for us, and we would think our existence continuous. Here, some philosophers would claim that this is in fact the case. But if it were the case how would we have learned of the physical world's quantum-jumping intermittency? We *are* aware of its intermittency, and we *feel* ourselves to be continuous, *not* to have lost our memory on account of the quadrillions of quantum gaps occurring at every tick of the clock. The scientific view, not that of some philosophers, seems more likely to be correct: the Seer, whether a fine matter Being or a spiritual Being, is not of the same essence as the seen.

We do not claim that our argument is absolutely infallible. It relies greatly on our own psychology. But is that not one of the main points in its favor? We are Beings, while tables and chairs are not. The argument *may* be circular, but if so it is *existentially* circular (like the anthropic principle) rather than *logically* unreliable because *logically* circular. We think the argument is probably valid, and will in due time be recognized as empirical fact.

Let us go over it, briefly, once more, and move on. A self-contained system, whether a strange loop or not, cannot make a static, permanent, record of itself. Gödel's theorems, crucial to the view we reached at the end of chapter 15, help us here too. Something that is outside a system is needed to remember the past or to foresee the future of that system. We are outside the physical system of our world-about in just this way, and we observe, remember, and predict the changes in that system. We are in the (physical) world, but not of it. We live and move and have our very Being elsewhere. The physical world *in itself* has neither knowledge nor memory *of itself*. It might even be defined as that base level of reality that is entirely *without* such consciousness as we show. When we edit a document on the computer without first making a copy, and then save the changed version, the original is absolutely lost. The computer itself

cannot remember it. It no longer exists in the computer, but we can recall it. The physical universe is like the computer. It has a present state, but it has lost its past states and doesn't know its future states.

We are different. We remember, and, in principle at least, we can often foresee the future with some reliability. We, our conscious selves, are not part of the physical universe—and this is shown to us (though we rarely notice) by the fact that we have memory and foresight. The point we are making here is that even though memory and consciousness, with their recollection and understanding, their foresight and their intention, operate "in" the world, *they are themselves nonspatial and nontemporal*. They are of a different nature, in a different category. They cannot be "in" the world in the same sense that tables and chairs and machines are "in" the world. Here, if in few other places, Gilbert Ryle would be right, though we note now, as we did before, that *this* category-difference is real, and the consequence is precisely what he set out to scorn, a chasmic *real* duality between what von Franz denoted as "spirit" and "matter."

We *are* the Ghost in the Machine, and (returning to matters arising earlier in this chapter) if consciousness itself, and the prayer that consciousness makes, are not of the *same* essence as the Great Being, who, rationally believed to have at least equal personness to ourselves, must be postulated as the spiritual Healer, the great maker of wholeness, then they are at least a step toward that higher way of Being, a step above the physical world. No wonder, then, that *our* intentionality, above the automatic quantum-jumping of the physical, sometimes succeeds in invoking a spiritual power that performs healing, and does so at huge terrestrial distances without loss of effect. Even the rather different experience of the person who suffered disturbance at the time his brother died, two hundred miles away, which we described in detail in chapter 15, is strongly suggestive of the real existence of such a structure behind the scenes of the everyday physical world.

In arguing for his view, Dossey takes the more cautious path, mentioned earlier, of assuming that in distant healing consciousness uses the interconnectedness of the physical world now established by Alain Aspect and his team. Dossey says, "Suggestions that consciousness is spatiotemporally extended are not new within science. . . . Nonlocal events have repeatedly been demonstrated experimentally within quantum physics, our most accurate science, for over two decades. . . . While the philosophical ramifications of quantum nonlocality are unclear, the experimental findings appear to be no longer in doubt."[26] This is a direct reference to Aspect's Paris experiment, and others of its type, of course, and Dossey is implying, though not proving, that Aspect's result suggests the possibility that what we have described is correct. We agree, while acknowledging that more research must be done. But Dossey goes further. He remarks that most of us are still bound by the idea that intentionality and prayer have to be directed somewhere, but points out that "If healing works nonlocally, there is no necessity for intentions, thoughts and prayers to be 'sent' anywhere because they are 'already there.'"[27] This seems closer to the view we have ourselves put forward, that consciousness functions outside the physical world, so, again, we agree even more strongly.

If correct, this view removes our considerations from the physical realm of space-time altogether: distance has been eliminated entirely and directionality has been superseded by *placelessness*. Everything is serene Being, even interdependency of being somehow now united into simple *Being*. Intentionality remains, in some sense, but there is now a question as to whose intentionality it is that remains. Nothing "reaches out," indeed there is no "out," or even "up" to reach out to. For Being at this level all is present-at-hand. Convolvement within the all-encompassing *Strange Loop of the Great Being's Being-in-the-greater-world-of-the-All* is total. Doubtless, this spiritual world is, in metaphorical senses, "higher" than the physical world, but it is not anywhere, or, at least, not anywhere in or relative to our physical world. It is a "space" of its own that is "beyond" (but not divorced from) our space. It may *contain* our space, yet be so different in its unlimitedness that it cannot be said to be in the same place as our space. It may also be beyond the quantum vacuum, full though that vacuum is of all potential for the spatiotemporal kind of existence that we experience in the world.

So perhaps we can say that there *is* a *limit* to the hybrid world of "As above, so below" or "As in the mind, so in the body," while *full* spirituality is *beyond* that, and not limited at all. The world of "As above, so below" is *our* world, yet a *part* of us, our conscious intending self, is *not* in the physical world, but in the world above, the

world of mind. This view does not devalue our bodies, as Descartes did, nor our consciousness, as the current biomedical model does, but stands firmly astride both worlds, proclaiming us a unified complex of mind and body that can be fully in touch with the world above even as it dwells in this lower world.

Dossey draws out a further possibility, familiar to the "religious" mind but not to the skeptical. Perhaps it is the Great Being, not ourselves, who *causes us* to use our tiny intentionality to request the power to heal, *because that power is about to act anyway,* and it is seeking a channel—a healer—"down here." If so, it may be our *duty* to discover how to align ourselves with that healing power and so see more healing in the world. As physicist Fritjof Capra stated in 1982, every practicing physician knows that healing, that is, "whole-making," is an essential aspect of all medicine. He says the phenomenon is considered outside the present scientific framework because it cannot be understood in scientific terms, but that medical science will have to extend its narrow view of health and illness. This does not mean it will have to be less scientific. On the contrary, by broadening its conceptual basis it will become more consistent with recent developments in science such as the recent recognition of electromagnetic phenomena in the body.

Dossey states that "If distant effects of mental intentionality exist, we shall have to deal with them sooner or later, whether we like it or not. If we acknowledge them up front, they may lend a comprehensiveness to our thinking about the dynamics of consciousness which otherwise would be sacrificed. Acknowledging these phenomena early on might spare us at some later date the difficulty of retrofitting our models of the mind in order to accommodate them, or perhaps having to scuttle our models altogether."[28] Herbert Dingle would approve, but perhaps upbraid us for taking a lifetime to grasp what he and Jung and Pauli were saying in the 1930s. When we look forward and upward (metaphorical directions, of course) we see how inadequate is the status quo. Descartes' science, and that of his immediate successors, has served us after a fashion, but *itself* now leads us to go beyond it. Physics is less mechanistic than it was, but medicine lags far behind, having ignored the pioneers of the twentieth century until recently. As we glance back at Newtonian mechanism and current mechanistic medicine we implore medicine to catch up and look up. There is more to healing than has ever been known in *its* philosophy.

Is any overall hypothesis available to explain healings, whether distant or not (since *that* earth-level question is apparently irrelevant)? What stares us in the face is a more mature version of Descartes' simplistic and discredited dualism. Totally fused though consciousness and the body normally are during embodied life, we are not *just* material beings. We have consciousness, intentionality, and memory, and experiences that are difficult to explain without recourse to notions of "spiritual" nonidentity with the physical body. But we *are* confused between our own intentionality and that of some higher Being. Are we confused only because we have not yet seen that our own Being, with its healing intentions, and the Great Healer are in some absolutely real sense one and the same Being? Tat twam asi. Or is it only the higher intentionality that has actual power to heal, while we merely *invoke* it, sometimes successfully, sometimes not? Do we use it or does it (now and then) use us? In the present state of our knowledge we have more questions than answers. Here are a few of the questions we have attempted to consider:

Is intentionality at work at the mundane, physical, and physiological level of any valid healing, by contrast with conventional medical practice where there is no requirement for intention to heal but only for technology applied to the physical body?

Is there any evidence that everyday human intending is effective in producing healing?

Is there an upper, nonphysical level of our being, and, if so, what can we say about it?

Is intentionality at work at such an upper level in healings (and in other life events)?

Is not any intentionality that is truly effective itself of the essence of some such upper level (which would explain its absence from conventional, technological medicine)?

Finally, the question posed a few paragraphs ago: Does the evidence for intentionality at a spiritual level that its attested effectiveness provides, and that physics merely underpins, enable us to put together a plausible inclusive theory of what (genuine) healing is and how it works?

Answers to such questions may come from studies of the effects of body-centered forms of mysticism shown in clinical cases observed under the prevailing clinical conditions. Professor Olga Louchakova has published a study of the effects of psychospiritual practices known as the "Prayer of the Heart" applied to persons suffering cardiovascular disorders.[29]

Prayer of the Heart

In chapter 6 we discussed the role of the heart in Sufi prayer. It may be possible for those without the experience itself to glean some further impression of what the "Prayer of the Heart" is from a phenomenological account given of his own experience in the writings of Theophanis the Monk (eighth century CE), which illustrates the prayer's developmental stages:

> *The first step is that of purest prayer,*
> *From this there comes warmth of heart,*
> *And then a strange, a holy energy,*
> *Then tears wrung from the heart, God-*
> *   given.*
> *Then peace from thoughts of every kind.*
> *From this arises purging of the intellect,*
> *And next the vision of heavenly mysteries.*
> *Unheard of light is born from this,*
> *   ineffably,*
> *And thence, beyond all telling, the heart's*
> *   illumination.*
> *Last comes—a step that has no limit*
> *Though compassed in a single line—*
> *Perfection that is endless . . .*[30]

An exoteric, structural account of the developmental stages in the Prayer of the Heart shows that it includes:

Vocal prayer

Mental prayer

Prayer of recollection

Perfume prayer (Latin, *per* "through," *fumum* "smoke," unceasing prayer that spontaneously exhales from the soul)

Illumination (spiritual enlightenment)

Theosis (self-realization, the deification of the person through union with God)

The techniques used in the study carried out by Olga Louchakova were drawn from several traditions, but all of them contained the following components:

Devotional repetition of the names of Goddess or God. Louchakova notes that an experienced teacher will advise the practitioner regarding which names will augment, and which will inhibit, certain qualities of character.

Simultaneous activation of various functions of the psyche: subtle spiritual states, experiences of faith, trust, and so on.

Focusing on the various somatic faculties: breath, sensations, degrees of awareness in the interior space of the body.

The qualitative analysis of Louchakova's study data demonstrated that, in cases of brain strokes and heart attacks, there were observable differences both in the course of the disease and in the recovery process between practitioners of body-centered forms of mysticism and nonpractitioners of such spirituality. Dr. Louchakova found that, in particular, the subjects practicing chest-centered forms of mystical prayer or chest-centered forms of meditation displayed a significant degree of psychological transformation, showing a more balanced and integrated personality structure, integration of the archetypal level of the psyche, and increased capacity for "letting go." She states that the recovery of such patients is faster, and missing anatomical functions are frequently totally restored.

These findings, she believes, suggest the "spiritual" nature of some cases of stroke or heart attack, where the disease can be brought into association with the activation of the particular centers of consciousness in the subtle body that are energetically connected with the affected areas of the heart or brain. This suggests that body-centered forms of spiritual practice can lead to the uncovering, activation, and release of the psychosomatic conflicts that underlie the development of some forms of cardiovascular pathology. Consequently, "psychosomatic" forms of prayer can also be used for the prevention and possibly the treatment of some forms of brain strokes and heart attacks. Dr. Louchakova's presentation at the biannual "Spirituality and Health-Care" conference at the University of Toronto, Canada, in October 2002

reviewed several cases of cardiovascular disorders where practices from the spiritual tradition of Hesychasm, an early Christian mysticism based on the cultivation of stillness that is used in the Eastern Orthodox Church, and similar Sufi practices, were successfully used for self-management of the health problem.

The first case history describes a male student of yoga in his late fifties, with a progressive, possibly hereditary, disturbance of the rhythm of the heart muscle. Used over the course of five years, the practice of a psychosomatic focusing upon the heart area allowed the patient to monitor the condition of his heartbeat, and to avoid inpatient treatment. The second case history describes the brain stroke of a long-term practitioner of the Hesychastic Prayer of the Heart. Dr. Louchakova believes that the use of the psychosomatic form of prayer reduced the damaging effects of the stroke. In a third case, that of a female student of kundalinī yoga in her fifties who suffered a brain stroke, the psychospiritual practice of focusing on the spiritual heart center allowed her to regain health, reducing the adverse consequences and complications of the stroke. Though the psychospiritual practice used in this case was from kundalinī yoga, it is similar to the Prayer of the Heart insofar as it follows a psychosomatic approach.[31]

A New Cosmology

Louchakova's survey is one of the myriad small-scale but essential scientific studies that contribute to the advance of understanding. Alain Aspect's famous experiment is akin to it, a naïve experimentalist's contribution, as he himself modestly described it, despite having huge importance for living Beings beyond its more immediate significance for physics. In another part of the circle of the human community are the theoreticians, the mathematicians, the contemplative cosmologists. The theologian, cosmologist, and cultural historian Thomas Berry is one of these. There is a sense in which he places humankind at the center of humankind's own small cosmos, as the ancients were content to do and had, perforce, to do, but with the infinitely wider view available today he sets that tiny cosmos of our Being-in-the-world within the greater Whole, and calls humankind's attention to some very sobering facts that demonstrate the self-damaging myopia of most humans on this planet.

He does not merely admonish from this small perspective, but warns us that we need to ground ourselves in a new cosmology that will encourage the growth of universal compassion and empathy for all forms of life. He says that humans will come to understand that they are but one manifestation of the dynamic creative energy of the cosmos, one species in the great community of life. Human health is but a subsystem of the earth's health, he says. You cannot have well humans on a sick planet.

> We are ensouled beings capable of reflecting on the deeper aspects of the universe. . . . [O]ur intention, therefore, must be to heal, to make whole, our connection *with* the whole, to renew the visionary imagination and the natural human need for relationship and connection.[32]

Our conscious intentions carry the power to change, and what we choose to change not only changes us but changes the world around us. To paraphrase David Hamilton, "Every intention changes the collective unconscious, vibrates the web and influences the world." And the role of the subtle body in our conscious Being-there in this world arises from the fact that the subtle body is greater than we in the West have ever thought. It is not merely that which "links us to God" but that which "extends our being all the way to the Great Being, and *is* the Great Being." We must become more aware of what we are.

SEVENTEEN

The Integral Body

*People are psycho-spiritual beings who are integrated and integrative systems with overlapping, but partly distinct, subsystems. The spiritual dimension . . . is one of the subsystems as well as the integrating force for all the subsystems.**

G. W. ELLISON, "SPIRITUAL WELLBEING:
CONCEPTUALISATION AND MEASUREMENT,"
JOURNAL OF PSYCHOLOGY AND THEOLOGY

In the image of the subtle body is written not only the history of past tradition but the knowledge of our future evolution, our emergent, *integral* consciousness.[1] One of the most important keys to our understanding of our own evolution is the notion that we have not only a subtle body but also a subtle *mind,* or perhaps it would be more accurate to say a subtle *body-mind.* Human history shows stages in our development, at each of which a new kind of consciousness emerged following a period during which we had pressed the preceding mode to its limits. It is recognized by some thinkers today that we are in the transition between the mental and integral stages, the fourth and fifth structures in Gebser's schema of the evolution of consciousness.

The main characteristic of integral consciousness is its "stepping out of" dualistic perspectives that characterized the mental-rational consciousness stage. Of course, this integration of formerly conflicting perspectives is not a reference to the wish on the part of some to abolish dualistic views of our nature as Beings, but the

integration of all our perspectives on the world-about. It is the embrace of a wider view that supervenes the merely intellectual with all its categorizings. Integralism *contains* the dualities and dualisms, and expresses itself in a fluid, lively understanding of the *multiplicity* of perspectives available, every one of which it attempts to honor in the context of the whole.[2] This applies not only to individual awareness but to our relationships with others and our concern for the future of our planet: in short, we are evolving a new worldview, which is already being referred to by some as *integralism.*

Integralism
The New Worldview

What exactly is *integralism* and how is it shaping the model of the subtle body as we are coming to understand it in the West? Sri Aurobindo, the Indian mystic and spiritual and political leader, was the first to claim that the transformation of consciousness was the fundamental and signal ongoing event of our time. He first published thoughts on the evolution of consciousness as

*What Ellison describes here is an example of the "strange loop." See chapter 15.

early as 1914–1916. His insights arose from his contemplation of problems relating to Indian life. In due time they evolved into *The Life Divine,* published in 1951, a philosophy of life designed to reaffirm the reality of the world from the ultimate standpoint, and the meaningfulness of sociopolitical action from the spiritual standpoint. Aurobindo set out his integral philosophy in the terms of the metaphysico-spiritual language of his native Indian tradition, but from the age of seven until he reached twenty-one he had been educated in England, and there is no doubt that "he imbibed a great deal of Western learning."[3]

Gebser acknowledges that the idea of integralism came from the East, through Aurobindo, whose writing Gebser first encountered about 1957.[4] Aurobindo's incorporation of the evolutionary perspective of the modern West with the traditional mystical outlook of India produced an enlightening wholeness. The process of evolution within the world manifests the creative energy inherent in ultimate reality, and provides visible evidence of the principle "As above, so below" at work.

Aurobindo's system, which he called Integral Yoga, was based on his conception of a simple linear hierarchy of eight levels of reality as perceived and experienced by humans, which he lists from highest to lowest. They are:

1. Existence, Divine Existence, Pure Existent, Ultimate Reality, Absolute Spirit, *sat-cit-ananda* (the Unmanifest)
2. Consciousness, Force, Conscious Force, Sakti
3. Bliss
4. Supermind, Gnosis
5. Mind
6. Psyche, Soul
7. Life
8. Matter[5]

The Bengali philosopher Haridas Chaudhuri, founder of the California Institute of Integral Studies, states that in Aurobindo's view, the universe in its essential structure is real, not from the standpoint of ignorance but from that of supreme knowledge, and it is so because it is the expression of pure energy (Sakti), which is one with pure existence (Siva, sat, puruṣa). Being (*Brahman*) as the ultimate ground of the universe is the indivisible unity of pure existence and pure energy. "This equation," Chaudhuri explains, "*existence = energy,* is central to the integral awareness of Being, which is the cornerstone of Aurobindo's integral philosophy. Actualization of man's supramental potential* is the ultimate goal of his yoga. Supramental transformation of human personality is considered essential to the reconstruction of our society in accordance with the principles of unity-in-diversity, peace-with-justice, love-with-freedom."[6]

Intellect, ever the left-brained analyst, is the source of dichotomous thinking, as the history of Gebser's consciousness structures has shown. The result hitherto has been that the mind has planned to establish unity, yet in pursuing that goal has resorted to the crushing of diversities, attempting to achieve peace by imposition of control and by ignoring justice, expressing only a debased love that in reality smothers freedom. By contrast, the principle of integral consciousness is to accept all opposites, and allow *them* to *find* their own harmony, so laying the foundation for a unified world order in which unity *and* diversity, peace *grounded in* justice, love *and* freedom coexist. The stance that this requires has been named the *supermind,* which is the fourth of Aurobindo's levels of reality. Chaudhuri says that "*Purna yoga* or *integral yoga* is the art of bringing forth into overt operation, in our life and society, the integral and all-integrating consciousness of the supermind."[7]

Integral philosophy today aims to achieve a "dynamic integration of the scientific, phenomenological, and dialectical methods of the West and the self-analytical, psycho-integrative, nondual values of the East. Integralism speaks to its very own evolution occurring on individual and collective levels."[8] Its proponents are coming to prominence among thinkers of today, revolutionizing earlier attitudes and beliefs. Among those influenced by Aurobindo's philosophy, besides Haridas Chaudhuri, are the psychologist, educator, and prolific author on Aurobindo's teachings Indra Sen, who coined the term "integral psychology,"[9] Michael Murphy, author and co-founder of the Esalen Institute, which promotes Eastern and Western studies in human potential,[10] psychologist-philosopher Ken Wilber,[11] the Yoga histo-

---

Supramental is Sri Aurobindo's term for the highest plane of our own essential dynamic being and consciousness, hence *supramental potential* means having the capacity to develop beyond ordinary consciousness.

rian Georg Feuerstein (see chapter 1), and many others. Millions are espousing similar beliefs as the result of *their own* thinking, for the ideas and the process are "in the air" of the twenty-first century, and no new world such as is envisaged could possibly ground itself in the sectarian following of human leaders or heros. The underlying assertion of integral theory is that, as transpersonal psychologist S. M. Saiter puts it, "There are powerful forces at work in the world that shape and mould our experience as human beings. It has been postulated that ever since humankind started to record this experience there have been attempts at grand, universal visions designed to explain and to help in comprehending and dealing with the mysterious dilemma of existence."[12]

Spiral Dynamics and the Subtle Body

The subtle body is one of these "universal visions" and, as such, retains its place in this scheme of things since integral theory begins by acknowledging and validating mystical experience, rather than denying its reality. Humans in all cultures and in all eras have these experiences, so they are accepted as valuable, not pathological. Integral theory claims that *both* science and spirituality are necessary for complete understanding of humanity itself and of the universe we inhabit. Indeed, the new science will, necessarily, include within its own wholeness a "science of spirituality itself." That this be accepted is particularly important for the present age, as a profound shift in consciousness is even now under way and mature steadiness is needed if this pivotal transition from one age into another is to be accomplished with minimal trauma to the new way of being human that is now coming to birth.

We need a comprehensive understanding of what may show itself to be the most refined manifestation of human potential in our species' history. The various images, from many cultures, of the facets of the subtle body map out stages of consciousness that transcend all the earlier levels of consciousness yet continue thereafter to include them, still functioning and alive. The integral vision expresses a multidimensional model encompassing perennial truth, unifying, timeless, spaceless, formless, as old as recorded history, yet able to accommodate continuous new growth. Ervin Laszlo calls it an "integral theory of everything."[13]

In the past two decades, some integral theorists,

especially the developmental psychologists, have extended the model of the subtle body to encompass new stages of growth. While many have worked with the subtle body in the traditional Eastern way as a "ladder of being" (see chapter 3), a concept of "ascent" to higher consciousness, others have found a new way to picture the way we develop to reach new stages. These researchers recommend that we visualize the stages not as ascending a staircase, a merely linear movement in which each step is left behind as the next is reached, but rather as a widening *spiral* movement that, as it completes each turn, *encompasses the previous stages within itself.* This model of human development has been given the name Spiral Dynamics and the concept was introduced by psychologists Chris Cowan and Don Beck in 1996, in their book of the same title.[14] They were inspired by ideas propounded by Professor Clare Graves, an American psychologist, which he named the theory of "Emergent Cyclical Levels of Existence."

Of course, the very essence of a process of widening that maintains its own earlier stages as it grows is that new concepts arise out of earlier, usually unnamed, notions. Each new stage is first known in the *experience* of being, to be *named* only when seen with a degree of detachment as the next stage of being arrives and the person, the human Being, looks back introspectively to analyze what that person has been, and to gain an appreciation of what he or she has now become. We are all constituted by our past even as we also look forward and move into our future. While this gradual widening of consciousness sometimes progresses quickly, and today seems to be advancing at an exponentially accelerating rate, the evolution began even before humans first became dimly conscious of being Beings who were conscious, first of the world-about, then, later, of themselves-in-that-world.

Spiral forms have been used throughout history by Hindus and others to signify processes that are *both* cyclical and progressive, and the term *spiral* commonly denotes *both* flat spirals, such as snail shells, and cylindrical spirals, such as corkscrews. Today, any concept of mental growth needs to illustrate both the widening of consciousness and the forward progress in maturity of awareness, and perhaps the best visual form would therefore be a spiral that both widens and moves forward from its narrow origin, forming an ever-widening cone. Our development as persons might thus be seen as following a widening helical path. The spiral has indeed become part of fashionable New Age lore, but often in so vague a form that in some modern schemata it is difficult to see what justifies their proponents' use of spiral representations. Whether apposite or not, we should always bear in mind that any illustration is only an aid to contemplation of the reality it represents. It is the reality that matters.

An example of a progressive helical structure is illustrated in plate 35. However, the figure also alludes to yet another terrestrial-world fact of our embodied life, the bicameral brain. The brain is a unity containing great diversity, the right brain more creative and intuitive, the left more analytical, both modes needed, in temporal alternation, if a wholeness—a healthiness—of embodied-human-beingness is to be achieved. We picture the process as the cyclical alternation of yin and yang operations within the human consciousness, first in the mode of one cerebral hemisphere, then in the mode of the other, the effect being a spiraling, progressive synthesis ever-moving toward greater awareness and maturity of mind. This progress we label broadly according to Aurobindo's schema, with further annotations after others who have contemplated our way of

being-in-the-world and have reached similar conclusions.

Saiter believes "The notion of the spiral is an elegant model in the context of this comprehension. It can be seen as both linear and cyclical."[15] He suggests that by looking into the Spiral Dynamics model we shall see that seemingly different phenomena, such as the perennial wisdom traditions, and certain complex modern problems, such as environmental degradation and the global infrastructure, relate to each other. There are important connections between all expressions of human existence. By perceiving and pondering these connections we create a space for the further expansion of consciousness at both collective and individual levels. Saiter suggests that "Gebser is proposing a whole new way of being," but offers the sobering thought that this requires "a level of understanding yet to be experienced by the vast majority of people on the planet." However, he says, "perhaps it is meant to be seen as a necessary variable in an attempt to push the evolutionary impulse that much further."[16]

According to the theory of Spiral Dynamics, we remain in each stage for however long it "works" for us, whether a few years, a few decades, or an entire lifetime. Change in our habits and thinking patterns occurs when we discover new information, find ourselves in a new situation, or experience something that our normal

The Gödelian View

A Gödelian world-view of the evolution of Beings-in-the-world as constituting a consistent system depending from a "place" or "state" that we are constrained to see as an "Above" suggests a multiplex of spirals, resembling the engineer's "multi-start thread," from which each and every part of the lower world, including the living Beings in it, subtends. The "threads" represent what, in mathematical logic, would be the unprovable axioms from which the consistent system depends. Thus, livingness itself, and the physical world itself, each instantiate the Gödelian structure, for each depends directly from the Above, and, as suggested in chapter 15, does so independently of the other. For as long as it continues, any life is necessarily *incomplete,* but also, by logical necessity, *consistent with its unique self.* When it ends it becomes, in Heidegger's view, a Whole, therefore *complete,* but,

in a vague sense, also *inconsistent,* for a nonliving body is an anomaly. Bodies have *meaning* when lived. A view based on Heideggerian and Gödelian notions, then, is that as long as life continues it depends from above, for the Above is the Source of both livingness and physics, and ipso facto the higher pole of the Being-to-thing duality we noticed in chapter 15. While making no claim that the structure we depict in plate 35 resembles, let alone constitutes, a mathematical proof, it is a clear pictorial analog of phenomena of our world-about that continually reveal themselves to us as ecstases out-from the Platonic world. The colors we show in the spiral are those of the seven main chakras, themselves the steps of a development from the physical toward the spiritual, adjusted a little in an attempt to maintain perspicuity in the finished diagram.

way of seeing the world cannot accommodate; then we grow, often in spite of ourselves. Gradually, a new, more inclusive view emerges and we evolve toward a more enlightened stage. But, as Gebser observes, "it is fitting that we recall from time to time the pains which we experience because of the tensions of these new realities, for without them there could be no preparation for the birth of a new mutation capable of liberating us from the earlier sufferings."[17] We note the close parallel with all valid forms of psychotherapy.

The Integrative Principle

The essence of any process of deep, personal development is the addition to what exists of something new, but the integration of the new into what already exists does not necessarily take place automatically. The elements to be combined, having never been brought together before, might resist their own integration. Herbert Dingle, reviewing such a situation, would say that the incompatible prior hypotheses must find valid modifications that bring them into agreement. This would be the only outcome able to claim a greater truth than the antecedent disunity. Physics itself, the grounding "hard science," is being evolved in precisely this way. Similarly, the evolution of consciousness, the soul, the spirit (many words have been used in the attempt to describe or label such ideas) has certainly required the human race to synthesize elements that might be seen as conflicting. Dingle, Jung, and Pauli all knew this was the situation in science, wherein even physics itself was not yet completely self-consistent, and psychology and physics were not yet able to share even a little ground.

But there is a third factor, the main agent, the human viewer, capricious and unpredictable (like Dingle's living fly). We do not obey the "laws of physics," so there may be other reasons for failure to integrate than an inherent mis-fit between the existing beliefs themselves. Undiagnosed unwillingness to change, the bias we saw afflicting science, or a lack of imagination in the human view of the problem might blight and delay the new synthesis. Saiter spoke of most people's perceptions being unready for the necessary changes, and others, too, have noted this. It is the person, probably more than the inconsistency of the existing beliefs, who foretells the outcome, especially as that which most requires change

is not in the unconscious world-about but in the human being's own mind, often thrust below consciousness, particularly when uncomfortable or when it demands an ethical change. No whole-world progress can be expected so long as these subconscious voices go unrecognized, or are deliberately swept aside in dishonest pride. Persons, even more than prior hypotheses (themselves the mental products of persons), must change.

Gebser explains that the integrating principle is polarity, on which notion we shall allow him to say more shortly. Polarity within the personal structure sets up a *tension within the person* that resolves as a *new* structure of consciousness arises, pressing toward a completion in which the complementary expressions will have found a transformative state of synthesis. This idea of polar opposites tending toward a unity is not new, for the Taoist notions of yin and yang are millennia old already, though perhaps we are now more aware of polarity *as it is in itself,* and as a motive force in spiral progression, needing less than heretofore to find its truth in the creative inspiration of symbolic pictures arising in our minds, strange and puzzling, arresting and intriguing. The very process is now an object of introspection for any reflective person. We can watch ourselves thinking. We need fewer myths, now, to explain matters to ourselves, fewer fantastical and ultimately obstructive "correspondences." We feel the resolution of polar tensions "in our bones," and enjoy the illumination of our inner being as the newly balanced opposites reveal themselves to us. We also have more facts from science to provide for new vision, and imagination is, in an important sense, now optional, no longer obligatory if we as a race are not to be bored unless waging war. Katavul might now plan the next step of his own evolution, rather than harass the demons. Imagination, no longer standing in for knowledge (as it did too often in the age of alchemy), but aiding our acquisition of knowledge, at least in the sphere of science, is now free to become itself and find honorable employment in every sphere of life.

Consciousness at Gebser's mental stage has enabled us to define many problems, and bring them into verbal formulation, though this has itself now proved dangerous, as we pointed out in our treatment of science and philosophy. We see expressions of polarity in the symbolism of pairs of opposites in numerous traditions: in the microcosm and macrocosm, in the Siva and Sakti of kundalinī yoga, in the yin and yang of Taoism, in the king and queen of Western alchemy, in body and soul, in life and death, and in contemporary language as the positive and negative poles of electromagnetic fields.[18]

Unlike a mere sign, a symbol thus has substance. "A true symbol," Gebser says, "always encloses two complementary poles; it is always ambivalent, ambiguous, indeed polyvalent, particularly if we focus on only one of its values or poles." Gebser reminds his readers that the word *symbol* comes from the Greek *symballo,* meaning "to roll together," "join," or "unify," and that every symbol, being a unity formed from a duality by such a "rolling together," contains two essences or possibilities that in fact are antithetic. The antithetical components may form a *complementary* whole, but ambivalence is never far away. "Only when we proceed from their complementarity and not from the individual poles, recognizing in each pole its polar complement, will the true symbol and the self-complementarity of the soul be revealed."[19]

The soul, or mind, or life (again many words have been used to name elusive entities) is the arena in which consciousness itself must forge and maintain what unity it can in the face of cognitive dissonances of many kinds, and symbolism has often been used, consciously or intuitively, as, for example, in certain psychotherapies. But the psychological is difficult to represent in graphic modes, as a quick survey of the illustrations in this book, and any intelligent graphic artist, will confirm, while a serious, introspective composer of music has a better chance of expressing it. Gebser discovered that the Chinese Tai Chi is one of very few such graphic symbolisms, though a very succinct one, being, as he puts it, "one of the manifest original configurations of the primal and invisible cosmic universal structure and formation . . . a preforming and primal paradigm of being, in short, the whole of reality."[20]

Gebser states that "at all times and in all places, many and diverse ways have led to the living knowledge of the soul's polar complementarity." He goes on to say that the soul and the body, in their mutually conditioning and complementing tension, have the same relationship to one another as time and space. The acute energy of the soul corresponds to the latent energy of the body. Whatever we can *understand* on the one hand, we must also *sense* or *experience* on the other. This sensing or experiencing is the living knowledge required to com-

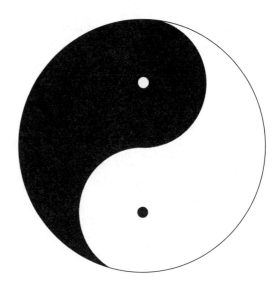

Fig. 17.1. The paradoxical Oneness of the Tao is expressed in the symbol of yin and yang. The dark yin contains a tiny spot of the light yang, and vice versa, signifying that, though opposite, yin and yang are complementary, and constantly flow into each other, being contained within one Whole. Taoists believe that we should learn to "go with the flow" of natural changes and cycles rather than resisting them.

plete our calculative, estimative knowledge, and without this process and achievement, no life is capable of reaching conscious integration.[21] In putting forward this view, Gebser rightly sets himself against the overly intellectual current stage of mental consciousness, exemplified by those recent philosophers who have scorned holistic thought, retreating into verbal analysis and shunning experience of reality.

This need to stand against intellectual unwholeness is also a main message of many other authors who advocate journeying beyond mental consciousness toward integral consciousness, among them Ken Wilber, Ervin Laszlo, John Holman, Drew Leder, and many others who will forgive us not attempting what would be an ever-lengthening list of names. It is also the unspoken message of every artist, in whatever medium, whose work is true expression rather than stylistic cliché expressed with merely competent technique. Creativity is for all of us, of course, for if we do not work as artists in any conspicuous sense, we may all work on one great work of art, ourselves.

Another example of a creative response in this process is readily available for the mental or rational consciousness: when self- or ego-consciousness reaches a certain degree of intensity or "condensation," it inevitably becomes involved in a struggle to resolve inherent conflict between itself and all others. It begins to develop strategies for restoring psychic harmony or equilibrium. This may be expressed in terms of a quest for new self-understanding (thus emphasizing the affective aspect). However, this struggle or search always implicates the total person, and once the quest has begun it shows itself to have many different dimensions. As Feuerstein notes, in the final analysis this search is always a movement not only toward self-integration but toward self-transcendence.[22]

The preconditions for the integral structure, Gebser explains, include "the concretion of time," the making-present *now* of all the historical stages of consciousness, simultaneously, in the human being of today. This requires work, for the various consciousness structures cannot be understood merely by contemplating them as intellectual abstractions. By their very nature they are *not* intellectual abstractions, indeed, they *cannot* be intellectual abstractions. They are self-aware experience. Consciousness cannot be words on paper, nor even the understanding grasp of those words by an intelligent reader. Consciousness *experiences* itself, for it *is* that *experiencing. Experiencing,* pure and strong, is *what consciousness is.* No one is entitled to speak of consciousness unless he *does* it, and, sadly, this is scarcely the risible and otiose admonition it might seem, for, as Ouspensky pointed out, and as Hermes taught many centuries ago, most people are asleep. The failure to recognize this is precisely the catastrophic error of those philosophers who analyze verbal statements instead of the experiences the verbal statements purport, or genuinely attempt, to convey or represent.

The Open Door

A person must, Gebser believes, *experience* the earlier modes of consciousness, and then, only then, will be able to know the integration of himself, first *with* or *within* himself, and then with the Whole. We have to learn to *see,* to become *seers,* to "lift the veil" between this world and the next, and we have to forge the spiritual technologies to do it. This integration is something known *within,* by *feeling.* In expounding his view Gebser shows himself a close ally of Heidegger, even using rather similar phraseology, for Heidegger characterizes our sense or

feeling of being Beings by using the word *Befindlichkeit,* translatable *literally* as "the state in which one may be found," but expressive of a *feeling-and-sensing* for which English has no satisfactory single word. Gebser's translators use the word *diaphanous* to convey the character of deep self-knowledge. Deriving from the Greek φαινειν, "to show," φαινομενον, "a thing appearing to one's view," δια, "through," the word *diaphanous* means somewhat more than its everyday usage as *transparent* for it describes a process of "revealing through," where something becomes a "phenomenon," emerging out-from its source beyond, and coming toward the viewer. It is *there* before us, though at first we may not see it. Indeed, it may "appear" by a gradual process, but the process is in us, as we begin to see it, not in *its* primordial ever-presence. It was always there to be seen, and now we must become Seers of the φαινομενον of the wholeness being offered us by the cosmos.

Self-knowledge thus becomes *a new way of being a Being,* with an altogether higher, wider, brighter feeling-sense and, the view-about being in the eye of the beholder, a clearer gaze, out upon itself-in-the-world, the world-about and the greater cosmos. It is as if, as we find ourselves in deep self-knowledge, the universe finds us. This is, again, the anthropic principle, but the Anthropos is now a larger Being. Gebser, as translated into English, thus lights upon the same meaning, that of *transparency,* that Heidegger (also in translation) uses to describe the direct, spontaneous flow of skilled performance or creativity of which we become aware only if we stumble on a difficulty, such as the breaking or unsuitability of the tool in the hand, which obstructs that creative, dreamlike flow and brings consciousness down again to the mundane until the meditation-like creative state supervenes once more. Like every person of experience Gebser struggles to find words that will express his subtly nuanced meanings. He suggests that the way to achieve personal integration is for the various structures of which the person is constituted to become *diaphanous to that person's own introspective view.* The person then sees the effects on his life and destiny and is able to master his own "deficient components" by insight.[23] Important for both Gebser and Heidegger are the sense of being a Being, of a spontaneity born of self-knowledge, of a wholeness of being that expresses itself in a flow of which the performer him- or herself does not need, or wish, to be made aware as if observing it from *out*side, for the performer and the performance, the liver and the life, have become one spontaneous living movement.

We have seen that this knowledge is already available to us. It has been making itself known throughout our development, era upon era, through the archaic, magical, mythical, and mental stages of consciousness. The archetypal symbols for this process, as Jung has pointed out, are now imprinted in our unconscious. It is the task of the integral stage of our evolution to bring up into consciousness this accumulation of prior work.

The transformative practice of integralism, as Ken Wilber phrases it, is the truth of the ever-present Self. Wilber, one of the most noted and popular integral theorists of our day, explains that while we can attain the related states by spiritual practice, these practices cannot, in and of themselves, be or produce enlightenment.[24] Even if the related state is itself achieved the experience can be ignored, bearing no fruit in the sitter's life. To claim that the practices are the mystical experience would be to misunderstand the process, for enlightenment is not "caused" or brought about automatically by assiduous carrying-out of the exercises. It is not a manufactured state, purposefully engineered by us by making a series of internal adjustments of the psyche. Rather, it is as already described, ever-present *before* us, but not yet present *within*. The notion is cognate with the ancient Indian conception of *Brahman* as the "Ground of Being." A "ground" is timelessly present, perhaps unseen, but simply there, supporting, ready to infuse those Beings who have perceived it and have paused to take notice. This, too, is the concretion of time referred to earlier. It can scarcely be described as a process. Enlightenment *is,* and we may enter *it. We* align with *it,* perhaps having erroneously thought it "over there" or "out there" (which in a sense it is *until* we find it) but we then *discover* it *within* ourselves. Like the earlier modes of humankind's consciousness, it can be ever-present to us.

This being the nature of the doorway into the *state* of *enlarged consciousness,* Wilber's Integrative Transformative Practice, the practical embodiment of Gebser's view, attempts to exercise the physical, emotional, mental, and spiritual dimensions of the *self,* first *within* the self, but then in relationship with others and with the larger world of human community and nature. However, the *practices,* as distinguished from the *state,* are transformative only in that *relational* sphere that involves ourselves and others in the world. Wilber therefore encourages the practitioner, the individual seeker of the enlightenment, to take the steps first of making the body-mind *increasingly transparent to itself,* just as Gebser and, in a related way, even Heidegger have advocated, and then increasingly receptive of the Divine φαινομενον, which has always been, and still is "there," waiting patiently to disclose itself and be seen. We need practices that involve the Absolute, the very source of the ever-present φαινομενον, though such words do not express it well. It is better, perhaps, to say that as the Divine is always "there" before *us,* we should make *ourselves* as ever-present to that Absolute Source as we can.

EIGHTEEN

The Subtle Body and the Transformed Being in Society

Transformation is the manifestation of the content of illumination, i.e. faith, in the life of the mystic, and hence the mediation of the fruits of illumination to the unillumined world. In the gift of illumination the devotee receives all she needs for her own salvation or liberation. And if, as some claim, mysticism is only an individual phenomenon which has no impact on society, then illumination is all that is necessary. But the teachings of mystics explicitly deny this claim. They maintain instead that the ultimate goal of mysticism is to transform society—to act within the world in such a way that every aspect of human existence will become a manifestation of illumination.

JOHN E. COLLINS, *MYSTICISM AND NEW PARADIGM PSYCHOLOGY*

The end of chapter 17 might have served as a fitting end to this book, but the aim of chapter 17, the opening up of our greater consciousness, is itself the reason for an eighteenth chapter. This final chapter sketches the means and says something of the ends of that endeavor.

In part 1 we looked at the main ideas, of many kinds, which together composed the notion of the subtle body in Eastern traditions. We discovered that what we term the *subtle body* was, in ancient Hindu, Tibetan, and Chinese cultures, regarded as a means to an end, that of achieving "liberation" from the sufferings of ordinary human life while in an ordinary state of consciousness that was still totally involved with the all-too-ordinary body. There was no transcendence, and that ordinary state of consciousness did not even produce analysis, in anything like our modern scientific sense, of what it was that the conscious thinker *was*. He had a body, and he

thought, and, somewhere in this prehistory of consciousness, he had stumbled upon meditation and liked the way it felt. More important than *what it was* that did the meditating (if "it," the person's own Being, was conceived as a "thing" at all) was what the *experience itself* achieved, which was enjoyed in memory, so encouraging the experiencer to seek the repetitions of it that initiated the millennia-long process of human enlightenment that lay ahead.

In that era's prevailing state of consciousness, as Gebser has now shown us, humans probably did not have a sense of *self*hood to explore. They were concerned more with getting the fruits-in-feeling of their meditation. This selfish satisfaction-seeking was a state of spontaneous action, and on that account a state to be desired, but it was innocent, too innocent. Awareness of self, of others, and of ethics, were probably all lacking, but the meditation itself was the source from which those more mature realizations would, in time, accrue. The sense of self that has become, today, almost a tyrant would come later, the introspection of it later still, bringing the recognition of the false, prideful, resentful, divisive, social, indeed utterly useless "ego-selves," which the wise discern and reject as such. By the spiral development we have often noted, a new spontaneity and innocence, as we saw in chapter 17, have at last become the *conscious goals* of the *already*-conscious.

As yogis, mystics, and other spiritual seekers confirm, by altering consciousness an experience that came to be known as samādhi or nirvāna was attained. It was a different state existing within, yet seeming to be greater than, the as-yet unchanged earlier state of being; it was a state of ecstasy, a standing out from a continuing ordinariness. It included a Self, of a very different sort from the usual, and was also known as "bliss," and gave a sense of safety and of joy, quite unlike everyday experience. It was recognized as oneness with "something higher," with the postulated Creator, Brahman, or "Great Being," for the "spacelessly huge" awareness of the presence of a non-material-beingness-*that-was-beingness-itself,* as it overcame the sitter, seemed to warrant its being so characterized and named.

Sometimes wonderful visions appeared before the sitter's closed eyes; sometimes magic powers (known as siddhis) operated. Teachers generally warned against allowing them attention, though in fact they are evidence of a true reality, whatever its nature, either within the body-mind or in some sense "flowing into it" from that "above." The warning, however, was wise, unless the meditator showed unusual moral maturity. It is rational to ask whether we have such maturity now. We need it! Recognizing this, we believe the most mature among humanity have made it attainable, for we seem to have discovered that a chief quality of the subtle body is its own intentionality. These thoughts, viewed from our place in the evolutionary history of consciousness, are a clue to the route this final chapter will take, and the reason for that direction.

In part 1 we saw that the desire for a state of union with the "above," transcending the material-minded quest for the perfection of the material body, eventually appeared. In part 2 we have seen that this desire is universal. It pervades the many systems that make up the tapestry of Western traditions, just as it informs some traditions in the East, and this spiritual search is not only present in most major religions but is also found more explicitly in the philosophia perennis, a set of metaphysical truths defining the nature of Reality and our relationship with the Divine.[1] However, following Hermeticism and Neo-Platonism, in the West, came skepticism and science. Sweeping imaginary correspondences aside it began to discover facts. A few centuries later it is discovering facts among the sweepings, too.

Having first been a good servant, and then become a bad master, science is now ready to be an equal cooperator. As we saw, while it has not achieved, nor ever set out to achieve, a grand unified theory of all past musings on what our inner being might be, it has nonetheless uncovered stubborn but very pleasing facts that support the old notions. The subtle body is not a physical body strangely lacking physical characteristics, but it does have a reality of its own. Science supports at least some of the intuitive dreams of the past, and sharpens their theory and vocabulary. It therefore provides us with a route into the future, not one that raises science above all history but one in which science is a part of the armory of consciousness *itself* with which further discoveries in consciousness will be made.

With itself as subject and object of research, both agent and recipient of attention, consciousness has found itself to be substantial, in some sense of the word, and can now expect to raise itself above the erstwhile level of its own mentality, into an integral way of Being-in-the-world. This, then, is our direction of, and the justification for, one more chapter. We want to find out *how* (quoting our own words) to "make *ourselves* as ever-present to that Absolute Source as we can." We want to build a new tower to reach the heavens, not of mud blocks, and not of Babel (for that word means "confusion"), but of spiritual contact for each person with the Source of safety and joy. This was pictured long ago, and we have, now, more tools, more *spiritual* tools, to achieve it than we had before. We want to transform ourselves, and, as so often, we set the scene for that building of a future by looking back.

The common notion in all the spiritualities, Eastern or Western, is that *transformation,* a metamorphosis of the personality, of the *self-as-sensed* by each "I," *is* possible. Joyful selfhood *can* be reached by the use of spiritual tools or techniques that have evolved and survived, been discovered, and rediscovered, over centuries. Despite great historical upheavals and cultural changes they have proved to be as useful and effective today in the Western world as they were five thousand years ago in the East. St. Ignatius of Loyola declared that "a single hour of meditation . . . had taught him more truths about heavenly things than all the teachings of all the doctors put together."[2] In Britain today, ten million people practice some form of meditation daily.[3] It would therefore be reasonable to ask at this point what changes these self-altering techniques produce in the individual and how the changes affect society as a whole.

The process of mystical transformation has four distinct stages, which professor of religion John E. Collins identifies in both Eastern and Western spiritual traditions:

Awakening
Purgation
Illumination
Transformation[4]

Awakening

Collins notes that in the stage of awakening, also known as "transcendent experience," "peak experience," or simply "mystical experience," the meditator, yogi, or spiritual practitioner "catches a glimpse of the nature of transformed reality, of transformed consciousness, of transformed self, and of the possibility of subjecting oneself to spiritual discipline which could result in *sustained* [my emphasis] transformation."[5] What is this transformed state like? What is it that the spiritual practitioner experiences?

In the Hindu tradition, the adept is said to have become the ānanda-maya-kośa, the "body of *bliss*," and many descriptions from the mystical traditions state that we experience *ecstasy*. St. Ignatius, for example, related how he felt one day when contemplating the Holy Trinity, saying that "the vision flooded his heart with such sweetness that the mere memory of it in after times made him shed abundant tears."[6] Another common feature is the admission that the experience is difficult to describe in words and it is therefore often communicated in metaphor, poetry, parable, or paradox.

William James states, "The kinds of truth communicable in mystical ways, whether these be sensible or supersensible, are various. Some of them relate to this world—visions of the future, the reading of hearts, the sudden understanding of texts, the knowledge of distant events, for example; but the most important revelations are theological or metaphysical."[7] For example, St. Teresa of Avila* writes that one day it was granted her to perceive in an instant how all things are seen and contained in God. "I did not perceive them in their proper form, and nevertheless the view I had of them was of a sovereign clearness, and has remained vividly impressed upon my soul . . . the view was so subtle [*sic*] and delicate that the understanding cannot grasp it." "On another day," she writes, "Our Lord made me comprehend in what way it is that one God can be in three persons."[8] Here we can compare similar experiences in the Indian tradition among contemplatives of the *Trimurti,* the three-fold aspects of God as Brahma the Creator, Siva the Destroyer, and Vishnu the Preserver. St. Teresa continues, "He made me see it so clearly that I remained as extremely surprised as I was comforted" and whenever she thinks or hears of the Trinity, she says, "I understand how the three adorable Persons form only one God, and I experience an unspeakable happiness."[9]

"The deliciousness of some of these states," comments James, "seems to be beyond anything known in ordinary consciousness. It evidently involves organic sensibilities, for it is spoken of as something too extreme to be borne, and as verging on bodily pain. But it is too subtle and piercing a delight for ordinary words to denote. . . . Intellect and sense both swoon away in these highest states of ecstasy."[10] Sometimes these states have been described as profound feelings of peace and serenity and awareness of the "presence of God." Such experiences have happened, and continue to happen, not only to "saints" and "religious people," but also to ordinary people who do not follow any organized religion or particular spiritual path, though it is noteworthy with regard to the latter class that the experiences are commonly followed by emotional and

*St. Teresa of Avila (1515–1582) was a reformer of the Carmelite Order whose mystical writings had a formative influence on later theologians. She was the first female to be named a Doctor of the Church, in 1970.

psychological transformation so profound that even if the experience lasts no more than a second it is often followed by the recovery or discovery of a deep faith. We ask why it is that, when ordinary life produces so much pessimism, experience we recognize as "different," and therefore designate as *spiritual,* gives such very great joy. We trust this chapter will go some way to answering this, step by step.

Purgation

However, the euphoric stage, of which the experiences of Teresa and Ignatius are instances, may not last very long. As John Collins states, "The awakening experience reveals that all are trapped within the conditions of totally unsatisfactory existence, *dukkha,*" and while some mystics may go through feelings of impotence, meaninglessness, and despair, for the mystic on the path of raja yoga "the awakening is the end of one kind of consciousness and the beginning of another." Collins gives the example of Gautama Buddha who, realizing that worldly pleasures can neither give ultimate satisfaction of human desire nor lead to the goal of liberation, embarked on a search for an effective spiritual discipline, which would involve severe austerity, self-denial, and, ultimately, renunciation.[11]

In the lives of ordinary people, the stage of purgation often starts with a spiritual search motivated by a subtle, unnamed longing or yearning. In her book *The Ecstatic Journey: The Transforming Power of Mystical Experience,* Sophy Burnham describes how her own mystical path began with an experience she recognized as samādhi when she glanced out of a window at a tree and "for an instant I became the tree. No separation. I was the bark, the wood, the fleshy summer leaves. Time stopped. The experience lasted hardly a second. But I have never forgotten that restful state of perfect peace. Time stopped, all feeling, analysis, all consciousness of self, all sense of being 'I.' I knew something precious had been given me. I didn't know it was a state that you could cultivate, or that it had anything to do with this word called 'God.'"[12] The next stage in Burnham's life came just as unexpectedly, with an intuitive flash of insight. She suddenly knew that she had to make changes in her life, which she had been resisting, a hard struggle that entailed giving up her home, her family,

and her friends. It brought her to the brink of despair, to a virtual purgatory. In Gebser's terms, she had experienced the "diaphanous" transparency of revealed clear insight.

Illumination

The third stage on the mystical path, says John Collins, requires cleansing and purification. "Anything that had given the former life meaning and purpose is to be exposed as devoid of ultimate value. He is not allowed to cling to the desires and devices of the past, but must surrender them all, especially" (as we saw in Burnham's case) "the ones which had been most dear to him. This psychological void is created so that nothing will inhibit the influx of truth which is given in illumination.[13] . . . Illumination is the process of rebirth of consciousness. . . . Through purification one kind of consciousness is systematically set aside; through illumination a radically different kind is acquired. In the story of Gautama this acquisition is made in one night" when the Buddha sat under a Bo tree and reached enlightenment in meditation. "For the ordinary seeker it takes years, perhaps lifetimes, of uncompromising discipline." Collins describes how Buddha searched for seven years and, despite having mastered the philosophical and theological teachings of his day, subjected himself to austerities to the point of threatening his life. Eventually, he reached a critical point. He fell into the trance in which he found peace and freedom from suffering.[14]

Abhayadatta, the twelfth-century chronicler of the lives of the Siddhas, the poet-philosopher-yogis and healers of South India, whose teachings survive in stories and songs intended to inspire others to achieve liberation, has this to say about the "critical point": "Turning from the ordinary life is the necessary first step to transformation, for if one is content with the usual run of life, there is little desire to change. Only when discontent arises does one begin to look for a different way of being. Such internal discontent often manifests as a life crisis." He observes that in some cases the crisis is brought on by an affliction that makes life almost unbearable. "The misery of *samsara* (the 'chain of rebirths') expresses itself in personal affairs."[15]

The critical or crisis point of severe stress in the

aspirant's life, with its breakthrough to ecstasy or serenity, is one of the ways by which the normal chemistry of the brain can be altered to produce a mental state of euphoria. This switching between stress and ecstatic experience can be found in the clinical profiles of people with disturbed or drug-dependent conditions as well as those of healthy people following a spiritual path. Collins states that the commonest way of inducing transcendent experience is through "intentional stress."[16] He explains that "The great variety of spiritual disciplines practiced in the various religious traditions have at least one thing in common—the intentional stressing of the organism. Each spiritual discipline calls upon its initiates to ask their bodies and brains to perform functions for which they are not normally adapted. *Hatha yoga,* fasting . . . concentration, trying to answer an unanswerable question, endless repetitions of a *mantra,* detailed inspection of one's sinfulness, etc., can cause considerable mental stress. One might easily conclude that the more vigorous the practice, the more severe the stress and the greater the likelihood of transcendent experience."[17]

We add that, while each person's experience is both unique and absolutely private to that individual, and comparison between experience and its results is therefore very difficult, it seems that some reach the required spiritual stance, or outlook, less by deliberate imposition of stress upon themselves than by simple long privation in a trying life.

Transformation

In his discussion of the life of Buddha, Collins states that transformed consciousness has three prominent characteristics:

> *Prajñā* (wisdom)
> *Karuna* (compassion)
> *Nirvāna* (passing away)[18]

Prajñā

Derived from the root *jñā,* meaning to know or understand, the Sanskrit word *prajñā* is usually translated as "intuitive wisdom" or "true knowledge," a state of consciousness that is not bound by space, time, causality, or identity. It is transcendental in relation to ordinary consciousness and may be experienced as extraordinary, miraculous, supernormal, as we saw from the descriptions of experiences related above.[19]

Karuna

We saw that the model of the ideal human in the Hindu and Tibetan traditions is the jīvan-mukta, the liberated or fully self-realized embodied being. Swami Bhajanananda points out that an ordinary person who has attained greatness in any field, for example social service, art, or science, can influence the lives of thousands.[20] But the great prophets and world teachers appear as the embodiment of the dominant ideal of a particular age whose lives affect millions for centuries. The ancient ideal of the jīvan-mukta, however, had its limitations. Swami Bhajanananda states that the great Indian teacher, Sri Ramakrishna,* taught that the ideal person, the perfected being, was one who not only strives for liberation for himself as the jīvan-mukta has successfully done, but for the liberation of others. Sri Ramakrishna was the first modern teacher to introduce into Hinduism a Vedantic counterpart of the bodhisattva ideal in Buddhism: one who turns away from nirvāna and works for the welfare of others. The ideal for our own age, Sri Ramakrishna believed, is the *vijñāni,* literally meaning one who "sees knowledge," that is, one who fully understands Reality.[21]

In the Western world, Pierre Pradervand, author and personal development facilitator in the field of social justice, says there are two types of people: those for whom the spiritual quest is no more than a search for personal development and well-being, and those who have reached a stage of illumination, through intense and disciplined practice, who are committed to "spiritual service."[22] The transformation from one stage

---

*Sri Ramakrishna (1836–1886), the rustic Bengali mystic who became the teacher of Swami Vivekananda and other influential Indian figures, was a Hindu priest, who was also initiated into Islam by Govinda Roy, a Hindu guru who practiced Sufism, then practiced Christian spirituality for a time, during which the culminating experience was of merging his body with that of Christ. The British historian Arnold Toynbee wrote that, like Mahatma Gandhi, Sri Ramakrishna realized that despite some differences, all religions lead to the same goal, an example of the spirit that makes it possible for the human race to grow together into a single family, which is the only alternative to destroying ourselves.

of being to the other seems to arise from the healing of the self at a deep level, from understanding and resolving conflicts that arise from fear, insecurity, difficult relationships, and the inability to express love and creativity. As we saw in chapter 1, Feuerstein believes that the tools for this transformation are contained within the many paths of Yoga and meditation. By focusing on the subtle bodies, on the planes of existence, the kośas, and the chakras, the energy centers associated with levels of development, we are able to understand how the conflicts in our lives induce crisis, and the prajñā, the wisdom or insight, the "clear seeing," that follows can enable us to change our ways of being and thinking.

Nirvāna

Nirvāna is a characteristic of "Buddha consciousness," the word itself derived from the root *va*, "to blow" and the negative prefix *nih*, which together mean "blowing out," usually translated as "passing away." Although in the life story of Buddha nirvāna referred to his final passing away or extinction, it is generally taken to mean the passing away of any person's desire and the death of his or her "old self." In many religious traditions, the aspirant may take a new name to indicate his or her newly acquired identity. The self that is experienced as the center of consciousness is the seat of energy and the generator of desire. However, since, according to Collins, there is no sense of self in the transformed state, there is also no sense of suffering from unfulfilled desire. While in Buddha's case this meant a final "passing away" with no rebirth into other lives, which would have brought the renewal of suffering, in the life of the ordinary person the passing away of the old life with its painful emotions and strong attachments brings moments of peace and contentment. And while the struggle goes on, freedom can be glimpsed through the sustained practice of meditation.

In her mystical writings, St. Teresa of Avila also describes the ascent of the soul. She sees four stages, and her account has features in common with Collins' description of the Buddha's experience:

> Heart's devotion: This is the stage of devout contemplation or concentration, which she describes as withdrawal of the soul from without and as

focusing on the devout observance of the passion of Christ, and on penitence.

> Devotion of peace: The human will is lost in that of God by virtue of a charismatic, supernatural state given of God, while the other faculties, such as memory, reason, and imagination, are not yet secure from worldly distraction. While a partial distraction is due to outer performances such as repetition of prayers and writing down of spiritual thoughts, the prevailing state is one of quietude.

> Devotion of union: An ecstatic state that she describes as characterized by a blissful peace, a sweet slumber of at least the higher soul faculties, a conscious rapture in the love of God.

> Devotion of ecstasy or rapture: Consciousness of being in the body disappears, sense activity ceases, memory and imagination are also absorbed in God, in a state she describes as "intoxicated," when body and spirit are in the throes of a sweet, happy pain, alternating between a fearful, fiery glow and such a state of ecstasy that she feels lifted into space.[23]

This last state is the climax of mystical experience, from which the trance state is produced. St. Teresa wrote in her *Autobiography* that from this state she often awakened in tears.

Meditation Studies

The practice of meditation, as hundreds of scientific studies over decades have shown, appears to be one of the most successful ways of effecting transformation in the individual and, ultimately, may have a long-term effect on the "crisis of consciousness" that Gebser predicted would awaken us to the need to go beyond our narrow personal concerns to serve the evolution of humanity and the survival of our planet.[24]

Let us now look briefly at the field of meditation to see how these states of transformation arise from particular spiritual practices. Since the early 1930s, empirical studies of meditation and other forms of contemplative experience have been a subject of scientific interest, particularly in Britain, Europe, India, Japan, and America. Recent surveys of the entire field by Michael Murphy of the Esalen Institute,[25] Jon Kabat-Zinn at the University of Massachusetts Medical Center,[26] and many others reveal that even today experiments in nonordinary experiences, religious or spiritual, tend to focus on the physical, neurological, or chemical changes effected, a narrow focus that dichotomizes the person. In these studies, spirit is associated with the brain while the body is separated from the manifestations of the spirit.

As research scientist Professor Olga Louchakova and transpersonal psychologist Dr. Arielle S. Warner have noted, in its attempts to demonstrate the neural basis for spiritual experience "science does not render a definitive scientific account," as it leaves "will, choice, desire, insight, revelation and capacity to act outside the reach of inquiry" and there is, therefore, "an emerging need for a new theory."[27] They have attempted to address this problem by positing a model of "Psychosomatic Mysticism" (PM), which designates those dimensions of spiritual traditions that observe, utilize, and focus on the various forms of spiritual insight associated with awareness of the lived body or, putting it another way, relate to the parts of mystical tradition that recognize the broad *body-related* manifestations of spirituality. The purposes of the PM model are:

> To recognize the common principles of somatospiritual experiences.
>
> To show through studies in neuroimmunology that the body does have the material faculties to mediate the higher expressions of consciousness.
>
> To show that the traditional transpersonal systems emphasize the development and use of these systems.
>
> To examine how a body-related phenomenology of consciousness, expressed as spiritual experiences and a spectrum of subtle energies and neuroimmunological findings, complement each other and open avenues to the wholeness of the self.[28]

Louchakova and Warner researched not only the main traditions of the East but also some recent and still-current Western traditions. See the comparison table starting on page 330, which summarizes their results. They also conducted extensive interviews with traditional teachers of Hesychasm (an early Christian mysticism), Taoist alchemy, kundalinī yoga, Sakta Vedanta, and Bektashi Sufism in Russia, India, and Turkey and with living practitioners and teachers of a number of other contemporary eclectic esoteric schools. These included the esoteric Christianity of Gurdjieff in Russia, France, and the United States, the psychophysical self-regulation of Vladimir Antonov in Russia, Estonia, and Eastern Europe, the "Diamond Heart of Almaas" in the United States and Europe, Kebza of Yagan in Canada, and the Arika system of Oscar Ichaso in Chile and the United States.*

In their analysis of these systems, Louchakova and Warner state that, in contrast to psychology and neuroscience, many spiritual traditions have long recognized the body as the locus of transformation of consciousness and that it is "body-based mysticism" that offers the technical knowledge required for practice through awareness of the subtle energies of the body. According to their theory of psychosomatic mysticism, "consciousness is the body (not only the brain) and the body is consciousness via the spectrum of subtle energies." The authors find that there are numerous health benefits, and a number of skills associated with energy-based health practices, and in the systems they looked at "the knowledge of the 'ensouled' spiritual body can lead to the understanding of subtle mechanisms underlying spiritual changes in perception, transformations of awareness, emergence of altered states, non-pathologizing characterological transformations and developmental shifts in self-identity constituting the core of spiritual growth and human completion."[29]

When one considers the opposition once mounted

---

*Most of these teachers are better known in the United States than in Britain, just as there are spiritual teachers in Britain and Europe who are probably unknown to the researchers. Louchakova and Warner's study omitted Celtic spiritual practices from all the Celtic countries: Scotland, Ireland, Wales, and Brittany, which also have a following in Belgium. They state that questions of classification regarding the genealogy of the various forms, their mutual enrichment, and the relationship between PM and mystical philosophies such as Persian Philosophy of Illumination or the Neo-Platonic thought of Pseudo-Dionysius remain to be researched. Shamanism, too, is not covered, as the forms of embodied awareness in shamanism are extremely complex and require special research attention. For those interested in shamanism Michael Winkelman's study of the physiological processes of altered states in shamanism might be a good place to start.

against it, it is gratifying that Louchakova and Warner observe that the Indian system of kundalinī tantra is particularly successful in giving deep appreciation of the spiritual structures through its theories of the subtle anatomy. They believe that kundalinī tantra describes, and offers methods of recognizing, seven chakras that correspond to seven segments of the body. Chakras are considered to operate as spatially represented domains of stable clusters of psychological experiences.[30] For example, the root chakra, identified as an interior space of consciousness appearing when the practitioner focuses attention inside the area between the pubic bone and the sacrum, is associated with survival and psychological-social stability. The throat chakra is associated with the development of capacity for discernment, moral sense, congruence of expression, sense of beauty and exaltation.[31]* Chakras also serve as entrances into the subtle states of consciousness, and as transformers of energy and emotions in the alchemical forms of kundalinī tantra. Louchakova and Warner give examples of how emotional or mental states may be transformed. By moving concentration between the solar plexus and heart chakras (a movement we noted in qigong practice), the practitioner can cause the transformation of the emotion of anger into the emotion of compassion. "In our study, we observed how by focusing in the various regions of the head chakra the practitioner can initiate the experiences of clairvoyance, absorption in pure consciousness, light, void, or interior silence."[32]

Louchakova and Warner found that, depending on which centers become actualized during the process of spiritual development, one can have a variety of psychological and spiritual experiences, accompanying different forms of spiritual awakening. These may range from gradual deep intrapersonal work to wide opening of empathetic connection to community, and to ascetic forms of spiritual life characterized by extreme detachment. In contrast to the example of kundalinī tantrism, Hesychasm—from *hesychia,* meaning "stillness, rest, quiet, silence," an eremitic tradition of prayer in the Eastern Orthodox Church—is presented as another example, though in less detail. Hesychasm does not involve all the centers of the body but, rather,

specializes in the knowledge of the centers of the chest in which its whole map of the psyche is contained.* It begins its exploration of consciousness with the focusing of the attention of practitioners on the inner space of the chest in the region where "all the powers of the soul reside."[33]

Most interesting for our purpose here, Louchakova and Warner also noted differences in the way that the different goals among the spiritual models shaped their outcomes. For example, they state that "Hindu Kundalinī Yoga focuses on individuation, while Christian Hesychasm focuses on interrelatedness, both requiring balancing of the type of self-to-community relationships congruent with their cultures of origin (e.g., the Hindu practice compensates or counterbalances the *inter*dependent Indian type of self while the Christian practice helps to neutralise the isolation of the *in*dependent Western type of self)."[34] This clearly shows the recognition of the value of "wholeness," of a balanced "roundedness" of character, and raises the broad question of what, in general and in regard to ethics, a transformation of a personality should achieve, the word *should* being used here in the sense of the *ethical* (not the logical) *ought*. If this were a book on ethics this question would have occurred at its beginning, but in this book it arises now, in a final chapter dealing, in part, with *our personal response to understanding,* and it demands to be dealt with, however briefly, before we continue. Some clarity with regard to it cannot but help our appreciation of the matters in hand.

Like all ethical judgments, the question of what personal transformation *ought* to achieve is a *value* judgment, which is *itself* a value judgment or choice among alternatives, *depending upon our valuation of ethics itself* and also on our *relative* valuations, within ethics, of particular ethical questions, their relationships, and the possible courses of action. This, we would contend, is how most of us use our ethical sense in practice. Ethics is thus recursive, self-referential, a strange loop. We sense its authority, yet when we try to explain it we find that its hierarchy of authority is confused. It is a

---

*A detailed study of the behavioral aspects of the chakras can be found in Swami Rama et. al., *Yoga and Psychotherapy: The Evolution of Consciousness,* 1976.

---

*Note that in the Sufi traditions it is taught that there are three centers, side by side, across the chest. This arrangement also corresponds with the arrangement in the Kabbalistic Tree of Life. Hinduism also recognizes them, as the *granthi* ("knots," or blocks in subtle energy), only one of which is counted among the seven principal chakras.

rational and wise whole, at least in the view of those who have given it honest thought, but its "truth" is unprovable by linear argument from any premises, and seems to be at least to some degree personal. Hence, no doubt, the ancient perception of karma, and hence also its relevance to questions of our relationship with the "above." We *choose* our ethics, according to our *ethical* principles (herein is the circularity), and it seems difficult to prove anything more than that a complete lack of ethics is obviously and self-demonstratingly destructive of both the victim and, though perhaps only later, the perpetrator. No one can prove to the selfish that it is "better" to share. The selfish person lives in his own world and sees with dazzling clarity that he is right and you a fool. The world itself will have to present him with the φαινομενον, the disclosure out-from the hidden, which will one day change his mind.

We all carry with us, whether conscious of the fact or not, a largely preconsidered set of values, which themselves show a hierarchy, some being always more important than others (such as giving up a pleasurable stroll beside the village pond to save a drowning child), some being invoked according to the individual facts of a case (such as whether or not to allow your child a pleasure she craves), yet others invoked only when it seems that all prior ethical claims upon us have been met, such as the search for our own pleasure or fulfillment. And since meditation is a source of "pleasure" for those with some skill in it, the question we set ourselves at the beginning of this final chapter, namely how we should place ourselves as close as possible to the Great Being, is an ethical question at all levels. Giving ourselves this pleasure is no less a pleasure on account of its also being a duty. It is part of the evolution of the world, a drawing down of sun and moon into a world that very much needs both. Yet duty should never be performed out of a sense of duty if it can be performed in love. But can it have moral worth if it is performed so easily as it is when we feel love? Ethical choices, too, need to be intuitively, rather than intellectually, determined. There is a hierarchy even among *them*.

James Austin's chapter "Consciousness Evolves when the Self Dissolves" in the symposium *Cognitive Models and Spiritual Maps* includes the chart below, pertinent to our concerns here. We must note that "duality" shown in this chart is not mind-body duality, but "I-thou" duality, the interpersonal, social, moral duality, and return to Louchakova and Warner. The tables on pages 330–32 appear in their article, and are reproduced here with their kind permission.

The Dissolution of	Means Subtracting	And Is Experienced As
I	The aggressive "doing self." Self-concepts in time.	Freedom from compulsive doing, from "shoulds" and "oughts." Timelessness.
ME	The besieged and fearful self.	Fearlessness. Deep peace.
MINE	The clutching self that 1. had possessed other persons and things. 2. had been captured by its own dualistic attitudes.	The world as *it* really is without self-referent attachments. The world's original diversity, coherence and unity.[35]

SUMMARIZED COMPARISON OF SPIRITUAL TRADITIONS

Name, Affiliation and History	Methodology: Body-Centers of Consciousness; Central Practices; Goals of Work	Major Achievements and Practical Implications
In Christianity: Hesychasm Appeared in Egyptian Desert in the first centuries A.D., spread to Byzantium, later to Greece and Russia. Declined around the 8th century, and became very active again around the 14–15th century.	Focus on Spiritual Heart Center; methods include specific type of mindfulness ("sobriety") inner silence and the psychosomatic Prayer of the Heart (Dubrovin, 1990); goal is Theosis, i.e. Union with God.	Described the association of thinking, imagination, archetypes, sense of self, various modes of awareness and emotions with the chest area. Developed methods of character transformation through the specific techniques of focusing in the centers of consciousness in the chest. Can have practical applications in the treatment and prevention of cardiovascular pathology (Louchakova, 2002).
In Islam: sections of Sufism which acknowledge the lataif (subtle body system of centers), such as the Northern African Sufism, the Naqshbandi order, or the system of Simnani. Emerge independently after 6th century in Middle Asia, Persia, and India.	Mainly centers of the chest. Practices: attitudinal, awareness, internal concentrations and variants of internal and external *dhikr*. Goal depends on the philosophy of the particular system, and the faculties of the adept. Goal: various degrees of Union.	Spiritual psychology, healing systems, and the methods of "engineering" the character. Lots of community-building practices, methods of dialogue and social healing. There is a significant cultural dimension.
In Hinduism: **Kundalinī** *Tantra*, originated around 3000 B.C., in Tamil Nadu, Southern India. Mainly active in 5th–8th century and around the 15th century.	Whole body system of chakras, centers and spiritual meridians; the emphasis is on the centers of the head and of the chest, and 3 major spiritual meridians; practices consist mainly of the internal concentrations with ritual visualizations. Goal is the union of all possible opposites, including the opposition of transcendent awareness and manifestation. Expressions of this goal may vary (Briggs, 1938/1998) depending on the individual predisposition and the type of "spiritual destiny" of the seeker.	The whole psyche is placed into the body, and the psychological and spiritual faculties are attributed to various centers of embodied consciousness. Developed elaborate philosophy of intentional consciousness, evolutionary Kundalinī theory, and body-based life-span oriented spiritual psychology. Has precise knowledge of the subtle energies. Can contribute to body-based psychological theory, clinical methods of character transformation, and to the understanding and treatment of the systemic diseases, such as multiple sclerosis or cancer. Hatha yoga, as the offspring of the system, has many health-related outcomes. Has a unique way of enhancement of human development and mental health due to methodology of working with psychological opposites.
Kashmir Shaivism; specific form of Kundalinī Tantra, which has independent scriptural and oral sources. Appears in Kashmir, Northern India, around the 15th century.	Chakra system, main focus on the centers of the brain. Extremely broad set of practices includes unique concentrations, visualization, awareness, group guided meditation (Muller-Ortega, 1989). Has a developed philosophy of recognition of Reality and aesthetics theory; goal is the recognition of the Ultimate Reality, personalized as Shiva.	Discovered how the individual differences affect spiritual development and meditation; developed more than a hundred meditative methods which can be used in psychological healing practice. Discovered the ego-harmonization- and ego-transcendence-related effects of beauty.

Name, Affiliation and History	Methodology: Body-Centers of Consciousness; Central Practices; Goals of Work	Major Achievements and Practical Implications
Some forms of Shakta Vedanta (Hinduism), such as the **teachings of Sri Ramana Maharshi** in the 20th century.	Focus on the center of I-consciousness on the right side of the chest; method of introspective self-inquiry leading to experiential self-knowledge. Goal is liberation/Self-realization.	Unique practice of *Samādhi*, i.e. absorption in the nondual consciousness. Our preliminary research suggests that this practice can help in managing and treating narcissistic personality disorder, psychosis, etc. Needs clinical trials and more research.
In Buddhism: Tibetan Tantra Vajrayana. Appears in Northern India around the 7th century A.D. (Lama Kunzang Rinpoche, August 24, 2002, personal communication).	Centers of the whole body with the focus on the abdomen, heart, and head. Practice involves breath techniques, concentration, visualization of the subtle forms of energy, and worshipful use of sacred rites. Goal is the union of opposites, with the female principle of manifested world (*Candali*) uniting with her Lord (awareness principle). Results in the experience of the uncreated light, *prabhasvara* (Sanskrit).	Specific contribution is the understanding of compassion, and development of psychological techniques intensively purifying the subconscious and causing integration of the self via work with embodied structures of the psyche (Lama Kunzang Rinpoche, August 24, 2002, personal communication). Successful attempts were made to use the practices of the Tibetan dream yoga in psychological work (Stefik, 1999).
Zen Buddhism. First text dated 11th century traces it back to Buddha. In Japan Zen was introduced from Korea in 6th century.	Hara center in the lower belly (Durkheim, 1962). Practice involves primarily concentration. Goal of the Hara training is re-rooting one's life in this center, associated with original Oneness.	The knowledge of "malformations" of the self. The original psychological system to be researched. Has potential to actualize latent faculties which seem near-"miraculous," very high productivity, focus, healthy self-esteem, adaptability, stress resistance etc.
In Taoism: Alchemy. First written evidence is found in 11th century China.	3 centers corresponding to the lower, middle and upper body. Dynamic internal concentrations, leading to integration of all the regions of the body and transformation of energies. Goal varies from recognition of Tao to individual immortality.	Developed large number of healing methods, unique system of energy-based medicine, methods of work with emotions and of actualization of hidden potential of human being, such as longevity. The energy knowledge of Taoism and Buddhism gave birth to martial arts systems and many movement systems such as *Bagua, Tai Chi, Wu-Shu, Qi-Gong* etc., transforming energy and mind.
Contemporary eclectic esoteric schools, adapted to local cultural contexts. Esoteric Christianity of Gurdjieff in Russia, France, U.S.A.; Psychophysical self-regulation of Antonov in Russia, Estonia, Eastern Europe; Diamond Heart of Almaas in U.S., Europe; Kebza of Yagan in Canada; Arika of Ichaso in Chili, U.S.[36]	Usually draws on PM in major religious tradition, and adapts practices cross-culturally. Often concentrates on relatedness, and brings in the ecological dimension.	Assist healing, development and transformation of the self in cultural context. Usually carry some kind of adaptation to an historical task and help to restore the healthy self.

MEANING-STRUCTURES ASSOCIATED WITH THE ZONES OF THE EMBODIED CONSCIOUSNESS IN PSYCHOSOMATIC MYSTICISM

Zones of the Body	Psychological Aspects	Spiritual Aspects
Head	Archetypes, unconscious; embodied awareness of deep characterological transformation.	Divine names, finding one's own spiritual family, uncreated light, void, opening of the space of pure consciousness, ego-transcendence.
Neck and collar zone	Changes of verbal expression and perception.	Rise of discrimination; impossibility of living an inauthentic life.
Trunk above the diaphragm, chest predominantly	Deconstruction of the false (narcissistic) self, rise of true psychological self.	Experience of oneself as pure consciousness, essential Self. Later, possibilities of experiencing cosmic Self.
Lower body below the diaphragm, trunk predominantly[37]	Beginning of work with subconscious.	Paranormal, psychic, non-normative experiences.

Note: The developmental process involves changes in perception, self-awareness, identification, values, and personality structure. Spiritual experiences are but landmarks amid the overall changes of the self. In the developmental process (the kundalinī process), the centers are actualized from the bottom upward.

Life after Illumination

As we saw in earlier chapters, the goal of many spiritual systems is to attain what Louchakova and Warner designate "the grand goals of human fulfillment—such as Enlightenment, Liberation or Union."[38] But out of this process other significant changes accompanying the actualizing of cosmic consciousness may have an important effect not only on the self of the individual but also on those with whom the person interacts personally and socially. For example, in Hinduism and kundalinī tantra, the practices that relate to the union of psychological opposites may lead to increased awareness of the effects of intentionality in resolving conflicts. Those forms of Sakta Vedanta that emphasize introspective self-inquiry can help reduce narcissistic behavior, and Tibetan Buddhist Tantra deepens the understanding of compassion and kindness as a way of relating to others through practices that promote ego-transcendence.[39] Many contemporary Western approaches are also believed to help the healing, development, and maturation of the self in their own cultural contexts. The writings of Alice Bailey and others of the Theosophy movement, for example, emphasize the importance of "spiritual service" both as a path to, and as a result of, personal growth. Each causes the other and brings new wholeness to the person.

According to Swami Bhajanananda, the most important quality in the spiritually evolved person is concern for the welfare of humankind.[40] Although many spiritual teachers in the past have been social or religious reformers, such as Swami Vivekananda and Sri Aurobindo, leading their nation out of the "dark ages" of foreign oppression to the independence of self-governance, not all meditators or spiritually aware people have the calling, inclination, or charisma for this kind of work. Whether recognizing this difference between individuals or not, many have taught that the ideal or perfected state comes not from limiting ourselves to fulfilling our own personal aspirations, but by striving for the liberation of others from pain, misery, isolation, and ignorance through loving, understanding, and compassionate use of whatever personal skills we have.

In her book *Serving Humanity*, Alice Bailey states that we are called to demonstrate spiritual activity in this age according to human need and in service of the Great Being or Higher Beings in the celestial hierarchy. She believes that in past ages it was the service of one's own soul (with the emphasis upon one's own individual salvation) that engrossed the attention of the aspirant. She also states that worship of, or service to, an incarnate spiritual master or teacher is no longer of dominant interest but that three great sciences will come to the fore in the "New Age" and will lead humanity from the "unreal to the real and from aspiration to realization." These are, she says:

> The science of Meditation, the coming science of the mind.
> The science of Antahkarana, or the science of the bridging which must take place between the higher and lower mind.
> The science of Service, which is a definite technique of at-one-ment.[41]*

She claims that "when men achieve illumination, intelligently precipitate the karmic quota of their time, and lift the subhuman kingdoms (with the reflex action of lifting the highest simultaneously), then they can and do share in the work of the Hierarchy."[42] Earlier she explains what she means by "illumination." She regards humanity as the "planetary light bearer, transmitting the light of knowledge, of wisdom and of understanding, and this in the esoteric sense. These three aspects of light carry three aspects of soul energy to the soul in all forms, through the medium of the anima mundi, the world soul . . . The downpouring spiritual Triangle and the upraising matter Triangle meet point to point in humanity, where the point of balance can be found. In man's achievement and spiritualization is the hope of the world."[43] (See plate 36.)

Bailey also points to meditation as the means of awakening consciousness, a process to which she refers as "bringing the lower man under the control of the spiritual man," which, she says, "will awaken the centers of force in the etheric body and stimulate into activity that mysterious stream of energy which sleeps at the base of the spinal column." Life should be lived in steady practice of "one-pointed intent" over a long period of time, with detachment and "in parallel with a life of loving service." When a person has done all this, she says, and

---

*The neologism *at-one-ment,* "making one with," is a pun on the English *atonement,* found in the Bible in passages relating to Mosaic Law, which probably arose as a conceit of preachers, but the Biblical *atonement* is quite different, meaning "expiation for sin," which required a blood sacrifice under Mosaic Law. *At-one-ment* means simply "reconciliation," and is, of course, opposite to Christianity, but Bailey's usage probably envisages *only* such "at-one-ment," such unification, without any reference to blood sacrifice.

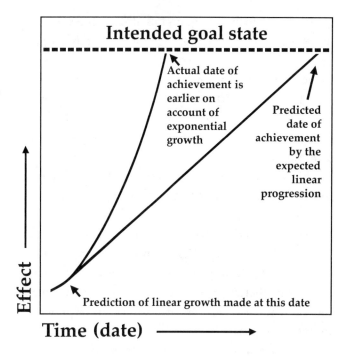

Fig. 18.1. Growth is often quicker than has been anticipated.

"built the necessary vibrating material into his three lower bodies . . . suddenly he may see, suddenly he may hear, suddenly he may sense [that] aspiration has become recognition. . . . Your meditation should now be regarded by you as a process of penetration, carried forward as an act of service, with the intent of bringing enlightenment to others.[44]

Transforming the Earth

The question of what the effect may be of some ten million people in Britain meditating every day, plus several billion others around the world, has intrigued British scientist Peter Russell. In his book *The Global Brain* he speculates on the effects of long-term meditation practice on individuals and on the consequences for society and the planet. He agrees with the contention that "What humanity urgently needs today are the means to bring about a widespread shift in consciousness. This will come about not through a revival of any particular religion but through a revival of the techniques and experiences that once gave these teachings life and effectiveness. We need to rediscover the practices that directly enable the experience of the pure Self and facilitate its permanent integration into our lives." Further, he believes that this integration is already under way. As we begin to combine the growing understanding of the brain and consciousness with the knowledge and techniques of mystics and spiritual teachers, he says, we will be better able to see how the teachings work, how they can be improved or developed, and how best to facilitate the transition from "experimental steam engine to mass transportation."[45]

However, Russell also points to the argument of some commentators that the number of individuals involved in inner growth is very small and, regardless of the effect of such efforts on the people themselves, they are unlikely to have any significant impact on humanity as a whole. He answers this by pointing out that when making predictions about the future we often unconsciously assume a linear growth pattern. If the growth is in fact exponential any goal will be reached much sooner, as illustrated in figure 18.1. He compares the movement for personal growth with the growth of information technology, and illustrates the facts graphically. "Rapid as the growth of the information industry is, it may not be the fastest-growing area of human activity. There are indications that the movement toward the transformation of consciousness is growing even faster. In terms of sheer numbers the movement may not at present be very significant, but it shows a doubling time of about four years, which makes it one of the steepest growth curves society has ever seen."[46]

The findings from several studies on changing social values conducted over the past twenty years* reveal a steady shift in the relative weight given to different values. As we remarked earlier, choices are being made among the available ethics, and it seems that at least some of those choices are being made on the basis of ethics itself, not of selfishness. The number of people referred to by Feuerstein (see part 1) as following the karma yoga path, who are motivated by "outer-directed values" such as the need to feel more materially secure, or to be in positions of power, is steadily decreasing. Meanwhile, there is a steady increase of those motivated by "inner-directed" values, which express themselves in several different ways. Among these are concern for health, growing support for ecological and environmen-

*For example, the Values and Lifestyle Study in the United States and the European International Research Institute's study on social change.[47]

tal groups, and a greater awareness of the need to act according to our sense of right and wrong.

Russell points out that only a proportion of those interested in raising consciousness actually work in what might be thought the most directly related professions, such as teachers, therapists, meditation guides, and so forth, but if the growth of general interest continues so will the number of people employed in the field. We could eventually reach a point where "consciousness processing" would have become the dominant area of human activity. We would have shifted from the Information Age into the Consciousness Age, and wisdom rather than knowledge would be society's goal. He adds that while this may sound like science fiction, the speculation that this evolution will occur is plausible since some of humanity is already traveling in the required direction.[48]

Effects on Society

What effects, then, would those involved in consciousness-raising have on the rest of society? Effects upon society as a whole will necessarily involve aggregates of effects brought about between individuals, and such effects are already well observed if not yet fully explained. One frequently cited study of the effects of collective meditation demonstrated an increase in the coherence of brain activity within the individual, but there was also an apparent entrainment of the brain rhythms of others throughout a group of three thousand meditators, and a further influence upon another, smaller, group meditating a thousand miles away. When the smaller group meditated unaware that the larger group was also meditating at the same time, entrainment of the rhythms of those in the small group intensified.[49] This provided evidence acceptable to science of the objective reality of some kind of collective consciousness and of mind-to-mind influence. In fact the process resembles that by which electromagnetic waves are brought into phase as a laser starts up. As so often, the central notion, that of coherence between minds, is far from new. The Vedic tradition posits a pervasive field of pure consciousness as the ground of all individual minds. The thoughts and perceptions of individuals are believed to be the fluctuations or modulations of this underlying ground state of a Field of Consciousness of which each Being is a part.

We might postulate that the more coherent, less

excited, state-of-brain produced in the smaller group of meditators when the larger group was itself already in this state will be inherently more peaceable than an uninfluenced state, and that the incoherent state, by contrast, is one and the same as the state we recognize as that of mental stress. Note what has been done here. We have suggested a physicalist mapping of or correspondence with the state of mental stress onto measurable, graphable, brain processes. Maharishi Mahesh Yogi was, with others, a prominent advocate of the view, implicit in that mapping, that as a nation's internal stress level increases it reaches a point when civil unrest or even large-scale violence and war with other nations (upon which a society's own faults can be projected) makes military action inevitable.

Despite the fact that the mechanisms are not yet fully understood, possible applications of the new knowledge soon became apparent, and have been tested. The aim of what we might call the "Jerusalem Experiment" was to demonstrate that a small proportion of meditators in a society can influence for the better the life of that society as a whole. In 1983 a much larger experiment was very carefully designed to quantify as accurately and as objectively as possible the effects of groups of meditators. The chosen real-world situation for the experiment was the millennia-long Arab-Israeli conflict that adversely affects the quality of life for all concerned. The testable hypothesis underlying the experiment was that a sufficiently large group of meditators, sitting in Jerusalem, would improve the quality of life in Jerusalem, in Israel as a whole, and even in Lebanon, with which Israel was actively at war at the time. The expected result was that the conflict would, to a measurable extent, be calmed. Naturally, any calming effect would also show in other areas of life. Road accidents and crime rates might be reduced. All these were measured, and even the incidence of fires.

The results naturally cannot be given in full here. A few of the changes were too small to reach statistical significance but a reduction in road accidents as high as 34.4 percent was recorded. The war with Lebanon, measured by deaths per day, showed a reduction of no less than 75.9 percent over the period of the experiment, from a mean of 40.1 deaths per day to 9.7 per day. Fires reduced by 30.4 percent. A Composite Index of Quality of Life showed a clear parallel with the size of the meditating group.[50]

Although scientific attempts to explain the results of this and other such investigations are complex, involving quantum field theory and quantum entanglement,* they seem to indicate that as more and more people experience higher states of consciousness, others gradually experience a similar, if weaker, effect, possibly through quantum interconnection, or via an even "higher" all-encompassing Being surrounding our whole universe. People influenced in this way, it is believed, eventually find it easier to reach the same altered states themselves. This connectivity within the human race clearly relates to the question of the extent and the range of influence of the subtle part of our being, that which, for example, showed Pat Price the gantry crane running to and fro over a factory in Russia ten thousand miles from where he sat.[51]

Peter Russell speculates about what such society-wide developments in consciousness would bring both for the individual and for human society. He suggests that while biological, chemical, and physical laws would not dramatically change, our individual functioning as conscious self-directing beings in the material world already shows the beginnings of a synergy that will alter our collective behavior, and the laws of sociology, economics, and politics that govern us. Humanity will begin to live in harmony with its planet-wide environment and with itself. Although he presents an optimistic view of the future, he reminds us that the problems facing us now—crime, pollution, hunger, unemployment, homelessness, and so on—would not magically disappear and would still require individual and collective willed action to resolve, but our attitudes would have changed and our worldview would have been transformed, effects that inherently tend toward that goal.[52]

As we become more socially responsible through "spiritual service," Russell believes, we could expect to see new abilities appearing as indications of greater interconnectivity and of a unitive level of consciousness.[53] These would include increased incidence of healing ability, synchronicity, telepathy, and clairvoyant states, faculties that some researchers, such as the physicists Russell Targ and Harold Puthoff, believe are latent in us all,[54] and which former Princeton professor and parapsychologist Dean Radin recognizes as those pragmatic consequences of meditation that mystics and spiritual teachers have long considered to be the result of transformation brought about by consistent and skillful spiritual practice.[55]

---

*See chapter 15.

However, just as practitioners in early Hindu society were cautioned by Patanjali not to be distracted by the appearance in their lives of spiritual powers, then known as siddhis and long afterward termed "glamours" by Alice Bailey, so today we need to remember that if and when they manifest they are merely tools. If, but only if, they are put to use in the service of humanity rather than to fulfill ego-desires they will help us transcend the problems of society, renew our planet, and bring about a more peaceful and sustainable world.

"Finding a positive direction for the next transformation of civilization is a challenging, but not an insuperable, task," Ervin Laszlo believes. "We know that a viable new civilization must evolve a culture and consciousness very different from the mindset that characterized most of the twentieth century. Such *lógos*-inspired civilization was materialistic and manipulative, driven by the search for wealth and power. The alternative to it is civilization centered on human development, and the development of the communities and the environments in which humans live their lives."[56]

In the final analysis, the essence of the esoteric worldview, bringing Eastern and Western into one, is that the many systems and paths to transcendence all lead to the highest normal experience of being human. There is evidence that the subtle body is a *real* but, by present definitions of physics, *nonphysical* entity, impossible to observe and impossible to experience except for the "owner" himself or herself. Introspective analysis is difficult, and perhaps only reliably possible in meditation, which is itself difficult if the meditator attends to such an objective instead of to the experience of pure consciousness itself. At that level of meditation the sitter is indeed self-observing, for there is nothing else to observe, yet even so is no longer external to the experience. The self-observer has to be quiet, detached, unobtrusive, if he or she is not to interfere with what is experienced, his or her own consciousness, a situation curiously parallel to that of the undisturbed propagation of waves and the subsequent "mutual measuring" by wavicles, which then condense into physical (unconscious) "reality." The spiritually aware mind-state seems analogous to wave propagation, the ordinary somatic state analogous to that of matter. How substantive such a parallel might be is a topic for speculation for which only meditators, perhaps not even they, are qualified.

However, even to the "outside" view, the Hermetic claim that "As things are above, so they are below" seems universally true of part-to-whole dualities. Madhva, denying Advaita, recognized that while we can hardly claim to be the whole of Brahman, we can each claim to be a small part of Brahman. As it must, our initial discovery of the subtle body takes place largely via its externally observable *effects,* which we have discussed throughout this book. We learn of it via the world-about, which is the ground not of spirituality but of physics. The known limitation of physics to the world of the *external* senses, discussed in chapter 15, shows that physics may not be able to extend in the way required to bring the subtle body within its realm except in regard to quantum interconnection. The subtle body's exact position in the hierarchy from the above down to the below is uncertain. Some believe it ranges over several levels, in effect having layers within itself. In any event there seems to be an interface of some kind between the stolidly physical and the highly spiritual. Physics may be able only to *assist,* from outside, the other means of discovering any entity that stubbornly shows itself to be *there,* yet to be nonphysical. That "other means" appears to be meditation, the attainment of states of consciousness that seem to put us in direct touch with the above. Nonetheless, physics itself gives strong support to hypotheses now emerging as to how we should describe the subtle body and as to how it "works."

While no more than a frame of reference or a map for the journey to a destination, the *concept* of the subtle body (as contrasted with the subtle body as it is in itself), is at least serviceable to that end and if we are to know and experience it at all, we have to "*go there,*" presumably, as we have said, in meditation, in one or other of its many forms. Then, no doubt, we shall also discover at least a little more of what the subtle body *is.* The science of the subtle body (which may, as many have thought, prove broader than any extended *physics*) can also then begin. "The only means of knowing what is, as opposed to knowing *ideas on* what is, is *gnosis,*" Holman says in *The Return of the Perennial Philosophy*. "There seems to be a broad consensus today that we need a new map—a new *Naturphilosophie* that, as Antoine Faivre says, 'would associate the flesh with the flame,'" a flame, we hasten to add, that does not consume, but enlivens what it touches. "Upon the dissemination and general acceptance of this," Holman continues, "the ideal society (or at least a better one) depends."[57]

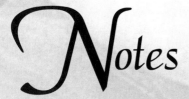

Notes

Preface

1. Collins, *Mysticism and New Paradigm Psychology*, 1.
2. Walsh, *The Spirit of Evolution*, 30.
3. Davidson, "Concomitants of Meditation: A Cross-Sectional Study," 227.
4. Collins, *Mysticism and New Paradigm Psychology*, x.
5. Feuerstein, "Foreword" in Govindan, *Kriya Yoga Sutras of Patanjali and the Siddhas*, xv.
6. Govindan, *Kriya Yoga Sutras of Patanjali and the Siddhas*, 186.

Introduction

1. White, *The Alchemical Body*, 15.
2. Tansley, *Subtle Body: Essence and Shadow*, 5.

Chapter 1. The Spiritual Enterprise

1. Eliade, *Yoga: Immortality and Freedom*, 4, 301.
2. Organ, *The Hindu Quest for the Perfection of Man*, 66.
3. Ibid., 148.
4. Feuerstein, *The Yoga Tradition: Its History, Literature, Philosophy and Practice*, 6.
5. Ibid.
6. Ibid., 350.
7. Gebser, *The Ever-Present Origin*, 45.
8. Feuerstein, *The Yoga Tradition*, 92–93.
9. Gebser, *The Ever-Present Origin*, 45.
10. Ibid., 45–60.
11. Ibid.
12. Ibid., 46.
13. Feuerstein, *The Yoga Tradition*, 93.
14. Gebser, *The Ever-Present Origin*, 67.
15. Ibid., 76–77.
16. Feuerstein, *The Yoga Tradition*, 198.
17. Gebser, *The Ever-Present Origin*, 102.
18. Aurobindo, *The Life Divine*, 891.
19. Seeman, *Individuation and Subtle Body*, 19.
20. Feuerstein, *The Yoga Tradition*, 56.
21. Feuerstein, *Tantra: The Path of Ecstasy*, 46.
22. Ibid., 53.
23. The Holy Bible, Revised Standard Version.
24. Nikhilananda, *The Upanisads*, 109.
25. Ibid., 146.
26. Sinha, "Human Embodiment: The Theme and the Encounter in Vedantic Phenomenology," 239–47.
27. Eliade, *Yoga: Immortality and Freedom*, 4.
28. Collins, *Mysticism and New Paradigm Psychology*, xi.
29. Sinha, "Human Embodiment: The Theme and the Encounter in Vedantic Phenomenology," 239–47.
30. Ibid.
31. Feuerstein, *Tantra: The Path of Ecstasy*, 53.
32. Feuerstein, *The Yoga Tradition*, 56.
33. Ibid., 48.
34. Ibid.
35. Feuerstein, *The Essence of Yoga: A Contribution to the Psychohistory of Indian Civilisation*, 192.
36. Ram-Prasad, *Eastern Philosophy*, 56.
37. Ibid., 139.
38. Raju, "The Concept of the Spiritual in Indian Thought," 195–213.
39. Deussen, *The Philosophy of the Upanishads*, 40.
40. Raju, "The Concept of the Spiritual in Indian Thought," 196.

Chapter 2. The Cosmic Person

1. White, "Why Gurus Are Heavy," 44.
2. Eliade, *Yoga: Immortality and Freedom*, 114–15.

3. Ibid.

4. Ibid., 115.

5. Ibid., 116.

6. White, "Why Gurus Are Heavy," 43.

7. Ibid.

8. Eliade, *Yoga: Immortality and Freedom,* 117.

9. Bosch, *The Golden Germ,* 230–31.

10. Mabbett, "The Symbolism of Mount Meru," 66.

11. Daniel, *Fluid Signs: Being a Person the Tamil Way,* 3.

12. Ibid., 4.

13. Ibid., 5.

14. Ibid., 6.

15. Hume, *Katha Upanishad* VI.I, 358.

16. Daniel, *Fluid Signs: Being a Person the Tamil Way,* 6.

17. Eliade, *Yoga: Immortality and Freedom,* 235.

18. White, *Tantra in Practice,* 9.

19. Eliade, *Yoga: Immortality and Freedom,* 235–36.

20. Deussen, *The Philosophy of the Upanishads,* 12.

21. Eliade, *Yoga: Immortality and Freedom,* 98.

22. White, "Why Gurus Are Heavy"; and White, *The Alchemical Body.*

23. Eliade, *Yoga: Immortality and Freedom,* 250–51.

24. Ibid., 250.

25. Beck, "Body Imagery in the Tamil Proverbs of South India," 27.

26. Tiruvalluvar, G. U. Pope, trans., *Tirukkural.*

27. Yogeshwarananda, *Science of Soul,* 4, 22.

28. Zysk, "The Science of Respiration and the Doctrine of Bodily Winds in Ancient India," 198–213.

Chapter 3. The Ladder of Being

1. Organ, *Western Approaches to Eastern Philosophy,* 50.

2. Feuerstein, *The Yoga Tradition,* 7.

3. Ibid., 3.

4. Ibid., 4.

5. Ibid., 5.

6. Ibid., 17.

7. Deussen, *The Philosophy of the Upanishads,* 262.

8. Ibid., 263.

9. Bjonnes, "Koshas: The State of the Mind," 1.

10. Feuerstein, *Tantra: The Path of Ecstasy,* 18.

11. Ibid., 51.

12. Rama, Ballentine, and Ajaya, *Yoga and Psychotherapy,* 218.

13. Hume, trans., *Taittiriya Upanisad* II.I, 283.

14. Feuerstein, *The Yoga Tradition,* 50.

15. Ibid., 133.

16. Kazlev, *Advaita Vedanta,* n1.

17. Niranjanananda, *The Koshas,* 1.

18. Ibid., 3.

19. Ibid.

20. Ibid.

21. Ibid.

22. Feuerstein, *The Yoga Tradition,* 144.

23. Shapiro and Walsh, *Meditation: Classic and Contemporary Perspectives,* 336.

24. Bjonnes, "Koshas: The State of the Mind," 1.

25. Parthasarthy, *The Nature of Man,* 329.

26. Ibid., 361.

Chapter 4. The Organs of the Soul

1. Woodroffe, *The Serpent Power,* 21.

2. Deussen, *The Philosophy of the Upanishads,* 264.

3. Ibid.

4. Zysk, "The Science of Respiration and the Doctrine of Bodily Winds in Ancient India," 205.

5. Ibid., 209.

6. Feuerstein, *Tantra: The Path of Ecstasy,* 149.

7. Ibid.

8. Wujastyk, "The Science of Medicine," 397–98.

9. Heilijgers-Seelen, *System of Five Cakras in Kubjikamatatantra,* 14–16.

10. Ibid.

11. White, *The Kiss of the Yogini,* 224–25.

12. Feuerstein, *Tantra: The Path of Ecstasy,* 149.

13. Flood, *The Tantric Body,* 158.

14. Goswami, *Layayoga,* 182.

15. Feuerstein, *Tantra: The Path of Ecstasy,* 150.

16. Rama, Ballentine, and Ajaya, *Yoga and Psychotherapy,* 221.

17. Ibid., 222.

18. Ibid., 224.

19. Feuerstein, *Tantra: The Path of Ecstasy,* 150.

20. Feuerstein, *The Yoga Tradition,* 356.

21. Ibid.

22. Schul, *The Psychic Frontiers of Medicine,* 211.

23. Krishna, *Kundalini,* 12.

24. Ibid., 13.

25. Woodroffe, *The Serpent Power,* 21.

26. Niranjanananda, *The Koshas,* 1.

27. Ibid., 2.

Chapter 5. The Yoga of the Subtle Body

1. Fields, *Religious Therapeutics*, 22.
2. Samuel, *The Origins of Yoga and Tantra*, 2.
3. Ibid., 271, 351.
4. Brockington, "Yoga in the Mahabharat," 14.
5. White, *The Kiss of the Yogini*, 143.
6. Bentor, "Interiorized Fire Rituals in India and Tibet," 595.
7. *Linga Purana*, II.713.
8. Gupta, Hoens, and Goudriaan, *Hindu Tantrism*, 196, 145.
9. Bentor, "Interiorized Fire Rituals in India and Tibet," 595.
10. Whicher, "The Integration of Spirit and Matter in the Yoga Sutra," 51.
11. Smith, "Adjusting the Quotidian: Ashtanga Yoga as Everyday Practice," 6.
12. Leder, *The Absent Body*, 4.
13. Morley, "Inspiration and Expiration: Yoga Practice through Merleau-Ponty's Phenomenology of the Body," 73–82.
14. Desikachar, *The Heart of Yoga: Developing a Personal Practice*, 23.
15. Baranay, "Writing, standing on your head," 246.
16. Alter, *The Wrestler's Body: Identity and Ideology in North India*, 95.
17. Matsuda, *A Phenomenological Study of the Imagining Body*, 35.
18. Morley, "Inspiration and Expiration: Yoga Practice through Merleau-Ponty's Phenomenology of the Body," 73–820.
19. Matsuda, *A Phenomenological Study of the Imagining Body*, 18.
20. Ibid., 86.
21. Morley, "Inspiration and Expiration: Yoga Practice through Merleau-Ponty's Phenomenology of the Body," 73–82; and Shapiro and Walsh, *Meditation: Classic and Contemporary Perspectives*, 8.
22. Hayes, "Metaphoric Worlds and Yoga in the Vaisnava Sahajiyā Tantric Traditions of Medieval Bengal," 165.
23. Sarukkai, "Inside/Outside: Merleau Ponty Yoga," 459–78.
24. Schmidt, *Dzogchen Essentials*, 168–69.
25. Ibid.
26. Ray, *Saints in India*, 38.
27. Rele, *The Vedic Gods as Figures of Biology*, ix.
28. Ibid., 13.
29. Brown and Gerbarg, *Yoga Breathing, Meditation and Longevity*, 54–62.
30. Hayes, "Metaphoric Worlds and Yoga in the Vaisnava Sahajiyā Tantric Traditions of Medieval Bengal," 178.

Chapter 6. The Subtle Body in Sufi Cosmology

1. Stoddart, *Sufism*, 61.
2. Godlas, *Sufism's Many Paths*, 16A.
3. Cole, "The World as Text: Cosmologies of Shaykh Ahmad al-Ahsa'i," 2.
4. Corbin, *Creative Imagination in the Sūfism of Ibn ʿArabī*, 187.
5. Nasr, "Al-Serat: The Interior Life in Islam," 16A.
6. Howell, "Sufism and the Indonesian Islamic Revival," 701.
7. Ibid.
8. Corbin, *History of Islamic Philosophy*, 188.
9. Ibid., 18, 28, 187.
10. Cole, "Individualism and the Spiritual Path," 10.
11. Ibid., 11.
12. Corbin, *Creative Imagination in the Sūfism of Ibn ʿArabī*, 4.
13. Stoddart, *Sufism*, 61.
14. Shah, *The Way of the Sufi*, 61.
15. John 5.24.
16. Touma, *The Music of the Arab*, 162.
17. Nasr, "Al-Serat: The Interior Life in Islam," 16A, n11.
18. Ibid.
19. Stoddart, *Sufism*, 62–64.
20. Ibid., 65.
21. Ibid.
22. Schuon, *Understanding Islam*, 37.
23. Chittick, "The Perfect Man as the Prototype of the Self in the Sufism of Jāmī," 135–57.
24. Austin, in the introduction to Stoddart, *Sufism*, 12.
25. Takeshita, Review of Chittick's "Ibn ʿArabī's's Theory of the Perfect Man and Its Place in the History of Islamic Thought," 707.
26. Elias, "Sufism: A Review of the Encyclopaedia Iranica," 595–613.
27. Chittick, "The Perfect Man as the Prototype of the Self in the Sufism of Jāmī," 138.
28. Ibid., 154.
29. Shah, *The Way of the Sufi*, 141.
30. Fusfeld, *The Shaping of Sufi Leadership in Delhi: The*

Naqshbandiyya Mujaddiyya, 1750–1920, quoted in Hermānsen, "Shah Wali Allah's Theory of the Subtle Spiritual Centers: A Sufi Model of Personhood and Self-Transformation," 2.

31. Corbin, *Creative Imagination in the Sūfism of Ibn ʿArabī,* 221–22.
32. Ibid.
33. Eliade, *Yoga: Immortality and Freedom,* 234.
34. Corbin, *Creative Imagination in the Sūfism of Ibn ʿArabī,* 221–22.
35. Ibid., 230.
36. Godlas, *Sufism's Many Paths,* 1.

Chapter 7. The Bodies of Buddha

1. Ram-Prasad, *Eastern Philosophy,* 8.
2. Sangharakshita, *A Guide to the Buddhist Path,* 28.
3. Ibid., 48.
4. Feuerstein, *The Yoga Tradition,* 168.
5. Tansley, *Subtle Body,* 49.
6. Yuasa, "The Body" in *History of Religions,* 151.
7. Ibid.
8. Sangharakshita, *A Guide to the Buddhist Path,* 51.
9. Hopkins, "Tantric Buddhism, Degeneration or Enhancement," 88.
10. Ibid., 90.
11. Ibid., 91.
12. Snellgrove, *Hevajra Tantra: A Critical Study,* 9.
13. Hopkins, "Tantric Buddhism, Degeneration or Enhancement," 96.
14. Ibid., n13.
15. Ibid.
16. Ibid., 91
17. Feuerstein, *Tantra: The Path of Ecstasy,* 70.
18. Dalai Lama, *How to Practise,* Audio CD.
19. Wikipedia, *Sand Mandala,* section 3, and *Kalachakra Mandala,* sections 1 and 2.
20. Feuerstein, *Tantra: The Path of Ecstasy,* 71.
21. Flood, *The Tantric Body,* 110.
22. Ashley-Farrand, *Healing Mantras,* 66.
23. White, *The Alchemical Body,* 43.
24. Feuerstein, *Tantra: The Path of Ecstasy,* 72.
25. Salzberg, *Lovingkindness,* 2.
26. Bjonnes, "Koshas: The State of the Mind," 1.
27. Ibid.
28. Ibid., 2.
29. Ibid., 5.

Chapter 8. The Taoist Body of Inner Alchemy

1. Irwin, "Daoist Alchemy in the West," 1.
2. Sullivan, "Body Works: Knowledge of the Body in the Study of Religion," 87.
3. Schipper, *The Taoist Body,* 141, 298.
4. Ibid., 142.
5. Ibid.
6. Ibid.
7. Köhn, *The Taoist Experience,* 11–12.
8. Köhn, "The Subtle Body Ecstasy of Daoist Inner Alchemy," 325.
9. James, *The Varieties of Religious Experience,* 38.
10. Underhill, *Mysticism,* 170.
11. Köhn, "The Subtle Body Ecstasy of Daoist Inner Alchemy," 326.
12. Köhn, *The Taoist Experience,* 191–92.
13. Robinet, "Metamorphosis and Deliverance from the Corpse in Taoism," 50.
14. Ibid.
15. Robinet, *Taoism: Growth of the Religion,* 195.
16. Ibid.
17. Ibid., 206.
18. Winn, "The Quest for Spiritual Orgasm," 20.
19. Winn, "Daoist Internal Alchemy," 13.
20. Köhn, "The Subtle Body Ecstasy of Daoist Inner Alchemy," 330.
21. Gyatso, *Clear Light of Bliss;* and Short and Mann, *The Body of Light;* and Winn, "The Quest for Spiritual Orgasm," 331.
22. Lu K'uan-yü, *Taoist Yoga,* 115.
23. Köhn, "The Subtle Body Ecstasy of Daoist Inner Alchemy," 328.
24. Shendelman, "The Vision of the Body: Primary Body Focus Zones in Qigong Practice," 1.
25. Ibid.
26. Ibid.
27. Lama Somananda Tantrapa, *Qi Dao: Tibetan Shamanic Qigong,* 7.

Chapter 9. East Meets West

1. Organ, *Western Approaches to Eastern Philosophy,* 16.
2. Deutsch, *Advaita Vedanta,* 4.
3. Organ, *Western Approaches to Eastern Philosophy,* 14.
4. Aurobindo, *The Life Divine,* 782.
5. Versluis, "Western Esotericism and Consciousness," 20–33.

6. Ibid.

7. Rensselaer, "Esoteric Wisdom East and West," 73.

8. Ibid.

9. Ibid., 74.

10. Ibid.

11. Ibid., 75.

12. Ibid.

13. Johnston, *Angels of Desire,* 10.

14. Ibid., 18.

15. Ibid., 22.

Part Two Introductory Text

1. Faivre and Voss, "Western Esotericism and the Science of Religions," 61.

2. Ibid.

3. Huxley, *The Perennial Philosophy,* vii.

4. Faivre and Voss, "Western Esotericism and the Science of Religions," 64.

5. Fanger, *Esotericism, Art and Imagination,* 277–87.

6. Riffard, *L'Esotérisme,* 45.

7. Faivre and Voss, "Western Esotericism and the Science of Religions," 50–51.

8. Ibid., 51.

9. Ibid., 52.

10. Riffard, *L'Esotérisme,* 45.

11. Faivre and Hanegraaff, *Western Esotericism and the Science of Religion,* 8.

Chapter 10. Symbolism and the Subtle Body in the Ancient World

1. Hall, *The Secret Teachings of All Ages,* 222.

2. Eliade, *The Myth of the Eternal Return,* 3.

3. Hall, *The Secret Teachings of All Ages,* 222.

4. Ibid., 228–29.

5. Eliade, *Yoga: Immortality and Freedom,* 97.

6. Ibid.

7. Ibid., 86–87.

8. Proverbs 4.1–9.

9. Hall, *The Secret Teachings of All Ages,* 273.

10. Numbers 21.5–9.

11. Mead, *The Orphic Pantheon,* 103.

12. Hall, *The Secret Teachings of All Ages,* 93.

13. Watson, *A Dictionary of Mind and Spirit,* 155–56.

14. Hall, *The Secret Teachings of All Ages,* 98.

15. Ibid., 99–106.

Chapter 11. The Forgotten Philosophy

1. Mead, *The Doctrine of the Subtle Body in Western Tradition,* 5.

2. Ibid.

3. Poortman, *Vehicles of Consciousness,* vol. 1, 108.

4. Hare, *Plato,* 11.

5. Lee, trans., *Plato: Timaeus,* 9.

6. Opsopaus, *The Parts of the Soul: A Greek System of Chakras,* 2.

7. Osborn, "Plato and the Chakras," 2.

8. Lee, trans., *Plato: Timaeus,* 7.

9. Sorabji, "Soul and Self in Ancient Philosophy," 14.

10. Robinson, "The Tripartite Soul in the Timaeus," 104; and Smith, "Plato's Analogy of Soul and State," 31.

11. Feuerstein, *The Yoga Tradition,* 56.

12. Feuerstein, *Tantra: The Path of Ecstasy,* 46.

13. Onians, *The Origins of European Thought About the Body, the Mind, the Soul, the World, Time, and Fate,* 44.

14. Osborn, "Plato and the Chakras," 2.

15. Feuerstein, *The Yoga Tradition,* 67.

16. Onians, *The Origins of European Thought About the Body, the Mind, the Soul, the World, Time, and Fate,* 126, n3.

17. Feuerstein, *The Yoga Tradition,* 352.

18. Robinson, "The Tripartite Soul in the Timaeus," 103.

19. Ibid., 107.

20. Ibid., 109.

21. Mead, *The Doctrine of the Subtle Body in Western Tradition,* 8.

22. Ibid., 36.

23. Ibid.

24. I Corinthians 15.35–58; and Philippians 3.21.

25. Mead, *The Doctrine of the Subtle Body in Western Tradition,* 59.

26. Hall, *The Secret Teachings of All Ages,* 160.

27. Mead, *The Doctrine of the Subtle Body in Western Tradition,* 62.

28. Fernel, *De Naturali Parte Medicinae,* Book IV, 1542, in Walker's "The Astral Body in Renaissance Medicine," 119–33.

29. Wallis, *Neoplatonism,* 170.

30. Ibid., 153.

31. Ibid., 107.

32. Ibid.

33. Ibid.

34. Ibid., 108–9.

35. Ibid., 113.

36. Mead, *The Doctrine of the Subtle Body in Western Tradition*, 2.

37. Wallis, *Neoplatonism*, 108–9.

38. Ibid., 178.

39. Meece, *Neoplatonism and Alchemy*, 9.

40. Inge, *Philosophy of Plotinus*, 15.

41. Place, *The Alchemical Tarot*, 289.

42. Holman, *The Return of the Perennial Philosophy*, 5.

43. Huxley, *The Perennial Philosophy*, 33.

44. Holman, *The Return of the Perennial Philosophy*, xvii.

45. Versluis, *Magic and Mysticism*, 166.

46. Huxley, *The Perennial Philosophy*, viii–ix.

Chapter 12. The Alchemical Body

1. Mead, *The Doctrine of the Subtle Body in Western Tradition*, 11.

2. Miller, *Introduction to Alchemy in Jungian Psychology*, 1.

3. Mead, *The Doctrine of the Subtle Body in Western Tradition*, 12–15.

4. Ibid.

5. Ead, *Arabic Influence on the Historical Development of Medicine*, 4.

6. Burkhardt, *Alchemy*, 221.

7. Ibid., 170–81.

8. Edwardes, *The Dark Side of History*, 47.

9. Debus and Multhauf, *Alchemy and Chemistry in the Seventeenth Century*, 6–12.

10. Schuler, "Some Spiritual Alchemies of Seventeenth-Century England," 293.

11. Ibid., 300.

12. Ibid.

13. Ibid.

14. Ibid.

15. Walker, "The Astral Body in Renaissance Medicine," 120.

16. Ibid., 121.

17. Ibid., 126.

18. Harvey, *Opera Omnia: a Collegio Medicorum*, 115–16.

19. Bertacchi, quoted in Walker, *The Astral Body in Renaissance Medicine*, fol. 21ʳ–22ʳ.

20. Walker, "The Astral Body in Renaissance Medicine," 130.

21. Smith, in von Franz, *Alchemy: An Introduction to the Symbolism and the Psychology*, back cover.

22. Miller, *Introduction to Alchemy in Jungian Psychology*, 1.

23. Spiegelman and Vasavada, *Hinduism and Jungian Psychology*, 59.

24. Coward, *Jung and Eastern Thought*, 143.

25. Ibid., 144.

26. Seeman, *Individuation and the Subtle Body*, 147.

27. Jung, *Alchemical Studies*, 122–23.

28. Jung, *The Archetypes and the Collective Unconscious*, 312.

29. Jung, *The Structure and Dynamics of the Psyche*, 345.

30. Spiegelman, quoted in Seeman, *Individuation and the Subtle Body*, 144.

31. Jung, *Psychology and Alchemy*, 427–28.

32. Ibid., 278.

33. Ibid.

34. Roth, *The Return of the World Soul*, 4.

35. von Franz, *Alchemy: An Introduction to the Symbolism and the Psychology*, 13.

36. Ibid., 237.

37. Ibid.

38. Ibid.

39. Ibid., 236–38.

40. Seeman, *Individuation and the Subtle Body*, 52.

41. Coward, *Jung and Eastern Thought*, 10.

42. Ibid., 114.

43. Seeman, *Individuation and Subtle Body*, 48.

44. Jung, *The Structure and Dynamics of the Psyche*, 67.

45. Seeman, *Individuation and Subtle Body*, 186.

46. Miller, *The Modern Alchemist*, 2.

47. Lockhart, *Siddha Medicine*.

48. Miller, *The Modern Alchemist*, 4.

49. Ibid., 9.

Chapter 13. Theosophy, Anthroposophy, and the Subtle Bodies

1. Snell, "Modern Theosophy in Its Relation to Hinduism and Buddhism," 200.

2. Ibid., 201.

3. Ibid.

4. Ibid., 203.

5. Bailey, *Esoteric Healing*, vol. IV, 2.

6. Ibid., 33.

7. Ibid., 34.

8. Ibid., 35–38.

9. Woodroffe, *The Serpent Power*, 14.

10. Ibid., 15.

11. Ibid., 16.

12. Ibid.
13. Ibid.
14. Williams, *The Chakras and Ancient Wisdom Traditions Worldwide,* 4.
15. Michaelson, *God in Your Body,* quoted in Williams, *The Chakras and Ancient Wisdom Traditions Worldwide,* 4.
16. Ibid.
17. Steiner, *Founding a Science of the Spirit,* 2.
18. Ibid.
19. Clemen, "Anthroposophy," 283.
20. Steiner, *The Inner Development of Man.*
21. Ahern, *Sun at Midnight,* 16, 35–36.
22. McDermott, "Rudolf Steiner and Anthroposophy" in Faivre and Needleman, *Modern Esoteric Spirituality,* 303ff.
23. Clemen, "Anthroposophy," 282–83.
24. Ibid., 283.
25. Steiner, *Founding a Science of the Spirit,* 5.
26. Ibid., 6.
27. Popper, and Eccles, *The Self and Its Brain,* 102–3.
28. Pitson, *Hume's Philosophy of the Self,* 196.
29. Steiner, *Founding a Science of the Spirit,* 143.
30. Ibid., 7.
31. Ibid.
32. Ibid., 10.
33. Clemen, "Anthroposophy," 292.
34. Cousins, ed., quoted by Versluis in "A Review of Modern Esoteric Spirituality by Antoine Faivre and Jacob Needleman," 425.

Chapter 14. Energy Healing and the New Age Body

1. Faivre and Voss, "Western Esotericism and the Science of Religions," 48.
2. Hanegraaff, "Introduction: The Birth of a Discipline," 3–21.
3. Ibid.
4. Albanese, "The Aura of Wellness: Subtle-Energy Healing and New Age Religion," 30.
5. Ibid.
6. Albanese, "The Subtle Energies of Spirit," 310.
7. Watson, *A Dictionary of Mind and Spirit,* 27.
8. Burr and Northrup, "The Electro-Dynamic Theory of Life," 332–33.
9. Karagulla and Kunz, *The Chakras and the Human Energy Fields,* 53.
10. LeShan, *The Medium, the Mystic and the Physicist,* 192–93.
11. Motoyama, *Theories of the Chakras,* 24.
12. Bruyere, *Wheels of Light,* 20–22.
13. Hunt, *Infinite Mind,* 9.
14. Tiller, *Science and Human Transformation,* 128–29.
15. Schlitz and Harman, "The Implications of Alternative and Complementary Medicine for Science and the Scientific Process," 361.
16. Albanese, "The Aura of Wellness: Subtle-Energy Healing and New Age Religion," 31.
17. Brennan, *Hands of Light: A Guide to Healing through the Human Energy Field,* 45.
18. Ibid., 76.
19. Ibid., 89.
20. Oschman, *Energy Medicine,* 83.
21. Ostram, *Understanding Auras,* 25.
22. Ibid., 29.
23. Ibid.
24. Ibid., 32–33.
25. Carroll, *Spiritualism in Antebellum America,* 120–51.
26. Jung, *Psychology and Alchemy,* 44.
27. Ibid., 375.
28. Payne and Bendit, "The Subtle Body and Countertransference," 210.
29. Judith, *Wheels of Life,* 308.
30. Carroll, *Spiritualism in Antebellum America,* 120–51.
31. Benor, *Healing Research: Holistic Medicine and Spirituality,* 35.
32. Carroll, *Spiritualism in Antebellum America,* 120–51.
33. Payne and Bendit, "The Subtle Body and Countertransference," 210.
34. Quoted in Mead, *The Doctrine of the Subtle Body in Western Tradition,* 2.
35. Watson, *A Dictionary of Mind and Spirit,* 139.
36. Albanese, "The Aura of Wellness: Subtle-Energy Healing and New Age Religion," 314.
37. Watson, *A Dictionary of Mind and Spirit,* 139.
38. Brennan, *Hands of Light,* 14.
39. Albanese, "The Subtle Energies of Spirit," 314.
40. Albanese, "The Aura of Wellness: Subtle-Energy Healing and New Age Religion," 48.
41. Pauli and Jung, *The Interpretation of Nature and the Psyche,* 1955.
42. Popper and Eccles, *The Self and Its Brain,* 105, 464, 494.

Chapter 15. Science, Philosophy, and the Subtle Body

1. Ayer, "The physical basis of the mind," 1109–10.
2. Dingle, *Through Science to Philosophy,* 112.
3. Ryle, *The Concept of Mind,* 17.
4. Ibid., 23–24.
5. von Franz, *Projection and Recollection in Jungian Psychology,* 54.
6. Pauli and Jung, *The Interpretation of Nature and the Psyche,* 38.
7. von Franz, *Projection and Recollection in Jungian Psychology,* 54.
8. Popper and Eccles, *The Self and Its Brain,* 134–35.
9. Heidegger, *Being and Time,* McQuarrie and Robinson trans., numbered section 9, numbered paragraph 2, 67ff.
10. Ryle, *The Concept of Mind,* 23.
11. Ibid.
12. Hofstadter, *I Am a Strange Loop,* 101.
13. Heidegger, *Being and Time,* McQuarrie and Robinson trans., 426.
14. Hume, *Treatise of Human Nature,* 1.4.6.
15. Heidegger, *Being and Time,* McQuarrie and Robinson trans., 426.
16. Ibid., 427.
17. Ibid., chapter 6, section 79.
18. Hofstadter, *I Am a Strange Loop,* 111.
19. Oschman, *Energy Medicine,* 110.
20. Aspect, "Bell's Theorem: The Naïve View of an Experimentalist," see the bibliography.
21. Ibid., 25.
22. Ibid., 31.
23. Penrose, *Shadows of the Mind,* 7–8, 238.
24. Puthoff and Targ, "A Perceptual Channel for Information Transfer over Kilometer Distances: Historical Perspective and Recent Research," 329.
25. Ibid.
26. Penrose, *Shadows of the Mind,* 408.
27. Ibid., 43.
28. Ibid., 26–33.
29. Dingle, *Through Science to Philosophy,* 166.

Chapter 16. Consciousness and the Subtle Body

1. ISSSEEM, *Subtle Energies and Energy Medicine* 17 (2008): 1.
2. Oschman, *Energy Medicine,* 83.
3. Laszlo, *Science and the Akashic Field,* xi.
4. Ibid.
5. Bache, *Dark Night, Early Dawn: Steps to a Deep Ecology of Mind,* 6.
6. Quoted in Benor, *Healing Research: Holistic Medicine and Spirituality,* 65.
7. Ibid., 66.
8. Ibid., 269.
9. Ibid., 12.
10. Schlitz, "Distant Intentionality and Healing: Assessing the Evidence," 11.
11. Laszlo, *Science and the Akashic Field,* 112.
12. Ibid.
13. Ibid., 113.
14. Tiller, *Science and Human Transformation,* 128.
15. Ibid.
16. Pert, *Molecules of Emotion,* 4.
17. Ibid., 137.
18. Ibid., 179.
19. Hamilton, *It's the Thought That Counts,* 36.
20. Ibid., 84.
21. Capra, *The Tao of Physics,* 102.
22. Dossey, *Healing Words: The Power of Prayer and the Practice of Medicine,* 233.
23. Ibid., 293.
24. Benor, "Survey of Spiritual Healing Research," 9–33.
25. Dossey, *Healing Words,* 10.
26. Ibid., 55.
27. Ibid., 179.
28. Ibid., 273.
29. Louchakova, "Psychospiritual Practices from the Prayer of the Heart in Monitoring Cardiovascular Disorders: A Case Study."
30. Quoted in ibid., 6.
31. Ibid.
32. Berry, *The Great Work: Our Way into the Future,* 159–65.

Chapter 17. The Integral Body

1. Gebser, *The Ever-Present Origin,* 97.
2. Saiter, "A General Introduction to Integral Theory and Comprehensive Mapmaking," 14.
3. Bolle, "Tantric Elements in Sri Aurobindo," 130.
4. Ibid., 102, n4.
5. Ibid., 131.

6. Chaudhuri, "The Philosophy and Yoga of Sri Aurobindo," 7.

7. Ibid., 10.

8. Schlitz, Amorok, and Micozzi, *Consciousness and Healing,* xxxviii.

9. Sen, "Sri Aurobindo's Theory of the Mind," 48–49.

10. Murphy, *The Future of the Body,* 553.

11. Wilber, *Integral Psychology,* 10, 83.

12. Saiter, "A General Introduction to Integral Theory and Comprehensive Mapmaking," 3.

13. Laszlo, *Science and the Akashic Field,* 1–2.

14. Beck and Cowan, *Spiral Dynamics,* 1996.

15. Saiter, "A General Introduction to Integral Theory and Comprehensive Mapmaking," 6.

16. Ibid., 16.

17. Gebser, *The Ever-Present Origin,* 136.

18. Ibid., 385.

19. Ibid., 220–21.

20. Ibid.

21. Ibid.

22. Feuerstein, *The Yoga Tradition,* xxvii.

23. Gebser, *The Ever-Present Origin,* 99.

24. Wilber, *The Eye of Spirit,* 231.

Chapter 18. The Subtle Body and the Transformed Being in Society

1. Holman, *The Return of the Perennial Philosophy,* 2.

2. Quoted in James, *The Varieties of Religious Experience,* 322.

3. BBC Documentary on "Meditation" in the Alternative Medicine Series shown on 31 March 2008.

4. Collins, *Mysticism and New Paradigm Psychology,* xx.

5. Ibid.

6. Quoted in James, *The Varieties of Religious Experience,* 322.

7. Ibid.

8. Quoted in ibid., 323.

9. Ibid.

10. Ibid.

11. Collins, *Mysticism and New Paradigm Psychology,* 9.

12. Burnham, *The Ecstatic Journey,* 12.

13. Collins, *Mysticism and New Paradigm Psychology,* 13.

14. Ibid., 14.

15. Robinson, trans., Abhayadatta's *Caturasiti-siddha-pravṛtti: Buddha's Lions, The Lives of the Eighty-Four Siddhas,* 12.

16. Collins, *Mysticism and New Paradigm Psychology,* 197.

17. Ibid.

18. Ibid., 22.

19. Ibid.

20. Bhajanananda, "Three Aspects of the Ramakrishna Ideal, Part 1," 1.

21. Ibid., 4.

22. Pradervand, *The Gentle Art of Blessing,* 279.

23. St. Teresa of Avila, *Autobiography,* 113.

24. Gebser, *The Ever-Present Origin,* xxvii.

25. Murphy, "Scientific Studies of Contemplative Experience: An Overview," Part 3, 23.

26. Kabat-Zinn, "Meditation Research at the University of Massachusetts Medical Center," 5.

27. Louchakova and Warner, "Via Kundalini: Psychosomatic Excursions in Trans-personal Psychology," 115–58.

28. Ibid., 116.

29. Ibid., 118.

30. Antonov and Vaver, *A Handbook of Complex System of Psychophysical Self-Regulation* quoted in Louchakova and Warner, "Via Kundalini," 117; Goswami, *Layayoga: The Definitive Guide to the Chakras and Kundalini,* quoted in Louchakova and Warner, "Via Kundalini," 123.

31. Antonov and Vaver, *Complexnaya systema psychophysicheskoi samoregulatsii* (A handbook of complex system of psychophysical self-regulation), quoted in Louchakova and Warner, "Via Kundalini"; and Tirtha, *Devatma Shakti (Kundalini)* quoted in Louchakova and Warner, "Via Kundalini," 122.

32. Louchakova and Warner, "Via Kundalini," 115–58; and Chia, *Fusion of the Five Elements I: Basic and Advanced Meditations for Transforming Negative Emotion,* 122.

33. Palmer, Sherrard, and Ware, trans. and eds., "St. Simeon the New Theologian: The Three Methods of Prayer," 73.

34. Louchakova and Warner, "Via Kundalini," 122.

35. Austin, "Consciousness Evolves when the Self Dissolves," 209ß.

36. Louchakova and Warner, "Via Kundalini," 121.

37. Ibid., 124.

38. Ibid., 119.

39. Salzberg, *Lovingkindness,* 35.

40. Bhajanananda, "Three Aspects of the Ramakrishna Ideal, Part 1," 2.

41. Bailey, *Serving Humanity,* 98.

42. Ibid., 99.

43. Ibid., 98.

44. Ibid., 151.

45. Russell, *The Global Brain,* 176, 181.

46. Ibid., 195–96.

47. Ibid., 197.

48. Ibid., 198–99.

49. Orme-Johnson, Alexander, Davies, et al., "International Peace Project in the Middle East: The Effects of the Maharishi Technology of the Unified Field," 326–46; and Schrödt, "A Methodological Critique of a Test of the Effects of the Maharishi Technology of the Unified Field," 745.

50. Orme-Johnson, Alexander, Davies, et al., "International Peace Project in the Middle East: The Effects of the Maharishi Technology of the Unified Field," 776–812.

51. Puthoff and Targ, "A Perceptual Channel for Information Transfer over Kilometer Distances," 329.

52. Russell, *The Global Brain,* 211.

53. Ibid., 211.

54. Targ, Puthoff, and Tart, *Mind at Large,* 70.

55. Radin, *Entangled Minds,* 233.

56. Laszlo, *The Chaos Point,* 40.

57. Holman, *The Return of the Perennial Philosophy,* 128.

Bibliography

Ahern, Geoffrey. *Sun at Midnight: The Rudolf Steiner Movement and the Western Esoteric Tradition.* Wellingborough, UK: The Aquarian Press, 1984.

Albanese, C. "The Subtle Energies of Spirit: Explorations in Metaphysical and New Age Spirituality." *Journal of the American Academy of Religion* 67, no. 2 (June 1999): 305–25.

———. "The Aura of Wellness: Subtle-Energy Healing and New Age Religion." *Religion and American Culture* 10, no. 1 (Winter 2000): 29–55.

Aldridge, David. *Spirituality, Healing and Medicine.* London: Jessica Kingsley Publishers, 2000.

Allchin, D. "Points East and West: Acupuncture and Comparative Philosophy of Science." *Philosophy of Science* 63, no. 3 (September 1996): S107–S115.

Alter, Joseph S. *The Wrestler's Body: Identity and Ideology in North India.* Berkeley: University of California Press, 1992.

Antonov, V., and G. Vaver. *Complexnaya systema psychophysicheskoi samoregulatsii* (A handbook of complex system of psychophysical self-regulation). Leningrad, Russia: Cosmos, 1989. (All books by this author are available from him directly: Do vostrebovania, Sanct Petersburg, Russia.)

Ashley-Farrand, Thomas. *Healing Mantras.* Dublin: Gateway, 1999.

Astin, J. A., and W. Astin. "An Integral Approach to Medicine." *Journal of Alternative Therapy and Health Medicine* 8, no. 2 (March–April 2002): 70–75.

Aspect, Alain. "Experimental Tests Of Bell's Inequalities in Atomic Physics." In *Atomic Physics* 8, edited by I. Lindgren, A. Rosen, and S. Svanberg. Proceedings of the Eighth International Conference on Atomic Physics held in Göteborg, Sweden, August 2–6, 1982. New York: Plenum Publishing, 1982.

———. "Bell's Theorem: The Naïve View of an Experimentalist." In *Quantum (Un)speakables—From Bell to Quantum Information,* edited by R. A. Bertlmann and A. Zeilinger. New York: Springer, 2002.

Aurobindo. *Supramental Manifestation Upon Earth.* Twin Lakes, Wis.: Lotus Press, 1949.

———. *The Life Divine.* Pondicherry, India: Aurobindo Ashram, 1955.

Austin, James. "Consciousness Evolves when the Self Dissolves." In the symposium *Cognitive Models and Spiritual Maps,* 209ß.

Austin, J. W. Foreword in *Sufism: The Mystical Doctrines and Methods of Islam,* by W. Stoddart. Wellingborough, UK: The Aquarian Press, 1976.

Avatamsaka Sutra (sixth century). *Atharva Veda Samhita,* vol. VII. Translated by Whitney William Dwight. Cambridge, Mass.: Harvard University Press, 1904.

Avila, St. Teresa of. *Autobiography* ca. 1567 (originally published in Salamanca in 1589). Available as *The Life of Teresa of Jesus: The Autobiography of Teresa of Avila.* Translated by E. Allison Peers. New York: Doubleday, 1991.

Ayer, Alfred J. *Language, Truth and Logic.* London: Victor Gollancz, 1962.

———. "The physical basis of the mind." *The Listener,* 30 Dec 1949, 1109–10. (See also Coppleston, F.C.)

Bache, Christopher. *Dark Night, Early Dawn: Steps to a Deep Ecology of Mind.* Albany, N.Y.: SUNY Press, 2000.

Bailey, Alice A. *Esoteric Healing,* vol. V. London: Lucis Press, 1953.

———. *Serving Humanity.* London: Lucis Press, 1972.

Baker, D. C. *Studies of the Inner Life: The Impact of Spirituality on Quality of Life.* Quality of Life Research (Supplement 1). Dordrecht, Netherlands: Kluwer Academic Publishers, 2003.

Baranay, Inez. "Writing, standing on your head." Griffith University, South Brisbane, Australia, *Griffith Review* 4 (2004): 245–49.

Beck, Brenda E. F. "Body Imagery in the Tamil Proverbs of South India." *Western Folklore* 38, no. 1 (January 1979): 21–41.

Beck, Don, and Christopher Cowan. *Spiral Dynamics: Mastering Values, Leadership and Change.* Oxford, UK: Blackwell, 1996.

Bennett, M. R., and P. M. S. Hacker. *Philosophical Foundations of Neurosience.* Oxford, UK: Blackwell, 2003.

Benor, Daniel J. "Survey of Spiritual Healing Research." *Complementary Medical Research* 4, no. 1 (1990).

———. *Healing Research: Holistic Medicine and Spirituality.* Deddington, UK: Helix, 1993.

Bentor, Yael. "Interiorized Fire Rituals in India and Tibet." *Journal of the American Oriental Society* 120, no. 4 (October–December 2000): 594–613.

Berry, Thomas. *The Great Work: Our Way into the Future.* Carmarthen, Wales: Crown Publications, 2000.

Bhajanananda, Swami. "Three Aspects of the Ramakrishna Ideal, Part 1." *Prabuddha Bharata* (March–April 1982) English monthly journal of the Ramakrishna Order. Kolkata, India: Advaita Ashrama.

Bible, The Holy. Revised Standard Version. Edinburgh: Thomas Nelson and Sons, 1957.

Bjonnes, Roar. "Koshas: The State of the Mind." *New Renaissance* 10, no. 1 (2000).

Blackburn, Simon. *The Oxford Dictionary of Philosophy.* London: Oxford University Press, 1996.

Böhm, David. *Wholeness and the Implicate Order.* London: Routledge Classics, 2002.

Bolle, K. W. "Tantric Elements in Sri Aurobindo." *Numen* 9 (September 1962): 129–42.

Bosch, F. D. K. *The Golden Germ: An Introduction to Indian Symbolism.* The Hague, Netherlands: Mouton & Co., 1960.

Brennan, Barbara Ann. *Hands of Light: A Guide to Healing through the Human Energy Field.* New York: Bantam Books, 1987.

Brockington, John. "Yoga in the Mahabharat." In *Yoga: The Indian Tradition,* edited by Ian Whicher and David Carpenter. London: Routledge Curzon, 2003.

Brown, Richard P., and Patricia Gerbarg. *Yoga Breathing, Meditation and Longevity.* Press Release, Columbia University College of Physicians and Surgeons, New York, August 2009. www.nebi.nim.nih.gov/pubmed/19735239.

Bruyere, Rosalyn L. *Wheels of Light: Chakras, Auras and the Healing Energy of the Body.* New York: Simon & Schuster, 1994.

Burkhardt, Titus. *Alchemy: Science of the Cosmos, Science of the Soul.* Translated by William Stoddart. Baltimore: Penguin, 1967.

Burnham, Sophy. *The Ecstatic Journey: The Transforming Power of Mystical Experience.* New York: Ballantine Publishing, 1997.

Burr, H. S., and F. S. C. Northrup. "The Electro-Dynamic Theory of Life." *Revolutionary Biology* 10 (1935): 322–33.

Cade, C. Maxwell, and Nina Coxhead. *The Awakened Mind: Biofeedback and the Development of Higher States of Awareness.* Shaftesbury, UK: Element, 1996.

Capra, Fritjof. *The Tao of Physics.* Flamingo edition. London: Fontana Paperbacks, 1983.

Carpenter, D. "Practice Makes Perfect." In *Yoga: The Indian Tradition,* edited by Ian Whicher and David Carpenter. London: Routledge Curzon, 2003.

Carroll, Bret E. *Spiritualism in Antebellum America.* Bloomington: Indiana University Press, 1997.

Chalmers, David J. *The Conscious Mind: In Search of a Fundamental Theory.* New York: Oxford University Press, 1996.

Chaudhuri, H. "The Philosophy and Yoga of Sri Aurobindo." *Philosophy East and West* 22, no. 1 (January 1972): 5–14.

Ch'en, Kenneth K.S. "The Chinese Tripitaka." In *Buddhism in China: A Historical Survey,* 365–68. Princeton, N.J.: Princeton University Press, 1964.

Chia, M. *Fusion of the Five Elements I: Basic and Advanced Meditations for Transforming Negative Emotion.* Huntington, New York: Healing Tao Books, 1991. (Reissued as *Fusion of the Five Elements.* Rochester, Vt.: Destiny Books, 2007.)

Chittick, William E. "The Perfect Man as the Prototype of the Self in the Sufism of Jāmī." *Studia Islamica* 49 (1979): 135–57.

Clemen, C. "Anthroposophy." *The Journal of Religion* 4, no. 3 (May 1924): 281–92.

Cole, Juan R. I. "The World as Text: Cosmologies of Shaykh Ahmad al-Ahsa'i. *Studia Islamica* 80 (1994): 1–23.

———. "Individualism and the Spiritual Path in Shaykh Ahmad al-Ahsa'i." *Occasional Papers in Shaykhi, Baha'i and Baha'i Studies* 4 (September 1997).

Collins, John E. *Mysticism and New Paradigm Psychology.* Lanham, Md.: Rowman and Littlefield, 1991.

Conway Smith, C. Quoted in *Alchemy: An Introduction to the Symbolism and the Psychology,* edited by M-L von Franz. Toronto: Inner City Books, 1980.

Coppleston, Frederick Charles. *Memoirs of a Philosopher.* Lanham, Md.: Rowman and Littlefield, 1993.

Corbin, Henry. *Creative Imagination in the Sūfism of Ibn ʿArabī.* Translated by Ralph Manheim. Princeton, N.J.: Princeton University Press, 1969.

———. *Temple and Contemplation.* London: Kegan Paul International, 1986.

———. *History of Islamic Philosophy.* London: Islamic Publications and Kegan Paul International, 1993.

Cousins, E. Quoted in "A Review of Modern Esoteric Spirituality by Antoine Faivre and Jacob Needleman," by A. Versluis. *The Journal of Religion* 75 no. 3 (July 1995): 423–25.

Coward, Harold. *Jung and Eastern Thought.* New Delhi: Sri Satguru Publications, Indian Book Centre, 1991.

Dalai Lama, H. H. *How to Practice: The Way to a Meaningful Life.* Translated and edited by Jeffrey Hopkins. New York: Simon and Schuster, 2003.

Daniel, E. Valentine. *Fluid Signs: Being a Person the Tamil Way.* Berkeley: University of California Press, 1984.

Davidson, Richard J. "Concomitants of Meditation: A Cross-Sectional Study." In *Meditation, Classic and Contemporary Perspectives,* by Shapiro and Walsh. Piscataway, N.J.: Aldine Transaction Publishers, 2008.

Davies, Paul. *God and the New Physics.* London: Penguin Books, 1984.

Debus, Allen G., and Robert P. Multhauf. *Alchemy and Chemistry in the Seventeenth Century.* Los Angeles: University of California, William Andrew Clark Memorial Library, 1966.

de Michelis, Elizabeth. *A History of Modern Yoga: Patanjali and Western Esotericism.* London: Continuum, 2004.

de Purucker, G. *The Esoteric Tradition.* Pasadena, Calif.: Theosophical University Press, 1940.

Descartes, Rene. *Discourse on Method and the Meditations.* Translated by F. E. Sutcliffe. Middlesex, England: Penguin Classics, 1968.

Desikachar, T. K. V. *The Heart of Yoga: Developing a Personal Practice.* Rochester, Vt.: Inner Traditions, 1995.

Deussen, Paul. *The Philosophy of the Upanishads.* New York: Dover Publications, 1966.

Deutsch, Eliot. *Advaita Vedanta: A Philosophical Reconstruction.* Honolulu, Hawaii: East-West Center Press, 1969.

Dingle, Herbert. *Through Science to Philosophy.* London: Oxford University Press, 1937.

Dossey, Larry, M.D. *Healing Words: The Power of Prayer and the Practice of Medicine.* New York: HarperCollins, 1993.

Dossey, L., and H. Koenig. "Health-Prayer Studies: The Future of Prayer Experiments." *Science and Spirit* 13 (2002): 46–47.

Ead, H. *Arabic Influence on the Historical Development of Medicine.* Faculty of Science, University of Cairo, 1998.

Edwardes, Michael. *The Dark Side of History: Magic in the Making of Man.* New York: Stein and Day, 1977.

Eliade, Mircea. *The Myth of the Eternal Return: Cosmos and History.* London: Arkana, 1954.

———. *Yoga: Immortality and Freedom.* London: Arkana, 1958.

———. *Shamanism: Archaic Techniques of Ecstasy.* London: Arkana, 1989.

Elias, Jamal J. "Sufism: A Review of the Encyclopaedia Iranica." *Iranian Studies* 31, nos. 3/4 (Summer–Autumn 1998): 595–613.

Ellison, G. W. "Spiritual Wellbeing: Conceptualisation and Measurement." *Journal of Psychology and Theology* 11, no. 4 (1983): 330–40.

Ellwood, Robert S. *Theosophy: A Modern Expression of the Wisdom of the Ages.* Wheaton, Ill.: Quest Books, 1994.

Faivre, A., and W. J. Hanegraaff, eds. *Western Esotericism and the Science of Religion.* Leuven, Holland: Peeters, 1998.

Faivre, A., and K-C. Voss. "Western Esotericism and the Science of Religions." *Numen* 42, no. 1 (January 1995): 48–77.

Fanger, Claire. Review of Faivre and Voss, "Western Esotericism and the Science of Religion" in *Esotericism, Art, and Imagination,* vol. III. Charleston, S.C.: MSU Press, 2001, 277–87.

Feinstein, David. "Subtle Energy: Psychology's Missing Link." *IONS Noetic Sciences Review* (June–August 2003): 21.

Ferrer, Jorge N. *Revisioning Transpersonal Theory: A Participatory Vision of Human Spirituality.* Albany, N.Y.: SUNY Press, 2002.

Fernel, J. *De Naturali Parte Medicinae,* Book IV, 1542, in "The Astral Body in Renaissance Medicine," by D. P. Walker. *Journal of the Warburg and Courtauld Institutes* 21, no. 1–2 (January–June 1958): 119–33.

Feuerstein, Georg. *The Essence of Yoga: A Contribution to the Psychohistory of Indian Civilisation.* London: Rider, 1974.

———. *Tantra: The Path of Ecstasy.* Boston, Mass.: Shambhala, 1998.

———. *The Yoga Tradition: Its History, Literature, Philosophy and Practice.* Prescott, Ariz.: Hohm Press, 2001.

———. Foreword in *Kriya Yoga Sutras of Patanjali and the Siddhas,* by Marshall Govindan. 2nd ed. Quebec: Kriya Yoga Publications, 2005.

Fields, Gregory P. *Religious Therapeutics: Body and Health in Yoga, Āyurveda and Tantra.* New Delhi: Motilal Banarsidass, 2002.

Flood, Gavin D. *The Tantric Body: The Secret Tradition of Hindu Religion.* New York: I.B. Tauris, 2006.

Fuller, R. C. "Unorthodox Medicine and American Religious Life." *The Journal of Religion* 67, no. 1 (January 1987): 50–65.

Fusfeld, Warren. *The Shaping of Sufi Leadership in Delhi: The Naqshbandiyya Mujaddiyya, 1750–1920.* Ph.D. diss., University of Pennsylvania, 1981.

Gebser, Jean. *The Ever-Present Origin.* Athens: Ohio University Press, 1985.

Gharote. M. L., and G. K. Pai, eds. *Siddha-Siddhanta-Paddati of Goraksanath.* Lonavla, India: Lonavla Yoga Institute, 1983.

Gödel, Kurt A. *On Formally Undecidable Propositions of Principia Mathematica and Related Systems.* Translated by B. Meltzer. New York: Basic Books, 1962. (Paperback reissue, Dover, 1992.)

Godlas, A. *Sufism's Many Paths.* Athens: University of Georgia, 2000.

Goswami, Shyam Sunder. *Layayoga: The Definitive Guide to the Chakras and Kundalini.* Rochester, Vt.: Inner Traditions, 1999.

Govindan M., ed. *Thirumandiram: A Classic of Yoga and Tantra by Siddha Thirumoolar.* Quebec: Kriya Yoga Publications, 2003.

Govindan, Marshall. *Kriya Yoga Sutras of Patanjali and the Siddhas.* 2nd ed. Foreword by Georg Feuerstein. Quebec: Kriya Yoga Publications, 2005.

Gregory, Richard L. *Mind in Science: A History of Explanations in Psychology and Physics.* New York: Cambridge University Press, 1981.

Grossinger, Richard. *Alchemical Tradition in the Late Twentieth Century.* New York: Random House, 1991.

Gupta, S., D. J. Hoens, and T. Goudriaan. *Hindu Tantrism.* Leiden, Germany: E.J. Brill Publishers, 1979.

Gyatso, Kelsang. *Clear Light of Bliss: Mahamudra in Vajrayana Buddhism.* Translated by Tenzin Norbu. London: Tharpa Publications, 1982.

Hall, Manly P. *The Secret Teachings of All Ages.* London: Philosophical Research Society/Duckworth and Co., 2006.

Hamilton, D. *It's the Thought That Counts.* London: Hay House, 2005.

Hanegraaff, Wouter J. "Introduction: The Birth of a Discipline." In *Western Esotericism and the Science of Religion: Selected Papers presented at the 17th Congress of the International Association for the History of Religions,* edited by Antoine Faivre and Wouter J. Hanegraaff. Mexico City, 1995.

———. "The New Age Movement and the Esoteric Tradition." In *Gnosis and Hermeticism,* by van den Broek and Hanegraaff. Albany, N.Y.: SUNY Press, 1998: 351–61.

Hare, Richard M. *Plato.* London: Oxford University Press, 1982.

Harvey, William. *Opera Omnia: a Collegio Medicorum.* London: W. Bowyer, 1766 (a presentation copy published more than a century after the author's death).

Hayes, G. A. "Metaphoric Worlds and Yoga in the Vaiṣṇava Sahajiyā Tantric Traditions of Medieval Bengal." In *Yoga The Indian Tradition,* edited by Whicher and Carpenter. London: Routledge Curzon, 2003.

Heidegger, Martin. *Being and Time.* Translated by John McQuarrie and Edward Robinson. Oxford, UK: Blackwell, 1995.

———. *Being and Time.* Unpublished translation by D. E. Walford.

Heilijgers-Seelen, Dory. *System of Five Cakras in Kubjikamatatantra 14–16.* Los Altos, Calif.: Indo-American Books, 1990.

Heisenberg, Werner K. *The Uncertainty Principle,* vol. 43 (Uber den anschaulichen Inhalt der quantentheoretischen Kinematik und Mechanik, in Zeitschrift fur Physik). Berlin: Julius Springer, 1927.

Hermānsen, M. K. "Shah Wali Allah's Theory of the Subtle Spiritual Centers: A Sufi Model of Personhood and Self-Transformation." *Journal of Near Eastern Studies* 47, no. 1 (January 1988): 1–25.

Hofstadter, Douglas R. *Gödel, Escher, Bach: An Eternal Golden Braid.* New York: Basic Books, 1979.

———. *I Am a Strange Loop.* New York: Basic Books, 2007.

Holman, J. *The Return of the Perennial Philosophy: The Supreme Vision of Western Esotericism.* London: Watkins Publishing, 2008.

Hopkins, Jeffrey. "Tantric Buddhism, Degeneration or Enhancement: The Viewpoint of a Tibetan Tradition." *Buddhist-Christian Studies* 10 (1990): 87–96.

Howell, Julia Day. "Sufism and the Indonesian Islamic Revival." *Journal of Asian Studies* 60, no. 3 (August 2001): 701–29.

Hume, David. *A Treatise of Human Nature.* Edited by David Fate Norton and Mary J. Norton. Oxford Philosophical Texts. Oxford, UK, and New York: Oxford University Press, 2001.

Hume, Robert Ernest, trans. *The Thirteen Principal Upanishads.* Oxford: Oxford University Press, 1931.

Hunt, Valerie. *Infinite Mind: Science of Human Vibrations of Consciousness.* Malibu, Calif.: Malibu Publishing, 1996.

Hunt, V., W. Massey, R. Weinberg, R. Bruyere, and P. Hahn. *Project Report: A Study of Structural Integration from Neuromuscular, Energy Field, and Emotional Approaches.* Los Angeles: U.C.L.A., 1977.

Huxley, Aldous. *The Perennial Philosophy.* New York: Harper Perennial Modern Classics, 2004. (First published in 1945.)

Inge, William Ralph. *The Philosophy of Plotinus: The Gifford Lectures at St. Andrews, 1917–1918,* vols. I and II. London: Longmans, Green and Co., 1918.

———. *Outspoken Essays,* vol. I. London and New York: Longmans, Green and Co., 1919.

Irwin, Lee. "Daoist Alchemy in the West: The Esoteric Paradigms from Western Esotericism, Eastern Spirituality and the Global Future." *Esoterica* 3 (2001): 1–47.

ISSSEEM, *Subtle Energies and Energy Medicine* 17 (2008). (Journal of the International Society for the Study of Subtle Energies and Energy Medicine.)

James, William. *The Varieties of Religious Experience: A Study in Human Nature.* New York: Collier, 1961.

Johnson, Mark. *The Body in the Mind: The Bodily Basis of Meaning, Imagination, and Reason.* Chicago: University of Chicago Press, 1987.

Johnston, J. L. H., Ph.D. *Angels of Desire: Subtle Subjects, Aesthetics and Ethics.* NSW, Australia: University of West Sydney, 2004.

Judith, Anodea. *Wheels of Life: A User's Guide to the Chakra System.* St. Paul, Minn.: Llewellyn Publications, 1987.

Jung, C. G. *The Structure and Dynamics of the Psyche.* Translated by R. F. C. Hull. Princeton, N.J.: Princeton University Press, 1931.

———. *The Archetypes and the Collective Unconscious.* Translated by R. F. C. Hull. Princeton, N.J.: Princeton University Press, 1950.

———. *Psychology and Alchemy,* vol. 12, Collected Works. Translated by R. F. C. Hull. Princeton, N.J.: Princeton University Press, 1952.

———. *Psychology and Alchemy,* vol. 12, Collected Works. Translated by R. F. C. Hull. Princeton, N.J.: Princeton University Press, 1952, reprinted 1980.

———. *Memories, Dreams, Reflections.* London: Flamingo Books, 1963.

———. *Alchemical Studies,* vol. 13, Collected Works. Edited by H. Read, M. Fordham, G. Adler, and W. McGuire. London: Routledge and Kegan Paul, 1967.

———. *The Portable Jung.* Edited by Joseph Campbell. E. Rutherford, N.J.: Penguin USA, 1976.

———. *Psychological Types,* vol. 6, Collected Works. Edited by G. Adler and R. F. C. Hull. Princeton, N.J.: Princeton University Press, 1976.

———. Commentary on "The secret of the golden flower" in *Alchemical Studies.* Princeton, N.J.: Princeton University Press, 1983. (Original work published in 1929.)

Kabat-Zinn, J. "Meditation Research at the University of Massachusetts Medical Center." In *The Physical and Psychological Effects of Meditation: A Review of Contemporary Research with a Comprehensive Bibliography,* by Michael Murphy and Steven Donovan. Petaluma, Calif.: The Institute of Noetic Sciences, 1999. research@noetic.org.

Kaltenmark, M. *La Mystique Taoiste.* Paris: Ravier, 1965.

Karagulla, Shafica. *Breakthrough to Creativity: Your Higher Sense of Perception.* Camarillo, Calif.: De Vorss and Co, 1969.

Karagulla, Shafica, and Dora van Gelder Kunz. *The Chakras and the Human Energy Fields.* Wheaton, Ill.: Quest Books, 1989.

Kazlev, M. Alan. *Advaita Vedanta.* www.kheper.net/topics/Vedanta.

Kenny, Anthony. *Descartes: A Study of His Philosophy.* New York: Random House, 1968.

Köhn, Livia. *The Taoist Experience: An Anthology.* Albany, N.Y.: SUNY Press, 1993.

———. "The Subtle Body Ecstasy of Daoist Inner Alchemy." *Acta Orientalia Academiae Scientarium Hung* 59, no. 3 (2006): 325–40.

Knowles F. "Experiments in the Relief of Pain." *Journal of the Society for Psychical Research* 33 (January–February 1946): 198–99.

Krippner, Stanley, and John White, eds. *Future Science: Life Energies and the Physics of Paranormal Phenomena.* Garden City, N.Y.: Anchor Books, 1977.

Krishna, Gopi. *Kundalini: Evolutionary Energy in Man.* London: Robinson and Watkins, 1971.

Kurin, Richard. *Person, Family and Kin in Two Pakastani Communities,* Ph.D. diss. University of Chicago, 1981.

Laszlo, Ervin. *Science and the Akashic Field: An Integral Theory of Everything.* Rochester, Vt.: Inner Traditions, 2004.

———. *The Chaos Point: The World at the Crossroads.* London: Piatkus Books, 2006.

Leadbeater, C. W. *The Chakras.* Adyar, Madras, India: Theosophical Publishing House, 1927.

Leder, Drew. *The Absent Body.* Chicago: University of Chicago Press, 1990.

Lee, H. D. P., trans. *Plato: Timaeus.* London: Penguin Books, 1965.

LeShan, Lawrence L. *The Medium, the Mystic and the Physicist: Toward a General Theory of the Paranormal.* New York: Viking, 1974.

Leonard, George B., and Michael Murphy. *The Life We Are Given: A Long-term Program for Realizing the Potential of Body, Mind, Heart and Soul.* New York: Tarcher, 1995.

Linga Purana. Ancient Indian Tradition and Mythology Series, vols. 5–6. Translated by a board of scholars. Delhi: Motilal Banarsidass, 1973.

Lockhart, M. *Siddha Medicine.* Lecture at the Body MA Residential Conference, University of Wales Lampeter, June 2006.

Louchakova, O. "Psychospiritual Practices from the Prayer of the Heart in Monitoring Cardiovascular Disorders: A Case Study." Paper presented at the 2nd Annual Spirituality and Healthcare Conference. Toronto, October 2002.

Louchakova, O., and A. S. Warner. "Via Kundalini: Psychosomatic Excursions in Trans-personal Psychology." *The Humanistic Psychologist* 31, nos. 2–3 (Spring 2003): 115–58.

Lu K'uan-yü. *Taoist Yoga: Alchemy and Immortality.* London: Rider, 1970.

Mabbett, I. W. "The Symbolism of Mount Meru." *History of Religions* 23, no. 1 (August 1983): 64–83.

Matsuda, Yoshiko. *A Phenomenological Study of the Imagining Body: Toward a Conception of Imagination as a Mode of Being in the Body.* Ph.D. diss., University of Toronto, 2001.

Mead, George R. S. *The Orphic Pantheon.* Edmonds, Wash.: Alexandrian Press, 1984.

———. *The Doctrine of the Subtle Body in Western Tradition.* New York: Cosimo Classics, 2005.

Meece, E. A. *Neoplatonism and Alchemy: The Forgotten Philosophy.* San Jose State University Alumni Philosophy Conference, San Jose, California, 23 April 2005.

Michaelson, Jay. *God in Your Body.* Woodstock, Vt.: Jewish Lights Publishing, 2006.

Miller, Iona. *Introduction to Alchemy in Jungian Psychology.* Grants Pass, Ore.: Rogue Community College Press, Spring Quarter, 1986.

Miller, Richard and Iona. *The Modern Alchemist: A Guide to Personal Transformation.* Grand Rapids, Mich.: Phanes Press, 1994.

Monroe, Robert A. *Journeys Out of the Body.* London: Souvenir Press, 1972.

Morley, J. "Inspiration and Expiration: Yoga Practice through Merleau-Ponty's Phenomenology of the Body." *Philosophy East and West* 51, no. 1 (January 2001): 73–82.

Morris, James, Michel Chodkiewicz, and William Chittick. *The Meccan Revelations.* With English introduction to the *Futūhāt al-makkiyya* from the English-French work originally published in Paris in 1988. New York: Pir Publications, 2002.

Motoyama, Hiroshi. *Theories of the Chakras: Bridge to Higher Consciousness*. Wheaton, Ill.: Theosophical Publishing House, 1981.

———. *The Theories of the Chakras: Bridge to Higher Consciousness*. New Delhi: New Age Books, 2003.

Murphy, Michael. *The Future of the Body: Explorations Into the Further Evolution of Human Nature*. New York: Jeremy Tarcher, 1993.

———. "Scientific Studies of Contemplative Experience: An Overview." In *The Physical and Psychological Effects of Meditation*. Petaluma, Calif.: The Institute of Noetic Sciences, 1999.

Nasr, Seyyed Hossein. "Al-Serat: The Interior Life in Islam." *American Physical Society Journal* III, nos. 2 and 3 (2009). www.publish/aps.org.

Nichol, Lee, ed. *The Essential David Böhm*. Introduction by H. H. the Dalai Lama. London: Routledge, 2003.

Nikhilananda, Swami. *The Upanisads*. New York: Ramakrishna-Vivekananda Center, 1977.

Niranjanananda, Swami. *The Koshas*. From talks presented at the Pratyahara Course conducted by Swami Niranjanananda at Satyananda Yoga Ashram, Mangrove Mountain, Australia, April 1995.

Onians, Richard Broxton. *The Origins of European Thought About the Body, the Mind, the Soul, the World, Time, and Fate*. Cambridge: Cambridge University Press, 1951.

Opsopaus, John. *The Parts of the Soul: A Greek System of Chakras*. Biblioteca Arcana, 1994. www.cs.utk.edu.

Organ, Troy Wilson. *The Hindu Quest for the Perfection of Man*. Athens: Ohio University Press, 1970.

———. *Western Approaches to Eastern Philosophy*. Athens: Ohio University Press, 1975.

Orme-Johnson, David W., Charles N. Alexander, John L. Davies, Howard M. Chandler, and Wallace E. Larimore. "International Peace Project in the Middle East: The Effects of the Maharishi Technology of the Unified Field." *Journal of Conflict Resolution* 32, no. 4 (December 1988): 776–812.

Osborn, David K. "Plato and the Chakras." In *The Principles of Greek Medicine*, 2008. www.greekmedicine.net.

Oschman, J. L. *Energy Medicine: The Scientific Basis*. London: Churchill Livingstone, 2000.

Ostram, J. *Understanding Auras: A Contemporary Overview of the Human Aura*. New Delhi: HarperCollins Publishers India, 1999.

Palmer, G. H., P. Sherrard, and K. Ware, trans. and eds. "St. Simeon the New Theologian: The Three Methods of Prayer." (From the tenth-century original, *The Philokalia,* vol. IV, 67–78.) Boston: Faber and Faber, 1995.

Parthasarthy, S. *The Nature of Man*. Mumbai: Vedanta Life Institute, 1984.

Pauli, W., and C. G. Jung. *The Interpretation of Nature and the Psyche*. London: Routledge and Kegan Paul, 1955.

Payne, Phoebe P., and Laurence J. Bendit. "The Subtle Body and Countertransference." In *Lifestreams: An Introduction to Biosynthesis,* edited by David Boadella. London: Routledge, 1987.

Penrose, Roger. *Shadows of the Mind*. London: Vintage, Random House, 1995.

Pert, Candace. *Molecules of Emotion*. New York: Touchstone Books, 1999.

Pitson, A. E. *Hume's Philosophy of the Self*. Routledge Studies in Eighteenth-Century Philosophy. London and New York: Routledge, 2002.

Place, Robert M. *The Alchemical Tarot*. London: Harper Collins, 1995.

Poortman, J. J. *Vehicles of Consciousness: The Concept of Hylic Pluralism (Ochema),* vols. I–IV. Madras, India: Theosophical Publishing House, 1978.

Popper, Karl R., and John C. Eccles. *The Self and Its Brain*. Berlin, London, New York: Springer-Verlag, 1977.

Pradervand, Pierre. *The Gentle Art of Blessing: Lessons for Living One's Spirituality in Everyday Life*. Fawnskin, Calif.: Personhood Press, 2003.

Pribram, K. In *Ancient Light: Our Changing View of the Universe,* by A. P. Lightman. Cambridge, Mass.: Harvard University Press, 1991.

Pseudo-Dionysius, the Areopagite. *The Complete Work*. Translated by K. Luibheid. Mahwah, N.J.: Paulist Press, 1987. (Original publication date unknown.)

Puthoff, H. E., and R. Targ. "A Perceptual Channel for Information Transfer over Kilometer Distances: Historical Perspective and Recent Research." *Proceedings of the IEEE* 64, no. 3 (March 1976): 329–44.

Radin, Dean. *Entangled Minds: Extrasensory Experiences in a Quantum Reality*. New York: Paraview Pocket Books, Simon and Schuster, 2006.

Raju, P. T. "The Concept of the Spiritual in Indian Thought." *Philosophy East and West* 4, no. 3 (October 1954): 195–213.

Rama, Swami, Rudolph Ballentine, and Swami Ajaya, *Yoga*

and Psychotherapy: The Evolution of Consciousness. Honesdale, Pa.: The Himalayan International Institute, 1976.

Ram-Prasad, Chakravarthi. *Eastern Philosophy.* London: Weidenfeld and Nicolson, Orion Publishing Group, 2005.

Ray, Reginald. *Saints in India.* New York: Oxford University Press, 2005.

Rele, Vasant G. *The Vedic Gods as Figures of Biology.* New Delhi: Cosmo Publications, 2001.

Rensselaer, R. "Esoteric Wisdom East and West." *Sunrise: Theosophic Perspectives* (June–July 1974).

Rhine, Joseph Banks. *Extrasensory Perception.* Dingle, Ireland: Brandon Books, 1983.

Riffard, Pierre A. *L'Esotérisme.* Paris: Laffont, 1990.

Robinet, Isabelle. "Metamorphosis and Deliverance from the Corpse in Taoism." *History of Religions* 19, no. 1 (August 1979): 37–70.

———. *Taoism: Growth of the Religion.* Palo Alto, Calif.: Stanford University Press, 1997.

Robinson, J. B., trans. Abhayadatta's *Caturasiti-siddha-pravṛtti: Buddha's Lions, The Lives of the Eighty-Four Siddhas.* Ratna Ling, Calif.: Dharma Publishing, 1979.

Robinson, James V. "The Tripartite Soul in the Timaeus." *Phronesis* 35, no. 1 (1990): 103–10.

Roth, Remo F. *The Return of the World Soul: Wolfgang Pauli, Carl Jung and the Challenge of the Unified Psychophysical Reality.* Zurich, Switzerland: Pro Litteris, 2002–2004.

———. *The Archetype of the Holy Wedding in Alchemy and in the Unconscious of Man.* Zurich, Switzerland: Pro Litteris, 2005.

Rubin, Vera C. "A Brief History of Dark Matter." In *The Dark Universe: Matter, Energy and Gravity,* edited by Mario Livio, 1–13. Proceedings of the Space Telescope Science Institute Symposium held in Baltimore, Maryland, April 2–5, 2001. New York: Cambridge University Press, 2001.

Russell, Bertrand, and Alfred North Whitehead. *Principia Mathematica.* New York: Cambridge University Press, 1910.

Russell, Peter. *The Global Brain: The Awakening Earth in a New Century.* Edinburgh: Floris Books, 2007.

Ryle, Gilbert. *The Concept of Mind.* London: Hutchinson, 1949; Penguin (Peregrine), 1966.

Sahtouris, E. "Living Systems in Evolution." From the "At Home In the Universe: A Dialogue Between Science and Religions" symposium held at the World Parliament of Religions, Cape Town, South Africa, 1999.

Saiter, S. M. "A General Introduction to Integral Theory and Comprehensive Mapmaking." *Journal of Conscious Evolution* (2005). www.cejournal.org.

Salzberg, Sharon. *Lovingkindness: The Revolutionary Art of Happiness.* Boston and London: Shambhala, 1995.

Samuel, Geoffrey. *The Origins of Yoga and Tantra.* Cambridge: Cambridge University Press, 2008.

Sangharakshita. *A Guide to the Buddhist Path.* Glasgow: Windhorse Publications, 1990.

Sarukkai, Sundar. "Inside/Outside: Merleau Ponty Yoga." *Philosophy East and West* 52, no. 4 (October 2002): 459–78.

Schipper, Kristofer. *The Taoist Body.* Translated by Karen C. Duval. Berkeley: University of California Press, 1993.

Schlitz, M., and W. Braud. "Distant Intentionality and Healing: Assessing the Evidence." Paper presented at the Fourth Annual Conference on Evolutionary Theory at the Esalen Institute in Big Sur, California, 2002.

Schlitz, M., T. Amorok, and M. Micozzi. *Consciousness and Healing: Integral Approaches to Mind-Body Medicine.* St Louis, Mo.: Elsevier, 2005.

Schlitz, M., and W. Harman. "The Implications of Alternative and Complementary Medicine for Science and the Scientific Process." In *Consciousness and Healing: Integral Approaches to Mind-Body Medicine,* 361. St Louis, Mo.: Elsevier, 2005.

Schmidt, Marcia Binder. *Dzogchen Essentials: The Path that Clarifies Confusion.* Hong Kong: Rangjung Yeshe Publications, 2004.

Schoeps, Hans Joachim. *Religionen: Wesen und Geschichte.* Translated from the German by Richard and Clara Winston as *An Intelligent Person's Guide to the Religions of Mankind.* London: Victor Gollancz, 1967.

Schopenhauer, Arthur. *The World as Will and Representation,* vol. 1. Translated by E. F. J. Payne. New York: Dover Publications, 1969.

Schrödinger, Erwin. "An Undulatory Theory of the Mechanics of Atoms and Molecules." *The Physical Review* 28 (1926): 1049–70. (*The Physical Review* is a publication of the University of Minnesota.)

Schrödt, P. A. "A Methodological Critique of a Test of the Effects of the Maharishi Technology of the Unified

Field." *The Journal of Conflict Resolution* 34, no. 4 (December 1990).

Schul, Bill. *The Psychic Frontiers of Medicine.* London: Coronet Books, 1977.

Schuler, R. M. "Some Spiritual Alchemies of Seventeenth-Century England." *Journal of the History of Ideas* 41, no. 2 (April–June 1980): 293–318.

Schuon, Frithjof. *Understanding Islam.* Translated by D. M. Matheson. Baltimore: Penguin Books, 1972.

Scott-Mumby, Keith. *Virtual Medicine: A New Dimension in Energy Healing.* London: Thorsons/HarperCollins, 1999.

Seeman, Gary M. *Individuation and Subtle Body: A Commentary on Jung's Kundalini Seminar.* Ph.D. diss., Pacifica Graduate Institute, Santa Barbara, California, 2001.

Sen, Indra. "Sri Aurobindo's Theory of the Mind." *Philosophy East and West* 1, no 4 (January, 1952): 45–52.

———. *Integral Psychology: The Psychological System of Sri Aurobindo.* Pondicherry, India: Aurobindo Ashram Trust, 1986.

Shah, Idries. *The Way of the Sufi.* London: Octagon Press, 1980.

Shapiro, Deane H., and Roger N Walsh. *Meditation: Classic and Contemporary Perspectives.* Piscataway, N.J.: Aldine Transaction Publishers, 2008.

Sheldrake, Rupert. *A New Science of Life.* Rochester, Vt.: Park Street Press, 1995.

———. *The Presence of the Past.* Rochester, Vt.: Park Street Press, 1995.

———. *Dogs That Know When Their Owners Are Coming Home: And Other Unexplained Powers of Animals.* London: Arrow, 2000.

Shendelman, E. "The Vision of the Body: Primary Body Focus Zones in Qigong Practice." *The Empty Vessel: Journal of Contemporary Daoism* (2001). www.abodetao.com.

Short, L., and J. Mann. *The Body of Light.* San Francisco: Fourth Way Books, 1988.

Sinha, Debabrata. "Human Embodiment: The Theme and the Encounter in Vedantic Phenomenology." *Philosophy East and West* 35, no. 3 (July 1985): 239–47.

Smith, Benjamin Richard. "Adjusting the Quotidian: Ashtanga Yoga as Everyday Practice" (post-doctoral research paper). Canberra: The Australian National University, 2004.

Smith, Nicholas D. "Plato's Analogy of Soul and State." *The Journal of Ethics* 3, no. 1 (1999): 31–49.

Snell, M-M. "Modern Theosophy in Its Relation to Hinduism and Buddhism." *The Biblical World* 5, no. 3 (March 1895): 200–205.

Snellgrove, David L. *Hevajra Tantra: A Critical Study.* London: Oxford University Press, 1959.

Sorabji, R. "Soul and Self in Ancient Philosophy." In *From Soul to Self,* edited by M. J. C. Crabbe. New York: Routledge, 1999.

Spiegelman, Marvin J. "Jungian Psychotherapy." *Psychological Perspectives* 18, no. 1 (Spring 1987): 127–64.

Spiegelman, M. J., and A. U. Vasavada. *Hinduism and Jungian Psychology.* Phoenix, Ariz.: Falcon Press, 1987.

———. *Founding a Science of the Spirit: Fourteen Lectures Given in Stuttgart between 14 August and 4 September 1906.* London: Rudolf Steiner Press, 1999.

Steiner, Rudolf. *The Inner Development of Man.* Herndon, Va.: Steiner Books, 1970.

———. *Founding a Science of the Spirit: Fourteen Lectures Given in Stuttgart between 22 August and 4 September 1906,* reprint ed. E. Sussex, UK: 2007.

Stoddart, William. *Sufism: The Mystical Doctrines and Methods of Islam.* Wellingborough, UK: The Aquarian Press, 1976.

Sullivan, Lawrence. "Body Works: Knowledge of the Body in the Study of Religion." *History of Religions* 30, no. 1 (August 1990): 86–89. (This is a special issue focusing on the body.)

Takeshita, Masataka. Review of William C. Chittick's "Ibn 'Arabī's's Theory of the Perfect Man and Its Place in the History of Islamic Thought." *Journal of the American Oriental Society* 109, no. 4 (October–December 1989): 707.

Tansley, David V. *Subtle Body: Essence and Shadow.* London: Thames and Hudson, 1977.

Tantrapa, Lama Somananda. *Qi Dao: Tibetan Shamanic Qigong, The Art of Being in the Flow.* Bloomington, Ind.: AuthorHouse; and Milton Keynes, Buckinghamshire, UK: AuthorHouse UK, 2007.

Targ, R., H. Puthoff, ed., and C. T. Tart. *Transpersonal Psychologies: Perspectives on the Mind from Seven Great Spiritual Traditions.* Charles T. Tart Homepage and Consciousness online: www.paradigm-sys.com.

Tart, C. T. , H. E. Puthoff, and R. Targ, eds. *Mind at Large: IEEE Symposia on the Nature of Extrasensory Perception.* Charlottesville, Va.: Hampton Roads, 2002. (Originally published in 1979.)

Tiller, William A. *Science and Human Transformation: Subtle Energies, Intentionality and Consciousness.* Walnut Creek, Calif.: Pavior Publishing, 1997.

Tiller, William A., Walter E. Dibble, and Michael J Kohane. *Conscious Acts of Creation.* Walnut Creek, Calif: Pavior Publishing, 2001.

Tirtha, V. *Devatma Shakti (Kundalini): Divine Power.* Rishikesh, India: Vigyan Press, 1993.

Tiruvalluvar. *Tirukkural.* Translated by G. U. Pope. Tiruvelli South Indian Saiva Siddhata Works. Reprinted 1962.

Touma, Habib Hasan. *The Music of the Arabs.* Translated by Laurie Schwartz. Portland, Ore.: Amadeus Press, 1996.

Underhill, E. *Mysticism: A Study in the Nature and Development of Man's Spiritual Consciousness.* London: Methuen and Co., 1911.

Versluis, A. Review of Ewert H. Cousins, ed., Antoine Faivre, Jacob Needleman, and Karen Voss, *Modern Esoteric Spirituality. Journal of Religion* 75, no. 3 (July 1995): 423–25.

———. *Magic and Mysticism: An Introduction to Western Esotericism.* Albany, N.Y.: SUNY Press, 2003.

———. "Western Esotericism and Consciousness." *The Journal of Consciousness Studies* 7 (2006): 20–33.

von Franz, M-L. *Alchemy: An Introduction to the Symbolism and the Psychology.* Toronto: Inner City Books, 1980.

———. *Projection and Recollection in Jungian Psychology: Reflections of the Soul.* Peru, Ill.: Open Court Publishing Company, 1980.

Walbridge, J. *The Leaven of the Ancients: Suhrawardi and the Heritage of the Greeks.* Albany, N.Y.: SUNY Press, 2000.

Walker, D. P. "The Astral Body in Renaissance Medicine." *Journal of the Warburg and Courtauld Institutes* 21, no. 1–2 (January–June 1958): 119–33.

Wallis, Richard T. *Neoplatonism.* London: Duckworth, 1972.

Walsh, Roger. *The Spirit of Evolution.* An overview of Ken Wilber's writings, 2007. www.kenwilber.com.

Watson, Donald. *A Dictionary of Mind and Spirit.* Calcutta: Rupa and Co., 1991.

Wettstein, Harri R. "On Pain, Palliative Care and Values." Presented at the *Wittgenstein Symposium,* Kirchberg, Austria, 1997.

Wheeler, E. In *The Non-local Universe: The New Physics and Matters of the Mind,* by R. Nadeau and M. C. Kafatos. New York: Oxford University Press, 1999.

Whicher, I. "The Integration of Spirit and Matter in the Yoga Sutra." In *Yoga: The Indian Tradition,* edited by Ian Whicher and David Carpenter. London: Routledge Curzon, 2003.

White, David Gordon. "Why Gurus Are Heavy." *Numen* 31 (July 1984): 40–73.

———. "Yoga in Early Hindu Tantra." In *Yoga: The Indian Tradition.* London: Routledge Curzon, 2003.

———. *The Alchemical Body.* Chicago: The University of Chicago Press, 1996.

———, ed. *Tantra in Practice.* Princeton, N.J.: Princeton University Press, 2000.

———. *The Kiss of the Yogini: "Tantric Sex" in its South Asian Contexts.* Chicago: University of Chicago Press, 2003.

White, J. "Enlightenment and the Body of Light." *What Is Enlightenment?* (Spring–Summer 2002). Evolution issue.

Whitmont, Edward C., M.D. *The Alchemy of Healing Psyche and Soma.* Berkeley, Calif: North Atlantic Books, 1993.

Wikipedia. *Sand Mandala* and *Kalachakra Mandala.* www.wikipedia.com. Accessed 2009.

Wilber, K. Foreword in *Coming Home: The Experience of Enlightenment in Sacred Traditions,* by Len Hixon. Burdett, N.Y.: Larson Publications, 1995.

———. *Integral Psychology.* Boston: Shambhala, 2000.

———. *The Eye of Spirit: An Integral Vision for a World Gone Slightly Mad.* 3rd ed., expanded. Boston: Shambhala, 2001.

———. Foreword in *Consciousness and Healing: Integral Approaches to Mind-Body Medicine,* by M. Schlitz, T. Amorok, and M. Micozzi. St. Louis, Mo.: Elsevier, 2005.

Williams, Patricia Day, M.D. *The Chakras and the Ancient Wisdom Traditions Worldwide.* www.patriciadaywilliams.com. Accessed 2008.

Winkelman, Michael. *Shamanism: The Neural Ecology of Consciousness and Healing.* Westport, Conn.: Bergin and Garvey, 2000.

Winn, M. "Daoist Internal Alchemy: A Deep Language for Communication with Nature's Intelligence." Paper presented at the Conference on "Daoist Cultivation," Vashon Island, 2001.

———. "The Quest for Spiritual Orgasm: Daoist and Tantric Sexual Cultivation in the West." Paper presented at the Conference on Tantra and Daoism, Boston University, 2002.

Wisneski, Leonard, and Lucy Anderson. *The Scientific Basis of Integrative Medicine.* London: Oxford University Press, 2005.

Wittgenstein, Ludwig. *Philosophical Investigations.* Translated by G. E. M. Anscombe. Oxford, UK: Basil Blackwell, 1958.

Woodroffe, John George, Sir. *The Serpent Power.* 9th ed. Madras, India: Ganesh and Co., 1973. (Originally published in 1928.)

Worrall, Olga, and Ambrose Worrall. *The Gift of Healing: A Personal Story of Spiritual Therapy.* Santa Cruz, Calif.: Ariel Press, 1989.

Wujastyk, D. "The Science of Medicine." In *The Blackwell Companion to Hinduism,* edited by Gavin Flood. Oxford, UK: Blackwell Publishing, 2003.

Yogeshwarananda, Sri. *Science of Soul.* New Delhi: Vedic Books, Yoga Niketan Trust, 1980.

Yuasa, Y. *The Body: Towards an Eastern Body-Mind Theory.* Translated and edited by Shigenori and Kasulis. Albany, N.Y.: SUNY Press, 1987.

Zysk, K. G. "The Science of Respiration and the Doctrine of Bodily Winds in Ancient India." *Journal of the American Oriental Society* 1133, no. 2 (April–June 1993): 198–213.

Index

Page numbers in *italics* indicate illustrations.

Books of Related Interest

Chakras
Energy Centers of Transformation
by Harish Johari

Kundalini
The Arousal of the Inner Energy
by Ajit Mookerjee

The Akashic Experience
Science and the Cosmic Memory Field
by Ervin Laszlo

Science and the Akashic Field
An Integral Theory of Everything
by Ervin Laszlo

Microchakras
InnerTuning for Psychological Well-being
by Sri Shyamji Bhatnagar and David Isaacs, Ph.D.

Vibrational Medicine
The #1 Handbook of Subtle-Energy Therapies
by Richard Gerber, M.D.

Decoding the Human Body-Field
The New Science of Information as Medicine
by Peter H. Fraser and Harry Massey with Joan Parisi Wilcox

The Three Secrets of Reiki Tao Te Qi
The Original Teachings of Master Huang Zhen Hui
by Idris Lahore

INNER TRADITIONS • BEAR & COMPANY
P.O. Box 388
Rochester, VT 05767
1-800-246-8648
www.InnerTraditions.com

Or contact your local bookseller